MEN IN TRANSITION

Theory and Therapy

MEN IN TRANSITION

Theory and Therapy

EDITED BY

KENNETH SOLOMON, M.D.

Adjunct Assistant Professor
Department of Psychiatry
University of Maryland School of Medicine
Associate Director for Education and Planning
Levindale Hebrew Geriatric Center and Hospital
Baltimore, Maryland

AND

NORMAN B. LEVY, M.D.

Professor of Psychiatry, Medicine, and Surgery
New York Medical College
Director, Liaison Psychiatry Division
Westchester County Medical Center
Valhalla, New York

PLENUM PRESS • NEW YORK AND LONDON

Library of Congress Cataloging in Publication Data

Main entry under title:

Men in transition.

Includes bibliographical references and index.
1. Men—Mental health. I. Solomon, Kenneth, 1947– . II. Levy, Norman B., 1931– . [DNLM: 1. Identification—Psychology. 2. Men—Psychology. 3. Psychoanalytic theory. 4. Psychotherapy. WM 460.5.M5 M266]
RC451.4.M45M46 1982 362.2′088041 82-15134
ISBN 0-306-40976-3

A Division of Plenum Publishing Corporation
233 Spring Street, New York, N.Y. 10013

Printed in the United States of America

Contributors

Jack O. Balswick, Ph.D., *Department of Pastoral and Family Ministries, Fuller Theological Seminary, Pasadena, California*

Teresa Bernardez, M.D., *Department of Psychiatry, Michigan State University, East Lansing, Michigan*

Jacqueline Boles, Ph.D., *Department of Sociology, Georgia State University, Atlanta, Georgia*

Alexandra Botwin, Ph.D., *Department of Medical Psychology, University of California, San Francisco, California*

David A. Dosser, Jr., Ph.D., *Department of Child Development and Family Relations, College of Home Economics, North Dakota State University, Fargo, North Dakota*

Jerry M. Friedman, Ph.D., *Department of Psychiatry and Behavioral Medicine, School of Medicine, State University of New York at Stony Brook, Stony Brook, New York*

Marvin R. Goldfried, Ph.D., *Department of Psychology, State University of New York at Stony Brook, Stony Brook, New York*

Robert E. Gould, M.D., *Departments of Psychiatry and Obstetrics and Gynecology, and Family Life Division, New York Medical College and Metropolitan Hospital Center, New York City, New York*

Richard L. Grant, M.D., *Southeastern Colorado Family Guidance and Mental Health Center, La Junta, Colorado, and Department of Psychiatry, University of Colorado Medical School, Denver, Colorado*

Ellen Halle, M.M.H., *Department of Psychiatry and Behavioral Sciences, Johns Hopkins University, Baltimore, Maryland*

Wolfgang Lederer, M.D., *Department of Psychiatry, University of California, San Francisco, California*

Norman B. Levy, M.D., *Psychiatric Liaison Service, Westchester County Medical Center, and Departments of Psychiatry, Medicine, and Surgery, Valhalla, New York*

Robert A. Lewis, Ph.D., *Department of Child Development and Family Studies, Purdue University, West Lafayette, Indiana*

John Money, Ph.D., *Department of Psychiatry, Phipps Clinic, Johns Hopkins University School of Medicine, Baltimore, Maryland*

Carol C. Nadelson, M.D., *Department of Psychiatry, Tufts-New England Medical Center, Boston, Massachusetts*

Theodore Nadelson, M.D., *Department of Psychiatry, Veterans Administration Medical Center, and Department of Psychiatry, Tufts University School of Medicine, Boston, Massachusetts*

Joseph L. Norton, Ph.D., *Department of Counseling Psychology and Student Development, State University of New York, Albany, New York*

James M. O'Neil, Ph.D., *Department of Education, University Counseling Center and Department of Counseling, University of Kansas, Lawrence, Kansas*

Craig L. Roberts, *Department of Sociology, University of Minnesota, Minneapolis, Minnesota*

Kenneth Solomon, M.D., *Levindale Hebrew Geriatric Center and Hospital; Department of Psychiatry, University of Maryland School of Medicine, Baltimore, Maryland*

Terry S. Stein, M.D., *Department of Psychiatry, Colleges of Human Medicine and Osteopathic Medicine, Michigan State University, East Lansing, Michigan*

Charlotte Tatro, Ph.D., *Institute for Women, Miami, Florida*

Martin R. Wong, Ph.D., *Psychology Service, Veterans Administration Medical Center Battle Creek, Michigan*

Preface

Every year the few hundred members of the Committees, Task Forces, and Councils of the American Psychiatric Association meet in Washington, D.C. to conduct their business. They deliberate on a wide variety of issues encompassed in the activities of each group. The psychiatrists constituting this mixed and somewhat elite group include some of the better-known and promising people in the profession, which makes the plenary session and cocktail party good occasions to meet old friends and to make new ones.

Several years ago one of us (N.B.L.) attended this gathering as a member of a soon-to-be defunct group, the Committee Liaison with the American College of Physicians, and met Ann Chappell, a member of the Task Force on Women. We were soon joined by Richard Grant. Ann impressed us with the work her group was doing on issues surrounding the Women's Movement as it relates to patients and the changing roles of the early 1970s. She was struck by the fact that although some women had been very active in this endeavor, nobody in American psychiatry was addressing issues which are arising in men as a result of the changing roles of women in society. Dick and Norm were moved by what she said and decided that they would make an effort to gather together people interested in the issue of the changing roles of males in society at the oncoming meeting of the American Psychiatric Association.

The initial occasion, in 1977, was a relatively informal Open Forum in which a variety of interested people spoke, some quite articulately, about the effects of the Women's Movement upon men. In subsequent years, sessions at the American Psychiatric Association were organized and chaired by the editors of this book. We were most impressed that this was a theme of active interest in a significant group of people. As we became further involved with this subject, we got to know a number of individuals who have actively addressed this theme. They were sociologists, psychologists, social workers, and psychiatrists. We thought that psychiatrists and other mental health workers, in particular, needed to know about the research on and effects of changing masculine roles.

Unlike other medical specialties whose concepts of normality are relatively fixed, mental health workers must adapt their concepts of illness and health to custom and social change. The consequences of the Women's Movement's examination of gender role stereotyping have produced profound social changes. For example, in judging illness vs. health, when considering a man's wish to stay at home and assume greater household responsibility in order to permit his partner greater freedom for outside work, mental health workers should respond differently now from the way they did in the 1950s. Issues of normality or abnormality in this area cannot be addressed with the certainties of the past. Mental health workers need to be sensitive to and aware of the changing spectrum of societal norms and its impact upon the people they see for diagnosis and therapy. In addition, they need to monitor themselves so that they do not bring outdated value systems into their work.

Two years ago we agreed to coedit a volume of the papers presented at past American Psychiatric Association meetings and selected new ones on changing masculine roles. Although this book is not the first volume with the general theme of the changing roles of males in society, it is the first that is edited by psychiatrists and has significant contributions by mental health workers. It is also the first not written just upon what changes have, will, or should occur, but also the pertinence of these changes for the practice of psychotherapy.

We were most pleased to find Plenum Publishing Corporation actively receptive and extremely interested in publishing this book. We are particularly thankful to Hilary Evans and Beth Kaufman of Plenum Publishing Corporation for their support. In addition, we wish to express our gratitude to a number of people who have helped in producing this volume. Special thanks goes to Ann Chappell, whose actions and continued perseverence began the entire process and whose continued support has been invaluable. Also, gratitude goes to the contributors of this book, as they have struggled with the editors' comments, critiques, demands, and deadlines and still wrote their chapters! We want to thank our secretaries, Camille Damiano (for N.B.L.) and Joyce Hammock (for K.S.) for their daily work on the manuscript, and Barbara Lazar, who indexed this volume. Finally, there is special gratitude for those too many to mention—our fathers, sons, friends, lovers, wives, patients, colleagues, men and women who have supported and critiqued this work and who have contributed to and shared with the joys and pains of our growth as men.

KENNETH SOLOMON
NORMAN B. LEVY

Contents

Introduction

JOHN MONEY

In the very term "male sex roles," there is a redundancy that usually passes unnoticed and that introduces a strong theoretical bias into what should more accurately be identified simply as male roles. A male role is one performed by a person classified as male, not female, on the basis of genital configuration. A male role, as compared with a male sex role, may or may not be one that can be performed by a female as well as a male. A male sex role, by contrast, is exclusively male insofar as its performance involves the sex organs, or more precisely, the erotosexual organs. A sex role that is male and that is genuinely a sex role is dimorphically coded as male and not as female. That is to say, it is *sex-irreducible.* There are three other grades of sexually dimorphic role, namely, those that are *sex-derivative, sex-adjunctive,* and *sex-arbitrary.*

The basic and *irreducible* difference between male and female is that men impregnate and women menstruate, gestate, and lactate. There are some species of fish in which sexual dimorphism is not absolute but situationally reversible, so that an individual fish is able to change and breed both as a male and a female in the course of its life. Once science discovers the sex-reversal secret of these ambisexual or hermaphroditic fish, then this newly discovered knowledge will undoubtedly become transferred from the science of fish to the science of mammals. The fictional science of today becomes the applied science of tomorrow. Thus one may hypothesize that some time in the 21st century humankind will tangle with the ethics of episodic and optional sex reversal. There is a contemporary relevance to this hypothesis insofar as there is in some of today's opposition to changing roles for males and females a vehemence that bespeaks fear lest change in any aspect of sex dimorphic roles will reverse in entirety the sexual status of men and women. Such, of course, is not the case. Not even the invention of infant feeding formulas and prepared baby foods makes a man less masculine by permitting him to feed an infant when the mother is not lactating. On the contrary, it adds to his repertory of masculinity.

A *sex-derivative* male role is classified as derivative insofar as its develop-

JOHN MONEY • Department of Psychiatry and Behavioral Sciences and Department of Pediatrics, The Johns Hopkins University and Hospital, Baltimore, Maryland 21205

mental origins stem in part from the same hormones that in prenatal life govern the differentiation of the sex organs as male or female. Prenatal anatomical differentiation as male or female follows, according to current knowledge, the Adam principle. The Adam principle signifies that the primary inclination of a fetus, regardless of its genetic status as XX or XY, is to differentiate as a morphologic female unless something is added. It is only a slight oversimplification to say that the something added is androgen, the male sex hormone. Ordinarily, the androgen of fetal masculinization is produced in a male fetus by its own testes. If the testes fail to develop, a fetus will develop the genital morphology of a female, minus ovaries. An obvious sex-derivative behavioral by-product of such a deandrogenized development is that the baby will grow up to urinate in the female urinary position. Other sex-derivative behavioral by-products of fetal deandrogenization are sex dimorphic not in any absolute sense of either/or, but rather insofar as they are sex-shared but threshold-dimorphic. Parentalism is an example. Parentalism is sex-shared insofar as it is exhibited by the father as well as the mother, but is threshold-dimorphic insofar as an infant or child evokes it more readily and more frequently in the mother than the father. For example, the sleeping mother is typically more sensitive to the stirrings of the neonate than is the sleeping father.

To date, there have been isolated nine phyletically basic behavioral dispositions that, though they might appear as sexually dimorphic, are actually sex-shared and dimorphic only in either threshold or frequency of manifestation. With the advent of new research, the list may well need to be revised.

First is kinetic energy expenditure which, in its more vigorous, outdoor, athletic manifestations, is typically more readily elicited and prevalent in males than females, even before males reach the postpubertal stage of being on the average, taller, heavier, and more lean and muscular than females.

Second is roaming and becoming familiar with or marking the boundaries of the roaming range. Whereas pheromonal (odoriferous) marking is characteristic of some small animals, in primates and humans vision takes the place of smell. The secretion of marker pheromones is largely under the regulation of male sex hormone and thus is more readily elicited in males than females. The extent of a sex difference in the threshold for visual marking in primates is still conjectural.

Third is competitive rivalry and assertiveness for a position in the dominance hierarchy of childhood, which is more readily elicited in boys than girls. A position of dominance may be accorded an individual without fighting or after a victory. Whereas fighting and aggressiveness per se are not sexually dimorphic, despite a widespread scientific assumption that they are, sensitivity to eliciting stimuli may or may not be. An example of the latter is retaliation against a deserter or rival in love or friendship, which is not sex specific.

Fourth is fighting off predators in defense of the troop and its territory which, among primates, is typically more readily elicited in males than females.

Fifth is fighting in defense of the young, which is more readily elicited in females than males. Females are more fiercely alert and responsive to threats to their infants than, in general, are males.

Sixth is a provision of a nest or safe place for the delivery, care, carrying, and suckling of the young. It is possible that this variable is associated with a greater prevalence of domestic neatness in girls than boys, as compared with the disarray which is the product of, among other things, vigorous kinetic energy expenditure.

Seventh is parentalism, exclusive of delivery and suckling. Retrieving, protecting, cuddling, rocking, and clinging to the young are more prevalent in girls' rehearsal play with dolls and/or playmates.

Eighth is sexual rehearsal play. Evidence from monkeys is that juvenile males elicit presentation responses in females and juvenile females elicit mounting responses in males more readily than vice versa. The taboo on human juvenile sexual rehearsal play and on its scientific investigation prohibits a definitive generalization regarding boys and girls at the present time.

Ninth is the possibility that the visual erotic image more readily elicits an initiating erotic response in males than in females, whereas the tactile stimulus more readily elicits a response in females. Here again, no definitive generalization can yet be made because of the effects of the erotic taboo and erotic stereotyping in our society.

Sex-derivative roles are, by definition, not sex exclusive, but sex-shared or interchangeable. Statistically there is overlap, so that extremely masculinized people of either sex resemble one another more closely than do men at either end of the scale of masculinization—and conversely, women. It is, in fact, a severe hardship for men to be forced by cultural tradition into an ultramacho sex-derivative role to a degree beyond which they are, by disposition, ill prepared.

Sex-adjunctive roles are those which bear a tertiary relationship to sex-derivative roles. To illustrate: Fetal androgenization has a primary effect in forming a penis instead of a clitoris (on even an XX female fetus should it be heavily androgenized). The same fetal androgen lays down a predisposition to sexually dimorphic play in infancy and childhood. When androgen reasserts itself again in boys at puberty, it governs the growth of bone, fatty, and muscle tissues in such a way that males—on the average, and despite much overlap with females—are more muscularly powerful than females, on the basis of being taller and leaner. Thus, in all the millennia prior to the modern age of industrial, farming, and domestic labor-saving devices, it made sense for societies to have a sex-based division of labor. This division of labor was, in ancient times, based on the greater mobility of the male as compared with the restricted mobility of the female while pregnant or breast-feeding. Women moved in closer proximity to the home base than did their men and they were chiefly responsible for feeding not only their babies but all members of their troop. The men ranged more widely in hunting, fighting, and trading. This ancient system of the division of labor survived the equalization of the sexes made possible first by the domestication of animals of transport and, more recently, by automotive transport and work on wheels or wings. Only now, in the 20th century, the age of birth control and the freedom of women from involuntary breeding, has the system begun to undergo extensive change. Most of the current feuding in the political debate regarding equal rights for men and women rages around issues of sex-adjunctive work roles and play roles.

To a visitor from another planet, this feuding could well seem incomprehensible, but the incomprehensibility would be nothing in comparison with that engendered by feuding over *sex-arbitrary* roles. Sex-arbitrary roles pertain to issues of sex-divergent body language, ornamentation, grooming, clothing, and etiquette. Often it is possible to conjecture some sort of connection between sex-arbitrary roles and sex-derivative roles. For example, the former Polynesian custom of restricting the amount of tattoo a woman might have on her face as compared with that of a man ostensibly reflected her lesser bravery as a warrior. In actual fact it signified her role as a lesser warrior who might fight only in defense of the tribal home territory when it was under attack by the enemy, whereas the male traveled far to maraud and initiate attack.

The ancient and widespread custom of the greater mobility of men is also reflected in the footwear of women. Until the 1949 victory of the Communist Revolution in China, families who aspired to wealth and prestige deformed the feet of their young daughters by binding them. These daughters were a living testament to their father's wealth, and also to that of their prospective husbands, insofar as their deformed feet rendered them incapable of working competitively with men, but only as courtesans or prostitutes. Today in our own society, we have an adumbration of this same custom of deformed feet in the fashion of high-heeled shoes for women which hobble their gait and enforce a method of locomotion which men interpret as needing their support.

The contemporary American customs of feminine decoration can be traced to an earlier era in which women were idle display models, exhibiting the wealth of their fathers or husbands. Now that women work and have their own wealth, there is a new fashion either for women to abandon cosmetic and jewelry decoration, or for their male partners to be decorated similarly to themselves. The furor in the 1960s regarding new long hair styles for males as well as females alienated many fathers from their own sons as effectively as if long hair were a badge of homosexual effeminacy—even though the new style dictated a macho moustache and beard as a badge of masculinity. Here is certain evidence of the pervasive extent to which the superficialities of the male role permeate the average man's perception, or rather his misperception, of his irreducible masculinity. Misperception is the correct term, for the average man, including the average physician or scientist, is not accustomed to differentiating his *sex role* from his *gender role.*

A person's sex role is a component of his/her gender role. A gender role is, like the obverse of a coin, the obverse of a gender identity. The identity is privately experienced. It is publicly manifested as the role. The role (and hence the identity) comprises everything that one says or does to manifest oneself as masculine, feminine, or androgynous. In toto, one's gender-identity/role (G-I/R) comprises the irreducible, the derivative, the adjunctive, and the arbitrary components of one's role on the basis of one's sexual status as male or female.

There are many variations of G-I/R compatible with sexual status as male or female in today's world. In yesterday's world there was no such variation. Cultural antiquity embodied as personal habit dies hard. That is why there is so much to say about male roles in contemporary science as applied to contemporary mental health, as exemplified in this book.

Chapter 1

Gender-Role Conflict and Strain in Men's Lives

Implications for Psychiatrists, Psychologists, and Other Human-Service Providers

James M. O'Neil

Introduction

Gender-role conflict and strain are part of contemporary society's gender reevaluation. This gender reevaluation includes a critical assessment of masculinity, femininity, and androgyny as norms for optimal functioning in a rapidly changing society. Gender-role reevaluation is the process whereby men and women assess, maintain, and redefine their feelings, thoughts, and behaviors about their masculine, feminine, and androgynous roles. Gender-role reevaluation is also part of society's concern with how the sexes interact and relate to each other. Currently, the sexes are asking questions about their gender-role definitions and how they have been emotionally affected or restricted by their socialization and sexism in their lives. From these gender reevaluations, many individuals are discovering gender-role conflicts and strains that emanate from early gender-role socialization and societal expectations related to the appropriateness of masculine and feminine roles. The reevaluation of gender roles is difficult for many to integrate into their emotional, career, and interpersonal lives and there is much struggle to incorporate new gender-role definitions without strain and conflict.

Gender-role conflict and strain has emerged for three central reasons. First, the public has assumed that biologic sex affects gender development in many more ways than has been scientifically documented. In other words, it has been assumed that one's sex dictates mutually exclusive roles of masculine and feminine behaviors. These assumptions have produced many unproven stereotypes

James M. O'Neil • University of Kansas, Lawrence, Kansas 66045; now at University of Connecticut, Storrs, Connecticut 06268

about men's and women's innate and behavioral options. These unproven stereotypes are a major source of gender-role conflict and contribute to the pervasiveness of sexism in our society.

Second, these stereotypes have contributed to parents' socialization of children and adolescents toward rigid gender roles of masculinity and femininity. In the past, healthly socialization was considered sex specific. Boys were to aspire to highly sex-typed masculine behavior and girls to highly sex-typed feminine behaviors. Boys learned to avoid and fear their femininity, while after puberty, girls were taught to suppress their masculine sides. This kind of rigid socialization has prohibited the sexes from developing both the masculine and feminine parts of their personalities. The outcome has been a restrictive behavioral repertoire and gender-role conflict and strain during life.

Third, gender-role strain has increased in response to societal, political, and technologic change. The Women's and Feminist Movements were major sources of change in the 1970s. Feminism affected all parts of society and the effects are still being felt at work and home, and in interpersonal relations. Although many of these changes have been positive, they have also caused considerable tension, role strain, and conflict for both men and women. A decade ago Toffler[1] warned that Future Shock was a major psychological problem for societies not able to adapt, understand, and integrate rapid changes in society.

Gender-Role Strain and Conflict in the 1970s: Effects on Men

Being male in the 1970s was full of insecurities, contradictory demands, and defensive behaviors. The Feminist and Women's Movements criticized many aspects of traditional male behavior as sexist, oppressive, and unacceptable. Traditional male courtesies and behaviors were attacked and repudiated by feminists who recognized that sexism was a destructive form of human oppression. Since many men have been socialized into these traditional behaviors, there were continual personal and interpersonal conflicts in the 1970s over male–female roles, attitudes, and behaviors.

A complete analysis of these gender-role conflicts is complex and still difficult for many men and women to understand. Nonetheless, both sexes are now attempting to piece together new definitions of masculinity and femininity. If men have learned anything about themselves from women feminists, it is that *men are also oppressed by rigid gender-role socialization processes (i.e., sexism) that limit their potential to be fully functioning, androgynous, human beings* (see Refs. 2–4, see also Chapter 2 in this volume, by Solomon).

The idea that men are oppressed by sexism and gender role socialization is difficult for men to accept. Many men have been socialized to behave in a sexist manner and their attitudes, values, and behaviors have never been challenged or analyzed. Additionally, few new roles that compliment women's demands for equality at work, home, and in interpersonal relations have emerged for men. As a result, many men have had difficulty developing and integrating new male roles that are compatible with nonsexist behavior.

Reactions to these gender-role conflicts are varied. Some men have few problems in adjusting to changes in women's roles and handle their life situations effectively without great stress.[5] Another group of men rigidly cling to sexist beliefs that once stablized their roles and therefore maintain control over women. Other men resist the inevitable social change that is necessary to equalize women's place in this democratic society. These men carefully conceal a defensiveness resulting from diminishing self-confidence. Some other men withdraw from gender-role conflicts at work and in the home in order to avoid resulting tensions which occur in interpersonal relations. Many of these reactions to changing roles are no longer healthy in a society where sex discrimination is against the law[6] and sexism is considered by many to be inhumane.

Although it is difficult to determine what the effects of these social changes will eventually be on men and women, it is apparent that gender role definitions are being discussed, debated, and changed. These discussions are part of our current gender-role reevaluation, and men are becoming aware of the effects of gender roles and sexism in their lives. Lewis and Pleck[7] indicate that "the investigation of male roles is now clearly established as part of the study of sex roles in the social sciences" (p. 429).

The purpose of this chapter is to discuss men's gender-role strain and conflict in the context of their socialized view of masculinity and femininity. It is hypothesized that the concepts of gender-role strain and conflict are central to understanding men's behavior and their common psychological problems. Secondly, it is hypothesized that the fear of femininity underlies much of men's current gender-role strain and conflict. It is also posited that the fear of femininity is learned during early gender-role socialization and can affect both psychological and physical health. Lastly, the fear of femininity and gender-role pat-

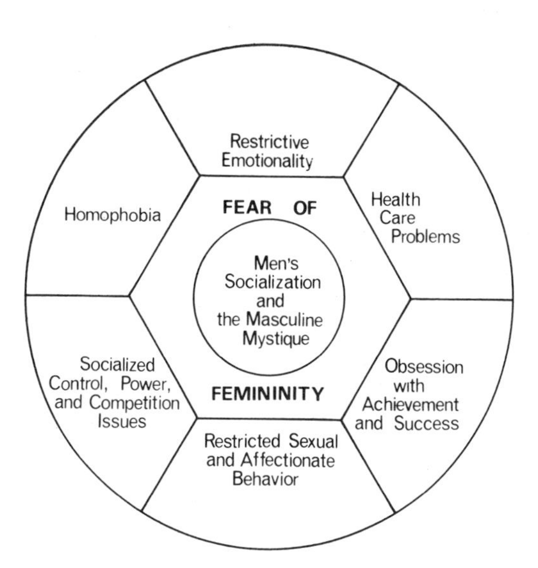

Figure 1. *Six patterns of gender-role conflict and strain emanating from men's socialization and the fear of femininity.*

terns and conflicts are identified as important concepts when working with men in counseling and psychotherapy. Figure 1 shows how men's socialization process and the Masculine Mystique and Value System relate to the fear of femininity. This fear produces six patterns of gender-role conflict and strain including: (1) restrictive emotionality, (2) homophobia, (3) socialized control, power, and competition issues, (4) restrictive sexual and affectionate behavior, (5) obsession with achievement and success, (6) health care problems. Each of these patterns of gender-role conflict will be discussed to better understand their value to psychiatrists, psychologists, and other human-service providers during these times of gender reevaluation.

RECENT LITERATURE ON MEN: COMMON THEMES OF GENDER-ROLE STRAIN AND CONFLICT

Recently there has been a substantial increase in literature about men and masculinity. Grady, Brannon, and Pleck[8] have synthesized much of the research literature in their annotated bibliography of over 250 entries. This bibliography demonstrates the growing amount of literature on the male sex role.

There are currently three kinds of literature providing printed information about men: (a) popularized, commercial books which summarize authors' opinions about men; (b) nonempirical journal articles, chapters, and books from the social sciences; and (c) journals and books that publish research on the male condition. Each of these sources is important to better understand men's lives and the gender-role conflicts and patterns that relate to masculinity.

The popularized books are usually available in paperback and often the most visible to the public.[9–26] These books describe the negative outcomes of adhering to a rigid masculine value system. Although these books outline men's problems and suggest solutions, they are replete with generalities that may fit a majority of men, but certainly not every man. These books provide readers with the basic issues of the men's liberation movement, and some[12,14,16,17,22] can be helpful for male clients experiencing masculinity and gender-role conflicts in counseling and psychotheray.

The second area of information on men is that the professional literature in the social sciences.[2,3,27–53] These sources include theoretical, speculative, and scholarly articles that synthesize past research and knowledge about men, masculinity, and male socialization. This literature provides greater scientific objectivity and fewer generalizations about men than in popularized books and offers support for the assumption that the masculine socialization process may contribute to men's emotional and physical problems.

The third source of information on men comes from experimental research and case studies in the social sciences. The empirical research is limited, and Pleck and Brannon[39] state that "...only recently have researchers begun to study systematically the impact on men of the powerful social expectations they face by virtue of being males" (p. 1). It is beyond the scope of this chapter to cite all the experimental research, but summaries are available elsewhere.[8,28,40,54,55] Additionally, four case studies of men have recently been reported in the literature[56–59] and provide important insights into men's lives. These case studies report interviews with men about their life experiences and the effects of these events on their physical and emotional lives. Levinson et al.'s results[58] are particularly important and valuable. They used intensive long-term interviews of 40 men to document the patterns that underlie men's lives. Levinson et al. found that men pass through predictable adult stages that are typified by change, stress points, ambitions, dreams, successes, and failures.

From popularized books, scholarly writings, and empirical research, we are learning more about the process of male socialization and the ways in which men can overcome restrictive notions of masculinity. The three sources of information on men vary in content, depth, and approach to understanding men's problems. There also appears to be a white middle class bias in reporting the state of men's lives. The popular literature periodically makes unwarranted generalizations about all men, but it does capture many aspects of the observable male condition. The theoretical articles from the social scientists go beyond the popular literature in depth by contributing sociologic and psychological meaning and respectability in the professions. The experimental and case studies are too few for a final evaluation, but future ones should provide a better scientific understanding of the male socialization process.

The literature reviewed suggests that primary outcomes of male socialization may produce conflicts for men, women, and children. Many men do experience physical and emotional stress from rigid adherence to masculine gender roles learned during socialization.[2,16,17,20,29,30,39,40,42,49,60,61] Unresolved gender role conflicts can potentially inhibit human maturity, affect overall emotional and physical health, and reduce happiness in life.[3,39–41]

GENDER- AND SEX-ROLE TERMINOLOGY

Gender- and sex-role conflicts are best defined by reviewing the terms "gender" and "sex role." Many psychologists and sociologists have used the terms gender and sex role synonymously. Both terms have implied the process where each sex learns their gender-related masculine and feminine roles and functions in society. Unfortunately, the term *sex* role has implied that gender learning is primarily affected by many biologically based, innate sex differences that predict and maintain stereotypic and sometimes sexist behavior.

Most researchers and theoreticians believe that even though biology may affect gender learning, the effects of family, peers, and society are more influential. Numerous authors indicate that cultural and societal learnings are likely to override *most* biological predispositions of men and women toward certain behavior patterns.[2,60,62,63] Moreover, how biological sex affects gender identity is controversial and a topic of intense research. Therefore, how biologic sex and gender relate and how they impact each other are both empirical and theoretical questions open to future research and speculation.

Unger[64] suggests that more concise and operational definitions are needed to explain sex and gender differences. Money (Foreword) and Solomon (Chapter 2 in this book) have addressed these definitional issues and provide sound rational for sex and gender as different but related concepts. Psychologists and many other writers have understood gender issues by researching psychological sex-role differences. Consequently, the research literature commonly uses the term "sex-role" to explain gender role behaviors. It is critical to have precise definitions if the professions are to better understand gender-role socialization and the causes of gender-role conflict. The following definitions are specified to facilitate understanding of the concepts and provide conceptual consistency throughout the chapter:

1. *Sex differences:* Differences in the average performance of the sexes in a given area of behavior due to either *biologic* or *psychological* factors.
2. *Biological sex differences:* Differences in human functioning between the sexes based on innate, *biologic* factors.
3. *Psychological sex difference:* Differences in human functioning between the sexes based on *psychological* factors. The psychological study of sex differences in personality is concerned with how the average female differs from the average male on a particular trait or behavior.[65,66]
4. *Gender identity:* An individual's subjective sense as to whether or not they are man or woman; masculine or feminine; or both man and woman and masculine and feminine.
5. *Gender role:* Those *nonphysiological* components of sex that are culturally regarded as appropriate to males or to females.[64] Behaviors, expectations, and role sets defined by society as masculine or feminine which are embodied in the behavior of the individual man or woman (Solomon, Chapter 2).
6. *Sex role:* Those physiological components of sex which determine different behaviors, expectations, and role sets for men and women.
7. *Gender-role socialization:* The process by which children and adults acquire and internalize the values, attitudes, and behaviors associated with either femininity, masculinity, or both.
8. *Gender-role conflict and strain:* A psychological state where gender roles have negative consequences or impact on the person or on others. These negative consequences occur when there is a discrepancy or conflict between the real self and the ideal self concept that is culturally associated with gender.[67] The ultimate outcome of this conflict is the restriction of the person's ability to actualize their *human potential* or the restriction of someone else's potential.
9. *Sex-role conflict and strain:* A psychological state where one's *biologic sex* has negative consequences or impact on the person or others.
10. *Sexism:* Any attitude, action, or institutional structure which subordinates, restricts, or discriminates against a person or group because of their biologic sex, gender identity or role, or sexual preference. *Personal sexism* is the subjective belief in the superiority of one sex, gender, or sexual preference over another and specific behaviors that maintain this superiority. *Institutional sexism* is the overt, covert, and subtle manifestations of personal sexism through institutional practices, structures, or policies.

These definitions attempt to specify the uniqueness and relationship of biologic sex and socialized gender identity. They also specify how biologic sex and gender socialization interact and affect human behavior and consequently have importance in understanding gender-role conflict and strain in contemporary society.

Gender-Role Conflict and Strain Explained

Many authors indicate that men's socialized adherence to rigid notions of masculinity and femininity contribute to emotional, interpersonal, and physical problems.[2,16,17,29,30,39,40,42,46,57,58,60,61] Many men do measure their manhood, masculine identities, and their personal value by how well they approximate the traditional male sex role. Society also has expectations and standards of masculinity that include such characteristics as strength, invulnerability, successfulness, toughness, self-reliance, aggressiveness, and daring. The pressures to meet these masculine norms produce gender-role strain and conflict.

Gender-role strain and conflict occur when rigid gender roles restrict a person's ability to actualize their human potential. Garnets and Pleck[67] define sex-role strain as discrepancies between individuals' perception of their personal characteristics and their standards derived from sex-role norms. Komarovsky[57] refers to sex-role strain as a lack of congruity between idiosyncratic personality characteristics and social roles. In a similar way, Turner [68] decribes one kind of sex-role strain as occurring when "a relatively uniform role is ascribed arbitrarily to a set of people with highly varied potentialities" (p. 292).

Garnets and Pleck[67] operationally define sex-role strain "as a discrepancy between the real self and that part of the ideal self concept that is culturally associated with gender" (p. 278). They believe that sex-role strain is in intrapsychic process that can lead to poor psychological adjustment, particularly low self-esteem. It is believed that when inflexible, rigid gender-role norms set standards that do not allow people to freely express themselves, these individuals will come to devalue themselves.[57,68] Garnets and Pleck[67] have recommended that further study and research be completed on the process of sex-role strain in men and women.

Researchers have discussed the effects of role strain on women,[65,66,69] on men,[3,38,53,57] and both men and women.[2] The extent to which sex-role strain negatively affects individuals is not well known and only a few studies have documented men's role strain.[56–58] An elaborate model explaining sex-role strain outcomes has been proposed.[67] Although it is beyond the scope of this chapter to describe this model, it does provide an example of how sex-role strain may be assessed and analyzed.

Gender-Role Socialization

Gender-role strain and conflicts are best understood in the context of a person's early gender-role socalization. The basis of gender identity is established in a person's childhood, particularly in the family, at school, and with peers. Between 18 months and 3 years nearly all individuals become sure that they are either male or female.[70,71] During this time, masculinity and femininity, as standards of behavior, are usually stereotyped and defined as polar opposites; and men and women develop sex or gender identities appropriate to their sex. This gender identity was once thought to be based on purely biological factors which produced many sex differences. It was believed that boys innately possessed masculine characteristics (strength, aggressiveness, rationality, independence, and task orientation), whereas girls innately possessed feminine characteristics (gentleness, passivity, intuitiveness, dependence, and relationship orientation). The polarization of gender attributes has incorrectly established ideas that sex differences are based entirely on innate, biologic differences rather than learned or socialized differences. This polarization of gender characteristics into dichotomous and dualistic categories (male and female) has attributed greater human differences to the sexes than really exist.

Although academicians and researchers have recognized that many gender roles are primarily learned, much of the public has believed that these roles are exclusively based on innate, genetic, and unchangeable biological differences. The dogmatic belief that men are exclusively the inheritors of one kind of gender identity and women inheritors of another kind has led to separatism between the sexes. This separatism (the battle between the sexes) has limited the perceptions, potentials, and possibilities for each sex and resulted in a restraining repertoire of attitudes, behaviors, and expectancies for both men and women.[63] This phenomenon is one basis of both personal and institutional sexism in our society.

Although research has not documented extensive psychological sex differences in humans,[72] sex-typing during socialization is very common. Many individuals have incorrectly generalized a few apparent biological or socialized sex differences to many unrelated skills, attitudes, and behaviors of males and females. Because of these unwarranted generalizations, children are taught the sex-typed communication styles and behavior patterns that traditionally represent their gender. As a result, men and women have usually learned only a portion of the skills and behaviors necessary to cope effectively in life.

Furthermore, traditionally held and unfounded beliefs about how the sexes should fulfill their biological destinies have been supported by the mass media. Since stereotypes that represent the ideal masculine and feminine types sell products, the media has commercialized, glorified, and helped the public internalize both a Masculine and Feminine Mystique. The cool, calm, commercialized "Marlboro Man" and the National Football League superstars typify the Masculine Mystique. The Total Woman,[73] the doorbell-ringing "Avon Lady," and the Dallas Cowboy cheerleaders solidify the attributes of the Feminine Mystique. The televised "Dating Game" brings together these two rigid sex role stereotypes and promotes them as the valued gender identities in our society.

ANDROGYNY—A POSITIVE BUT STILL UNPROVEN ALTERNATIVE. Currently, there is much discussion, debate, and research on a unifying gender role category called androgyny.[74–76] It is hypothesized that the androgynous personality (possessing and expressing both masculine and feminine attributes appropriately) will be better adjusted psychologically. Bem[77] speculates that the androgynous individual is a person who is able to remain sensitive to the changing conditions of situations and engage in whatever behavior seems most effective at the moment, regardless of sex-role stereotypes. The androgynous individual is someone who is both independent and tender, aggressive and gentle, assertive and yielding, masculine and feminine, depending on the situational appropriateness of these various behaviors. For effective and healthy functioning, masculinity and femininity must each be tempered by the other; and the two must be integrated to form a more balanced, fully human, androgynous personality.[75]

Positive empirical support for the concept of androgyny is accumulating in the literature. Androgynous self-concepts are associated with greater maturity in moral judgments[78] and higher self-esteem.[79,80] Additionally, evidence has shown that androgynous persons are flexible in their social behavior and that they can vary their behavior according to situational demands, rather than according to sex role stereotypes.[77,81,82]

Androgyny is not without criticism and debate.[83–85] Pedhazur and Tetenbaum [85] point out major weaknesses of the *Bem Sex Role Inventory* (BSRI) which proposes to measure psychological androgyny. The logic, validity, and utility of research on psychological androgyny has also been questioned.[84] Other researchers provide additional suggestions, guidelines, and cautions for future research on androgyny.[86–89]

The debate and interest in psychological androgyny is one of the many positive outcomes of the Feminist Movement of the 1970s. As noted above, there are many unanswered questions about androgyny from both theoretical and empirical perspectives. Worell[89] comments that the theoretical and empirical problems with androgyny are common to "other areas of virgin research." Future research and debate should help therapists better understand androgyny and its implications for therapy and positive mental health. Until more research is generated, androgyny will be a positive theoretical ideal but not an empirically validated construct.

THE RESEARCH LITERATURE AND THE POPULAR AND PROFESSIONAL LITERATURE ON MEN. The research and theory on gender-role socialization, gender roles, and socializing practices was extensive in the 1970s and emerged mainly from the psychology of women's literature written by women feminists.[2,31,60,63–66,69,72,78] These authors have significantly advanced the "psychology of gender roles" but there remain numerous problems in collectively interpreting their theory and research. Besides the definitional problems mentioned earlier,[64] there are also differences of opinion. For example, Maccoby and Jacklin's[72] classic and authoritative review of over 1600 studies on sex differences has been questioned and criticized.[63,78] Even with these problems, some common themes and tentative conclusions can be drawn from the research literature:

1. Research on sex differences, gender roles, and gender-role socialization is controversial and strongly debated.[63,64,66,69,72]

2. The effects of biology, cultural socialization, and combinations of both on gender development are not well known.
3. Research on sex differences, gender roles, and gender socialization is far from conclusive. It is unlikely that any work on the topic of sex differences will be accepted as definitive in the near future.
4. There are few documented psychological sex-role differences between the sexes that have empirical backing.[72]
5. Those psychological sex-role differences that do exist appear to be learned mainly through socialization, but researchers have documented at least two biologic (hormonal) sex differences in behavior patterns.[2,63,65,72]
6. Numerous authors have indicated that some of the literature on sex differences reflects the societal biases and the personal stereotypes of the researchers.[2,63,65,66,72]
7. Only a few differential socialization practices between the sexes have been documented in the research.
8. The research does suggest that boys seem to (a) have a more intense socialization experience than girls and (b) experience more pressure to conform to an unclearly defined masculine role.[72]

These *tentative* conclusions are still open to debate and controversy. It is expected that research on gender issues will be maintained in the 1980s. Much of the work completed has emanated from the psychology of women literature and there is only minimal research and scholarship on the psychology of men and gender roles.[7,8,30,39,46,57,58] Through additional research efforts, the effects of growing up male will be better understood and integrated into the psychology of gender roles.

The popular literature has recently criticized the male socialization process as a primary cause of men's physical and emotional problems.[14–17,19–21,23,24,90] In essence, these authors imply that men's socialization and adherence to rigid masculine sex-role stereotypes pose serious threats to their psychological health. The professional journals, books, and other scholarly works also suggest that the male socialization process may have serious negative outcomes for men.[6,30,38,40,51,91]

Although the popular literature contains many overgeneralizations, it does provide examples of problems emanating from the masculine socialization process.[14–17,21–23] Goldberg[16] describes 19 masculine binds that may emerge out of male socialization. These binds are summarized in the following conflict situations for men: (a) conflicts over integrating socialized male behaviors with new behaviors that are necessary to fulfill adult roles; (b) conflicts between traditionally defined feminine needs and external social pressure to be masculine; and (c) conflicts between the numerous, diverse roles to be fulfilled. Olson[23] discusses how men are programmed towards potentially negative outcomes that are directly related to the masculine socialization. Nichols[22] develops his criticism of the male socialization on the idea that roles are central in the average man's self-concept and, therefore, critical to understanding men's problems.

Mayer[21] and Levinson et al.[58] describe the potential long-term effects of male socialization during the midlife crisis in terms of physical health, emotional happiness, work patterns, and marital and family relations. Farrell's[14] synthesis describes the male socialization process as emanating from (a) 10 rigid commandments of masculinity, (b) masculine stereotypes learned at an early age, and (c) fear of femininity and, most of all, feminine values.

The professional literature, taken as a whole, suggests that the masculine socialization process underlies many of men's problems with themselves, other men, women and their work and leisure.[29,30,39,40,44,92] Men socialized into a restraining masculine gender role may demonstrate emotional and physical problems that are self-defeating and self-destructive. This view is based on the belief that exclusive adherence to socialized male values may be confining, insufficient for a healthy life, and oppressive to self and others.

Popular and professional literature suggests that beyond this recognition of restrictive male socialization is another problem. This is the problem of male awareness and acceptance of the ways past socialization and societal expectancies maintain restrictive and unhealthy attitudes, behaviors, and values for men. The imprint of early childhood learning and standards of masculinity are well established in adult males. Also, there is little societal reward for men to change during this period of gender reevaluation. Men may, therefore, experience difficulty understanding how internalized male values maintain their problems and limit their growth.

To understand how the male sex role may be limiting, men need to be open to introspection, ongoing self-evaluation, and feedback from others. Traditional masculine norms and values may prohibit men from openly and intimately examining life's emotional problems, expressing vulnerability, and giving up control. Therefore, the process of gender role reevaluation may be difficult for many men to start. Some men need a crisis that forces them to reevaluate themselves and build a new life structure without the past burdens of a narrowly defined role.[21] One of the first steps for men who are trapped in a rigid masculine gender role is to understand the values of the Masculine Mystique.

THE CULMINATION OF MEN'S SOCIALIZATION: THE MASCULINE MYSTIQUE AND VALUE SYSTEM. The Masculine Mystique and Value System is a complex set of values and beliefs that define optimal masculinity in a given society. The values and assumptions of the Masculine Mystique are based on rigid sex and gender role stereotypes. From these stereotypes emerge numerous assumptions, expectancies, and attitudes about what American manhood really means. Historically, the male value system has been considered positive and to produce normal and healthy development in men. There is little doubt that men's values have contributed positively to our growth as a nation and as a culture. Nonetheless, these values have recently been criticized as having negative outcomes for men, women, and children. Although nearly all men have been affected by the Masculine Mystique, the degree of negative effect will vary from man to man, depending on the situation, his social class, race, and early socialization.

The values of the Masculine Mystique in this country emerged within our early agrarian society which tamed the wilderness and started the American experiment in democracy. These particular male values were considered necessary to establish our economy before and after the Industrial Revolution, incorporate the principles of capitalism, and stablize the nuclear family. These values have changed little as our society has become more urbanized and computerized. The Feminist Movement of the 1970s was the primary stimuli for examining the Masculine Mystique, and other authors[14,21,29,32,93] have discussed individual aspects of these values. An expansion and synthesis of these assumptions follows:

1. Men are biologically superior to women, and therefore men have greater human potential than women.
2. Masculinity, rather than femininity, is the superior, dominant, more valued form of gender identity.
3. Men's power, dominance, competition, and control are essential to proving one's masculinity.
4. Vulnerabilities, feelings, and emotions in men are signs of femininity (weakness) and to be avoided.
5. Masculine control of self, others, and environment are essential for men to feel safe, secure, and comfortable.
6. Men seeking help and support from others show signs of weakness, vulnerability, and potential incompetence.
7. Masculine thinking, including rational and logical thought, is always the superior form of intelligence to understand life.
8. Interpersonal communications that emphasize human emotions, feelings, intuitions, and physical contact are considered feminine and should be avoided.
9. Men's success in relationships with women is contingent on subordinating females by using power, dominance, and words to control interactions.
10. Sexuality is a primary means of proving one's masculinity. Sensuality and intimacy are considered feminine and should be avoided.
11. Vulnerability and intimacy with other men are to be avoided because (a) being vulnerable with another male competitor may cause him to take advantage; (b) being intimate with other men may imply homosexuality or effeminacy.
12. Men's work and career success are measures of their masculinity.
13. Self-definition, self-respect, and personal worth are primarily established through achievement, success, and competence on the job.
14. Male power, control, and competition are the primary means to becoming a success and ensuring personal respect, economic security, and happiness.
15. Men are vastly different and superior to women in career abilities; therefore men's primary role is that of breadwinner or economic provider; women's primary role is that of caretaker of home, children, and men.

Male assumptions, expectancies, roles, and behaviors are usually shaped from the socialized values of the Masculine Mystique. Although the degree of effect will vary from man to man, most men will be affected in some way by masculine roles, expectancies, and values. For some men, proof of masculinity is situationally defined, and they must continually prove their masculinity through traditional male behaviors. Mayer[21] traces the development of the Masculine Mystique across male adult life stages and concludes that the myths about masculinity may self-destruct at midlife. Tolson[51] believes that masculinity is institutionalized and that our social, political, religious, and economic systems operate exclusively on masculine norms. To the extent that the values of the Masculine Mystique dominate our institutions, the same restrictive and unhealthy values will be a part of our institutions. Tolson[51] believes that one-dimensional masculinity is too simplistic. According to his analysis, normative masculinity varies according to social class. There exist working class, middle class, and progressive middle class definitions of masculinity. Each of these social class distinctions may have unique socializing effects on the man and shape his masculine attitudes, values, and feelings about himself.

Men who fail to conform to the Masculine Mystique are sometimes punished and labeled immature, unmasculine, and effeminate.[21] O'Leary and Donoghue[94] indicate that there is little research on how individuals react to males who deviate from the stereotypically defined masculine roles. However, their review does indicate: (1) sex-role deviance is more severely punished when displayed by boys than girls; (2) men are severely penalized for demonstrating incompetence and failing; (3) men who violate traditional masculine behavior risk devaluation; (4) early childhood deviation from the prescribed male role works against psychological adjustment. As a result, men may learn to punish and devalue themselves and others when they do not meet the Masculine Mystique and Value System.

It is believed that the strength of the Masculine Mystique helps explain the pervasiveness of sex-role stereotypes and sexism in our society.[11,14,30,41] This sexism violates women because the Masculine Mystique and Value System subordinates and restricts feminine attitudes, values, and behaviors. It violates men by denying them the opportunity to express their femininity and therefore denying them important parts of themselves.

SUBORDINATION OF FEMININE VALUES: OUTCOMES OF THE MASCULINE MYSTIQUE AND VALUE SYSTEM

Many assumptions of the Masculine Mystique reflect the implicit inferiority of femininity compared to masculinity as gender orientations. In other words, a direct outcome of men's socialization is the subordination of feminine values, attitudes, and behaviors. This subordination of femininity is central to an understanding of the conflict between the sexes in many life areas. It also explains much of men's gender-role strain and conflict in contemporary society.

The subordination of feminine values is defined in two ways: (1) to consider feminine characteristics, attitudes, and behaviors inferior compared to masculine characteristics, (2) to believe that women, men, and children who display feminine characteristics are inferior, inappropriate, and immature. The subordination of feminine values represents an attempt by men to solidify and express their masculinity as part of adult development and identity.

Numerous authors have described how men's aversion to femininity is central to understanding the male problems and masculine psychology.[17,22,30,58,95,96] The subordination of femininity will vary considerably depending on the man's early gender-role socialization, age, race, and social class. In varying degrees, many men develop a fear of femininity while trying to prove the superiority of masculinity.

Fear of Femininity: The Cradle of Gender-Role Conflicts and Strain

The fear of femininity is a strong, negative emotion in self or others associated with feminine values, attitudes, and behaviors. These emotional reactions are primarily learned in early childhood when gender identity is being formed by parents, peers, and the societal values. The dynamics of fearing one's femininity are not well understood and many times are unconscious to the man. When a man fears his feminine side, he really fears that others will see him as stereotypically and negatively feminine (i.e., weak, dependent, submissive) rather than positively masculine. This is not an unreasonable fear since femininity is subordinated and depreciated in many parts of society. Like most women, men fear that expressing their feminine sides will result in devaluation, subordination, and the appearance of inferiority in front of others. Men are aware that women's femininity is devalued by other men and attempt to avoid situations where their femininity could be observed and also devalued. The cost of showing stereotypic feminine qualities could be disrespect, failure, and emasculation and these are high costs for a man who wants to fulfill the Masculine Mystique.

Although the fear of femininity has gone unlabeled, numerous authors have written about how femininity threatens men during gender-role socialization and over the life cycle.[14,17,22,23,30,58] This author's review of the literature identified four principal authors who have contributed to the development of the concept of fear of femininity.[17,30,58,95,96] These authors discuss the fear and subordination of femininity from different but overlapping perspectives. Their writings span psychologic and sociologic theory and include both popular and professional literature.

JUNG'S ANIMA AND ANIMUS. Jung's explanation of the anima and animus is related to the fear of femininity. Jung believed that men and women possessed *both* feminine and masculine archetypes. Archetypes are defined as a universal thought form (idea) that contains a large element of emotion. The feminine archetype in man is called anima, the masculine archetype in woman is called animus. Specifically, the anima is the personification of all feminine qualities in a man's psyche. These feminine characteristics include a man's capacity for relatedness, emotionality, involvement with people, spontaneity, unplanned activities, and sensuality.

The anima represents an inherited, collective image of femininity and women in the man's unconscious. This image is first understood by the man's relationship with his mother. When the child grows older, his bonds with his mother and her femininity become more limited, restrictive, and frustrating. Consequently, the needs of the anima and the man's feelings about his mother and femininity are then repressed in the unconscious. The feminine characteristics and attitudes of the anima are also later repressed because they are alien to the masculine role that society expects from men. From this time on, the man's perceptions, feelings, and behaviors are affected by his unconscious and repressed notions of femininity through the anima. If the man's anima is not integrated into his personality, the man will appear detached, abstract, rational, and lacking in typically feminine ways. The anima-possessed man will be swayed by moods, depressions, anxieties, and fears.

After decreasing his identification with his mother, the man seeks out a mother replacement to fulfill the needs of the anima. If the man chooses a woman who is incompatible with his unconscious model of femininity experienced as a child, he will be disturbed by unconscious negative feelings. These emotions will make him dissatisfied with the woman and he will find faults and shortcomings but not be aware of the real reasons for his discontent. The more unaware the man is of his undeveloped anima, the more likely he is to be attracted to and conflicted with a woman who represents his unconscious ideals of femininity. The man may experience antagonism and conflict as he projects his unconscious, feminine side on to women who most directly remind him of his repressed femininity. Jung believed that much maladjustment and unhappiness is due to the inability of people to integrate the feminine and masculine parts of their personalities. For men, the antagonism toward women may largely be a projection of their repressed femininity and the threat that women pose during intimate and interpersonal encounters.

Maslow[97] summarizes Jung's thoughts on the anima. He indicates that the man who is unconsciously fighting against those qualities he and his culture defines as feminine, will fight these same qualities in the external world. He will simply be afraid of his own femininity and those who manifest it directly to him. This will result in the rejection of feminine values, attitudes, and behaviors and the subordination of women and feminine men in society. Maslow[97] speculates about the individual man by indicating: "If he can make peace with his female inside, he can make peace with the females outside, understand them better, be less ambivalent about them, and even admire them more as he realizes how superior their femaleness is to his own much weaker version" (p. 162).

The man who can resolve and accept his own femininity will be much better able to accept women's femininity and not be threatened or afraid of it. Jung's theory of the anima in men provides an intrapsychic and theoretical foundation for the fear of femininity in contemporary culture.

DAVID AND BRANNON'S NO SISSY STUFF. Another major theory defining the male sex role and explicating the fear of femininity has been described as No Sissy Stuff: The Stigma of Anything Vaguely Feminine.[30] This theme suggests a stigma associated with all stereotypically feminine characteristics and qualities.

Specifically, this theory suggests that the fear of femininity is learned by: (1) early anxiety of being considered a girl, sissy, or feminine; (2) a rule dictating that a "real man" must never resemble a woman or possess feminine characteristics; (3) openness and vulnerability being considered unmasculine; (4) fear of being seen as a homosexual.

These authors indicate that a boy learns these themes with difficulty because they must identify with a father who is usually absent and because it is difficult for the young boy to understand a culturally defined masculine role which is restrictive and unclear. Parents are concerned about how well boys conform to the masculine role and fathers are particularly concerned if their sons manifest feminine qualities. Boys learn to avoid most stereotypic feminine characteristics since both parents express displeasure at these qualities. Consequently, the male socialization process can produce: (1) a life-long aversion to any quality thought to be feminine; (2) constant striving for the ways to be masculine; (3) an inexpressive male image that prohibits open expression of feelings and feminine characteristics; and (4) an emotional and physical distancing between men because of feared homosexuality. The stigma of anything feminine is reinforced by parents and society. Consequently boys learn to reject and repress the feminine side of their personalities at an early age.

Research on male socialization does suggest that boys have more intense socialization experiences than girls.[72] Feminine qualities and characteristics in boys are discouraged and discredited. For example, boys receive "...more pressure against engaging in sex inappropriate behavior, whereas the activities that girls are not supposed to engage in are much less clearly defined and less firmly enforced" (p. 348).[72] It appears that boys are under pressure to manifest masculine characterisitcs and receive reprimand, particularly from fathers, when they deviate from the expected male behaviors. Growing up male seems to have some unique and direct negative consequences and pressures.

Hartley[98] grasped this fact two decades ago. Her review of the literature suggests that early male behavior is rarely defined clearly and that young boys must learn appropriate male behavior by trial and error. Many boys experience repeated reprimand and embarassment when deviating from masculine gender role norms. Her analysis indicates that the outcome of this process is anxiety because: (1) The boy is expected to behave in a certain way which is not clearly defined. (2) The expected behavior is based on reasons that the boy cannot understand. (3) The expected behavior is enforced by direct and indirect threats, punishment, and anger from important parental models. These conditions may force boys into early masculine behavior to avoid parental or peer punishment. In addition, Hartley indicates that boys will experience gender-role anxiety to the degree that: (1) pressure to be manly is exerted on the boy; (2) the boy is pressed to conform to rigid sex-role standards; (3) a good role model is available to the boy; and (4) the boy is successful in achieving the expected role. Hartley[98] concludes that these issues, as well as the influences of peers and society, can produce many male conflicts that may potentially affect later adult life. Although more research is needed, David and Brannon's "No Sissy Stuff" theme does have some empirical backing in the research literature.

Goldberg's Analysis. Goldberg addresses ways men cope psychologically with their femininity. He indicates that socialized masculinity is largely a psychologically defensive process rather than an authentic and organic process. Many men use their energy to prove and defend their masculinity and deny any feminine characteristics. Many men are motivated to prove that they are *not* feminine, vulnerable, emotional, helpless, afraid, weak, impotent, and unmanly.

Goldberg's analysis described men's psychological core as being repressed. This repressed core consists of men's forbidden parts, including their dependency, fear of emotions, and anything else that might be equated with femininity or unmasculine behavior. Since men's earliest identification is through a relationship with their mothers, femininity is therefore a natural part of their psychological core. The stronger the feminine identification, the more it may threaten the man or the more powerful his denial may be of his feminine parts. Goldberg[17] states "the more powerful and threatening this core is, the more rigid the defenses against it will be and the more he will need constantly to prove his autonomy, ability to perform, rationality, unemotionality, lack of dependence, hunger and other human needs" (pp. 149–150). Goldberg's analysis of men's psychological problems due to repressed femininity and rigid male sex roles needs further conceptualization in the psychiatric and psychological professions.

Levinson's Masculine/Feminine Polarity. Levinson et al.'s[58] research provides some direct support to substantiate the fear of femininity. Levinson and his associates have conducted case studies of 40 men between ages 35 and 45 in four different occupations. Their intensive and long-term interviewing of these men contributes to our understanding of how gender affects men over the lifespan and particularly how they respond to their femininity. One of Levinson et al.'s major findings was that all men experienced a masculine/feminine polarity that caused varying degrees of conflict over the life span.

From Levinson et al.'s case studies, it appears that boys learn what masculinity and femininity are from mothers, fathers, siblings, peers, and society at large. Attitudes, wishes, fantasies about masculinity and femininity are formed about self and through relationships with others. Masculine feelings and attitudes develop into a gender identity and men conclude that masculinity and femininity are separate polarities. In other words, men are masculine, women are feminine, and no one can be both. The integration of the masculine/feminine polarity is a principle task of midlife individuation and most men at midlife must come to terms with the coexistence of masculine and feminine parts of self.

The masculine/feminine polarity splits the concepts of masculinity and femininity into two separate categories. Stereotypic masculine and feminine characteristics are considered by many men to be opposite and therefore mutually exclusive. Levinson et al. summarize the masculine/feminine polarity found in their sample by describing the men's prescriptions of each gender orientation:

Masculinity is associated with:

1. power, exercising control over others; being (and being recognized as) a person of strong will, a leader who "gets things done";

2. strength, bodily prowess, toughness, and stamina to undertake long, grueling work and endure severe bodily stress without quitting;
3. logical and analytical thought, intellectual competence, understanding how things work;
4. achievement, ambition, success at work, getting ahead, earning one's fortune for the sake of self and family.

Femininity is associated with:

1. weak, frail, submissive, and unassertive behavior; victimization by others who have more power and are ready to use it exploitatively; limited bodily resources to sustain a persistent effort toward valued goals;
2. emotions, intuition; likelihood of making decisions on the basis of feelings rather than careful analysis;
3. building a nest, taking care of needs of husband and children;
4. homosexuality.

From their research, Levinson et al. suggest three reasons for the masculinity/ femininity split described above. First, the split is strongly reinforced by cultural traditions and norms in society. Second, the personal immaturity and problems of the men also contributed to their difficulties in integrating their feminine sides. Third, the magnitude and pressure of evolving life tasks in early adulthood required that masculinity be the driving force in the men's lives. Levinson et al. describe the resolution of the masculine/feminine polarity as a principal task of midlife individuation and an issue that spans much of the adult life cycle. Levinson et al.[58] summarized their research by indicating:

> The Masculine/Feminine polarity was of great importance to all the men in our study, though the specific content and conflicts varied enormously. Every man has his own identity. It is plain from their lives that the effort to attain one's manhood is at its peak in early adulthood. As a young man starts making his way in the adult world, he wants to live in accord with the images, motives, and values that are most central to his sense of masculinity, and he tends to neglect or repress the feminine aspects of his self. Any part of the self that he regards as feminine is experienced as dangerous. A young man struggling to sustain his manliness is frightened by feelings and interests that seem womanly. One result of this anxiety is that much of the self cannot be lived out or even experienced in early adulthood (p. 230).

Levinson et al. summarize the masculine/feminine polarity by indicating that, first, the male qualities observed are a multifaceted pattern of masculinity in opposition to a complementary pattern of femininity. Second, a unifying theme in the subjects' masculine patterns was doing, making, and having. Third, many men have difficulty utilizing their feminine sides in early adulthood. Fourth, there were developmental gains in middle adulthood in resolving the masculinity/femininity polarity particularly in a man's relation with his mother, peer women, and his role as a mentor. Lastly, Levinson et al.'s initial results clearly imply that the masculinity/femininity polarity is part of men's fear of femininity and that it exists in varying degrees in the sample studied.

Comment and Criticism on the Fear of Femininity

The fear of femininity has been presented by reviewing the psychologic and sociologic theory and the limited research available. Jung's concept of the anima postulates the psychological processes implied in the fear of femininity. Even though Jung's anima–animus concepts are open to criticism,[99,100] these concepts do provide a theoretical explanation of the fear of femininity as well as the way it operates as an intrapsychic process. David and Brannon's No Sissy Stuff is comprehensive in nature, has sociologic meaning, and has some empirical support in the literature. Goldberg's analysis lacks theoretical coherence and depth but does echo both Jung's anima concept and David and Brannon's postulates. Although Levinson et al.'s research methodology will be questioned, his case studies do provide direct evidence for the fear of femininity as manifested in the masculinity/femininity polarity. His results indicate that all the men studied experience their gender growth as a split between masculine and feminine characteristics. The predominant theme appearing for all men was an emphasis on their masculinity and varying degree of conflict with their femininity. Additional research is needed on the masculinity/femininity polarity as it relates to the fear of femininity and men's gender-role conflict and strain.

Patterns of Gender-Role Conflict and Strain Identified

The fear of femininity has been hypothesized to cause gender-role conflict and strain for men. Figure 1 depicts men's socialization and the Masculine Mystique and Value System producing the Fear of Femininity. The Fear of Femininity produces six patterns of gender-role conflict and strain including (1)restrictive emotionality, (2) homophobia, (3) socialized control, power, and competition issues, (4) restricted sexual and affectionate behaviors, (5) obsession with achievement and success, (6) health care problems. Each of these patterns will be defined and discussed since they have implications for counseling and psychotherapy with men.

Restrictive Emotionality. Skovholt[5] describes restrictive emotionality as a major problem for men. Goldberg[16] believes that men have not been socialized to communicate their feelings, be vulnerable, and express intense emotions directly. Nichols[22] points out that a man who expresses feelings too openly is usually judged as immature, unstable, or unreasonable. Vulnerability and direct expression of feelings would look feminine in the eyes of others. It would also mean giving up control emotionally, opening up the inner self to others, and admitting human weakness. Men reason that being honest, open, and expressive is dangerous because expression of feelings rather than fact can lead to loss of control. Some men reason that, if they give up control, people will take advantage of them, and they are moved to a "one down" position.

Restrictive emotionality is defined as having difficulty appropriately expressing one's own feelings or denying others their rights to emotional expressiveness.[101] Restrictive emotionality implies that men will have difficulty expressing feelings openly, giving up emotional control, and being vulnerable to self, others, and new experiences. These deficits imply that some men will have difficulty with self-disclosure, recognizing feelings, and processing the complexities of interpersonal life. Other times anger, hostility, and rage can result from repressed and unexpressed emotions. Explosions of anger sometimes result in aggressive and uncontrollable behavior. Family violence including wife battering, child abuse, incest, and rape can be the extreme consequences of restrictive emotionality.

To compensate for restrictive emotionality, men develop intellectual and rationalistic patterns of communication using words to explain reality, control situations, and express self. Restrictive emotionality may inhibit emotional, expressive, and intimate exchanges with other men, women, and children. Goldberg[17] indicates that for some men confronting one's inner emotions is a dreadful threat.

The fear of femininity contributes to men's restrictive emotionality and their difficulties in accepting and expressing emotions. These difficulties are related to the socialized values of the Masculine Mystique. Men restrict their emotions because they fear that their feelings will be associated with femininity and this will threaten their masculine roles. The fear of femininity and restrictive emotionality are related to four dubious assumptions:

1. Emotions, feelings, and vulnerabilities are signs of femininity and therefore to be avoided.
2. Men seeking help through emotional expression are immature, unstable, weak, dependent, and therefore feminine.
3. Interpersonal communication emphasizing emotions, feelings, and intuitions are considered feminine and to be avoided.
4. Emotional expression may expose inner fears and conflicts that could portray the man as feminine.

These assumptions are the basis for men's fears about expressing emotions. Men aspire to live out their socialized masculine values over the adult life cycle[58] and emotional expressiveness has usually been considered part of the feminine value system. Men fear that their emotionality will be associated with femininity and consequently they will be discredited by others. Consequently, men develop a cognitive–rationalistic approach to people and life in general.

Nichols[22] believes that the deprivation that men suffer from their restrictive emotionality can distort their perceptions of others and negatively affect their interpersonal relationships. For most men, the capacity for accurate recognition and communication of feelings is a prerequisite for growth and coping with life's problems. Levinson et al.[58] summarize this well by noting that "feelings are important to the whole sense of who the man is, who he wants to be, and who he is terrified of being" (p. 229). For many men, it is their femininity that they are most terrified of discovering and expressing to others.

Many authors describe men having difficulty communicating emotions, establishing trust, being vulnerable, and openly expressing feelings.[5,14,16,17,21,23,40,51,102] These authors believe that men are not taught to recognize and acknow ledge emotions, but to deny and fear them. Men may intellectualize their feelings and be preoccupied with logical reasoning and problem solving rather than the emotional impact of interpersonal communication. This socialized use of rational and logical thought has reduced men's ability to communicate intimately. It has also hindered men from understanding their feelings and generally distanced them from human emotion. If men are overdeveloped in the rational domain, they usually are underdeveloped in the affective domain.

Research in patterns of self-disclosure has shown that men typically reveal less personal information about themselves than women.[103] If self-disclosure is an empirical index of openness or presentation of real self, then the research would suggest that men are more prone to hide feelings about themselves and their emotional lives. Since self-disclosure, trust, and vulnerability are essential to the development of intimacy, men may have difficulty establishing close interpersonal relationships. Men's inability to disclose feelings, to be vulnerable, and to give up control, impedes the experiencing of pleasure in emotional growth and experiences.

Restrictive emotionality has caused men difficulties in their interpersonal relations. Many authors have written about men's limitations and difficulties in interpersonal communication.[2,14,16,22,23,30,104,105] Since gender-role socialization has supported the division of people into two categories, it is not surprising that men and women have developed different and sometimes conflicting interpersonal styles of communication. These conflicting styles of communication may limit intimacy and constructive problem solving in interpersonal situations. Socialized differences in communication may also offer some explanation for dysfunctional relationships between the sexes as well as for the spiraling divorce rates. Many women feel alone with their need to express, experience, and integrate their emotional lives. Over time, some women adopt the male model and also begin to doubt the legitimacy of emotional expression with men and others. This can cause interpersonal distance between men and women, limit full communication, and ultimately restrict intimacy and depth in relationships.

The popular literature has discussed men's differences and difficulties in interpersonal communication.[14,16,22,23] These authors believe that men's communication styles are based on the masculine value system and directly conflict with women's feminine style of communication. Additionally, many men believe that their style of communicating is superior to women's. Olson's[23] description of the specific differences in male and female communication patterns includes two different levels of communication each emphasizing important but sometimes conflicting parts of a communication exchange. Olson's analysis parallels Parsons and Bales'[106] description of two levels of communication associated with either masculinity or femininity.

The first level of communication is called *instrumental* and describes the stereotypically masculine approach to interpersonal communication. This approach emphasizes the content of the message by using logic, reason, and facts to explain the issues. It deemphasizes the dynamics of the interpersonal relationship and is concerned with the problem-solving, goal-oriented outcomes of the communication. This pattern of communication parallels the masculine socialization process that emphasizes objective information, task orientation, and outcomes. However, when used exclusively, it may restrict male/female relationships since women may see the instrumental approach to communication as impersonal or see men using it to maintain control of the relationship.

The second level of communication is called *expressive* and describes the feminine approach to communication. This approach is more concerned with how the interpersonal messages affect the relationship. It is also more subjective, intuitive, and more involved with the interpersonal process than specific solutions to conflicts. It is believed that women are socialized toward the expressive level of communication and are more effective at using it in interpersonal conflicts and situations. Since women are believed to be more aware of the subjective, expressive aspect of the message, they tend to use this information to effect desired changes in their relationships. Since many women have not been socialized to compete with men in instrumental communication exchanges, they are sometimes unsure about how to be assertive, express themselves, and use their expressive skills. Under these circumstances, the potential for miscommunication and misunderstanding is usually high.

These two different, socialized approaches to communication can obstruct the formation of intimate relationships based on openness, compromise, and the ability to solve problems. Sometimes these two levels of communication do not always break down according to sex. However they occur, differing levels of communication are enough to cause misunderstandings, conflicts, and control struggles that can inhibit and destroy intimacy. Both feeling and reason are needed to label the complexities of cognitive and affective experiences in interpersonal life. In the final analysis, both instrumental and expressive communication patterns are necessary for a fully functioning human relationship. If gender-role socialization continues to support sex-typed communication patterns for males and females, difficulties in interpersonal communication will also continue.

HOMOPHOBIA. Homophobia has also been described as negatively affecting men and their relationships with each other.[15,102,107–109] Morin and Garfinkle[108] define homophobia as any belief system which supports negative myths and stereotypes about homosexual people. These authors indicate that homophobia is (1) a belief system which justifies discrimination on the basis of sexual orientation; (2) the use of offensive language or slang (e.g., "queer") which characterizes gay people; and (3) any belief system which does not value homosexual life styles equally with heterosexual life styles. Lewis[102] defines homophobia as a fear of homosexuals or the fear of one's being or appearing to be homosexual. Lehne[107] defines homophobia as an irrational fear or intolerance of homosexuality and a socially determined prejudice much like sexism and racism rather than a medically recognized phobia. Homophobia does not exist in most cases as an isolated prejudice but is characteristic of an individual who is generally rigid and sexist.

The fear of femininity is central to understanding male homophobia. Men's stigma about femininity is directly associated with their fears about homosexuality[30] Levinson's[58] case studies revealed that men's aversion to femininity is in part due to their fears of homosexuality. If a man associates with gays, there is an automatic conclusion that he is feminine, effeminate, and a homosexual. This erroneous deduction equates homosexuality with femininity. Consequently, femininity, labeled as homosexuality, breeds homophobia and threatens men and their masculine roles. In this way, homophobia may be regarded as (1) an expression of the man's fear of his femininity and (2) his fears about his own sexual or interpersonal attraction to other men. A man who is afraid of his own femininity or his attraction to other men may attempt to reassure himself and others that he is heterosexual by vigorously suppressing all feminine, interpersonal, and intimate feelings or impulses.[108] When this fear turns to anxiety, the homophobic man, unable to handle his feared femininity or homosexuality, will project his fear by negatively labeling others as homosexuals. In the process, he denies his femininity and usually denies others their right to be themselves.

Morin and Garfinkle[108] reviewed eight psychological studies on the personality correlates of homophobia. They found those who are more negative in their attitudes toward homosexuality are more authoritarian, dogmatic, cognitively rigid, intolerant of ambiguity, status conscious, sexually rigid, guilty and negative about their own sexual impulses, and less accepting of others in general. They conclude that these personality characteristics might be expected of any highly prejudiced group of people. Their review also assesses homophobia from the standpoint of socialized belief systems within the culture and from the perspective of individual personality characteristics. They concluded that social and cultural learning is a powerful force associated with the dread, fear, and hatred of homosexuals. In summarizing the research available on homophobia, Morin and Garfinkle[108] describe the homophobic personality as one which is rural, white, male, first-born, reared in the Midwest and the South, more religious, and more conforming. Additionally, Lehne[107] specifies three social attitudes that are the basis of homophobia: (1) religious beliefs that homosexuality is morally wrong, (2) scientific theories of homosexuality as an illness or deviance, and (3) social beliefs that homosexuality is damaging to society.

Homophobia has been described by several authors as a powerful and central dynamic in the maintenance of traditional male roles.[107,108,110] Although there is little experimental evidence to show that homophobia prevents interpersonal and emotional intimacy between heterosexual men, it has been assumed to be a significant barrier to male self-disclosure, companionship, and touching. Homophobia is also a significant contributor to reinforcement and restriction of masculine roles.[38,108] Lehne[107] suggests that homophobia is used by men to enforce social conformity to the male role and maintain social control. When feminine behavior is shown by men and noticed by homophobic males, these behaviors will be ignored while also discredited and categorized as inappropriate, immature, and unacceptable. Men who are exclusively committed to the Masculine Mystique and rigid masculine gender roles will discredit or punish other men who deviate from the established male role. In this way, homophobia acts as a vehicle to maintain traditional male norms, values, and power. Lehne[107] indicates that homophobia (1) exists as a device of social control to maintain male behavior appropriate to the social situation, and (2) to control all men, not just male homosexuals. Homophobia is a gender-role conflict that limits and prohibits interpersonal closeness among men. The dynamics of homophobia are also part of the overt repression of male femininity and the oppression of both gay and straight males in our present society.

SOCIALIZED CONTROL, POWER, AND COMPETITION ISSUES. Most men are socialized to actualize controlling behaviors that relate to power and competition. *Control* implies to regulate, restrain, and to have others or situations under one's command. *Power* is authority, influence, or ascendancy over others. *Competition* is the act of striving against others to win or gain something.

The fear of femininity focuses men's attention on control, power, and competition issues. The controlled or impotent man is considered feminine and less of a man than one who is in charge, powerful, and competitive. The socialized Masculine Mystique suggests that power, dominance, and control are essential proof of one's masculinity. Control and power are vital to a man's positive self-image and competition is the vehicle to obtain both. Men's biologic predisposition toward aggressiveness and dominant behavior[72] interact with a learned fear of femininity that cause patterns of gender-role conflict.

Many authors believe that men are socialized to use power, control, and competition to validate their masculinity.[2,21,22,29,40,91,111–114] Men learn at an early age to compete for power and to establish their place in the home, school, or work setting. Young boys are biologically more aggressive than girls and, more importantly, are reinforced to be active, dominant, powerful, and in control of situations.[72] Additionally, boys receive more punishment, praise, and encouragement from their parents than girls.[65] Through this feedback from parents, boys have more opportunities to learn how to compete, to win, and feel in control. Also boys learn the value of power by modeling from adult men in work and family roles.[51] Boys often see men as more powerful than women and believe that being powerful is an essential part of being a man. They learn that power is important to control others, to establish and maintain priorities, and to meet most of their needs. Boys also learn to use power by observing family members who are struggling for independence, autonomy, and self-control. Men sometimes believe that power is a goal in itself to be continuously sought after. In many cases, power is viewed as something that is external to the self which must be taken from others. Since it sometimes appears that there are limited amounts of power, methods of manipulation may be learned to obtain it.

Closely related to the issues of control and power is the concept of competition.[30,57,91,102] Competition involves the comparison of self with others to establish superiority of one person over another in a given situation or activity. As a result, competition is less concerned with the innate abilities or qualities of the individual than with how those abilities stack up against the abilities of others. There are usually varying degrees of depersonalizing others in competitive situations.

Numerous authors believe men are socialized to be competitors during boyhood and that the need to compete is responsible for much role strain felt by the average male.[15,22,55] These authors imply that, when a man competes, winning becomes his primary objective and other issues become less important. Under the threat of defeat, emasculation, and loss of male self-esteem, sensitivity to others may be subordinated to one goal—winning.

In adult life, men find outlets for power, competition, and control issues in several ways. Competitive games and sports are outlets for learned competitiveness.[55] Sports are also ways for men to safely revitalize relationships with each other. Men also go to work to compete for power, position, and dollars. Since capitalism is based on competition, the work setting is a meaningful place to actualize competitive yearnings. Competition at work provides another way to validate one's masculinity through earning higher pay, gaining advancements, and prestige. Sometimes, men's intense competition with others can produce stressful work environments, work anxiety, and dysfunctional human relations.

Many authors believe that men's control, power, and competition issues can cause serious problems for men in their interpersonal relations.[2,21,22-29,40,91,111–114] Many men have learned to handle their interpersonal relations by using control, power, and interpersonal competition as a means of establishing their superiority. Some men have difficulty giving up power and control during interpersonal conflicts. This would appear to be feminine and pose threats to their masculinity. Safilios-Rothschild[41] suggests that men have turned love and sexuality into means for gaining power and control over women. She reports that men's "power trip" has interfered with their ability to love, disclose feelings, and be compassionate. Nichols[22] theorizes that before men can learn to give up control of others, they must learn to trust themselves and others in unstructured interpersonal and social settings.

The costs of always being powerful, dominant, controlling, and competitive are usually high. The man who justifies his masculinity through power and control makes himself vulnerable in many ways. Usually without knowing it, the man concentrates on his position or control in the relationship rather than on important communication and interpersonal dynamics that can make the relationship more intimate and, therefore, secure. Nichols[22] points out, the controlling man forfeits self-awareness, sensitivity to others, and freedom to be honest, vulnerable, spontaneous, emotional, playful, and socially adept. The tragedy of this is that these noncompetitive, uncontrolling characteristics are essential for open communication, conflict management, and intimacy which can sustain and revitalize interpersonal relations.

RESTRICTIVE SEXUAL AND AFFECTIONATE BEHAVIOR. Restricted sexual and affectionate behavior is defined as having limited ways of expressing one's sexuality and affection to others. For men, this is partly caused by their inability to accept the feminine sides of their nature. The fear of femininity limits men in sexual and affectionate encounters because they are socialized to (1) inhibit emotions and limit self-disclosure, (2) view touching and sensuality as feminine and inappropriate, (3) regard sex as an achievement, performance, or control situation, (4) view sex as separate from love and intimacy, (5) regard expression of sexual need and passive sexual behavior as feminine. These socialized realities limit men from expressing their feelings through touching and limit the range of sexual behavior in intimate relationships. Some men do not recognize the difference between affectionate and sexual behavior and, therefore, misunderstand and discredit *other people's* physical expressions.

The men's literature indicates that male sexuality is a product of the masculine socialization process.[14–16,21–23,40,41,111,115,116] Although there is no comprehensive theory to explain sexual preference and behavior,[117] numerous authors believe that men's problems with sexuality are related to rigid adherence to masculine sex-role norms and stereotypes.[16,21,41,50,111] Gross[111] reviewed the literature on the male role and heterosexual behaviors and offers three conclusions: (1) human sexual behavior is largely acquired through experience and socialization; (2) factors such as goals and success orientations, control and power, aggression and violence are socialized and can negatively affect male sexuality; and (3) influences of a restrictive sex-typed socialization process can be sexually maladaptive for men. These conclusions have important implications for understanding men's sexuality and interpersonal functioning.

Some authors[15,16,41] indicate that rigid adherence to stereotypes about masculine behavior may be incompatible with the interpersonal, sexual, and emotional needs of most women. As noted earlier, men have been socialized towards limited vulnerability, self-disclosure, intimacy, and expression of feelings. In many ways, sex for some men has been intellectually and emotionally separated from intimacy, sensuality, and love during adolescence. Stereotypically, women have been socialized differently and expect intimacy, sensuality, sex, and love to be integrated. Because of these different socialization experiences, men's interpersonal–sexual behavior may be too rigid and limited to fully satisfy the emotional, interpersonal, and sexual needs of others. Men who are not able to communicate feelings verbally, give up control emotionally, experience intimacy and sensuality, and show vulnerability may forfeit depth and meaning in their interpersonal–sexual experiences. Since many men will view these human characteristics as feminine and conflicting with the Masculine Mystique, they may have difficulty integrating them into the context of an intimate relationship with a woman. Fasteau[15] points out that the sexual act may be the closest many men come to intimate contact with women and their own femininity. Goldberg[16] sums up this conflict by stating:

> Only with the integration of his feminine, passive side will the male be able to liberate himself sexually, allowing himself to experience the totality of his feelings and freeing himself from concerns about performance and dominance. The macho male is an incomplete, dull, heterosexual partner because he clings to his stereotypical ways of responding (p. 40).

Numerous authors have discussed how men's socialized needs to achieve, perform, and control the interpersonal dynamics of a relationship may negatively affect sexuality and intimacy.[15,16,21–23,111] These authors indicate that the masculine socialization process may shape men's sexual attitudes and behaviors in ways that produce interpersonal distance during sex and, sometimes, sexual dysfunction. The literature points out at least five common themes that potentially restrict men's sexuality in interpersonal intimacy:

1. the conceptualization of sex and orgasm as a goal and conquest rather than an intimate communication process between two human beings;
2. the use of sex as a means of measuring performance, achievement, and one's masculinity;
3. the view of sex as an objective, impersonal process rather than as a subjective, intimate process;
4. the separation of sex from the interpersonal, affectionate, intimate, and loving parts of a human relationship; and
5. the view of sex as a situation where male control, dominance, and power are essential to obtaining mutual gratification.

Many authors believe that these themes emanate directly from the masculine socialization process. Also, they believe that interpersonal problems in sex, as well as sexual impotence, may be due to a sex-typed socialization process that is maladaptive in heterosexual relationships. Men who have become strangers to their sexual–sensual responses have found decreasing satisfaction in their sexuality because their important feminine qualities have been systematically extinguished during early social conditioning. Spontaneous, sensual, playful sex that emphasizes process rather than outcome is a difficulty for the macho lover. The sensual man who relies on process rather than sexual technique will be able to become less of a stranger to his inner emotions and needs. Goldberg[17] summarizes this point by writing:

> The male who is in touch with his inner experience will come to realize that he doesn't *have sex,* but rather that he *is sex,* which simply means that his so-called sexual response is *his* response and as such is one of the deepest, least consciously controllable, most powerful truth-telling expressions of who he is and what he feels (p. 132).

The literature, taken as a whole, suggests that men's gender socialization, adherence to the Masculine Mystique, and the fear of femininity are central factors in men's restricted sexuality and affectionate behavior.

Obsession with Achievement and Success. The obsession with achievement and success is defined as a man's persistent and disturbing preoccupation with work, accomplishments, and eminence as a means of substantiating and demonstrating his masculinity. The fear of femininity is a primary emotion that stimulates and shapes much of a man's obsessive work behavior particularly in early adulthood. Levinson et al.[58] point out that a man's work is his primary base for his life and represents his status in the occupational, cultural, and social matrix of society. Work, achievement, and success also become of great psychological importance and a vehicle for fulfillment or negation of central aspects of self.

Many men associate masculinity with competition, achievement, ambition, success at work, status, wealth, power, and influence. Conversely, femininity becomes associated with cooperation, unassertive and submissive behavior, minimal advancements and status, lack of drive towards success, influence, and wealth. To avoid being labeled feminine, men must be powerful, controlling, competitive, aggressive, achievement oriented, and successful. Stereotypically feminine qualities such as cooperativeness, emotionality, sensitivities toward others are considered counterproductive to achieving position, status, and success at work. Goldberg[17] enumerates the masculine ingredients for success: basic distrust, need to control, manipulation, and repression of human needs. These characteristics can twist men's lives into combative, competitive struggles that leave little time or energy for relaxation, pleasure, and a healthy nonwork life.

O'Neil[101] has discussed how male socialization and values affect men's career and personal development. The degree of validity of these assumptions will vary from man to man, depending on social class, race, and early gender-role socialization. A synthesis of these assumptions is found below:

1. Men are socialized to work by families, peers, and schools.[11,15,16,23]
2. Men are socialized to be competitive, achievement oriented, and competent.[11,23,91]
3. Men incorrectly learn that males and females have many sex-role differences (abilities, interests, and aptitudes) that dictate different jobs for men and women.[118]
4. Men learn that measures of masculinity are calculated by each man's success, achievement, and climb up the career ladder.[11,22,30,40]
5. Men learn that measures of manhood and masculinity are determined through career successes, achievement, and failures.[15,16,51]
6. Men learn that being masculine and a career success means being competitive, powerful, and in control of self and environment.[22]
7. Men learn that others will measure their masculinity in terms of their career success, achievement, power, and control. David and Brannon[30] call this the "big wheel, success, status, and the need to be looked up to" theme.
8. Men's breadwinner role is the exclusive domain of males unless it is economically necessary for women to work.[16]
9. Men look to work as the primary way to define personal and self-worth.[5,11,40,119]
10. Men believe that personal happiness and security will be assured by hard work, success, and achievement.[22,30]
11. Men may aspire for *personal rewards and satisfactions* that sometimes cannot be fully realized at work.[21]
12. Men who fail to obtain the expected personal rewards and satisfactions on the job believe that working harder will yield the desired outcome.[15]
13. Men may experience fear of failure, lack of confidence, uncooperative behavior with co-workers, and emotional problems due to unresolved masculinity problems that emerge at work.[21]
14. Men may work so hard to demonstrate success that they sometimes neglect their families and important relationships with spouses, friends, and their children.[16]
15. Men may experience overwork, fatigue, and stress at work that result in serious threats to physical and psychological health.[16,21]

These assumptions explain how men are socialized to become obsessed with achievement and success as well as how the obsession can produce gender-role strain and conflict. Goldberg (1977) discusses three career development binds that may emerge out of these assumptions. They include the breadwinner, success, and career-ladder binds.

The *breadwinner bind* is operative when the man is pulled between his worker–career role and his roles as husband, father, and family man. In order to fulfill the male adult role, a man must work as hard as possible to provide the best life for his family. Every advancement and salary increase is a measure of masculine career success. The more the man provides for his family, the more secure the man feels about his masculinity. Nichols[22] describes the "provider syndrome" through the following formula: job = money = possessions = security. Many times this formula dictates that more time, energy, and attention be directed toward work at the expense of family, children, and friends. Some men are criticized for neglecting family responsibilities because of their work or leisure activities. If a man decides to spend his extra time with his family at the expense of his job, he may lose out at improving his ability to make more money. Sometimes, allowing career advancements to slip away, the man may be resented by his family members or feel a lack of achievement in his career. Either way the breadwinner moves, he is caught between the male role that makes him the primary breadwinner and the tension of potentially neglecting his family. Masculinity issues, family responsibility, and male achievement needs conflict and may produce considerable stress and strain.

The *success bind* also pulls men in opposing directions. Many men are programmed to be successful and base their success on masculine norms and behaviors. To be a success means becoming competitive, goal-oriented, and driven. Many times this means that men must become impersonal and detached from others to accomplish tasks. At the same time, men are told that to be a success (leader, boss) they must be a good human being (warm, open, caring, and intimate). These humanist qualities are sometimes incompatible with the competitive, goal-oriented, success syndrome that men have been socialized towards.

Goldberg[16] indicates that men lose either way. If the man chooses to achieve and be successful, he must be competitive, which inevitably means distancing himself from others and not expressing feelings. If he chooses to be an emotional, open, noncompetitive, intimate human being, he may see himself as disadvantaged, unsuccessful, or even a failure. Success cancels out humanism and humanism cancels out success.

The *career-ladder bind* represents another bind for men. Upward mobility, promotions, and greater responsibility are critical in the masculine definition of success. Many times this means a man must give up the initial work that attracted him to the job for greater supervisory functions or administrative work. As the man moves up the ranks, it usually means greater distance from his friends and co-workers whom he either now supervises of with whom he has little contact. If the man contents himself with the work he enjoys and does not work towards climbing the career ladder, he may be passed by when promotions are made. As others climb the career ladder, the man may feel unappreciated, unsuccessful, and like a potential failure. On the other hand, if the man climbs the career ladder, it may take him away from his satisfying work and relationships.

There are three other career dynamics that relate to men's obsession with achievement, success, and work. First, if a man uses his work to verify his masculinity, then work may stimulate pressure and tensions. Since the capitalist system is based on profit, power, and competition, men are frequently pitted against each other at work. The demands of this system, coupled with past socialization, solidify men as competitors. Competition teaches men that success is contingent on using resources well, identifying and using power to their advantage, and showing constructive outcomes for their labors, usually as compared to their fellow workers. Under these circumstances, work may become a process of obtaining an advantage over co-workers in terms of position, rank, organizational prestige and respect, raises, and promotions.

Second, if work is one of the primary places for men to validate their masculinity, knowing how to use power and control in the work setting is usually as issue, if not a periodic obsession. Taken to the extreme, pressure to be successful and intense competition may compel some men to work at making their competitors look unsuccessful, incompetent, inferior, and without influence. Since many men see success as situationally defined, men may need continual successes as a means of proving their masculinity. It is not enough to succeed once; men must keep on succeeding.[40] This phenomenon may partially explain the classic work addict or workaholic who needs continual successes with each being superior to the last one.

Third, since male socialization emphasizes an outcome and task orientation, work relationships are usually directed at task completion rather than relationship maintenance. Some men feel that interpersonal relations and people's feelings get in the way of doing the job.[40] In some cases, intense emotions and interpersonal conflicts occur and are avoided in order to complete tasks. This restrictive emotionality may inhibit effective communication and problem solving when there are work conflicts between employees or with the boss. Temporarily, emotions can be transferred to tasks, but they can also build up and be expressed as frustration, anger, and career anxiety and work problems.

Some men who do not express their emotions at work take feelings home and express them inappropriately at family members. Family violence, including child abuse, incest, rape, and wife battering, may be stimulated by these intense outbursts of feelings. Other men use food, alcohol, and drugs to sedate themselves and reduce work tension. These work-related tensions can produce physical and psychological problems that affect the longevity and quality of a man's life.

HEALTH CARE PROBLEMS. These problems are defined as difficulties in maintaining positive health care in terms of diet, exercise, relaxation, sickness, and stress management. Many men have been socialized to ignore the physical symptoms that lead to acute illness or chronic health problems. The male gender role and its stereotypic rigidities promote men's projection of themselves as tireless, invincible workers with superhuman capabilities. Fasteau[15] characterized this stereotype as *The Male Machine*. Some men have limited body awareness which prevents them from understanding and being sensitive to their somatic functions, changes, or physiological processes. Many men are socialized to ignore their inner feelings in order to pursue ideas, tasks, and achievement. When a man is not able to read the "all is not well" signals of his body, he is a candidate for sickness, strokes, heart attacks, exhaustion, and early death.

Men's fear of femininity is related to their health care problems. When a man is sick, he has to admit his helplessness, vulnerability, and weakness in front of others. Since femininity has been typically associated with these characteristics, many men deny their physical problems to escape the label feminine. Goldberg's[17] analysis indicates that the basic processes, attitudes, and behavior patterns that are life sustaining and health maintaining are commonly identified as feminine, while body-destructive attitudes are considered masculine. Goldberg enumerates the feminine characteristics that diminish men's health problems. Femininity is associated with emotional expression, giving in to pain, asking for help, paying attention to diet, alcohol abstinence, self care, dependency, and touching. Goldberg[17] concludes that masculinity means

> The less sleep I need,
> The more pain I can take,
> The more alcohol I can hold,
> The less I concern myself with what I eat,
> The less I ask anybody for help or depend on them,
> The more I control and repress my emotions,
> The less attention I pay to myself physically,
> *The more masculine I am.* (p. 52)

The relationship between rigid, socialized masculine values and poor physical health has been discussed by many authors.[3,15,17,21–23,92] Harrison[3] reviews the literature on how the male sex role may be dangerous to men and shorten their life expectancies. In this review it is noted that, compared to females, males have

> a higher perinatal and early childhood death rate, a higher rate of congenital birth defects, a greater vulnerability to recessive sex linked disorders, a higher accident rate for males during childhood and all subsequent ages, a higher incidence of behavioral and learning disorders, a higher suicide rate and a metabolism rate which may result in greater energy expenditure and a consequent failure to conserve physical resources (p. 66).

Harrison's review attributes these male problems and higher mortality rate to either the biogenetic or psychosocial perspective. The biogenetic perspective attributes men's greater mortality to genetic factors, whereas the psychosocial perspective attributes men's greater mortality in large part to the lethal aspects of the male role. Harrison's critical review of available evidence concludes that the psychosocial perspective contributes more to higher mortality rate of men than the biogenetic approach. These results are similar to Waldron's[120] estimate that three-fourths of the difference in life expectancy between males and females can be accounted for by gender-role related behaviors which contribute to the greater mortality of men.

When men are socialized to constantly ignore feelings and their internal body signs, poor health can seem to emerge suddenly and unexpectedly. Many men who ignore messages from their bodies do not recognize internal stresses, strains, symptoms of sickness. Even when the inner signals of poor health are recognized, some men do not accept these distress signals and continue working.

Additionally, since males have not been socialized to express emotions, men often keep their stresses to themselves. Fears, anxieties, conflicts, and other painful emotions usually need to be expressed for growth and positive action. Emotions that are not expressed in words or actions may be released through physical pains and illness.[21] There is a growing body of evidence that shows that social pressure (especially stress) not only causes disease but also lowers life expectancy.[3,121] In addition, some men experience serious disappointments when their life goals and dreams appear to be beyond their reach.[58] Sometimes, there are feelings of despair and loss, as well as a general feeling that their life is out of control. Marital boredom, fears of unemployment, and other life realities can add stress and strain to the middle-aged adult male.

Goldberg[16] believes that sickness and emotional stress contribute to early deaths in men. His analysis indicates that stress is caused through (1) overuse of intellectualizations rather than expression of true feelings, (2) macho rigidity in terms of living out the Masculine Mystique and Value System, and (3) guilt about not measuring up to the male role. These factors emanate from early gender socialization and, in the final analysis, have life and death implications for the gender conflicted male.

Patterns of Gender-Role Conflict and Strain: A Critique

The popular and professional literature reviewed indicates that patterns of gender-role conflict and strain characterize men's changing roles in American society. The degree to which individual men experience the fear of femininity and gender-role strain remains an empirical question. The six patterns of gender-role conflict identified are not an exhaustive list of men's problems due to the fear of femininity and the masculine socialization process. Additionally, the cause–effect relationship between the fear of femininity and the patterns of gender role conflict has not been empirically established by research. Future research and further conceptualization of the concepts shown in Figure 1 are needed. Such research and discussion would help therapists and the public better understand the implications of gender-role conflict in men's lives. Attention also needs to be given to how the fear of femininity is learned in early boyhood and how it develops over the adult life cycle. A measure of fear of femininity is currently being developed and may assist therapists in assessing gender-role conflicts and strain in counseling and psychotherapy.

Implications of Gender-Role Conflict for Psychiatrists, Psychologists, and Other Human-Service Providers

The gender-role conflicts and strain described in Figure 1 have implications for the work of the therapist in counseling, psychotherapy, and preventive mental health interventions. Specifically, the patterns of gender-role conflicts have implications for

1. counseling and psychotherapy with men and women;
2. developing preventive outreach programming around gender-role issues for both sexes;
3. establishing in-service and continuing education about gender-role strain and conflicts for new and seasoned professionals; and
4. incorporating into the curricula and training of psychiatrists, psychologists, and other human-service providers information about gender-role socialization, sexism, and possible gender-role conflicts in counseling and psychotherapy.

The assessment of men's gender-role conflicts and strains in counseling and psychotherapy is recommended. Numerous authors have suggested the need to assess, conceptualize, and intervene around the gender-role conflicts of men and women[101,122–130] (see the chapters in this book by Solomon, Goldfried and Friedman, Stein, Dosser, and Bernardez). Helping professionals can help men examine the degree to which gender-role conflicts limit their emotional, interpersonal, and physical lives. Therapists working with couples, families, or individual women may need to examine how rigid adherence to masculine and feminine stereotypes may cause and maintain relationship problems.

The assessment and treatment of these gender-role conflicts needs further conceptualization and examination. Some important questions include the following: (1) How might therapists intervene to help men experiencing restrictive emotionality; problems with control, power and competition issues, restricted communication patterns, and difficulties in initiating and maintaining intimacy with women, other men, and children? (2) How can therapists help men explore and resolve gender-role strains and conflicts related to sexuality, homophobia, and career and family conflicts? (3) What traditional interventions will be useful in solving these problems and what new approaches are needed? Initial ideas of how to help men around gender-role issues need to be expanded.[44,45,49,52,53,114,122] Readers are referred to chapters in this book by Solomon, Dosser, Goldfried and Friedman, Bernardez, and Stein, which describe various approaches to helping men with gender-role conflict and strain.

There is a need for educational and preventive programming concerning gender-role strain and conflicts. Programs need to be developed for men only, women only, and also for mixed sex groups. Specifically for men, there is a need for factual information about restrictiveness and hazards of growing up male. Printed information, instructional materials, and multimedia presentations need to be developed to explain how sexism and past gender-role socialization may restrict men's options.

On a more emotional and personal level, men will need consciousness-raising experiences to explore their fear of femininity and its effects on their emotional and physical well-being. Numerous authors have described the content and process of men's liberation groups.[9,14,131–134] Additionally, there have been some valuable gender-role exercises and interventions developed[33,34,42,133,135,136] that could be used in men's groups as well as in individual counseling.

Wong's[133] list of 44 potential activities or topics of discussion are particularly valuable for men's groups and preventive programming.

In-service and continuing education programs may be needed for therapists to better understand male socialization and possible gender-role strains and conflicts. Some professional therapists may benefit from examining their own feelings and beliefs about masculinity in order to effectively help other men. This examination could be started in men's groups, through reading the men's literature, or through individual counseling and psychotherapy.

Formal course content about sexism, male socialization, and gender-role conflicts is recommended in psychiatric and psychological training programs. Required coursework, seminars, and specific units in the established curricula are needed to sensitize therapists-in-training to the problems that may occur as a result of restrictive notions of masculinity and femininity. These courses could also address how institutional sexism may perpetuate and support restrictive and discriminatory policies through their male-dominated values, attitudes, and organizational structures.

Some Final Thoughts and Personal Disclosures

The author's personal–emotional journey while writing this chapter is not evident from the narrative. What the author learned about his own socialization was intellectually stimulating, exhilarating, and also depressing and painful. It also opened up dialogues with other colleagues experiencing gender conflict in their personal and professional lives.[136–140] There were times when the author sensed a loss of objectivity due to heightened sensitivity to how gender conflicts have (or do) affect him. There were other times when the research and psychology of gender roles left him confused, dissatisfied, and cautious. Also, the literature accurately described most of what his clients and personal friends have expressed to him.

Gender-role reevaluation and conflict appear to be evident in the lives of many. However, the author believes that any generalities about gender conflict are doubtful and premature. The array of variables and dynamics that make gender conflict an important psychological construct is complex and need further explanation and thought. This chapter specified gender-role strain and conflict for men and hopefully will stimulate further analyses and empirical research on how gender-role socialization affects both sexes.

No doubt some of his thinking will be questioned and controversial, particularly to those who believe that defined and limited gender roles for the sexes are conducive to psychological health. There is little doubt that some individuals with rigidly defined gender roles are healthy and productive. It is also evident that gender-conflicted individuals develop psychological and physical problems that can negatively affect the quality of their lives.

One central theme emerged during those private days while integrating this information. It consisted of understanding the mutual relationships of the definitions noted earlier in this chapter. How do sex differences, gender-role socialization, and gender-role conflict relate to sexism? An answer to this question is critical to understanding how gender-role conflict and sexism operates in our society. It appears that perceived, but scientifically unproven, sex or gender differences have been used to justify rigid gender socialization practices and differential treatment of the sexes. This socialization has limited the sexes from developing all parts of their personality (masculine and feminine) needed to cope with the complexities of human experience. Restricted socialization of the sexes has produced gender-role stereotypes, behaviors, and conflicts for men, women, and children. These limitations in socialization have caused the sexes to subordinate and depreciate the others' gender-role socialization and values. The outcome of these exchanges between men and women is gender-role conflict and sexism.

Money,[141] in an important and controversial analysis of gender socialization, states that

> all behavior that is sex-classified or sex coded, regardless of its genesis, ultimately impinges on pair-bonding and the failure or the success of men and women in their relationship together (p. xii).

The author's analysis is similar and suggests that much gender conflict, between and among the sexes, is due to rigid gender socialization and orientations that result in dysfunctional attempts at communication, problem solving, and loving others. Men have learned through the Masculine Mystique and Value System to subordinate women, depreciate their femininity, and fear their own feminine sides. Women have also learned to subordinate men, depreciate their masculinity, and to fear their own masculine sides. Personal and institutional sexism as well as gender-role conflict have emerged in response to these gender dynamics. Men have justified their dominance, control, and subordination of women and feminine values to fulfill the Masculine Mystique. Women, as victims (unknowingly or willingly), have also used their roles and sexism to control and manipulate men. Much of this gender-role conflict between the sexes has gone unlabeled and unresolved. The outcome has been emotional pain for men, women, and children. The psychological, physical, and spiritual costs to humankind have been negative and great.[101]

The outcomes of gender- and sex-role oppression in contemporary society needs further conceptualization and attention. Sue's[142] analysis of how cultural oppression operates against Third World clients is relevant. From his perspective, cultural oppression occurs when a world view is blindly imposed upon the culturally different client. Gender oppression, by the same analysis, occurs when gender values, attitudes, and behaviors are blindly imposed on others resulting in a restriction of gender identity and sexual freedom. Gender oppression in this democratic society produces gender-role conflict, sexism, and a sexual dictatorship.[141] Heterosexual, homosexual, and bisexual lifestyles as well as other gender–sexual orientations are negatively affected by this oppression.

The process of gender-role reevaluation is still difficult for much of the public to consider, understand, and implement in their lives. Psychiatrists, psychologists, and other helping professionals can assist the public by more actively exploring and researching the psychological problems caused by rigid and sexist gender-role socialization. Further study and empirical research on patterns of gender-role conflicts would allow therapists to speak more authoritatively to the public on the dangers of restrictive gender-role socialization for men, women, and children.

ACKNOWLEDGMENTS

The author appreciates the helpful comments of students and colleagues in the Departments of Counseling and Counseling Psychology at the University of Kansas. Jan Muchow, Linda Hedrick, and Chris Meinecke were particularly helpful with the final stages of this manuscript. The clerical assistance of Cindi Hodges is also appreciated.

REFERENCES

1. Toffler A: Future Shock. New York, Random House, 1970
2. Forisha B: Sex Roles and Personal Awareness. Morristown, New Jersey, General Learning Press, 1978
3. Harrison J: Warning: The male sex role may be dangerous to your health. Soc Issues 34:65–86, 1978
4. Guttentag M, Bray H: Undoing Sex Role Stereotypes. New York, McGraw-Hill, 1976
5. Skovholt TM: Feminism and men's lives. Counseling Psycho 7:3–10, 1978
6. P.L. 92–318: The Education Amendment of 1972, Title IX, Prohibition of Sex Discrimination, 20 USC, 1681.
7. Lewis RA, Pleck JH: Men's Roles in the Family. Fam Coordinator 28:429–646, 1979
8. Grady KE, Brannon R, Pleck JH: The Male Sex Role: A Selected and Annotated Bibliography. Washington, U.S. Department of Health, Education and Welfare, 1979
9. Bradley M, Danchik L, Foger M, et al.: Unbecoming. New York, Times Change Press, 1971
10. Brenton M: The American Male. New York, Howard McCann, 1966
11. Bucher GR: Straight, White, Male. Philadelphia, Fortress, 1976
12. Cooke C: The Men's Survival Resource Book: On Being a Man in Today's World. Minneapolis, M.S.R.B. Press, 1978
13. Chesler P: About Men. New York, Simon and Schuster, 1978
14. Farrell W: The Liberated Man. New York, Bantam, 1974
15. Fasteau MF: The Male Machine. New York, McGraw-Hill, 1974
16. Goldberg H: The Hazards of Being Male, New York, New American Library, 1977
17. Goldberg H: The New Male: From Self-Destruction to Self-Care. New York, Morrow, 1979
18. Korda M: Male Chauvinism: How It Works and How to Get Free of It. New York, Berkley, 1972
19. Kriegel L: The Myth of American Manhood. New York, Dell, 1978
20. Lyon HC: Tenderness in Strength: From Machismo to Manhood. New York, Harper and Row, 1977
21. Mayer N: The Male Mid-Life Crises: Fresh Start After 40. New York, New American Library, 1978
22. Nichols J: Men's Liberation: A New Definition of Masculinity. New York, Penguin Books Inc., 1975
23. Olson K: Hey Man! Open Up and Live. New York, Fawcett, 1978
24. Robertiello RC: A Man in the Making. New York, Marek, 1979
25. Snodgrass J: A Book of Readings for Men Against Sexism. New York, Times Change Press, 1977
26. Wagenvoord J, Bailey P: Men: A Book for Women. New York, Avon, 1978
27. Balswick JO, Peek CW: The inexpressive male: A tragedy of American society. Fam Coordinator 20:363–368, 1971

28. Biller HB, Borstelmann, LJ: Masculine development: An integrative review. Merrill-Palmer Quart 13:253–294, 1967
29. Canavan P, Haskell J: The American Male Stereotype, in Exploring Contemporary Male/Female Roles: A Facilitator's Guide. Edited by Carney, CA, McMahon, SL. La Jolla, University Associates, 1977, pp 150–166
30. David DS, Brannon, R: The Forty-nine Percent Majority: The Male Sex Role. Reading, Massachusetts, Addison-Wesley, 1976
31. Denmark FL: Growing up male, in Exploring Contemporary Male/Female Roles: A Facilitator's Guide. Edited by Carney CA, McMahon SL. La Jolla, University Associates, 1977, pp 125–138
32. Dubbert JL: A Man's Place: Masculinity in Transition. Englewood Cliffs, New Jersey, Prentice-Hall, 1979
33. Moreland JR: A humanistic approach to facilitating college students' learning about sex roles. Counseling Psychol 6:61–64, 1976
34. Moreland JR: Facilitator training for consciousness raising groups in an academic setting. Counseling Psychol 6:66–68, 1976
35. Pleck JH: Masculinity–femininity: Current and alternate paradigms. Sex Roles 1:161–178, 1975
36. Pleck JH: Men's response to changing consciousness of women, in Women and Men Roles, Attitudes, and Power Relationships, Edited by Zuckerman, EL. New York, The Radcliff Club of New York, 1975, pp 102–112
37. Pleck JH: Male–male friendship: Is brotherhood possible? in Old Family/New Family: Interpersonal Relations. Edited by Blazer, M. New York, Van Nostrand Reinhold, 1975, pp 229–224
38. Pleck JH: The male sex role: Definitions, problems and sources of change. J Soc Issues 32:155–164, 1976
39. Pleck JH, Brannon R: Male roles and the male experience. J Soc Issues 34:1–4, 1978
40. Pleck JH, Sawyer J: Men and Masculinity. Englewood Cliffs, New Jersey, Prentice Hall, 1974
41. Safilios-Rothschild C: Love, Sex, Sex Roles. Englewood Cliffs, New Jersey, Prentice Hall, 1977
42. Sargent AG: Beyond Sex Roles. St. Paul, West, 1977
43. Scanzoni J: Sex Roles, Women's Role and Marital Conflict. Lexington, Heath, 1978
44. Scher M: On counseling men. Personnel Guidance J 57:252–254, 1979.
45. Scher M: The little boy in the adult male client. Personnel Guidance J 57:537-539, 1979
46. Skovholt T, Gormally J, Schauble P, et al.: Counseling men. Counseling Psychol 7:2, 1978
47. Skovholt T, Hansen A: Men's development: A perspective and some themes, in Counseling Men, Edited by Skovholt T, Schauble P, Davis R, Menlo Park, Brook/Cole, 1980, pp 1–29
48. Solomon K: Sexism and professional chauvinism in psychiatry. Psychiat 42:374–377, 1979
49. Solomon K: Therapeutic aspects of changing masculine role behavior. World J Psychosynthesis 11:13–16, 1979
50. Steven BS: The sexually oppressed male. Psychotherapy: Theory Res Practice 11:16–21, 1974
51. Tolson A: The Limits of Masculinity: Male Identity and Women's Liberation. New York, Harper and Row, 1977
52. Toomer JE: Males in psychotherapy. Counseling Psychol 7:22–25, 1978
53. Wong MR, Davey J, Conroe RM: Expanding masculinity: Counseling the male in transition. Counseling Psychol 6:58–61, 1976
54. Babl JD: Compensatory masculine responding as a function of sex role. J Consult Clin Psychol 47:330–335, 1979
55. Stein PJ, Hoffman S: Sports and male role strain. J Soc Issues 34:136–150, 1978
56. Komarovsky M: Cultural contradictions and sex roles: The masculine case. Am J Sociol 78:873–884, 1973
57. Komarovsky M: Dilemmas of Masculinity: A Study of College Youth. New York, Norton, 1976
58. Levinson DJ, Darrow CN, Klein EB, et al.: The Seasons of a Man's Life. New York, Knopf, 1978
59. Vaillant GE: Natural history of male psychological health. Arch Gen Psychiatry 31:15–22, 1974
60. Deaux K: The Behavior of Women and Men. Monterey, Brooks/Cole, 1976
61. Marlowe M: The assessment and treatment of gender-disturbed boys by guidance counselors. Personnel Guidance J 58:128–132, 1979

62. McCoy NL: Innate factors in sex differences, in Beyond Sex Roles. Edited by Sargent AG. St. Paul, West, 1977, pp 157–167
63. Tavris C, Offir C: The Longest War: Sex Differences in Perspective. New York, Harcourt Brace Jovanovich, 1977
64. Unger RK: Toward a redefinition of sex and gender. Am Psychol 34:1085–1094, 1979
65. Frieze IH, Parsons JE, Johnson PB, et al.: Women and Sex Roles: A Social Psychological Perspective. New York, Norton, 1978
66. Williams JH: Psychology of Women: Selected Readings. New York, Norton, 1979
67. Garnets L, Pleck JH: Sex role identity, androgyny, and sex role transcendence: A sex role strain analysis. Psychol Women Quart 3:270–283, 1979
68. Turner RH: Family Interaction. New York, Wiley, 1970
69. Blick-Hoyenga KC, Hoyenga KT: The Question of Sex Difference. Boston, Little, Brown, 1979
70. Kagan J: Acquisition and significance of sex-typing and sex role identity, in Review of Child Development Research, Vol I. Edited by Hoffman ML, Hoffman LS. New York, Russell Sage Foundation, 1964, pp. 137–167
71. Kohlberg L: A cognitive developmental analysis of children's sex role concepts and attitudes, in The Development of Sex Differences. Edited by Maccoby EE. Stanford, Stanford University Press, 1966, pp. 82–173
72. Maccoby EE, Jacklin CM: The Psychology of Sex Differences. Stanford, Stanford University Press, 1974
73. Morgan M: The Total Woman. Old Tappan, New Jersey, Revell, 1975
74. Bem SL: The measurement of psychological androgyny. J Consult Clin Psychol 42:155–162, 1974
75. Bem SL: Probing the promise of androgyny, in Beyond Sex-Role Stereotypes: Readings Toward a Psychology of Androgyny. Edited by Kaplan AG, Bean JP. Boston, Little, Brown, 1976, pp 47–62
76. Kaplan AG (Ed): Psychological androgyny: Further considerations. Psychol Women Quart 3:221–319, 1979
77. Bem SL: Sex role adaptability: One consequence of psychological androgyny. J Personality Soc Psychol 31:634–643, 1975
78. Block JH: Debatable conclusions about sex differences. Contemporary Psychol 21:517–522, 1976
79. Schiff E, Koopman EJ: The relationship of women's sex-role identity to self esteem and ego development. J Psychol 98:299–305, 1978
80. Spence JT, Helmreich R, Stapp J: Ratings of self and peer on sex role attributes and their relationship to self esteem and conception of masculinity and femininity. J Personality Soc Psychol 32:29–39, 1975
81. Bem SL, Lenney E: Sex-typing and avoidance of cross-sex behavior. J Personality Soc Psychol 33:48–54, 1976
82. Bem SL, Martyna W, Watson C: Sex-typing and androgyny: Future exploration of the expressive domain. J Personality Soc Psychol 34:1016–1023, 1976
83. Jones WH, Chernovetz ME, Hansson RO: The enigma of androgyny: Differential implications for males and females. J Consult Clin Psychol 46:298–313, 1978
84. Locksley A, Colten ME: Psychological androgyny: A case of mistaken identity? J Personality Soc Psychol 37:1017–1031, 1979
85. Pedhasur EJ, Tetenbaum TJ: Bem sex role inventory: A theoretical and methodological critique. J Personality Soc Psychol 37:996–1016, 1979
86. Kelly JA, Worell J: New formulations of sex role and androgyny: A critical review. J Consult Clin Psychol 45:1011–1115, 1977
87. Lenny E: Androgyny: Some audacious assertions towards its coming of age. Sex Roles 5:703–719, 1979
88. Lenny E: Concluding comments on androgyny: Some intimations of its mature development. Sex Roles 5:829–840, 1979
89. Worell J: Sex roles and psychological well-being: Perspectives on methodology. J Consult Clin Psychol 46:298–313, 1978

90. Lindner CE: Maleness and heterosexuality, in Straight, White, Male. Edited by Bucher GR. Philadelphia, Fortress, 1976, pp 66–88
91. Crites JO, Fitzgerald LF: The competent male. Counseling Psychol 7:10–14, 1978
92. Fein RA: Examining the nature of masculinity, in Beyond Sex Roles. Edited by Sargent GA. St. Paul, West, 1977 pp 188–200
93. Steinem G: The myth of masculine mystique, in Men and Masculinity. Edited by Pleck JH, Sawyer J. Englewood Cliffs, New Jersey, Prentice-Hall, 1974, pp 134–139
94. O'Leary VE, Donoghue JM: Latitudes of masculinity: Reactions to sex-role deviance in men. J Soc Issues 34:17–28, 1978
95. Jung CG: Concerning the archetypes, with special reference to the anima concept (1954), in Collected Works, Vol 9, Part I. New York, Pantheon, 1959, pp 54–72
96. Jung CG: Animus and Anima, in Collected Works, Vol VII. New York, Pantheon, 1953, pp 188–211
97. Maslow AH: The Farther Reaches of Human Nature. New York, Viking, 1971
98. Hartley RE: Sex role pressures and the socialization of the male child. Psychological Reports 5:457–468, 1959
99. Jones E: Free Association. London, Hogarth, 1959
100. Glover E: Freud or Jung. New York, Norton, 1950
101. O'Neil JM: Male sex role conflicts, sexism, and masculinity: Psychological implications for men, women and the counseling psychologist. J Counseling Psychol 9:61–80, 1981.
102. Lewis RA: Emotional intimacy among men. J Soc Issues 34:108–121, 1978
103. Jourard SM: The Transparent Self. New York, Van Nostrand, 1971
104. Aries E: Male–female interpersonal styles in all male, all female, and mixed groups, in Beyond Sex Roles. Edited by Sargent AG. St. Paul, West, 1977, pp 292–299
105. Henley N, Thorne B: Womanspeak and manspeak: Sex differences and sexism in communication, verbal and nonverbal in Beyond Sex Roles. Edited by Sargent AG. St. Paul, West, 1977, pp 201–218
106. Parsons T, Bales RF: Family, Socialization and Interaction Process. Glencoe, Free Press, 1955
107. Lehne GK: Homophobia among men, in The Forty-nine Percent Majority. Edited by David DS, Brannon R. Reading, Addison Wesley, 1976, pp 66–88
108. Morin SF, Garfinkle EM: Male homophobia. J Soc Issues 34:29–47, 1978
109. Stokes J, Fuehrer A, Child L: Gender differences in self disclosure to various target persons. J Counseling Psychol 27:192–198, 1980
110. MacDonald A: The importance of sex role to gay liberation. Homosexual Counseling J 1:169–180, 1974
111. Gross AE: The male role and heterosexual behavior. J Soc Issues 34:87–107, 1978
112. Henley NM: Body Politics: Power, Sex, and Nonverbal Communication. Englewood Cliffs, New Jersey, Prentice-Hall, 1977
113. Lofaro GA, Reeder CW: Male competition: An issue in counselor training. Counseling Psychol 7:20–22, 1978
114. Rice DG: The male spouse in marital and family therapy. Counseling Psychol 7:64–66, 1978
115. Lewis R, Casto R, Aquilino W, et al.: Developmental transitions in male sexuality. Counseling Psychol 7:15–19, 1978
116. Reed DM: Male sexual conditioning, in Kelmer's Counseling in Marital and Sexual Problems. Edited by Stahmann RF, Hiebert WJ. Baltimore, Williams and Wilkins, 1977, pp 205–220
117. Gagnon H, Simon W: Sexual Conduct: The Social Sources of Human Sexuality. Chicago, Aldine, 1973
118. Wesley F, Wesley C: Sex Role Psychology. New York, Human Sciences Press, 1977
119. Morgan JI, Skovholt TM, Orr JM: Career counseling with men: The shifting focus, in Career Counseling: Theoretical and Practical Perspectives. Edited by Weinroch, SG. New York, McGraw-Hill, 1979, pp 260–266
120. Waldron I: Why do women live longer than men? J Human Stress 2:1–13, 1976
121. Friedman M. Rosenman R: Type A Behavior and Your Heart. Greenwich, Fawcett, 1974
122. Bear S, Berger M, Wright L: Even cowboys sing the blues: Difficulties experienced by men

trying to adopt nontraditional sex roles and how clinicians can be helpful to them. Sex Roles 5:191–198, 1979

123. Berzins JI: Therapist–patient matching, in Effective Psychotherapy: A Handbook of Research. Edited by Gurman AS, Razin AM. New York, Pergamon, 1971, pp 222–251
124. Berzins JI: Discussion: Androgyny, personality theory and psychotherapy. Psychol Women Quart 3:248–254, 1979
125. Doster JA: Sex role learning and interview communication. J Counseling Psychol 23:482–485, 1976
126. Highlen PS, Russell B: Effects of counselor gender and counselor and client sex role on females' counselor preference. J Counseling Psychol 27:157–165, 1980
127. Kaplan AG: Androgyny as a model of mental health for women: From theory to therapy, in Beyond Sex-Role Stereotypes: Readings Toward a Psychology of Androgyny. Edited by Kaplan AG, Bean JP. Boston, Little, Brown, 1976, pp 352–362
128. Kaplan AG: Clarifying the concepts of androgyny: Implications for therapy. Psychol Women Quart 3:223–230, 1979
129. Kenworthy JA: Androgyny in psychotherapy: But will it sell in Peoria? Psychol Women Quart 3:231–240, 1979
130. O'Neil JM, Ohlde C, Barke C, et al.: Research on a workshop to reduce sexism and sex role socialization on women's career planning. J Counseling Psychol 27:355–363, 1980
131. Karsk R, Thomas B: Working with Men's Groups. Columbia, New Community Press, 1979
132. Kravetz DF, Sargent AG: Consciousness-raising groups: A resocialization process for personal and social change, in Beyond Sex Roles. Edited by Sargent AG. St. Paul, West, 1977, pp 148–156
133. Wong MR: Males in transition and the self-help group. Counseling Psychol 7:46–50, 1978
134. Washington CS: Men counseling men: Redefining the male machine. Personnel Guidance J 59:462–463, 1979
135. Carney CG, McMahon SL: Exploring Contemporary Male/Female Roles: A Facilitator's Guide. La Jolla, University Associates, 1977
136. Collison B: A procedure for sex role sensitization for men. Paper presented at the 88th Annual Meeting of the American Psychological Association, Montreal, Que, Sept 5, 1980
137. Skovholt T: Psychological services and male clients: How wide is the gap? Paper Presented at the 88th Annual Meeting of the American Psychological Association, Montreal, Que, Sept 5, 1980
138. Scher M: Men and intimacy: Implications for the counseling psychologist. Paper presented at the 88th Annual Meeting of the American Psychological Association, Montreal, Que, Sept 5, 1980
139. Birk J: Sexism, relevancy, and training in counseling psychology. Paper presented at the 88th Annual Meeting of the American Psychological Association, Montreal, Que, Sept 5, 1980
140. Hanson G: Impact of childhood sex role socialization on men's career choice. Paper presented at the 88th Annual Meeting of the American Psychological Association, Montreal, Que, Sept 5, 1980
141. Money J: Love and Love Sickness: The Science of Sex, Gender Differences, and Pair Bonding. Baltimore, John Hopkins Press, 1980
142. Sue DW: Eliminating cultural oppression in counseling: Toward a general theory. J Counsling Psychol 25:419–428, 1978

Chapter 2

The Masculine Gender Role

Description

KENNETH SOLOMON

How does an author begin a chapter on the gender roles of men? It seems like a simple problem, but for the author of this chapter, it became almost insurmountable. Gender role issues and change are usually considered the province of women, as institutionalized in the Feminist Movement. Men and their behaviors are usually discussed *vis-à-vis* those of women, as part of a feminist analysis of individual and society.

But this is a chapter on men in their own right. There is no frame of reference to use for an introduction. There is no history of a men's liberation movement to review. There are no spokespersons known to the public to quote. There are no dramatic research findings to cite. Most men and many women do not even acknowledge that there are men's issues worthy of examination. There is not even a consensus that the traditional masculine role is changing to any appreciable degree.

Having briefly presented this dilemma, the author has solved his problem. By doing so in this fashion, he shared a small bit of "unmasculine" behavior with the reader. He was open and sharing about his vulnerability and lack of omni-competence, and admitted, to those who know him, that his writing, albeit prolific and reasonably polished, is not always an easy process.

With this departure from the traditional masculine role, the author will move to his subject.

HISTORICAL OVERVIEW

Over fifty years ago, Allen published the first of three papers reviewing the available literature on sex differences.[1–3] In each of these three papers, he reached the same conclusion. On the basis of his evaluation of the literature on

---

KENNETH SOLOMON • Levindale Hebrew Geriatric Center and Hospital; Department of Psychiatry, University of Maryland School of Medicine, Baltimore, Maryland 21215

sex differences available to him, he concluded that there were certain innate physiologic and anatomic differences between men and women. Aside from obvious genital differences, these included such biologic parameters as the amount of fat tissue, muscle mass, or the concentration of different substances in the blood. He also concluded, on the basis of this same literature, that all behavioral differences between men and women are societally and culturally determined. He hypothesized that these behaviors were a function of both societal expectations for men and women as well as the individual's integration of these expectations into his/her own idiosyncratic cognitive patterns, personality, and behaviors. Although few of his peers acknowledged what he was saying and there are still frequent arguments over the source of behavioral differences between men and women (see, for example, Maccoby and Jacklin[4] and Wilson[5] for a more biological viewpoint and Money and Ehrhart[6] and Money[7] for an attempt at integration), his belief that gender-role behaviors, regardless of their sources, are mediated by society and are not innate in the biology of the individual has progressively become the more accepted point of view. However, it still remains largely hypothesis, as it was in 1927, as much needed data have yet to be collected.

In the fifty years since Allen wrote, there have been successive trends in the study of gender-role behaviors. For the first twenty years, research was almost exclusively conducted on children. Consistent with the sexist bias of the time, these data were usually interpreted in a way that reinforced the notion that behavioral differences were biologically innate. The evidence was that traditionally sex-stereotyped behaviors were seen in children as young as three and four years of age.

A forced change in gender-role behaviors occurred during World War II. Women began to work in factories and take on many traditionally masculine roles in the family, as husbands, brothers, and fathers were overseas. This cataclysmic change led to the beginning of the modern Feminist Movement and a subsequent change in the focus of gender-role research. Over the last twenty years, there has been a rapid increase in the number of studies on gender-role behavior in adolescents and young adults. There have also been occasional studies of people in middle age and over. Most of this research has concentrated on the gender-role behaviors of women in an attempt to clarify and understand the conflicts women face as they attempt to change their gender-role behavior. Another purpose of this research has been to note the psychologic and social sources of these role conflicts and strains. Other studies have attempted to identify the coping skills of women or to put the behaviors of women into various theoretical perspectives.

There have also been three major conceptual models that have shaped research on gender roles over the past three generations. Pleck[8] discusses these in terms of men's roles, but they seem to mirror the evolution of research in the field as a whole. The earliest model, called the "traditional perspective" by Pleck, evolved from the descriptive research in the area. In a time of minimal societal change, roles were defined *per se* and given inherent value, usually for perservation of the status quo. Deviations from traditional roles were considered pathologic and were examined by students of the processes of deviance (clinicians and nonclinicians alike). In this model, subtle harbingers of future role changes were occasionally noted, but their importance minimized. For example, in 1950, Rabban[9] predicted that the latency age girls he observed would demand more autonomy and a wider range of allowable role behaviors and be more assertive once they reached adulthood. Less than 2% of his paper is devoted to a discussion of this prediction. These girls became the vanguard of the Women's Movement a decade and a half later.

A second model, which developed along with the beginnings of the postwar Feminist Movement, is the "exploitation perspective." This model had the advantages of fostering political activity but transferred blame. It is a model of oppression that dealt with issues of power, control, and harsh economic realities. The positive aspects of womanhood were largely ignored. Men were uniformly seen as villains. This model led to a polarized literature, with men and women arguing for either radical change or the status quo. A few men took on the role of the oppressed in a twist to this model. This model generated various sociologic hypotheses and a renewed interest in the social factors that led to the development of gender roles.

The third model in the literature is the "changing role perspective." This is a recent conceptualization that grew out of the human potential movement. It is responsible for new empirical studies of the actual behaviors of men and women in the workplace, family, and interpersonal relationships. Studies on the psychologic effects of different role attributes on behaviors such as adaptation, sexuality, self-concept, and psychopathology have also emerged in the few years since this model has begun to evolve. The theoretical rumblings of the "exploitation perspective" are being clarified, revised, and tested.

Only recently has there begun to be a study of men and masculine gender role *per se*. For example, in 1976, Brannon[10] estimated that of the approximately 2.5 million books in print devoted to the behavioral sciences, there were no books on the masculine gender role. In the mid 1970s however, several books examining men and their behavior began to be published. At first, these books examined behaviors from a feminist point of view; men's behavior was discussed by how it impacted upon the liberation of women (e.g., Ref. 11). Shortly thereafter, other books began to examine men as an entity separate from women. Men had their own individual and group psychology and sociology. In these books, the negative results of the masculine role upon men themselves were emphasized (e.g., Refs. 12–15). Although they served an important function, most of these books were written for the lay public and have been noted for their relative superficiality and a lack of cohesive theory or research and academic emphasis. In addition, there has been no more than a minimal discussion of the rewards of being a man. There has been little published to help the graduate student, researcher, and clinician with their interest and work in the field. The Men's Liberation Movement has been developing with a notable lack of theory, political ideology, quality research, and clarity of direction. Indeed, as of 1980, it also seems to have taken a strong antifeminist direction.

Why study men? The author believes it is important to study men because some men are changing. The Feminist Movement, changes in the affluence of American society, the effects of the Vietnam era, Watergate and other national crises, the Sexual Revolution, and other changes over the past twenty years have been forcing men to change. The Humanistic Psychology and Human Potential Movements have developed a framework and expectation for some men to determine the nature and rate of their own growth. Thus, some men are changing because they want to change; they see personal advantages to changing some traditional masculine behaviors. Others are changing because they are forced to change either by the women who are close to them or by society. Still others are fighting a battle to keep things the way they are and the way they always have been; they are fighting to retain the traditional role that men have had. In this time of change and flux, they find newspaper photographs of very "unmasculine" behaviors such as football players crying at the same time that the veneration of John Wayne reaches the halls of Congress, which approves a commemorative medal upon his death. Role conflicts and strains lead to clinically manifest symptoms that require that clinicians have the therapeutic skills necessary to work with these men (Refs. 16–20, and chapters in this book by O'Neil, Solomon, Stein, Dosser, Goldfried and Friedman, Bernardez).

Because men are changing, it is important to know what they are changing from, the biologic, psychologic, and social roots of this change, and the impact of masculine behavior on various realms of human endeavor. These roots cannot be understood from a feminist perspective, although much can be learned from that. The childhood experiences, adult lives, and self-concepts of men are markedly different from those of women. For example, power, dependency, sexuality, intimacy, work, and sports have different meanings for men than for women. The understanding of men requires its unique conceptual foundation. With this foundation, one can then speculate upon the nature of future changes as well as be able to intervene in an appropriate therapeutic, educational, or political way to aid those men in society who are changing.

This chapter will describe the traditional American masculine gender role. This role is complex and has many dimensions, some of which will also be discussed in other chapters in this book. In this chapter, the author will attempt to clarify certain dimensions of the masculine role and describe some of the behaviors that are subsumed under each dimension. His conceptual bias is that all social roles, including gender roles, are primarily socially learned and are integrated into the psychosexual, psychosocial, and cognitive development of the child. He will examine some of the positive and negative effects of this role on both the individual and society. Although he strongly believes that the masculine role must change, both to ensure the growth and happiness of individual men as well as for societal and humanistic reasons, he will attempt to be as value-free as possible in his description of the role and its effects. If, perhaps, the negative aspects of the role are emphasized, it is because recent psychologic and sociologic research in the area of masculine roles have led professionals to become more aware of the negative impact of traditional masculine role behavior and the positive value of androgyny. Any emphasis on the negative does not necessarily reflect a value judgment on his part but rather is an attempt to present a balanced view of the masculine role.

DEFINITIONS

There are four concepts that are frequently confused in the literature on gender roles. These concepts are *biologic sex* (gender), *gender identity*, *gender role*, and *sexual object choice*. Even in this book, the terms "male," "man," and "masculine" are used somewhat interchangeably, reflecting the confusion over the use of these terms. This confusion has helped perpetuate the "nature–nurture" conflict over the development of gender roles. It also helps explain some of the contradictory results reported in the literature on masculine roles. For example, this semantic confusion may lead to unclear and inappropriate methodologies for the research paradigms adopted. An attempt will be made to simplify and clarify these concepts at this time.

Biologic sex, or *gender*, consists of the physiologic and anatomic attributes of a man or a woman that are derived from his/her genetic endowment and subsequent biologic factors (e.g., disease) acting upon this endowment. It is defined at conception, although the biologic environment may modify the phenotypic display of these qualities. For men, biologic sex includes the XY chromosome pattern, high levels of testosterone and other androgens, and low levels of estrogens. It also includes secondary sex characteristics such as the beard, distribution of pubic hair, presence of a penis and testes, fat/muscle ratio, height, weight, and distribution of head hair. Gender includes physiologic differences between men and women, such as the concentration of acid phosphatase in the blood and contents of seminal fluid and the other bodily fluids. Finally, biologic maleness includes the lack of menstruation and the specific physiologic parameters of biologic femaleness.

These biologic differences also include the biologic imperatives discussed by Money (Refs. 7, 21 and Foreword to this book). As he points out, the only biologic imperative facing a man is that of impregnation. Only men can impregnate women; men cannot impregnate other men nor can women impregnate other women. Man cannot lactate, gestate, or menstruate. However, even these imperatives are mediated by societal norms, as our society allows a man the choice of whether or not he wishes to impregnate. In addition, the choice of sexual position or reason for impregnation is psychosocially, not biologically determined.

Gender identity is the internal and subjective sense in an individual's psyche as to whether he or she is a man or woman. This is a core belief and a major component of a person's total identity. It includes such other subjective concepts as body image, self-esteem, and self-concept. *Ur*-delusions, conflict-free ego functioning, and the existential sense of wholeness also contribute to one's gender identity. Gender identity is hypothesized to be unchangeable by age 2 or 3. Knowledge about a person's gender identity is indirect, coming through what that person tells us about him/himself and through the behaviors associated with gender roles.

Gender roles consists of those behaviors, expectations, and role sets defined by a society as masculine or feminine which are then embodied in the behavior of the individual man or woman. It includes the norms, values, and cultural beliefs associated with the behaviors. These behaviors are objectively verifiable and follow certain consistent patterns that others can identify as being an integral part of a particular role. Gender role may be internalized as part of one's gender identity, although it is less part of the individual's core; therefore, it is more easily modified. Gender role will be discussed in more depth shortly.

Sexual object choice is the biologic sex of the person with whom one chooses to have sexual relationships. One can identify five possible sexual object choices. The most common is heterosexual, in which a person chooses to have sexual activity with a person of the opposite sex. The next most common is the homosexual choice, in which a person chooses to have sex with a person of the same sex. The third is bisexual or ambisexual, in which a person chooses to have sexual activity with members of either sex, and which some theorists believe to be the innate sexuality of humans. A few individuals are primarily autosexual, that is, the person prefers sexual behavior with him/herself (via masturbation or with vibrators, for example). Finally, there are those who are asexual, preferring to be involved in no sexual activity and rarely feeling sexual impulsions. Differences in sexual object choice have led to much discussion in the literature as to whether these behaviors are pathologic or normal. This chapter will not enter into this debate. Sexual object choice is a part of gender identity and the behaviors associated with it part of gender role.

Another set of concepts that are frequently confused in *gender role* and *sex role*. The author objects to the broad use of the term "sex role" on the same grounds as does Money in his Foreword. The behaviors discussed in this book relate to the total man and his masculinity rather than those that relate only to his sexuality and sexual behaviors; thus, sex roles are only a part of gender roles. In addition, the author believes that the term "sex role" leads to a mistaken association between role behavior and biologic sex. This in turn, leads to the mistaken hypothesis that one's biologic sexuality and genetic endowment are the responsible agents for the development of gender-defined social behaviors (gender role) in adult life.

Goffman[22] defines role as "the activity the incumbent would engage in were he to act solely in terms of the normative demands upon someone in his position." Brannon[10] has defined role as "any pattern of behaviors which a given individual in a specific set of situations is both (1) expected, and (2) encouraged and or trained to perform." Other definitions also emphasize that all roles have both important social and behavioral components. Roles do not develop in a social vacuum, for they are defined by society. The individual, as he/she matures, learns the behavioral characteristics and role expectations of various roles he/she must perform. The person then may opt for or opt out of any of these particular roles, depending upon his/her social, psychologic, and sociologic state. In these situations, the individual usually substitutes other societally defined roles in adopting new behaviors. A common example in the use of the sick role, which has several dimensions that allow individuals to divest themselves of work and family roles at times of physical illness.[23,24] Another example is the role of the bereaved. A major part of the socialization process in human development requires the internalization of role expectations and behavioral norms, so that they become an integral part of the individual's conflict-free ego functioning and identity.

These roles include not only gender roles, but also occupational, parenting, deviant, and sick roles. Goffman[22] also points out that roles are composed of multiple subroles, smaller bits of the behavioral repertoire that are characterized by their own role expectations that combine to make up the larger role. Thus, when the author writes of the masculine gender role, he is actually writing about many different behaviors in many different social contexts. However, because there are so many commonalities in the behaviors, expectations, and norms associated with the roles, they can be subsumed as dimensions of the masculine gender role. The behaviors of such seemingly disparate men as George Patton, Walter Mitty, Warren Harding, Muhammed Ali, the local grocer, the Dean of the Graduate School, and Woody Allen can then be seen to demonstrate many of the attributes of the traditional American masculine role.

The author will mention many of the subroles that comprise the masculine gender role. These subroles include roles that impact upon the three aspects of human behavior: cognition, affect, and action. They include subroles related to work, family, sexuality, intimacy, affective communication, and status of the individual. These subroles are fairly clearly defined in American society, and although minor deviations from the norm are allowed, major changes from the norm cannot occur without the creation of another role with its consequent labeling and interpersonal consequences (e.g., deviant roles).

Other important dimensions of role relate to the clarity of the role expectations and the institutionalization of the status of the role. Rosow[25] has suggested a typology of role that incorporates these parameters (Table I). Institutionalized roles are those roles which have clear role definitions and an institutionalized status. Much of the masculine role falls into the category of institutionalized roles. This category includes much of masculine work, family, parental, and sexual roles. Informal roles include roles with clearly defined behaviors and expectations, but without an institutionalized status. These roles include many interpersonal behaviors and are particularly important to the maintenance of the primary group. This category includes such roles as scapegoat in group therapy, social butterfly, and neighborhood "nice guy." Tenuous roles, on the other hand, are roles with an institutionalized status, and ill-defined behaviors and expectations. These roles include such roles as honorific positions and many of the roles that are defined by society as deviant. Those include being mentally ill, criminal, beatnik, eccentric, and other similar roles. Frequently, deviant subcultures develop their own role behaviors and status hierarchies, including role definitions and role expectations. This has been discussed for psychiatric in-patients by Goffman,[26] Stanton and Schwartz,[27] and Caudill et al.,[28] and for the single-room-occupancy

Table I. Role Typology[a]

Role type	Role expectations/behaviors	Status
Institutional	Clear	Clear
Tenuous	Vague	Clear
Informal	Clear	Vague
Nonrole	Vague	Vague

[a]Adapted from Rosow (Ref. 25).

aged by Cohen and Sokolovsky.[29,30] Rosow's fourth type is the category of nonrole behaviors which have neither clear behavioral definitions nor clear status. Solomon also includes rolelessness as a role type[31], defining it as a state without role behaviors, role expectations, and associated status. Rolelessness differs from nonrole by the absence of these role dimensions, rather than their vagueness, which is a part of nonrole behavior.

THE DEVELOPMENT OF GENDER ROLE

Biologic sex, gender identity, and gender role are usually well intercorrelated. The biologic male usually has sex-appropriate secondary sex characteristics, considers himself a man, and behaves in a way society considers masculine (including being heterosexual). In both the child and the adult, the biologic, psychologic, sociologic, and interpersonal aspects of role behaviors interact at all times. For example, the man's biologically deeper voice (by virtue of genetically programmed and hormonally created enlargement of the larynx) may be labeled by society as more powerful and authoritative. This may put the man in a potentially superior position over a woman when competing for a job requiring vocal (but not verbal) skills, such as newscasting. Or, a man whose height is less than average (although not unusually small) may have a poor body image and poor self-esteem because of taunting by parents and peers in adolescence. This may contribute to a belief that he can never be successful at anything; therefore he never tries.

Deviations from this intercorrelation are possible in each dimension. For example, some men deviate in terms of biologic variables. They are born with X and Y chromosomes, but develop the genitals and secondary sex characteristics of women; this is the testicular feminization or androgen insensitivity syndrome. These people are usually identified as female at birth and are reared as women. They consider themselves women. Their behaviors are usually feminine, although they may be more active and aggressive than female peers. They are biologic and psychologic, but not genetic women. Other examples of dissonance between sex genotype and phenotype are cases of pseudohermaphroditism.

Other biologic males have a gender identity in which they do not consider themselves men. Although they have XY chromosomes, a beard, a penis, and male secondary sex characteristics, these individuals (who are diagnosed as having transsexual or a gender dysphoria disorder), believe that they are truly women who are unfortunately trapped in a man's body. It is interesting to note that both these biologic and identity deviations are societally labeled as illnesses. By doing so, society allows these individuals to take on a new and sanctioned role, the sick role, that may be used in transition from one gender role to another. It also gives these "deviations" a label (diagnosis) and "etiology" that helps diminish collective anxiety about a set of events that threatens a masculine-dominated society.

The final area for deviation from the expected correlation of role, identity, and gender is gender role, which this book is about. The author believes that men are questioning traditional masculine gender-role behaviors and reexamining their values, choosing to accept more "feminine" behaviors, and moving toward a position more aligned either with femininity or androgyny. Androgyny can be considered the interdigitation of the positive aspects of the masculine and feminine roles. It is a mixture of gender-role behaviors that can be chosen to aid coping and adaptation and to increase the intimacy of one's interpersonal relationships (see Chapter 4 in this book, by Boles and Tatro). Until recently, androgynous women were considered deviant by society and in many ways, androgynous men still are. These men are frequently mislabeled "homosexual," which has many negative connotations. However, as society changes, it is hoped that these behaviors will be seen not only as less deviant, but also as more positive and adaptable.

Aside from the four biologic imperatives, Money (Introduction to this book) has noted nine sets of human behaviors that he considers to be innately and biologically different between men and women. They are:

1. Activity levels
2. Roaming behaviors
3. Dominance behaviors
4. Behaviors defending troop and territory
5. Behaviors defending the young
6. Nesting behaviors
7. Parental behaviors
8. Sexual rehearsal behaviors
9. Response to erotic stimuli

Although these behavioral differences are consistently noted in published research, the biologic basis of these behaviors is not proven at this time. Even if these behaviors do have biologic roots, they may be modified by society, culture, and parents. Cultural expectations and norms can extinguish or reinforce virtually any innate behavioral differences among individuals. Furthermore, gender-role expectations and behaviors are noted and integrated into the personality of all stages of psychosexual, psychosocial, and cognitive development. Social learning, mediated through parents, family, peers, school, and the media, is the mechanism by which the growing boy internalizes the masculine role.

Even before birth, the individual's social roles and gender roles are being molded by the parents' fantasies. These fantasies, with their expectations and behavioral proscriptions begin during the nesting process. The color of the nursery and clothes, the toys that are bought, and the attachment of the parents to the fantasies set the stage for their interactions with the baby.

These behaviors intensify at birth, immediately constructing a framework for societal expectations. For example, boys are dressed in blue (to identify them as boys to others in society, who can relate to them as boys*) and are given more active toys and more toys to manipulate. Boys are given strong-sounding, un-

*A delightful fantasy of a child raised without any gender role stereotyping is "X: A Fabulous Child's Story," by Lois Gould.[32]

ambiguously masculine names. Biological traits that fit the traditional role (such as size and strength) are reinforced; those that do not are ignored. Temperamental attributes noticeable at birth[33] that fit the traditional role are also reinforced; those that do not are extinguished. These neonatal parental inputs may be extremely subtle, such as the degree of bouncing or cuddling a baby gets from his/her parents, but they are part of a developmental pattern that will determine future role behavior.

As the boy grows up, he is given sports equipment, toy guns, and other toys that require active mastery, movement, manipulation, and manual dexterity. Boys are encouraged and expected to play games that are devised to require competitiveness, aggression, and violence. Affective displays are discouraged. Peers grow up with similar expectations and by virtue of both the joys and cruelties of childhood behavior, mold the behavior of their peers to act according to masculine rules. Advertisements, television, movies, school, and family all reinforce certain images that men are supposed to be a certain way and women are supposed to be another. Thus, it is not surprising that behavioral differences between boys and girls can be described by age 3.[34]

Schools further reinforce these expectations and norms. For example, young boys hear romantic versions of great adventurers such as Christopher Columbus in elementary school. They learn that "brave" Christopher Columbus chanced upon the Americas on a trip across the "great" Atlantic Ocean in his search for the Indies. They do not learn that Columbus' encyclopedic knowledge of Ptolemy and other ancient astronomers made him certain that the world was round. They hear of Columbus skirting mutiny with his own crewmen, but not that his knowledge allowed him to predict where land was and that he could risk mutiny because he knew that land would arrive prior to rebellion. They do not learn that Columbus was a manipulative, calculating politician who was cynically attempting to find a way to improve his own family fortune. Schoolboys learn about Benjamin Franklin, the "poor-boy-who-made-good" hero, a true version of a Horatio Alger story in American history. But they do not learn that Benjamin Franklin cynically used women to attain his own ends. These examples are not given to diminish the many accomplishments of Columbus or Franklin or other men, but to illustrate how the image of man is portrayed in elementary school.

Imitation and modeling are important mechanisms that allow children to learn how to behave and how to do certain things. Boys practice being little men; indeed they are frequently called "little men." Little men or big boys don't cry, they fight for themselves, they do not do needlepoint, and they fantasize themselves as kings, generals, and presidents. Molded by parents, peers, school, the media, neighbors, and the world-at-large, little boys integrate the masculine role and gradually grow up to become big boys, then little men, then adult men.

Once appropriate role behaviors are demonstrated, the boy/man remains under pressure to perpetuate these behaviors. In adulthood, they are the only roles he knows. To experiment with new role behaviors is costly and may lead to failure as there are no alternative role models. Nontraditional role behaviors may lead to social ostracism or loss of job. The old role has many rewards. Behavioral expectations and norms are clear and consistent. Success brings money, interpersonal contacts, and power. Sex is easy to get. The negative consequences of the role, such as stress-related diseases or lack of intimacy, are in the distant future and are not felt as a present affective experience; therefore, they are not integrated into the individual's psyche. Because of that, most men are not motivated to change traditional masculine behaviors.

Furthermore, society has labeled men in certain ways, the dimensions to be discussed later in this chapter. This label and its associated attributes are cognitively integrated by men and may be mistaken by them as objective data. This leads to a "Catch-22" situation for men. If they act according to the label, they prove the rule; if they act at variance to the label, they are the exception that proves the rule. In either case, the traditional role is reinforced by society.

(What about the boy who does not conform to these rules? One seven-year-old active, athletic, bright, manually manipulative and loud boy loved to do needlepoint with his parent's blessings and mother's teaching [his father had never learned how]. One day, he came home crying after being admonished by his grandfather about how "bad" a thing it was to do. One twelve year old was repeatedly assaulted by classmates because he was afraid to be involved in contact sports. He was being prepared for a career as a concert pianist and did not wish to risk hurting his hands. The behavior of his peers changed only when he became a member of his school's cross-country team [a sport he discovered after he learned that he could outrun his pursuers!]. One adolescent with artistic interests and a "feminine" demeanor had a very lonely adolescence until he attended a prestigious New England liberal arts college. The pain of not being socialized in the traditional way may last for a lifetime.)

Culturally defined variations of the masculine role are infinite. A few examples of these cultural differences in gender roles will serve as examples of this variety. In many European cultures, men kissing upon greeting each other is considered the norm. That behavior would raise eyebrows in the United States. There are differences in nurturing behaviors among Japanese, German, and American fathers. Mexican men touch each other more than do Anglo men. Italian men are more expressive than are Irish or Jewish men.

The most telling example of cultural variations of gender role behaviors comes from the work of Mead.[35] She examined three tribes in New Guinea, all of whom live within a fairly short distance of each other. Although her distillation of her data is somewhat naive and simplistic, the framework of the roles she describes is probably valid.

In one tribe, the Arapesh, the men and women behave in a way that would be considered feminine in our culture. Both men and women Arapesh tend to be passive, cooperative, peaceful, nurturing individuals. Their language, that royal road to a culture, shares the cultural belief that fathers as well as mothers bear children. Fathers participate in all aspects of child care from pregnancy to adulthood. Sexual interest in both partners is relatively low and their sexual style is relatively passive. Neither men nor women tend to be authority figures and specific children are selected to be trained to be more assertive so that leadership in the society is assured. War, except as self-defense, is uncommon.

Another tribe is the Mundugumor, who might be considered caricatures of "macho" men. Both men and women are aggressive, belligerent, violent, competitive, sexually aggressive, jealous, active, and fighting individuals. Their entire social system is pervaded by hostility. Children are virtually ignored both by mothers and fathers. Any contact that occurs between children and parents almost exclusively relates to biologic aspects of nurturing rather than psychosocial aspects of nurturing. The tribe is warlike and is a constant threat both to its neighbors and to its own members.

The third tribe is the Tchambuli, whose members behave akin to a role reversal for American men and women. The men are sensitive, artistic, passive, and independent. They gossip and are particularly fond of adorning their body and making up their hair. They walk with mincing steps and utilize the world as an audience for their various artistic activities. Women in the Tchambuli culture are competent, dominating, practical, and efficient. They run both house and society. They are the sexual aggressors and tend to be the active pursuer of sex. It is the women who take up leadership positions in that society.

These three cultures highlight the fact that the American pattern is not an immutable pattern nor is it the only pattern of gender-role behavior. Furthermore, all behaviors, with the exception of the four biologic imperatives defined by Money, have been seen in either men or in women in some society somewhere in history.

From a different perspective, Woods[36] has identified four psychodynamic conflicts leading to the development of male chauvinism. In a previous paper,[19] the author of this chapter has suggested that these psychodynamic issues were primarily operative in men with severe chauvinistic behaviors and that social learning was primarily operative in the development of the masculine role of men without psychopathology. He now believes that the interaction between social learning and different stages in the psychosexual development of men reinforce each other's effects in all men.

The four psychodynamic parameters identified by Woods are infantile strivings, power and dependency conflicts, Oedipal anxiety, and a hostile envy of women. It has been suggested that male infants are held less, are more actively manipulated and less passively nurtured, and are allowed to cry longer than are female infants. If so, many infantile needs remain unmet. True to the instinctual underpinnings of much of human motivation, these strivings become overvalued as the child matures and the resolution and integration of them into the ego remain incomplete. These include strivings for bodily closeness, nurturance, and relief from emotional discomfort. However, seeking relief as an infant does not always lead to relief, but rather more emotional discomfort and *angst*, so that the boy during the anal phase of psychosexual development becomes ambivalent about allowing these needs to be satisfied without controlling the person (mother) who can supply them. Dependency needs develop with the same pattern, leading to ambivalence and control. Because of the way others manipulate his body as well as his own self-discoveries, the boy during this stage (Paiget's stage of sensorimotor development[37]) has begun to integrate schemata of active mastery, activity, self-pleasure, and a narcissistic self-image.

The lack of response from the mother is interpreted by the infant from a paranoid position, which reinforces a life pattern of mistrust, as described by Erikson.[38]

As the boy enters the next phase of development, issues of power and control come to the fore. The boy has already learned a cognitive mode of active mastery and uses this in power and control struggles with the mother. His activity is ambivalently reinforced, leading to further struggles. Often, the boy has been able to get his more infantile needs met in a disguised way, but at the cost of becoming hostile and angry at the mother, who is now seen as an "all bad" object. The push for autonomy, separation, and individuation is ambivalently experienced as this push is correctly perceived to bring the boy further from the mother with whom he seeks intimacy. At this same time, he begins to cognitively integrate the world around him. He is able to affectively appreciate how girls are treated differently (and sometimes differentially). As preoperational cognitions allow the symbolic generalization and categorization of experience, he is able to attach these experiences to the anger he feels toward his mother. His envy toward girls and women begins to develop and his anger is further reinforced.

In the Oedipal period, a major task of the child is identification with the same-sex parent. As the boy views his father as a powerful rival for mother, the child can symbolically get mother (and satisfaction of infantile needs) by becoming like father. Many of the outward manifestations of the masculine gender role are adopted by copying the father and other significant men in the boy's life. Castration anxiety is experienced as a fear of being overpowered by significant men and the boy competitively manipulates father to avoid this end. Because father is a rival, the boy cannot get too close, although he also has desires to be intimate with the man he loves most. Sensory and intellectual input from the world at large frequently show male figures violently competing with and winning over superior rivals (as in many Saturday morning television cartoons); the boy vicariously integrates these experiences to help him best his father and stand out as "champion" over other significant men.

In latency, the boy receives his first heavy dose of socialization from others. Boys and girls are frequently separated in many activities reinforcing the developing gender-role dichotomy. Peer pressure and consensual validation are important socializing reinforcers. Cognitively, the boy is able to categorize behaviors and see similarities among disparate behaviors and expectations that comprise masculine and feminine roles. Chum relationships, as described by Sullivan,[39–40] serve as models for peer relationships. Although they may be the most intimate relationships the prepubertal boy has, these relationships tend to revolve around a nucleus of active competition, mutual aggression, and developing inexpressiveness as the boys integrate the masculine role. Schools teach much of the role, both from the content of the educational material, as noted in the examples of Columbus and Franklin, but also in a process that emphasizes active mastery and competition among boys in the same class.[41]

By adolescence, the boy has integrated all dimensions of the masculine role into his ego. Much of this is integrated into the realm of conflict-free ego functioning, although for individual boys, some dimensions may be sources of future conflict. For boys, much of the anxiety of adolescence is related to the behavioral manifestations of the masculine role, especially in the areas of sexuality and career. The educational system makes the job easier for boys at this age, by opening up many opportunities (with increased expectations) for them, opportunities not available to adolescent girls. There is an emphasis on formal cognitive operations for boys at this age, as they are channeled into career areas that require this cognitive mode, such as science, engineering, law, or business. This process continues in college. Peer pressure becomes increasingly important in maintaining previously learned role behaviors, in contrast to teaching these behaviors in latency. By adulthood, the role is integrated so thoroughly, with constant reinforcement from society (through peers, spouse, superiors, the media, advertising, and entertainment, among other ways), that it is virtually impossible for the man to make any changes in the dimensions of the masculine role unless he is willing to experience conflict, confusion, anxiety, and social sanctions.

Dimensions of the Masculine Role

Earlier in this chapter, several past and contemporary men were mentioned as examples of men who displayed the traditional masculine role. There are more similarities than differences in their masculinity. George Patton was reported to be an aggressive, inexpressive, rational, problem-solving, ambitious, manipulative, success-oriented, and successful person who used people for his own ends. Warren Harding was a similar kind of man, only his arena was the political, not the military. Harding and many other politicians have used women not to satisfy intimacy needs, but for sexual gratification and as steps to and symbols of power. Woody Allen, in his films, is obsessed with success and power in work and bed. To him, every human interaction is a like a chess game, a symbolic war, in which he, like Patton and Harding, is the aggressor. In his films, he never cries; indeed, he is extremely inexpressive. Walter Mitty does in his fantasies what Woody Allen does in his films.

The masculine role has many dimensions to it. These dimensions serve as a skeleton only. Within the rules bounded by the masculine role, a man has many options, options which are carefully chosen to keep the role intact and to preserve the role. In an attempt to clarify these behavioral roles, Farrell[12] has humorously listed the "Ten Commandments of Masculinity," which are paraphrased here:

1. Thou shalt not cry or expose other feelings of emotion, fear, weakness, sympathy, empathy, or involvement before thy neighbor.
2. Thou shalt not be vulnerable; thou shalt honor and respect the logical, practical, and intellectual as thou defineth them.
3. Thou shalt not listen except to find fault.
4. Thou shalt condescend to women in all ways, big and small.

5. Thou shalt control thy wife's body and all its relations, occasionally permitting it on top.
6. Thou shalt have no other egos before thee.
7. Thou shalt have no other breadwinners before thee.
8. Thou shalt not be responsible for housework before anybody.
9. Thou shalt honor and obey the straight and narrow pathway to success: job specialization.
10. Thou shalt have an answer to all problems at all times.
11. And, above all, thou shalt not read *The Liberated Man* or commit any other form of introspection.

In this simplified form, Farrell has emphasized the negative dimensions of these behavioral expectations. However, the dimensions of the masculine role are more complex and have positive and negative consequences, which will be described later in this chapter.

One of the major ways of examining roles is to analyze institutionalized roles, their expectations and behavioral norms, and status. This has the advantage of allowing the examination of specific issues for men, such as occupational and career roles and man as breadwinner, husband, father, grandfather, brother, or lover. However, the author believes that as the informal roles are an interdigitating matrix of behavior upon which the institutionalized roles are built, the masculine role is better analyzed from examination of these informal roles. Certian specific aspects of the institutionalized roles will be examined by other authors in this book (e.g., Lewis and Roberts, Nadelson and Nadelson), and the author will refer to aspects of these roles as appropriate. But he is choosing to emphasize the informal role matrix as more relevant to the study of the behavior of men than institutionalized roles.

In their book, David and Brannon[10] define four major dimensions of the masculine role which they label (1) "No Sissy Stuff," (2) "The Big Wheel," (3) "The Sturdy Oak," and (4) "Give 'Em Hell." The author will add two more dimensions to this: Homophobia and Sexual Dysfunctioning. He will discuss each of these dimensions in turn.

"NO SISSY STUFF." "No Sissy Stuff" is the avoidance of anything that is remotely or vaguely feminine, whether it be in cognition, affect, or behavior. As noted above, there is a societal dichotomy of the sexes that becomes established at birth. In adulthood, according to Farrell,[12] the dichotomy has become so pervasive that it permeates all aspects of gender role. To summarize the dichotomy, it means that the boy becomes a good talker and articulator rather than a good listener. He uses logic as opposed to emotion. He emphasizes visible conflict rather than behind-the-scenes incremental growth. He displays self-confidence in place of humility, quick decisionmaking rather than thoughtful pondering, charisma and dynamism rather than long-term credibility, and active striving for power rather than a general thrust to achieve even if power does not accompany the achievement. Politics or business becomes a Machiavellian end in itself rather than a means toward expressing human concern. The boy learns a hard, confident, and aggressive approach to people instead of a soft, persuasive approach. He learns a responsiveness to concrete, resolute ends and external, tangible rewards rather than less concrete, or internal satisfaction. He experiences genital sexuality rather than a total body sensuality.

This dichotomy has been supported by research data from several investigators. Harford et al.[42] noted that masculinity was negatively associated with warmth, brightness, emotional stability, and sensitivity and positively associated with suspiciousness, guilt, anxiety, and toughness. Bem et al.[43] noted that men were less nurturant than women although self-reports of nurturance feelings were the same in both sexes. Bem and Lenny[44] noted that men and women avoided activities traditionally associated with the other gender.

This dichotomy displays itself in many areas of childhood life. Boys prefer toys that allow for the expression of aggressive impulses and manual dexterity[45–48] and are drawn to occupations that emphasize active mastery over the environment and manual manipulation .[49,50] Children accept the dichotomy early in life and behave according to its rules. Parents, peers, and schools reinforce the dichotomy throughout the preschool[34,45–47,49–53] latency[9] and adolescent years.[54–57] The dichotomy is often cruelly enforced by peers, through the use of the one word that is so powerful that it inspires awe in all boys: "sissy."* No boy dares to chance being called by this most horrible of taunts, even if it is not accompanied by physical violence or social ostracism.

The lifelong hold of the word on a man with feminine interests can be seen in the following example. It also demonstrates the active avoidance of the feminine that characterizes this chauvinism. A 53-year-old biologist gave up a promising career as a classical pianist in adolescence because of peer pressure. He cringed whenever he heard the word "sissy" and was angry at himself for unsuccessfully pursuing a place on his high school football team at the expense of his instrument and career. His teens, twenties, and thirties were characterized by a need to prove to all his peers that he was not a "sissy." He was an aggressive and competitive grants-seeker and was reknowned in his field. He became the editor of a prestigious journal in his mid-thirties. He was an aggressive womanizer and had fathered several illegitimate children without caring about them. He was active in contact sports in spite of frequent injuries. But he was unhappy until be began to reexamine the role the word "sissy" played in his life. Only when he understood the impact of this word and the dimension of "No Sissy Stuff" in his life was he able to begin to have intimate relationships with women, share with colleagues, and again, take up the practice of music as an enjoyable pastime.

Another example is a 33-year-old man, a paranoid schizophrenic. Although he was not psychotic and was on medication, he remained quite anxious and phobic. His major fears were that other people were going to hurt him, men were trying to harm him, and unless he acted like a man, something dreadful would happen to him. He had difficulty controlling his aggressive impulses

*The origin of this word is unknown. However, it is hypothesized to have developed in Renaissance or Elizabethan England as a derogatory derivative of the word "sister."

(which made him intensely guilty), and he avoided any contact with other men. Another part of his personality, however, was that of a highly sensitive, artistic, creative man. In spite of admitting that he wanted to become an artist, he tended to deny this part of his personality. The first task in working with him was having him define what he meant by being a man and by being a woman. His definition of woman included expressing feelings, being creative, admitting weakness, being intuitive, and allowing himself to enjoy experiences of the moment. His definition of man included avoiding physical contact with men, not expressing one's fears and feelings, being aggressive, and having power. He felt that he was in a bind because he could not act according to his definition of being a man because it led to his phobias. Nor could he act as a woman because that meant being homosexual (the consequences of which he could not describe). In therapy, he realized that being creative and having feelings did not make him any less of a man and he was able to start to seriously develop his artistic talent.

The avoidance of feminine role behavior leads to an active avoidance of all role behavior associated with stereotypic feminine characteristics. It is socially advantageous for the male adolescent to mature early, for he becomes bigger, stronger, hairier, and has a deeper voice that clearly distinguishes him from his female peers. In our society, this also means that men avoid artistic endeavors, as did the men noted above, endeavors in which they must express their sensitivity and sensuality; this is considered feminine. Chass[58] notes that although male ballet dancers are in better physical condition than the average football player, their masculinity (usually subsumed under sexual object choice) is highly suspect. Sportswriters, coaches, truck drivers, and military men are automatically seen as masculine regardless of their physical condition because these occupations involve behaviors that are diametric opposites of feminine behaviors. Men in the 1960s began to grow their hair long, but a simultaneous event was the growth of beards; men were still clearly masculine and different from women. The range of colors, textures, styles, materials, etc., for men's clothing is sharply reduced as compared to those for women; men do not wear makeup. To be a "peacock" is to be like a woman.*

Not only are feminine qualities actively avoided, but masculinity is manipulated to promise a man that he will not turn into a woman or become feminine. The Marine Corps, seeking "a few good men," does this with extensive chains of command, overly aggressive training, avoidance of intimacy and affect, and the manipulation of shame and guilt.[59] In a more mundane world, colognes for men do not sell unless they have names like Command, Tackle, or Hai Karate. In a recent workshop that the author facilitated, he found that men were most attracted to colognes that had certain "masculine," i.e., leather or woody, scents. English Leather, one of the most popular men's colognes, was originally marketed as a woman's cologne. It failed miserably on the market until the name was changed and the market altered. Cars do not sell without model names such as Cougar, Mustang, or Eldorado.

*It is ironic that it is the male peacock, similar to the males of most birds, that has the colorful plumage.

Along with the avoidance of the feminine roles is the avoidance of affect and its outward display. As noted by Balswick and co-workers (see Refs. 60 and 61, and the chapters in this volume by Balswick and Dosser), the American man is unable or unwilling to express his feelings. Emotionality is the province of women. Expressiveness is evidence of vulnerability, weakness, and femininity. It means that one can "break down" under stress. Men who are upset are usually told to "get themselves together" rather than to ventilate their feelings about the source of their upsetting feelings. The British phrase, "stiff upper lip" is very apt in this situation. "Big boys don't cry" is a lifelong credo.

This inexpressiveness is not a total inexpressiveness because feelings of anger, contempt, hostility, and aggression are not commonly avoided by men. Indeed, expression of these affects, especially by physical means, is an expected part of the masculine role. However, these are not considered "feminine" feelings. Feelings of love, tenderness, trust, fear, shame, and vulnerability are kept to oneself. Men do not cry in public because that is feminine. Even in "safe" situations, where affective display is encouraged or expected, men may not be expressive. Men cry less frequently than women at funerals. In movement workshops facilitated by the author, men, generally including many athletic men, do not know how to move the fine muscles of their face (the muscles of expression) or fingers, but limit themselves to gross motor movement. In psychotherapy, a common problem faced is alexithymia, in which a man is unable to identify what he is feeling and translate it into words that can be utilized in the therapeutic process. Alexithymia is thought to be an important component in the development of psychosomatic disorders[62,63] and narcotic abuse.[64]

Along with the lack of expressivity is the inability of men to experience their sensuality and bodily sensations. Men are frequently totally unaware of their bodily sensations. If aware, they frequently do not know what these sensations mean. They are unable to identify concomitants of anger, happiness, stress, or joy in their bodies. If they identify a feeling, they frequently mislabel it. Again, in movement workshops, men frequently report experiencing nonspecific muscle tension when told to fantasize scenes of disappointment, anger, or joy.

Men are unable to relax, lie back, and experience what their senses are telling them. This is considered feminine, as it means becoming passive, which is not usually allowed men. The avoidance of passivity leads men to be constantly active. Men have difficulty sitting still when not doing anything. Men have great difficulty relaxing, even when their minds are not preoccupied. Even men's leisure time activities involve work. Mowing a lawn, painting a house, or playing softball do not allow for passive relaxation. A lifetime of activity makes it difficult for the man at any age to stay still for more than a few minutes.

A characteristic of women is a willingness to become emotionally or physically dependent on other people when necessary. When extreme, it is a problem of the feminine role and when caricatured, it may be a factor in the development of the hysterical cognitive style.[65] But in the well-functioning individual, regression to a dependent state may be useful for aiding psychological growth and adaptation. Woods[36] considers dependency and a denial of dependency to be a major source of the dynamic development of male chauvinism. He couples these unresolved dependency conflicts with an unresolved envy and anger at women for their ability to be open and vulnerable and survive in spite of it. However, dependency is seen as distinct from masculinity by most men, and is avoided, leading to solitary activity and problem solving, especially under stress.

Thus, American men avoid being feminine. Unfortunately, avoidance of feminine role characteristics does not necessarily lead to the development of masculine role characteristics that may be useful and adaptive. There are no positive opposites to expressiveness, sensuality, adaptive dependency, and interpersonal openness. Activity may be a positive opposite to passivity but purposeless activity may be inappropriate and destructive.

"The Big Wheel." The second dimension of the masculine role is "The Big Wheel." Men are expected to be successful, seek higher status, and be looked up to. The American man must achieve wealth, fame, or recognition. The records listed in the Guinness Book of World Records are usually accomplished by men. This is especially true for those records that are tests of physical endurance. For example, setting the record for continuous riding of a roller coaster meant putting up with the physical discomfort of nausea, dizziness, blood pressure and temperature changes, and exposure to the elements. Horatio Alger stories are another example of "The Big Wheel" socialization at work; schoolboys learn how only in the USA can a boy make his dream of becoming a self-made millionaire or President of the United States come true.

Even the man who cannot become the "World's Greatest" or the "World's Richest" is expected to do the best he can and achieve some recognition. The acquisition of material goods is the external manifestation of success. By emphasizing material goods, men can be sure that others recognize their success. Many men seek out a profession, such as medicine, law, or business that will, through its attendant high status, automatically qualify them as a success. They then seek out the external accoutrements of this successful profession. Men in other occupations seek and accept whatever blandishments they can acquire. For example, a skilled laborer who owned a one-man business was billed as the president of his company when his daughter's wedding announcement was published in the newspaper. As Willy Loman, in *Death of a Salesman,* told his brother, "A man can't go out the way he came in Ben, a man has got to add up to something."[66]

Early in life, boys realize that they all cannot be great doctors or another Babe Ruth or George Washington. They learn to compensate by channeling their drive for success and status into narrower but ego-syntonic activities. Compensation continues in adulthood. One may be the champion bowler on the bowling team, the policeman who has handed out the most tickets, or the clerk with the best sales record. Recognition (and therefore, some measure of success) occurs within the confines of their social stratum.

The American society assures success for some groups, whom Navarro[67] calls the "corporate class." Status is assured by birth and wealth. Further recognition, however, is still a goal, and men in this social class actively pursue power, frequently on a national or international scale. The rest of American men actively strive for higher status; this drive is constant, and never diminishes in intensity, as one can (and does) see beyond one's present state to a better one. This cognitive dissonance ("the grass is always greener in the Joneses' yard, especially when you have to keep up with and surpass the Joneses") makes the American man perpetually conscious of status and its accoutrements. He then frequently uses and manipulates other people to achieve his upward mobility. In return, he is manipulated in the competitive dash to fill fewer and fewer positions at the top of the pyramid.

A 42-year-old manager was promoted to a high executive position in his firm. At first, he enjoyed the increased income, the contact with government officials, and the travel. After several months, he noted that he was more fatigued, his wife was more irritable, and he had less time with his children. Travel became a chore. He felt pressured to compete with his closest friend for the next promotion; only one of them could have the position. He withdrew from his relationship with this friend until he reexamined what his new position had done to his life. He felt that his friends and family were more important to him than was his income. He chose to resign his position rather than continue the unhappy life he had been leading.

The striving for success and status underscores the importance of competition in men's lives. If it is not how you play the game but whether you win or lose, the man must have the behavioral tools necessary to win. Even leisure activities for men, such as sports, are either actively or passively competitive. To win, the man must manipulate others and mistrust others' motives. This precludes intimacy and caring. As the number of slots becomes fewer, it becomes harder to be successful and easier to fail; the man usually redoubles his efforts at that stage. Winning or losing precludes sharing and cooperation.

Adler[68] defined one aspect of masculinity as the will to power. Power is a masculine perogative in our society. Power is a direct result of success. The greater one's success, the more power is available to him. Men actively seek out power to be able to manipulate others to achieve more success. Power does not need to be physical force or economic holdings. It may be charismatic, such as the destructive power of a Jim Jones or the constructive power of Martin Luther King. It may simply be the power of words. A common complaint of many single women is that men manipulate the power of words and act open and "cool" until they are in bed.

This power and control extends to the family where the man is breadwinner and carries the label of head of household. It is the man who determines the economic and social status of the family as a unit and of each of its individual members. It is the man who gives the woman her share of the paycheck for food or household needs. The breadwinner role is the one institutionalized masculine role in the family that the man considers of primary importance. As noted by Lein,[68] men begrudgingly allow their wives to work and are usually threatened if their paychecks are greater. Men do not reciprocate with parenting or housekeeping roles except when those activities require masculine strength, like painting the house or mowing the lawn. It is the man who usually sits at the head of the table and who determines when people will eat. In one family, it is the father who determines whether or not his adolescent children can have second portions, depending upon their response to his question, "Do you need it?"

A final attribute of "The Big Wheel" is the meaning of work for American men. The Protestant ethic, based on the teachings of John Calvin, states that one must do good deeds and work hard to reach salvation. This is necessary to show others that you are one of the "elect," those destined to go to Heaven. This "ethic" has become a hallmark for most men; they must do work that assures them status, success, recognition, and power. Most men would work in the absence of economic necessity to do so.[70] Men so define themselves by their work that they may have no identity other than their occupational identity. For example, in meeting a man at a party we do not ask, "Who are you?" and "What kind of food do you like?" or "Who's your favorite singer?" or "Are you expressive?" Rather, we ask, "Who are you?" and "What do you do for a living?" or "What is your profession?" We immediately know something of that person's status which tells us whether or not we will be willing to interact with that person and whether or not we are willing to let him in our world, however superficially and momentarily. It does not tell us what kind of a person he is and whether or not we can form a relationship with that individual. The importance of work is underscored by the data that demonstrate that morbidity and mortality rates for men skyrocket one year after mandatory retirement. Depression, most common psychopathologic syndrome in the elderly, is frequently precipitated by mandatory retirement.[71]

"THE STURDY OAK." The third dimension of the masculine gender role is "The Sturdy Oak." Man carry themselves with an air of toughness, confidence, and self-reliance at all times. The poems of Rudyard Kipling glorify this type of man. Many of the characters played by John Wayne, Humphrey Bogart, Paul Newman, Marlon Brando, or Montgomery Clift are examples of "The Sturdy Oak" in action. No matter what the stress is, and no matter how difficult the stress is to cope with, the man is expected to stand up to it and survive. If he does not survive, he is expected to go down fighting, like Davy Crockett at the Alamo. That man will be a hero will be tested in a trial by fire. The man does not need to use physical force; moral force, such as that of Sir Thomas More or Soviet dissident Andrei Sakharov, may suffice if the risks are great enough.

In the more mundane world of most men, the expectations are the same. Men do not share the frustrations of work with their families for their heroism is winning the daily battle against traffic, supervisors, and an organizational system that makes them feel neglected and manipulated. They strive for their success alone, competing against all colleagues, with the same toughness and confidence that they see in their heroes on television. Part of the image of "The Sturdy Oak" is inexpressiveness and an inability or refusal to show evidence of fear or vulnerability. Another part of this image is the man exuding an aura of invulnerability in case he must dish out (and be prepared to take) tougher things to another man, in the competition for success. Heroism is an important component of this dimension, something discussed in more detail by Lederer and Botwin (Ref. 72 and Chapter 12 in this book).

Part of invulnerability is omnicompetence. This is the belief that man is expected to solve all problems. The American man places a premium on rational problem solving and his sense of omniscience. The American man, as part of this expectation of being always competent, always has the answer, even if the answer is not necessarily relevant to the problem. For example, when lost, men are more likely to continue to drive around rather than stop and ask directions. If a car won't start, men are more likely to putter around and come up with some statements about possibilities rather than seek out help. In the author's experience as an academic psychiatrist, he has noted that men residents are less likely to ask for help or advice in supervision than are women residents. Being competent assumes knowing the answers; and knowing the answers assumes having the information; not having the answers or knowledge assumes having the interpersonal skills to show that others also do not have the answers or to cover up one's own ignorance.

Coupled with this expectation of omnipotence and omniscience is the need for a man to be self-reliant. Man must be his own man, and if necessary, stand by himself. He must be a hero. If necessary, he must stand against an entire system, regardless of the danger, such as Doctor Stockmann in *An Enemy of the People*.[73] Men are also more dogmatic than women, as Heyman[74] has noted; this dogmatism, usually associated with hostility, is well integrated into the man's personality.

This dimension also includes the need for men to prove their athletic prowess and to demonstrate their physical strength. Many men become weekend athletes, although they are overweight, smoking, beer-drinking men who try to play the games the way they did at age 20. If athletics are not directly indulged in, they are to be enjoyed vicariously, through enjoyment of spectator sports. Competent Monday morning quarterbacking (in which men indirectly compete with by second guessing the athletes and their peers) is an expected part of this behavior. That sports monopolize weekend television and use several pages, if not a complete section, of every major daily newspaper, speaks to its importance for men. That popular sports include violent sports such as boxing, hockey, or football, attests to the close relationship between "The Sturdy Oak" and the next dimension ("Give 'Em Hell") of the masculine role. The sports that emphasize bodily skills, such as gymnastics, are relegated to lesser importance.

"GIVE 'EM HELL." The fourth dimension of the masculine gender role is "Give 'Em Hell." Daring, violence, aggression, and risk-taking are part of this dimension. That men are the more aggressive and violent of the sexes has been known for millenia. But the aggression may not necessarily be violent; it may be a component of negotiation, grants applications, competition in business, or a lack of sensitivity during sex. It means being ruthless and insensitive to the needs of others in a destructive way, frequently while in the process of working toward success.

Men are the war-makers. Men are the murderers. Men are the rapists. Men ravish the environment. Men kill themselves. Boys are told never to start fights, but they are taught how to violently defend themselves. Boys are taught that once confronted with a potentially violent situation, they are expected to use violence rather than other methods of potential problem solving in response. Kenny Rogers' hit song, "The Coward of the County," states that "sometimes you *have* to fight when you're a man." One is always expected to fight to protect an external part of one's masculinity, including one's money, business, or wife. Jimmy Connors, tennis star and "macho" hero, has fought tennis rivals, umpires, fans, and, in February, 1980, fought with a man who dared to speak to Connors' wife at a tennis match. His aggressiveness also makes him the tennis star that he is.

This dimension forces the man to always prove his masculinity. The success of today's role behavior is not sufficient proof for tomorrow. The man must begin to do more to prove his masculinity, each one a little riskier. Gradually, personal behavioral norms develop in which interpersonal, financial, or professional risk-taking becomes the expectation. As a result, intelligent politicans accept bribes. A majority of men have extramarital affairs,[75] often at the risk of losing a spouse. A whole frontier culture developed in the USA based on aggression and risk-taking, a culture still glorified in country and western music, movies, and television.

HOMOPHOBIA. The fifth dimension of the masculine role is the fear of homosexuality, or homophobia. The stereotypic homosexual is believed to be effeminate. The drag queen is believed to be the norm, although this is purely a myth (see Ref. 76 and Chapter 6, by Norton). Homosexuality, effeminate demeanor (a caricature of feminine behavior), and femininity are equated in American society. Through fear of becoming homosexual, the American man practically avoids all nonstructured social contact with other men. This taboo on man-to-man human contact is so complete that there is a minimum of touching and virtually no emotional intimacy between men for fear that this may lead them down the path to "perversion." The behavioral norms are that men can only touch each other in certain "safe," structured situations. There is the handshake, which is a highly ritualized way of breaking down territoriality between individuals. On the sports field, there may be a pat on the buttocks after a good play or a hug after a score, but certainly never a kiss. Medical students and physicians are reluctant to do rectal exams on their patients, a simple technique that can lead to the detection of over 50% of rectal cancers. The homophobia is expressed in a wide range of behaviors, from jokes to police raids on gay bars. Homophobia is common in the gay community as well. Locker rooms abound with scatological humor, comments about the size of women's breasts, and tales of men's sexual prowess with women, as a defense against the awareness of naked bodies of other men. Men are presumed to be straight unless effeminate, unless they are known to be "out of the closet." The lack of expressiveness and competition is in part related to homophobia, for one cannot get intimate with someone with whom one cannot share.[77] In addition, power and control issues, fears of being labeled as "homosexual," and a lack of intimate relationships with men in childhood tend to further inhibit the development of intimacy among adult men.

When asked about their homophobia, men at first deny it. They are heterosexual and know that their sexual object choice will not change. They may be friendly with gay men. On deeper exploration, however, the homophobia is admitted, but without explanation. The author has yet to meet a man who is able to identify the source of his homophobia. The author believes that this is because of the primitive, preverbal origins of homophobia. In the author's opinion, sexual object choice is intimately associated with gender identity and issues of separation and individuation from mother and is pre-Oedipal in nature. To love a man is to be like mother. One of the developmental tasks of the boy is to divest himself of the infantile relationship with his mother. Since this is generally incomplete, as evidenced by unresolved dependency issues, the only way the boy can create the *ur*-delusion of individuation is by refusing to love another man. This would help to explain the pervasive homophobia seen in the gay community as well as the reason men in general cannot identify the reason for their homophobia. It also helps explain the lack of intimacy (love) between men.

SEXUAL DYSFUNCTIONING. The final dimension of the masculine role is masculine sexual behavior. This dimension was summarized by one woman who said to the author, "Why is it that men think that the only sexual enjoyment occurs in the final one and a half centimeters of their erect penis?" Men's sexuality is limited in the areas of physical enjoyment as well as in intimacy. Many men do not allow themselves to experience their sensuality both as part of and separate from sexual pleasure. Most other men do not know how to enjoy their bodies and their sexuality. Activity precludes the mental and physical passivity necessary to experience one's sensuality. If genital orgasm is the only goal, all else along the way becomes something to be endured, not enjoyed. Litewka[56] has humorously described the adolescent male sexual evolution; in doing so, he dramatically shows how each bit of sexual behavior develops separate from all others, so that the adolescent boy never experiences sensual pleasure. Social pressure orients the boy for intercourse and ejaculation, so that each step is another battle and conquest, precluding intimacy and pleasure. This pattern continues throughout life.[78] Even men who are athletes are frequently out of touch with the messages they receive from their special senses and from their fine muscles, although they may revel in gross motor movement. Furthermore, enjoying skin sensations, nipple stimulation, or massage may be considered too feminine, bringing the dimension of "No Sissy Stuff" into a man's behavior. Of course, Masters and Johnson[79] have shown that the sexual response cycles of men and women are quite similar in many ways. However, most men focus on the specific penile sensations during sexual encounters.

Men also confuse ejaculation with orgasm. They are not necessarily synonymous, although they usually occur concurrently. Men may have orgasms without ejaculation, as when multiorgasmic, "dry" after repeated frequent ejaculations, or because of neurologic disease. In premature ejaculation, there may be ejaculation without orgasm or even erection, and rarely with any pleasure; the man is frequently distressed. This confusion between physical response and psychological experience may lead to stress in older men, who are unaware of diminished ejaculatory needs and ability as they age[79], and who then label themselves as having a sexual dysfunction (see Chapter 11 of this book, by Solomon).

Success drives are frequently brought from the boardroom to the bedroom and performance remains important for the man. He must get it up, keep it up, and give the woman her orgasms. He must be the "world's best lover." Men concentrate on control of their own feelings, holding back their own orgasms, and trying to interpret the nonverbal responses of their partners. Because of this conscious work and activity, they are rarely able to experience pleasure in the sexual encounter. On the other extreme, a hostile control of the woman's sexuality may lead the man to narcissistically concentrate on his own penile sensations and ejaculatory control, denying the woman sexual pleasure in the pursuit of his own. This quite frequently occurs during the preorgasmic and orgasmic phases of the sexual response cycle, in which many men become totally immersed in their penile sensations.

When carried to an extreme, the man who emphasizes success and control during sexual encounters will develop a promiscuous sexual lifesytle that manipulates sex partners as hedonistic and fetishistic objects. The Don Juan conquers women; he behaves in a way that is both demeaning and seductive. He does not accept the woman as a person in her own right, but as a vagina for the night. The more women with whom he has had sex, the better a lover he believes he is. The number and beauty of partners is another measure of masculine success. The association between power and sexuality is quite intimate and many men in power positions, including Jacques Casanova[80] and Benito Mussolini,[81] had enormous sexual appetites.

Furthermore, men do not have the behavioral tools that allow them to become intimate with member of the opposite or same sex. They are unable to develop the closeness that frequently accompanies gratifying relationships. Intimacy requires a willingness to risk vulnerability with and show imperfections to another person. Intimacy is a matter of egalitarian relating, which requires that the man give up power and control of the woman. Intimate relationships also require privacy for personal growth and autonomy from each other,[82] something difficult for men to allow themselves or others, as this too means giving up control. Empathy is an important aspect of intimacy, and, as shown by Hoffman,[83] men are less empathic than women. They are more likely to do active problem solving for another person rather than listen to and existentially be with the other person. Brody[84] has suggested that intimacy requires the ability to fantasize being a member of both sexes; this requires empathy. The fantasy of being a woman may stimulate homophobia and "No Sissy Stuff" fears that are integral components of the masculine role. Because of the lack of intimacy, men frequently find themselves dissatisfied with a few intimate partners and may seek a series of individual sexual relations, which gives them a pseudointimacy, such as that which pervades the singles lifestyle.

These various dimensions of the masculine role are constantly interdigitating with each other. For example, not being intimate with a woman is predicated on being relatively inexpressive and preserving invulnerability. To be expressive would mean that one is not acting like a man; the expressive man may be seen as a man who would be passive and therefore, effeminate, and perhaps homosexual. Being intimate would mean giving up power and being vulnerable. It requires means of relating that lead to cooperation, not competition. The man who changes cannot be assured that other men will share their power or fears with him. Not following the traditional masculine script leads to the risk of being socially ostracized and losing one's chance for success and status. For example, to cry in front of one's boss may be devastating for a man's career. To become a full-time father during the child's preschool years may lead to a loss of career or interpersonal opportunities that may never again arise. Conversely, pursuing a career during that time may lead the man to lose sharing important experiences with his children. Because of the complex interaction of these roles and the depth to which they permeate the performance of institutionalized roles, the cultural prescriptions and proscriptions become very difficult to separate from each other. The role is too much of a spider's web to perform only part of the role; like the action potential of neurophysiology, it is an all-or-nothing phenomenon. Thus, the man must attempt to fulfill the entire role and to fulfill it as an idealized role. This is an impossible task.

THE EFFECTS OF THE MASCULINE ROLE

The average life span of men is eight years less than that of women. In 1977, the life expectancy of white men was slightly less than 73 years. For white women it was just over 81 years. Indeed, throughout the twentieth century, the life expectancy of men has been considerably less than that of women. These differences have consistently ranged between eight and ten years. Some researchers consider the genetic endowment of an animal to be the major determinant of life expectancy.[85] Thus, the data on differential survival have been interpreted as evidence that man are constitutionally inferior to women and that innate biologic or genetic differences between men and women account for these differences in longevity. This might be true for boys in the first years of life, as they are more likely to die from major genetic diseases that are linked to the presence of a Y chromosome or absence of a second X chromosome. Well-known examples of these diseases include Duchenne muscular dystrophy and hemophilia.[86]

The author previously noted some of the flaws in conceptualizing life expectancy in a monolithically genetic way.[87] In addition, an examination of the causes of death of adult men also makes the hypothesis of biologic inferiority somewhat suspect. For example, men are nearly twice as likely to die from a myocardial infarction than are women (Table II).[88–90] It has been estimated that one out of every five men will die of a heart attack before the age of 65. Men die in combat roles, although war may affect all segments of the population. Men frequently kill men, and homicide is a major cause of death of younger men. The suicide rate of men is over two and one half times that of women. Automobile and occupational accidents take their toll, as do environmentally caused malignancies, because men are more frequently exposed to both unsafe conditions and a multitude of toxins in the workplace. Alcoholism, with its consequent cirrhosis of the liver and other disorders, hypertension, and stroke are other diseases that kill men more frequently than women. Indeed, with the exception

Table II. Sex Ratio and Cause of Death[a]

Cause of death	Ratio (M:F)
Myocardial infarction	1.75:1
Cancer of respiratory system	4:1
Stroke	1.2:1
Motor vehicle accidents	2.75:1
Other accidents	2.5:1
Cirrhosis of the liver	2:1
Suicide	2.5:1
Homicide	4:1
Peptic ulcer	2:1

[a]Data from Nathanson (Ref. 88) and Harrison (Ref. 89).

of diseases which cannot occur in the other sex, such as uterine or prostatic malignancies, only diabetes is an equal cause of death of both men and women.

An overview of the diseases noted above reveals that some of the underlying factors in the development of these diseases directly relate, at least in part, to traditional masculine gender-role behavior. Myocardial infarction is a stress-related disease and tends to occur in men who have a Type A personality.[91–92] These are very success-oriented and status-oriented, extremely active and aggressive individuals who are quite tense and inexpressive. They are impatient and have a sense of urgency about time. They are controlling, hostile individuals who are frequently workaholics. They do not know how to relax. They tend to deny most, if not any and all, dependency needs. Men with the Type A personality could be considered caricatures of the traditional masculine role if this personality pattern was not so common and so highly reinforced in American society. The similarities between the masculine role and the Type A personality forge the linkage between society's expectations of men, the masculine role, and death from myocardial infarction.

The stress that men experience frequently manifests itself in self-medication with drugs, particularly nicotine and caffeine. Caffeine intake has been hypothesized to be related to an increased frequency of cardiovascular disease. Nicotine intake, through cigarette smoking, causes lung, lip, and laryngeal cancer, all of which occur four times more frequently in men than in women and is another major factor in the development of cardiovascular disease. Self-medication for men commonly involves the use of alcohol. Alcoholism is a major contributor to automobile-related death as well as to occupational death and injury, laryngeal malignancy, malnutrition, and psychiatric disorders involving homicide and suicide. Illegal drugs are also primarily abused by men as a form of self-medication with subsequent morbidity and mortality. Indeed, Malinow[64] has noted that alexithymia, the inability to both express and label emotions, is a frequent concomitant of drug abuse in younger men. Alexithymia is an extreme of the inexpressiveness that is part of the "No Sissy Stuff" dimension of masculine gender role.

Two other stress-related diseases that increase mortality and affect men more than women are peptic ulcer disease and hypertension with its resultant renal disease and stroke. In addition, Nathanson[88] has shown that men are less likely than women to perform routine preventive health and dental health behaviors such as immunizations, teeth brushing, and getting adequate sleep. This may be a rejection of the dependency of the sick role as well as a risk-taking that defies illness and death. This denial of bodily vulnerability is another way the masculine role leads to patterns of behavior that further undermine the health of men.

Men are frequently killed by the violence of the masculine role. Men serve as combat soldiers. Risk-taking behavior manifests itself in repeated accidents and injuries both in the workplace and in automobiles. Homicide is largely a behavior of men.

Finally, men have a higher suicide rate than women. Suicide is a cause of death that increases with the age of the population.[93] Men are more likely to see themselves as failures and become severely depressed when they are unable to live up to their social role. They are more likely to kill themselves using violent methods such as weaponry, hanging, or jumping off a building than more passive and less successful methods which are more likely to be used by women.

Besides limiting life expectancy, the masculine role has other negative effects. Men frequently displace their frustrations and unhappiness onto their families. When this is done in a physical way, it results in spouse- and child abuse. While this may be a common extreme, the "loving suitor–angry mate" syndrome, in which the caring intimacy of courtship gives way to anger and hostility between spouses after marriage, is not.[94] The author[95] has suggested that this is a direct result of gender-role socialization prior to marriage. It is a frequent cause of divorce, as are sexual dysfunctions which may be the result of "spectatoring," performance fears, and lack of intimacy that occurs in the masculine role.

The social networks of men are marked by a lack of intimacy.[96] The poverty of this network may be a factor in the development and prognosis of major psychopathological syndromes and suicide, as the networks of people with neurotic and psychotic problems are quite impoverished.

The effects of the traditional masculine role on society may also lead to negative consequences. Competition, aggressiveness, risk-taking, and the need for status and success, when played out on an international scale may lead to rivalries which are involved in the development of economic or military war. Politics, based on this striving for power and success, is intimately related to this process. Politics require men to manipulate other men, not for genuine human concerns, but to seek and reach the power for which they strive. Politics has been called a cut-throat business. It is frequently a corrupt occupation, and one's success in one's political career must mean the ruination of another's. Maintaining a position of power requires that the man be autonomous, independent, and active, minimizing his feminine needs. It is also a lonely position, increasing the isolation men experience when stressed, with the negative consequences noted above. A similar situation may occur in the academic or office setting.[97]

Business concerns in a capitalist economic system frequently mirror the competition and aggression of the political world. Companies try to outdo each other and may lie and steal technologic secrets in an attempt to maximize profits at the expense of other people. Emphasizing human concerns may be cynically done to gain tax advantages or to sell more products. For example, one business owner told the author that he advertises his charitable donations at Christmas (part of the price of each toy goes to the local children's hospital) so that he may gain more customers (more profit) and get an end-of-the-year tax break. He also hopes the hospital will name a new wing for him. Businesses waste the environment. They also waste individuals through a lack of occupational safety or the sale of unsafe products in the continual striving for financial power and success. As business is one of the high-status professions in our society, these behaviors are frequently rewarded. John D. Rockefeller, Andrew Carnegie, and even Jay Gould, the archetype of the Robber Barons, are idolized in many high school history texts. Richard Nixon is still revered by many individuals in spite of the Watergate scandal, for he symbolizes making it to the top, inexpressiveness, independent activity, and courage for many men.

In the sexual realm, a major societal problem is rape. Many men have difficulty separating their sexual impulses from thier aggressive ones. When coupled with the need to devalue women and express one's power and aggression, this results in women being taken sexually at will. In a less physical way, one can include psychological rape. The dynamics and results are the same. However, women frequently collude with psychological (as opposed to physical) rape. It is a physically nonviolent behavior that tends to devalue both the men and women participants.

On the positive end, however, the masculine role brings a measure of happiness to many men. Success is rewarding in itself, whether it be becoming Chairman of the Board or adding to a stamp collection. Work may bring satisfaction if the job gives meaning to a man's life goals. Power can mean power to constructively change things for oneself, one's family, or one's community. Heroism has saved many lives and has led men to risk their lives for abstract ideals that still guide societies. Problem-solving skills and rationality are major personality assets, especially when an individual is under stress.

Conclusion

This chapter has attempted to review the dimensions of the masculine gender role in its traditional form. These role behaviors are changing in our society. What the final product will be is something that no one knows. The author hopes it will be androgynous, so that some of the positive aspects of power, success, activity, risk-taking, and problem-solving skills can be coupled with expressiveness, passivity, interdependency, caring, listening, with subsequent positive changes in both the individual and in society.

References

1. Allen CN: Studies on sex differences. Psychol Bull 24:294–304, 1927
2. Allen CN: Recent studies in sex differences. Psychol Bull 27:394–407, 1930
3. Allen CH: Recent research on sex differences. Psychol Bull 32:342–354, 1935

4. Maccoby E, Jacklin C: The Psychology of Sex Differences. Stanford, Stanford University Press, 1974
5. Wilson EO: Sociobiology: The New Synthesis. Cambridge, Harvard University Press, 1975
6. Money J, Ehrhardt A: Man and Woman, Boy and Girl. Baltimore, Johns Hopkins University Press, 1972
7. Money J: Love and Love Sickness: The Science of Sex, Gender Difference, and Pair-bonding. Baltimore, Johns Hopkins University Press, 1980
8. Pleck JH: Men's family work: Three perspectives and some new data. Fam Coordinator 28:481–488, 1979
9. Rabban M: Sex-role identification in young children in two diverse social groups. Genetic Psychol Monographs 42:81–158, 1950
10. David DS, Brannon R: The male sex role: Our culture's blueprint of manhood and what it's done for us lately, in The Forty-Nine Percent Majority: The Male Sex Role. Edited by David DS, Brannon R. Reading, Massachusetts, Addison-Wesley, 1976, pp 1–45
11. Steinmann A, Fox DJ: The Male Dilemma. New York, Jason Aronson, 1974
12. Farrell W: The Liberated Man. New York, Bantam Books, 1975
13. Fasteau MF: The Male Machine. New York, McGraw-Hill, 1974
14. Goldberg H: The Hazards of Being Male. New York, New American Library, 1977
15. Goldberg H: The New Male: From Self-Destruction to Self-Care. New York, Morrow, 1979
16. Stevens B: The sexually oppressed male. Psychother: Theory Res Pract 11:16–21, 1974
17. Wong MR, David J, Conroe RM: Expanding masculinity: Counseling the male in transition. Counseling Psychol 6:58–61, 1976
18. Maffeo PA: Conceptions of sex role development and androgyny: Implications for mental health and for psychotherapy. J Am Med Womens Assoc 33:225–230, 1978
19. Solomon K: Therapeutic approaches to changing masculine role behavior. Am J Psychoanal 41:31–38, 1981
20. Stein TS: The effects of the women's movement on men: A therapist's view. Presented at the 132nd Annual Meeting of the American Psychiatric Association, Chicago, Illinois, May 16, 1979
21. Money J: Nativism versus culturalism in gender-identity differentiation, in Sexuality and Psychoanalysis. Edited by Adelson E. New York, Brunner/Mazel, 1975, pp 48–66
22. Goffman E: Encounters. Indianapolis, Bobbs-Merrill, 1971, p 84
23. Parsons T: The Social System. New York, Free Press, 1951, pp 428–473
24. Wilson RN: The Sociology of Health: An Introduction. New York, Random House, 1970, pp 13–32
25. Rosow I: Status and role change through the life span, in Handbook of Aging and the Social Sciences. Edited by Binstock RH, Shanas E. New York, Van Nostrand Reinhold, 1976, pp 457–482
26. Goffman E: Asylums. New York, Doubleday, 1961
27. Stanton AH, Schwartz MS: The Mental Hospital: A Study of Institutional Participation in Psychiatric Illness and Treatment. New York, Basic Books, 1954
28. Caudill W, Redlich RC, Gilmore HR, et al.: Social structure and interaction processes on a psychiatric ward. Am J Orthopsychiat 22: 314–334, 1952
29. Cohen C, Sokolovsky J: Health-seeking behavior and social networks of the SRO aged. J Am Geriatrics Soc 27:270–278, 1979
30. Cohen CI, Sokolovsky J: Social engagement versus isolation: The case of the aged in SRO hotels. Gerontologist 20:36–44, 1980
31. Solomon K: The depressed patient: Social antecedents of psychopathologic changes in the elderly. J Am Geriatrics Soc 29:14–18, 1981
32. Gould L: X: A fabulous child's story (1972), in the Forty-Nine Percent Majority: The Male Sex Role. Edited by David DS, Brannon R. Reading, Massachusetts, Addison-Wesley, 1976, pp 321–330
33. Thomas A, Chess S: Temperament and Development. New York, Brunner/Mazel, 1977
34. Hartup WW, Zook EA: Sex-role preferences in three- and four-year-old children. J Consult Psychol 24:420–426, 1960

35. Mead M: Sex and Temperament in Three Primitive Societies. New York, Morrow, 1935
36. Woods SM: Some dynamics of male chauvinism. Arch Gen Psychiat 33:63–65, 1976
37. Piaget J: The stages of the intellectual development of the child. Bull Menninger Clin 26:120–128, 1962
38. Erikson EH: Childhood and Society, 2nd edition. New York, Norton, 1963
39. Sullivan HS: Personal Psychopathology. Early Formulations. New York, Norton, 1972, pp 157–181
40. Mullahy P: Psychoanalysis and Interpersonal Psychiatry. The Contributions of Harry Stack Sullivan. New York, Science House, 1970, 119–190
41. Levitin TE, Chananie JD: Responses of female primary school teachers to sex-typed behavior in male and female children. Child Dev 43:1309–1316, 1972
42. Harford TD, Willis CH, Deabler HL: Personality correlates of masculinity–feminity. Psychol Rep 21:881–884, 1967
43. Bem SL, Martyna W, Watson C: Sex-typing and androgyny: Further exploration of the expressive domain. J Personality Soc Psychol 34:1006–1023, 1976
44. Bem SL, Lenny E: Sex-typing and avoidance of cross-sex behavior. J Personality Soc Psychol 33:48–54, 1976
45. Benjamin H: Age and sex differences in the toy-preference of young children. J Genetic Psychol 41:417–429, 1932
46. Vance TF, McCall LT: Children's preferences among play materials as determined by the method of paired comparisons of pictures. Child Dev 5:267–277, 1934
47. Hattwick CA: Sex differences in behavior of nursery school children. Child Dev 8:343–355, 1937
48. Kagan J: The child's sex role classification of school objects. Child Dev 35: 1051–1056, 1964
49. Banham Bridges KM: Occupational interests of three-year-old children. J Genetic Psychol 34:415–423, 1927
50. Banham Bridges KM: The occupational interests and attention of four-year-old children. J Genetic Psychol 36:551–570, 1929
51. Fauls LB, Smith WD: Sex-role learning of five-year-olds. J Genetic Psychol 89:105–117, 1956
52. Hartley RE: Children's concepts of male and female roles. Merrill-Palmer Quart 6:83–91, 1959
53. Barry RB, Barry A: Stereotyping of sex roles in preschool kindergarten children. Psychol Rep 38:948–950, 1976
54. Komarovsky M: Cultural contradictions and sex roles. Am J Sociol 52: 184–189, 1946
55. Rosenkrantz P, Vogel S, Bee H, et al.: Sex-role stereotypes and self-concepts in college students. J Consult Clin Psychol 32:287–295, 1968
56. Litewka J: The socialized penis (1972), in Human Sexualities. Edited by Gagnon JH. New York, Scott, Foresman, 1977, pp 176–177
57. Komarovsky M: Cultural contradictions and sex roles: The masculine case. Am J Sociol 78:873–884, 1973
58. Chass M: A gut issue: Who shapes up best, athletes or dancers? NY Times, Sec 2, pp 1,25, Aug 18, 1974
59. Shatan CF: Bogus manhood, bogus honor: Surrender and transfiguration in the United States Marine Corps, in Psychoanalytic Perspectives on Aggression. Edited by Goldman GD, Milman DS. Dubuque, Kendall/Hunt, 1978, pp 77–100
60. Balswick JO, Avertt CP: Differences in expressiveness: Gender, interpersonal orientation, and perceived parental expressiveness as contributing factors. J Marriage Fam 39:121–127, 1977
61. Ward D, Balswick J: Strong men and virtuous women. A content analysis of sex roles stereotypes. Pacific Sociol Rev 21:45–53, 1978
62. Nemiah JC: Alexithymia. Theoretical considerations. Psychother Psychosom 28:199–206, 1977
63. Flannery JG: Alexithymia. Vol II. The association with unexplained physical distress. Psychother Psychosom 30:193–197, 1978
64. Malinow K: Doc, my meth isn't holding me: An analysis of the narcotic withdrawal syndrome. Presented at a scientific meeting of the Maryland Psychiatric Society, Towson, Maryland, Mar 6, 1980
65. Shapiro D: Neurotic Styles. New York, Basic Books, 1965, pp 108–133

66. Miller A: Death of a Salesman (1949), in Contemporary Drama: Eleven Plays. Edited by Watson EB, Pressey B. New York, Scribner's, 1956, p 286
67. Navarro V: The underdevelopment of health in working America: Causes, consequences and possible solutions. Am J Public Health 66: 538–547, 1976
68. Adler A: Understanding Human Nature (1927). Trans by Wolfe WB. New York, Fawcett, 1965
69. Lein L: Male participation in home life: Impact of social support and breadwinner responsibility on the allocation of tasks. Fam Coordinator 28:489–495, 1979
70. Morse NC, Weiss RS: The function and meaning of work and the job. Am Sociol Rev 20:191–198, 1955
71. Solomon K: Psychosocial crises of older men. Presented at at the 133rd Annual Meeting of the American Psychiatric Association, San Francisco, California, May 7, 1980
72. Lederer W: The decline of manhood: Adaptive trend or temporary confusion? Psychiatr Opinion 16:14–17, 1979
73. Ibsen H: An Enemy of the People (1882), in Plays of Henrik Ibsen. New York, Modern Library, 1950, pp 175–288
74. Heyman SR: Dogmatism, hostility, aggression, and gender role. J Clin Psychol 33:694–698, 1977
75. Hunt M: Sexual Behavior in the 1970's. Chicago, Playboy Press, 1974
76. Bell AP, Weinberg MS: Homosexualities, A Study of Diversity Among Men and Women. New York, Simon and Schuster, 1978
77. Lewis RA: Emotional intimacy among men, J Soc Issues 34:108–121, 1978
78. Lewis R, Casto R, Aquilino W, et al.: Developmental transitions in male sexuality. Counseling Psychol 7:15–19, 1978
79. Masters WH, Johnson VE: Human Sexual Response. Boston, Little Brown, 1966
80. Greenblatt RB: Casanova. Med Aspects Hum Sexuality 8:78, 82–84, 1974
81. Greenblatt RB: Benito Mussolini: Satyr. Med Aspects Hum Sexuality. 6:54, 56, 61, 65, 1972
82. Solomon K, Minor HW: The need for privacy in marriage. Med Aspects Hum Sexuality, 16:104, 106–107, 111, 1982
83. Hoffman ML: Sex difference in empathy and related behaviors. Psychol Bull 84:712–722, 1977
84. Brody EB: Intimacy and the fantasy of becoming both sexes. J Am Acad Psychoanal 6:521–531, 1978
85. Sacher GA: Longevity, aging and death: An evolutionary perspective. Gerontologist 18:112–119, 1978
86. McKusick VA: Simply inherited disorders, in The Principles and Practice of Medicine. Edited by Harvey AM, Cluff LE, Johns RJ, et al. New York, Appleton-Century-Crofts, 1968, pp 447–469
87. Solomon K: Is there a genetic basis to aging? Gerontologist, 19:226–228, 1979
88. Nathanson CA: Sex roles as variables in preventive health behavior. J Community Health 3:142–155, 1977
89. Harrison J: Warning: The male sex role may be dangerous to your health. J Soc Issues 34:65–86, 1978
90. Solomon K: The masculine gender role and its implications for the life expectancy of older men. J Am Geriatrics Soc 29:297–301, 1981
91. Friedman M, Rosenman RH: Type A Behavior and Your Heart. New York, Knopf, 1974
92. Kimball CP: Psychological aspects of cardiovascular disease, in American Handbook of Psychiatry, Vol IV, 2nd edition. Edited by Reiser MF. New York, Basic Books, 1975, pp 609–617
93. Weiss JAM: Suicide, in American Handbook of Psychiatry, Vol III, 2nd edition, Edited by Arieti S, Brody EB. New York, Basic Books, 1974, pp 743–765
94. Elcox KM, Everett HC: Loving suitor—angry mate: "Personality" changes which occur after marriage. Med Aspects Hum Sexuality 13:69,73,83–84, 1979
95. Solomon K: Commentary [to article by Elcox and Everett]. Med Aspects Hum Sexuality 13:87,93, 1979
96. Solomon K: Viewpoint: Do men have better relationships with each other than women do with other women? Med Aspects Hum Sexuality 13:39,43, 1979
97. Solomon K: Sexism and professional chauvinism in psychiatry. Psychiatry 42:374–377, 1979

Chapter 3

Psychoanalytic–Developmental Theory and the Development of Male Gender Identity

A Review

MARTIN R. WONG

INTRODUCTION

The concept of identity has been a central preoccupation of philosophers for centuries—perhaps since humankind developed consciousness of self. At one level, identity has come to be considered by psychologists to be synonymous with the "self" or "self system."[1] At another level, the self is a dynamic process within which each individual lives—partly serendipitous, depending on the vagaries of heredity and fate, and partly purposive as each individual works at developing toward an elusive goal.[2,3] Taken together then, identity consists of two elements, one a continuing integrated core of personhood, and the other a process of adaptation and change.

One need only be a casual observer of human behavior to realize that men and women act differently. Anthropologists have extensively documented that in most cultures there are definite differences in the way men and women behave. It is not unreasonable to hypothesize that there is a subset of percepts, ideas, expectations, and emotions that are a part of the self system because one identifies with one sex or the other.

Researchers in sexual identity development generally refer to this subset as "gender,"[4] or "gender identity."[5] Stoller sees it as psychological or cultural and created postnatally as a result of environmental influences.[4] It refers to the amount of masculinity or feminity in a person, and is complicated by the possibility of degrees of gender. One may see himself not only as a male, but perhaps as a macho male, as a male who sometimes fantasizes being a woman,

---

MARTIN R. WONG • Psychology Service, Veterans Administration Medical Center, Battle Creek, Michigan 49016

or even, as in the case of transsexuals, as a male who is locked in the body of a female and may choose to make the switch to the other sex.

Money and his colleagues[5] define it as "the sameness, unity, and persistence of one's individuality as male, female, or ambivalent, in greater or lesser degree, especially as it is experienced in self awareness and behavior" (p. 4). They further acknowledge the interrelatedness of gender identity to behavior by defining "gender role" as the public expression of gender identity, "everything that a person says and does to indicate to others or to the self the degree that one is either male, female, or ambivalent" (p. 4). Current heightened consciousness of the effects of sexism has occasioned the dominant male gender role to be held up to scrutiny. It is often found to be wanting and, to some writers, even dysfunctional as it relates to mentally healthy functioning.[6–10]

In this chapter, the author will attempt to review the writings of some of the more prominent psychoanalytic scholars, looking for ideas that are specifically relevant to the development and dynamics of male gender identity. The author's cursory review can in no way begin to do justice to all these writings, nor can he expect to review them all. However, an attempt will be made to highlight issues related to the development of male gender identity wherever they are found.

SIGMUND FREUD

In Freud's many writings, psychosexual development is used as a backdrop for the development of personality itself. In Freud's view, biologic factors play a major role in the development of gender identity with each person carrying the imprint of both female and the male within. Thus, the impetus toward sexual identification with one gender or the other springs from a common root which is in its very nature bisexual. He asserts that "without taking bisexuality into account, I think it would scarcely be possible to arrive at an understanding of the sexual manifestations that are actually observed in men and women" (Ref. 11, p.220).

Freud understood that root to be at least an anatomical one. It appears from some of his writings[11,12] that he saw a logical extension from the anatomic to the psychologic, although his attempts to extrapolate were not well developed.

In Freud's model of psychosexual development, instincts act as original drives, activated by a need to reduce tension. Development proceeds through a sequential series of stages, each centered around an erogenous zone (oral, anal, phallic, and genital), which successively assume importance in the individual's development. It is in the relative success of the resolution of conflicts, frustrations, and anxieties centered around tasks related to these erogenous zones that personality, as prepresented by the relative structure and contents of the three parts of the psyche, the id, ego, and superego, is developed.

At birth, only the id exists. It serves as the drive source, the primary energy pool. As the infant matures, the ego and superego develop by trapping and holding libidinal energy from the id for their own use. The predominant mode of energy attainment is through an identification process, a matching of a mental representative with an object or action in the real world. This matching involves an investment of energy—a cathexis. It is this identification process that enables the ego to grow in power so that it can take on its function of acting as rational executive for the personality and its secondary processes of perceiving, discriminating, judging, etc. It is in this same manner that defense mechanisms are also developed to control the undirected power of the id.

The superego also develops through processes of identification as the dependent infant forms object cathexes on his/her primary caretaker(s). He/she identifies with and cathects the ideals and prohibitions of the primary caretakers and develops his/her own superego in the process. Personality ultimately lies in the dynamic interplay of the energies of these three systems, their forces, cathexes, and anticathexes in their transactions with objects in the external world.

In the first few years there are only minor internal differences in the development of the personality of males and females. Between the ages of three and six, however, a very crucial event initiates the split which is seminal in defining the gender path that the developing human will take. The psychosexual energies of the child are said to become highly focused on the parent of the opposite sex. Thus, the male child normally develops a strong sexual cathexis for his mother and feelings of hostility for his imagined rival, his father. The female child normally develops a strong sexual cathexis for the father and a corresponding negative valence toward the mother. These cathexes, in which the child becomes the rival of the parent of the same sex, were named Oedipal and Electral by Freud, after the Greek myths. He recognized that the cathexes were of variable relative intensity and created developmental crises of relative strength. It is in the resolution of these crises that lies much of the directionality and appropriateness of development for the child. Freud realized what has been upheld by biological science, that each person has both masculine and feminine influences. He hypothesized that it was the relative strength of each that determined the outcome of the Oedipus situation—whether the child will identify with the father or the mother:

> the more complete Oedipus complex is twofold, positive and negative, and is due to the bisexuality originally present in children: this is to say, a boy has not merely an ambivalent attitude toward the father and an affectionate object choice toward his mother, but at the same time he also behaves like a girl and displays an affectionate feminine attitude to his father and a corresponding jealousy and hostility toward his mother (Ref. 13, p.33).

So it is on the relative profundity of the positive and negative valences established during the Oedipal period, and in the resolution of the crisis, that much of the direction and strength of gender identification is based.

The male's incestuous cravings for the mother bring him into conflict with the father, a much larger and more powerful object than himself. The resulting fear and anxiety, centered especially around what the father will do to his genital organs, causes him to repress his sexual feelings toward his mother. Since he cannot fight his father, he chooses instead to switch allegiances and begins to identity with his former rival. This intense repression allows the superego of the male to develop to a fully functioning level.

The path and resolution of the Electra complex is different in that, for girls, the primary love object and the ultimate identification figure are the same, the mother. The female child *temporarily* exchanges her original primary love object for the father. This, in part is caused by disappointment in her discovery of her "inferior," nonsalient sex organ. She transfers her love to her father in order to share the valued organ with him. In time, her envy of the penis and her realization that she may never have the male organ for her own weakens this transfer and she turns again toward the mother as a figure with whom to identify.

Of particular importance to the development of gender identity, in this scenario, are the lack of trauma produced by fear and anxiety in the development of the female gender identification, and the relative continuity in the sex of the identification object, the mother. There is no permanent switching of identification objects. Except for the brief period during the Oedipal crisis, the developing female follows a relatively smooth path in gender identification. No strong repression need occur.

The boy, on the other hand, emerges from the Oedipal conflict infused with tenuous feelings of his superiority, a heightened superego, and part of his self, his feminine side, repressed. The implications of these differences in the resolution of the Oedipal conflict are the bases for many of the supposed differences in functioning between the sexes. Freud sees the biological primacy and the superior anatomy of the male as providing him with a more solid foundation on which to build gender identity. The initial heterosexual relationship with the mother and the later trauma of the Oedipal period are seen as buttresses to this healthy beginning.

It is interesting to note that Freud's man becomes a man by rejecting his first lover who happens to be female. His orientation toward other love objects, female and male, depends on the successful resolution of his first love affair. If he cannot master the associated conflicts of the Oedipal crisis, and/or if his mother is too loving and too erotic, the developing boy may become overly concerned about penis loss, and fixate on or identify with his mother. Thus, he may choose to thereafter love as she does, those who have penises. This homosexual orientation is particularly probable if the boy's father is somewhat passive or altogether absent during the childhood period. True to his stance on the underlying bisexuality of humans, homosexuality is thus considered to be a learned preference. It is the early life experiences as they interact with biologic predispositions that determine for Freud the development of maleness, femaleness, or sexual ambivalence.*

Following the relatively stormy trauma of the Oedipal conflict, the child enters into a latency period during which time psychosexual development lies somewhat dormant. The direction of male or female personality has been set and the child moves along a relatively smooth developmental path, incorporating strong identifications, preparing for the heavy demands to come.

*Other interpretations of these events have led other theorists to different conclusions. The author will be reviewing those of Robert Stoller,[4,14] for example, in a later section.

The onset of puberty, with its new rush of hormones, thrusts the child once again into the psychosexual arena. Sexuality emerges from dormancy to again become the principal driving force. It is in this adolescent period that the most exaggeration and intensification of gender behavior occurs as the developing human girds her/his loins for the final surge into full adult genital sexuality.

At this time, there is a further differentiation of the sexes. Boys experience an enormous accession of libido. For girls, this period is, according to Freud, marked by a fresh wave of repression. The clitorally related aspect of her sexuality is affected most by this repression. Since clitoral sexuality is to Freud the masculine aspect, it is the masculine parts of her sexuality that are repressed. Freud asserts that somehow, this "brake upon sexuality brought about by pubertal repression in women, serves as a stimulus to the libido in men and causes an increase of its activity" (Ref. 15, p.87). In puberty, the girl is repressing and denying her sexuality and, in so doing, is putting aside her "childish masculinity" (Ref. 15, p.87). At the same time, the boy is engaged in a heightening and overvaluation of his sexuality, further differentiating the sexes. The corresponding male repression of the female aspects of personality occurred earlier during the Oedipal period.

In Freud's view, the cathexes of the earlier stages of development, oral, anal, and phallic, are fused and synthesized with these new strong genital attachments formed in the pubertal period. The personality consolidates into a firmer mold that will undergo only minor change as the individual moves through life.

Freud saw masculinity and femininity as concepts which needed to be clarified in order to have meaning. He did not rigidly accept the standard associations to masculine activity, largeness, and aggressiveness—because he was aware that there were animal species in which these qualities were assigned to the female (Ref. 15, p.86). He also noted that in human beings, pure masculinity or femininity is not to be found either in a psychological or biological sense. It was his contention that in every individual one could find the display of character traits belonging to his own and to the other sex. Furthermore, he felt that every human being shows a combination of activity and passivity.

In Freud's perspective, however, anatomy was still destiny. The "superior" male anatomy, coupled with the all-important Oedipal events, brings about the development of the masculine identity. The primary mechanisms that further this process are identification with other male objects and repression of the femaleness in himself. In becoming a male, the boy must identify with another male and repress much of what is female in himself.

Many of Freud's constructs have been challenged, especially those regarding the female developmental pattern.[16–18] Often some of his constructs have not been supported by results of scientific experimental investigation. Yet the basic tenets of the theory have proved to be extremely robust. The theory survives and serves as the basis of elaborations by many later theorists. Two in particular, Jung and Sullivan, have modified and extended the theory, paying closer heed to the environment as an interactive factor.

CARL GUSTAV JUNG

Although Freud never accepted it, Jung, first as a follower, then as a colleague, and later as an adversary, began the elaboration and opening-up process on Freud's closed-energy, instinctual drive theory. He posited a larger number of factors to explain human behavior.[19,20] Some are posited to be instinctive, such as hunger, sexuality, activity, reflection, and creativity; others are psychological, such as the conscious–unconscious continuum, the introversion–extroversion continuum, and the dichotomy of spirit and matter. He also added some other modalities such as sex, age, and hereditary disposition to explanatory factors in the theory. Finally, Jung gave the individual human a will to help ameliorate and direct the pressures of the drives. Developmentally, he extended Freud's theory into adulthood, positing a breaking point in the late 30's or early 40's when men's pursuits of youth tend to lose their value and be replaced with more generative interests. This idea is a forerunner to those of Erikson and other investigators of lifespan stages that continue throughout the life cycle.

According to Freud, the unconscious was filled with personal content derived from repression. Jung was convinced that not all of the unconscious could have been derived in this way. He found evidence that at least part seemed to emanate spontaneously from some impersonal source. He, therefore, hypothesized that there was a general division of the unconscious, one part derived from repressed personal experience; the other part he called the collective unconscious. He envisioned the contents of the collective unconscious to be a residue of much that has gone on before in the history of the lineage. It was made up of individual instincts and inherited patterns of behavior he called archetypes.[21,22] These archetypes can be thought of as inherited tendencies, not fixed responses.

Among the most highly evolved of the archetypes are those related to gender: the anima and the animus. As did Freud, Jung believed that humans are basically bisexual with each sex containing both feminine and masculine characteristics. The anima archetype represents the feminine characteristics in the universal unconscious; the animus represents the masculine characteristics. These two archetypes provide the basis for masculine and feminine gender identity. As with the "Yin" and "Yang" (female and male) constructs of earlier Eastern philosophies, characteristic tendencies are attributed to each.

Jung posited that the female archetype was primarily a "connecting" one; it has a tendency toward the development of interpersonal relationships. The male archetype represented a tendency toward abstract, analytic thought.[21] Jung stressed, however, that wholeness comes only through the development of both parts of the psyche. An overriding understanding in this construction is that the two archetypes are complementary to each other; they fit neatly together and are not adversarial.

There is then, according to Jung, a basic difference between the psychology of male and female that lies deep in the inherited genetic structure that is carried in the collective unconscious and is part of the natural order of life. In the male, the animus is dominant. The anima is presumably a psychic representation of the minority of female genes. It is an imprint, an image of the ancestral experiences related to femininity. On the basic foundations laid by the animus and the anima, the boy child builds his conception of what is masculine and what is feminine. In his relations with men and women, he builds on the archetypes. They affect his view of what he comes to experience as male and female as he projects his anima and animus onto his object relations in the interactive process of building gender identity and receives an idea of what to expect from the other sex.

For Jung, it is these archetypeal collections of experience of humankind that provide the basis for the establishment of gender identity. Which is dominant in a given individual, and in the individual's interactions with the world, will determine the unique expression of his/her maleness and femaleness.

Harry Stack Sullivan

Sullivan also made major contributions to the broadening of psychoanalytic thinking. Where Freud saw biology as destiny, Sullivan stressed the role of interpersonal relationships. He saw that personality could not exist except within relationships, and thus elevated interpersonal contact to the level of an innate biological need, alongside the need for air, water, food, and elimination.[1] Personality development was understood by Sullivan to be dependent in large measure on shaping by experience in interpersonal relationships. These experiences play on the unfolding maturational pattern of the growing child.[23] Sullivan's wider vision also included the effects of the culture within which development occurs as it defines and structures interpersonal experiences. He recognized that each culture may tend to encourage the development of some human capacities and discourage others.

From the moment of conception, the first and paramount human interaction is with the mother. It is she who carries the developing fetus, gives birth to it, and usually assumes the role of primary caretaker. It is most likely that the infant's first "personification" will be of the mother—the primary object of his/her beginning experience of object relationships.

Sullivan's explanation of the Oedipal complex was also less genetic and more experiential. As the infant grows, there occurs a development of "empathy" between the parent and child of the same sex. This empathic process somehow works to allow the child to take on the characteristics appropriate to his/her own sex and the attitudes of that sex toward the other sex. It is also the parent of the same sex who passes on the distressing aspects of reality to his/her offspring. Thus, the other parent is more distant and so retains more of the "all satisfying divinity" of infancy.[1] The child comes to identify with the parent of the same sex, and through this empathy process also retains more of the idealization of the parent of the other sex. To the degree that the parent of the same sex is oversensitive to this relative antipathy directed toward him/her, the Oedipus/Electra conflict and its associated fear, anger, and guilt will appear.

Later, in a period Sullivan identified as "preadolescence," the boy's familial interpersonal relations expand to take on "chums." In these close, intimate relationships, boys may experience, for the first time, the feelings of contributing to the growth of self-esteem of another person. They come to realize a greater awareness of being interaction objects in a relationship. Continuing interacting with others builds self and gender identity as the child accumulates a storehouse of information based on this experience. Some of this information remains untested; it is personally, subjectively valid. A second type of information accrues because it is supported through a process of "consensual validation." Sullivan describes this process as one of education through contact with multiple sources of experience with other people and things.[1]

These chum relationships provide a continuing stream of experiential possibilities for consensual validation and the corresponding formation of ideas, values, and attitudes that make up gender identity and the self. Chum relationships later widen into "gang" relationships which provide an even deeper experiential base for consensual validation. Development proceeds on a relatively predictable path and expands into relationships with the other sex. Again, the emphasis is on learning acquired in interpersonal interaction, as each previous relationship lays the groundwork for the ones to follow as the individual moves through life.

MARGARET MAHLER

Sullivan stressed the developmental pattern of growth of self-identity through a series of interpersonal relationships. The first interpersonal relationship children must experience is with the mother. This relationship has been closely studied by the theorist Mahler, and her colleages, who are primary contributors to the understanding of its relationship to continuing self-growth.

Mahler and her colleagues, in two painstaking observational studies of mother–child interaction, describe the developmental processes involved in movement toward what they refer to as the "psychological birth" of the human infant.[24,25] "Psychological birth" is a term used to describe the awakening of a sense of separateness, of individuality—the beginnings of self-identity. Mahler's scheme outlines the development of this sense of self through three main phases and four subphases: (1) Normal Autism; (2) Normal Symbiosis; and (3) Separation–Individuation with its four subphases: (a) Differentiation; (b) Practicing; (c) Rapprochement; and (d) Consolidation of Individuality and Beginnings of Emotional Object Constancy.

Normal Autism begins in the earliest moments of extrauterine life. The "symbiotic" phase begins somewhere between two and four weeks of age, when the neonate "develops a dim awareness that need satisfaction cannot be provided by oneself, but comes from somewhere outside the self" (Ref. 25, p.42). The infant in this stage, however, "behaves and functions as though he and his mother were an omnipotent system—a dual unity within one common boundary" (Ref. 25, p.44).

The phase she calls Separation–Individuation begins around six months of age and continues until around the third year of life. In the first two subphases of Separation–Individuation, the child becomes more and more outwardly directed. When the child attains the ability to walk, he/she becomes able to physically separate from the mother. Walking also brings the dawning awareness that the mother is missing and, with it, the beginning experience of object loss and associated anxiety. It is behavior associated with the desire for autonomy and independence, in conflict with anxiety and fear of object loss, that Mahler chronicles. She describes, for example, characteristic behavior of infants moving away from the mother and then "darting back for emotional refueling," as part of the Separation–Individuation process. Mahler sees the mother's response to this stage of Separation–Individuation as crucial to the child's later emotional well-being. She describes healthy mothers' responses as reinforcing individuation—moving away—and concurrently always being available for the emotional refueling that provides strength for the next movement away.

In the final subphase of Separation—Individuation, "Consolidation of Individuality and Beginnings of Emotional Object Constancy," Mahler sees the achievement of a definite individuality and the attainment of emotional object constancy as the main tasks. The attainment of emotional object constancy, along with the earlier establishment of Piaget's object permanence[26] makes possible the establishment of mental representations of the self. Being able to represent the self and the object makes self-identity formation possible.

According to Mahler, developmental difficulties during the crucial phases of Separation–Individuation can lead to pervasive separation anxiety, loss of love-object anxiety, narcissistic rage, the beginnings of infantile neuroses, and, in severe cases, borderline symptomatology. Thus, the role of the mother in responding to her male or female child takes on immense portent. Upon birth, it is the mother who provides the motivation to reverse what might be an inborn tendency toward a vegetative state, and turn the infant toward increased contact with the environment. During the Symbiotic phase, it is the fairly constant presence of the mother object that provides the holding and nursing—the human contact—that allows the infant to develop. It is the mother's face that is the first meaningful percept and the elicitor of the social smile. It is the person of the mother who is cathected, providing a basis for later differentiation. It is the mother whose interaction with the child in later stages either prompts, aids, or provides emotional support of individuation or hampers the infant's striving. Mahler sees the mother's role as critical in the beginnings of gender identity development. She comments that mothers report the bodies of their girl babies feel different from those of their boys. She also observes that boys on the whole were more "stiffly resistant to hugging and kissing" (Ref. 25, p.104). One can only suspect that these differences result in a different kind of interaction between mother and son, as compared with that between mother and daughter, beginning in the first moments of life.

The boy child's discovery of his penis she reports as taking place earlier than the girl's discovery of her genital organs, and quite a bit earlier than the discovery of the anatomical sexual difference in general. She hypothesizes that this much earlier recognition of the sensory–tactile–emotional components of the genitals may lead to the boy's greater cathexis of the organ. She also reports behavioral evidence of penis envy upon discovery by the girl children of anatomical differences. She summarizes that

> The task of becoming a separate individual seemed, at this point, to be generally more difficult for girls than for boys because the girls, upon discovery of the sexual difference, tended to turn back to mother, to blame her, to demand from her, to be disappointed in her, and still to be ambivalently tied to her. . . . Boys, on the other hand, seemed to find it more expedient than girls to function separately; they were better able to turn to the outside world or to their bodies for pleasure and satisfaction (Ref. 25, p. 106).

Differences between the sexes are noted throughout Mahler's work. In general, she uses the construct "mood" to help summarize a primitive sense of identity. Boys she details as having more active, aggressive strivings, and "gender determined motor mindedness" to help them maintain more belief in self during the Separation–Individuation crises. She describes girls on the whole as more prone to depressed mood on the realization of separateness. Boys, while having a generally less stormy rapprochement period, were more vulnerable than girls to the fear of reengulfment by the "dangerous mother after separation." This she relates to that fear of merging sometimes seen in adult male patients. As for gender identity specifically, she reports the impression that identification with the father, or an older brother, facilitates an early beginning of the boy's identity. Overidealization of the father seems to help protect against fears of reengulfment and merging.

Mahler emphasizes "constitutionally predestined gender-defined differences" (Ref. 25, p. 224) such as the boy's possession of and pride in his penis and girl's narcissism. Her reliance on the mother and the child's interaction with the mother as explanatory mechanisms in personality development leads us to consider them also as powerful forces, likewise in the development of gender identity. If mothers are such an all-important factor, the differences in their responses to their boy children as compared with their girl children must account for some of the differences in gender identity. Other research is supportive of this thesis, especially as it relates to the development of boys.

ERIK ERIKSON

While Mahler attempted to tease out the effects of early interactional patterns in later development, Erikson's contribution was in building a more lifelong model of stages of life. Erikson, following Jung's cue, recognized that development was more open-ended than Freud had outlined, and began the task of defining further crises that would take the organism through adulthood. He stressed the unity of what he referred to for the first time in 1959 as the "human life cycle" and pointed out that while a lasting ego identity cannot begin to exist without the trust developed in the first stage, it cannot be completed without the promise of fulfillment developed in adulthood. "It is the unity of the human life cycle and the specific dynamics of each of its stages, as prescribed by the laws of individual development and of social organization..." (Ref. 27, Preface).

As with Sullivan, who laid out his need-related tensions as polar continua, Erikson defines his eight life psychosocial crises as possible polar outcomes: the best and the worst. Thus, he attempts to define the healthy personality as well as the neurotic personality based on the relative success or failure in the resolution of eight conflicts. Erikson sees these conflicts as logical extensions of the same epigenetic principle which governs the growth of organisms in utero. After birth, the maturing organism continues to unfold,

> by a prescribed sequence of locomotor, sensory, and social capacities. . . the healthy child, given a reasonable amount of guidance, can be trusted to obey the inner laws of development, laws which create a succession of potentialities for significant interaction with those who tend to him. . . . Personality can be said to develop according to steps predetermined in the human organism's readiness to be driven toward, to be aware of, and to interact with a mother and ending with mankind. . . (Ref. 27, pp. 53–54).

These eight life psychosocial crises are not meant as replacements for Freud's psychosexual stages, but rather as a social overlay and extension defining a series of critical periods of development, the resolution of which results in ego qualities—relative strengths and weaknesses—that persist throughout life. The resolution of each of its resulting ego qualities affect the adaptation to and resolution of each later crises.

The eight ages are (1) Basic Trust vs. Basic Mistrust; (2) Autonomy vs. Shame and Doubt; (3) Initiative vs. Guilt; (4) Industry vs. Inferiority; (5) Identity vs. Role Confusion; (6) Intimacy vs. Isolation; (7) Generativity vs. Stagnation; and (8) Ego Integrity vs. Despair.[28]

The first three roughly correspond in developmental time with Freud's three pregenital stages. Thus, while Freud's child is deriving infantile sexual pleasures from sucking, biting, and incorporating, Erikson's perspective on the same child is that it is learning a relative mix of basic trust and mistrust. The degree to which the child incorporates these will set the tone for much of later development. The child at Freud's anal stage is undergoing first experiences with attempted external regulation of an instinctual impulse, learning to postpone pleasure, and to hold on or let go; psychosocially, the child is learning the ego qualities of autonomy and/or relative shame and doubt.

Erikson's third crisis overlaps with Freud's phallic stage and the encompassed Oedipal crisis. Freud focuses on the burgeoning sense of initiative. Infantile sexual feelings, curiosity, and the child's growing sense of autonomy and power lead to the jealousy, rivalry, and conflict of the Oedipal period. Erikson sees gender differences as underlying development. For example, Erikson's boy senses his "intrusive" power. Erikson's girl senses her "inclusive" power. It is in the resolution of the acting out of their rivalry and fantasy that relative initiative—assertiveness—and guilt are potentially established as basic patterns. The struggle on the part of the boy may take on greater proportions since it seems necessary for him to reject entirely the introjected mother-object who has first been part of himself, then a primary identification figure, then a fantasized lover, then a relatively less powerful member of the other sex. For the boy, the fear of the power of the father and other male figures leads him to reject and repress both his fantasy love wishes and his own female strivings and identifications. As with Freud, it is to the degree that these fantasies and strivings are squelched that guilt, and with it the superego—the cornerstone of morality—is developed.

During the latency period, before the reblooming of sexuality, Erikson stresses the learning of Industry and/or Inferiority. In the modern world this is the period of school entry and represents the beginning of time devoted to learning cognitive skills, acquiring knowledge, and accomplishing tasks under the direction of and for the reward or punishment of others. For boys, it is usually a continuation of the time when the major directors, rewarders, and punishers are female. It is not an unreasonable hypothesis to make that at this level knowledge may to some degree come to be associated with femaleness, and activity with maleness. It certainly seems to be true that for a few years after this period, the identity of many male children is directed more at instrumental actions as in sports, than toward knowledge. Erikson's opposition possibility to industry is the development of a sense of inadequacy and inferiority—a sense of not being able to do what is required as well as others. Certainly, male children's average developmental lag time of 27 months behind their female counterparts may be a contributing factor to the development of such feelings.

With the onset of adolescence, Erikson sees the formation of a coherent ego identity as

> more than the sum of the childhood identifications. It is the accrued experience of the ego's ability to integrate all identifications with the vicissitudes of the libido, with the aptitudes developed out of endowment, and with the opportunities offered in social roles. The sense of identity then, is the accrued confidence that the inner sameness and continuity prepared in the past are matched by the sameness and continuity of one's meaning for others... (Ref. 27, p. 261).

Again, it is not that at this stage identity becomes cast in rock, never to change, but that the mold that has been forming throughout the development of the human responds to the last internal physiological revolution and the new external pressures. By working toward some momentary resolution, it may set the tone for the rest of life.

It is at this stage that the question of career suddenly becomes very important, especially for the male (although much less especially today in this era of liberation and raised expectations for females). The identity of many adult males seems to lie more in what they do, what they are doing, and what they are going to do next rather than in *who* they are. This perhaps may be a result of society's stress for the male on initiative and industry being integrated for males with instrumentality, as identity.

Erikson's next two stages speak to adult crises: the need to establish a capability for real intimacy with another person(s), and the need to accept the task of reproducing and guiding the fruits of reproduction in responsible generativity. The alternative he sees as malfunctioning, a partial closing down of the system which was epigenetically programmed to carry out this trust, and in so doing to grow. When true intimacy and its concomitant openness to others is blocked, the alternative is closing down, self-absorption, a looking inward rather than an opening up. When true responsible generativity is denied or rejected, the alternative is stagnation, a further closing down, and an unnoticed preparation for death.

The traditional American male role stereotype involving a stress on physical achievement, suppression of affect, lack of development of interpersonal and emotional skills, prohibition of feelings of tenderness and vulnerability, and a limitation on intimacy as a potential source of vulnerability,[29–31] seems to work against the successful positive resolution of these two of Erikson's adult psychosocial crises.

The result of the successful resolution of earlier crises, what Erikson calls "the fruit of the (first) seven stages" (Ref. 27, p. 104), is a gradual growth toward integrity—an acceptance of self, responsibility, and life. The alternative is despair, and "a thousand little disgusts" which hide despair (Ref. 28, p. 269).

DANIEL LEVINSON AND GEORGE VAILLANT

Erikson's schema built on Jung's earlier extension of life stages into adulthood. His was the first exploration into life-span development and led the way for two major works on the adult life cycle. Erikson did not speak specifically to the development of gender identity, but stressed that identity was a process that continued throughout life. This realization has led other present-day researchers to elaborate further the stages on this path through life. The two documents that stand out as the most elegant and well documented are by Levinson et al.[32] and Vaillant.[33] Both of them are based on extensive data collected from the lives of men, and both synthesize their data into sequences of life experience, with related generalizations. They are of particular relevance to this review in that they study normal, not mentally troubled, men during an adult period of their lives.

Vaillant presents data from an extensive in-depth study of 95 men who were closely monitored by self-report and face-to-face intervews over a 35-year period beginning around 1940. The men were selected while in college because they were men who seemed to have done well up until that point and were expected to do well by people who were their superiors. In comparison to Vaillant, Levinson et al. intensively studied 40 men selected from four diverse occupational groupings: hourly workers in industry, business executives, university biologists, and novelists. The men ranged in age from 35 to 45. Levinson et al. interviewed each man for ten to twenty hours over a span of two to three months. Based on these intensive interviews, detailed biographical sketches were built retrospectively for each man portraying his individual life as it evolved over the years. From these 40 biographies, Levinson et al. derived generalizations about the life cycle of men in general.

While their data were collected in quite diverse ways, both Levinson et al. and Vaillant find that they uphold the general precepts of earlier developmental psychologists. Levinson et al. comment on similarities in their findings to the earlier ideas of Erikson and Jung. Vaillant reports that his systematically collected data also correspond in both ego and psychosocial development to many of the ideas put forth earlier by Freud, Jung, Erikson, and Piaget. He sees his data as supporting the concept of development as a step-by-step negotiation of stages in the life cycle. Vaillant views this development of his men from an ego perspective and sees it as particularly dependent upon development from within, a result of the "unfolding patterns of mastering and making sense of our own inner experience" (Ref. 33, p. 335). Becoming a more mature man is the result of learning more mature ways to adapt to life. How these mechanisms evolve and mature seem to him to be in large part a result of biological factors divorced from social history and good fortune, but also amenable to apprenticeship and absorption in relationships with others. In Freudian terms, the mechanism of introjection becomes the mechanism of identification as the ego matures. For Vaillant, absorption, internalization, and identification are the means to growth. The rediscovery of internalized parents during midlife became a source of strength and an impetus to growth.

Both research reports uphold Jung's and Erikson's basic idea that psychological development is a lifelong process. There is clear evidence in both studies that the development of purpose, meaning, and of identity in general did not stop with arrival at majority age, but continued at least through the age of fifty, the age at which the men being studied had arrived at the time of reporting.

Levinson et al. see life development as a "cycle," a process or journey from a starting point to a termination point that has within it various "seasons." The process of development is not continuous:

> There are qualitatively different seasons, each having its own distinctive character. . . The life course . . . evolves through a series of definable forms, . . . relatively stable segment(s) of the total cycle. (Ref. 32, p. 6–7)

They see these "seasons of men's lives" as developmental periods in the evolution of "life structure." They further maintain that the periods they describe are relatively universal, in that "everyone lives through the same developmental periods in adulthood, just as in childhood" (Ref. 32, p. 41). They deny that evidence exists that they stem simply from an unfolding of a biological, genetic program, but rather they see the periods as "grounded in the nature of man as a biological, psychological, and social organism, and in the nature of society as a complex enterprise extending over many generations" (Ref. 32, p. 322). They comment that the major influences that come into play are the individual's (1) sociocultural world as it impinges on him, e.g., the society in which he lives, his class, religion, ethnicity, family political system, occupational structure; (2) self as it includes a complex patterning of wishes, conflicts, anxieties, fantasies, moral values and ideals, talents, skills, character traits, modes of feeling, thought, and action; and (3) the man's participation in the world, his transactions between himself and the world.

While for Levinson et al., masculine and feminine are conceptualized as polarities, opposing tendencies, they somehow are also complementary, and it is the integration of the feminine and the masculine within each man that is one of four principal tasks of life. This polarity continues to exist throughout life, never to be fully resolved, but always a partially successful, strived-for integration. For Levinson et al., each human being starts life with a biological potential to be male or female and not both. This meaning of gender, however, goes beyond the purely biological and encompasses the social and psychological. In becoming a man, the boy selectively draws on and "adopts the gender images of his culture" (Ref. 32, p. 229). Through his relationship with mother, father, siblings, and others, he develops an internal cast of characters who represent the forms of masculinity of significance to him.

Vaillant's painstaking analyses of his 95 men over 35 years builds a case for five motifs: (1) that while early childhood events have a role to play, they are clearly not as powerful as Freud had supposed; (2) lives changes, and the course of life is filled with discontinuities; (3) what he calls "adaptive mechanisms" are the key to making sense of mental illness and mental health. (Many of these adaptive mechanisms are the same as those referred to by Anna Freud[34] and her followers as "defense mechanisms.") Vaillant feels that these can be arranged on a continuum that correlates with health and maturity. As the lives of men evolve, if they mature psychologically, the defensive styles also evolve predictably into more healthy mechanisms; (4) human development is a lifelong process in which truth remains relative and can only be discovered longitudinally; and (5) positive mental health exists and can be operationally discussed in terms that are, at least in part, free from moral and cultural biases (Ref. 33, p. 29).

Although these two studies collected and analyzed their data in different ways, taken as a whole they do not contradict each other. From their data, one can draw certain generalizations. Development of identity as it is represented in life structure is a lifelong process. While the child may be in part the father of the man, life is dicontinuous and only to a degree predictable. There is strong evidence for adult developmental periods such as those talked about first by Jung, and then by Sullivan and Erikson. There is evidence of a tendency, a drive toward integration and more positive mental health. The mechanisms for maturation in adulthood may lie in identification and introjection just as they did in childhood.

JOHN MONEY AND ROBERT STOLLER

These two scholars, introduced in the beginning of the chapter, have independently spoken to the question of the major factors which play a part in the determination of male gender identity development. Money is a researcher in the area of sexual development; Stoller approaches the research question from the position of a psychoanalytically trained practitioner and clinical researcher.

Both men agree on the basic determinants of gender identity, but, predictably, differ a little in their relative stress of the factors. Both agree that gender identity is the outcome of the interaction of three factors: (1) the effects of biologic forces; (2) the effects of anatomy, especially the genitalia; and (3) the effects of sociocultural influence.

Money[5] stresses the importance of the biologic influence, lying primarily in the relative amounts of, and timing of, androgens and estrogens distributed and incorporated in the developing human. He points out that the zygote will develop into a female structure unless interrupted during the sixth week of gestation by testicular hormones. According to Money, the presence or absence of testicular secretions

> accounts not only for the shape of the external genitals, but also for certain patterns of organization in the brain, especially, by inference, in the hypothalmic pathways that will subsequently influence certain aspects of sexual behavior (Ref. 5, p. 2).

Money's contentions about in-utero hormonally induced brain differences have been readily demonstrated in animals. Other experimentation seems to infer that there is a critical period during embryonic development during which the introduction of testicular hormones creates a change in the physical brain itself which differentiates males and females. Given the workings of these prenatal hormones, Money infers that the central nervous system passes on a program of behavioral traits which are traditionally and culturally classified as predominantly boyish and girlish.

While he stresses the workings of these hormonal factors, he recognizes that they take on their power as their outcomes, primarily those in anatomy, interact with the sociocultural influences brought to bear after the child is born. Money cites numerous situations where children born chromosomally of one sex have been successfully changed to the other sex. He contends that it is possible to assign the sex of a given child, regardless of chromosomal sex, given on-going treatment with externally administered hormones in conjunction with societal response which is appropriate to the sexual assignment. He feels that this sexual assignment or reassignment will have a good chance of success if done before the age of two and a much poorer prognosis if attempted after that age.

Stoller merges evidence gleaned from experimental with that obtained through clinical research. With a primary focus on attempting to understand transsexualism he uses this "natural experiment . . . as a fixed point for measuring variables contributing to gender development" (Ref. 4, p. 281). Perhaps because of his psychoanalytic background, he lays special stress on environmental events, especially those occuring just after birth. He feels that the newborn presents a "most malleable" central nervous system on which the environment can write. He goes on to explain his contention that, although humans may be "organized prenatally in a masculine or feminine direction," the effects of those biological systems are almost always too weak in humans to withstand the more powerful forces of the environment (Ref. 4, p. 281). Nevertheless, he reports a number of cases that apparently support the conclusions that occasionally biological forces break through the more powerful forces of environment and produce males who feel themselves to be females in the wrong bodies, and vice versa. These biological forces may be, for example, the presence or absence of hormonally induced central nervous system changes.

For Stoller, the first and most profound of the environmental forces is the mother. In Stoller's model, the appearance of an infant's genitals at birth starts the process that will, more than any other factor, lead to the determination of gender identity for that child. Thereafter,

> the child is named, clothed, held, and dealt with in innumerable exchanges, subtle and gross, all of which express, via mother's body impinging on her infant's perceptions, her attitudes and wishes in regard to *this* male, or *this* female (Ref. 4, p. 291).

As if to sum up his position, Stoller states that "anatomy is not really destiny; destiny comes from what people make of anatomy" (Ref. 4, p. 293). The little boy begins with an anatomical heterosexual relationship with his mother, but true psychological heterosexuality comes only after much developmental interactional struggle with her. Stroller refers to Mahler's description of the separation–individuation process as one which prepares the boy for true psychological heterosexuality which leads to the Oedipus conflict.

The account Stoller outlines disagrees with Freud's version in at least three primary ways: first, Freud's contention that maleness is the biologically natural state; second, that the male has a healthier start because of his heterosexual relationship with the mother; and third, that the presence of a penis is of primary importance to the development of male gender identity.

The biologic evidence reported by both Money and Stoller seems to indicate that, in fact, the resting baseline of the human sexual tissues is female until the male hormone is applied to these tissues. Stoller sees the male as having a more difficult path to follow than the female. He contends that the baby girl's homosexual relationship with the mother can only serve to augment a girl's identity: "If a mother can lay down *that* foundation in her daughter, then a strength—a permanence, a part of identity—is well situated. . ." (Ref. 4, p. 292). He thus argues that "femininity has a more stable basis in primary identification with the mother than does masculinity—penis envy notwithstanding. . ." (Ref. 4, p. 292), and uses the higher prevalence of non-normal sexual developments in the male as evidence of this more difficult path.

The role that the presence or absence of a penis plays seems also to be somewhat lessened by Stoller's clinical evidence suggesting that chromosomally male children who have been born without penises sometimes grow with an undeniable sense of maleness despite the defect. Stoller cites cases where this occurs in the face of mistaken efforts on the part of parents to feminize the children. More recent studies[35] indicate further evidence that even boys mistakenly raised as girls until the onrush of pubertal hormones can quickly make the adjustment to become heterosexual males.

RECAPITULATION

In the foregoing, a number of issues have been raised about the major contributing components of gender identity formation. Freud stressed underlying bisexuality, the role of the anatomy (more specifically the primacy and superiority of the male anatomy, and the special role of the penis), the mechanism of identification, the enduring importance of early life experiences, the resolution of the conflict of the Oedipal triangle, and the concept of stages of development. Other additions to Freud's original structure include Jung's consideration of the more mysterious collective unconscious with its anima and animus, and Sullivan's stress on the interpersonal and the mechanism of consenusal validation. Erikson extended Freud's idea of stages in life development throughout the human lifespan and proposed that the search for identity and meaning was a lifelong process. Levinson et al. and Vaillant attempted to refine the scheme based on more systematically accumulated data. Finally, two different modes of research by Money and Stoller brought the two to similar conclusions regarding the basic interacting forces that work to form gender identity.

White it would require a work of greater scope to analyze each of the foregoing concepts in great detail, the author will try to highlight how most stand up in relationship to present developments.

Freud's assertion that there is an underlying bedrock of bisexuality—that the human zygote can go either way depending on the forces that impinge—seems to be holding up well. According to experiments cited by both Money and Stoller, the developing fetus will take on a female form, despite the original chromosomal sexual assignment, unless there is a well-timed intrusion of the male hormone. These experiments seem to lay to rest Freud's assumption of the primacy of the male anatomy. It appears that, rather than the female anatomy being that of a defective male, the anatomy of the male is a modification built on to the basic form.

How important is the presence or absence of a penis to the developing infant? Freud felt that it played a primary part in the development of gender identity. While Stoller cites cases in which children developed a masculine gender identity, even in the absence of a penis, these cases may be exceptions. It is likely, however, that the penis is a signal for the parents and society in general to set in motion a sometimes subtle but definite pattern of behavior—feedback—to the child who wears a penis that is different from that which the female child receives. From birth on, the developing boy will be interacted with differentially and confronted with specific behaviors, expectancies, and reactions that are different from those communicated to the girl.

During the Oedipal period, the penis takes on a new dimension of meaning in psychoanalytic theory as conceptualized by Freud. The fear of what might happen to his penis leads the boy to repress his desires for his mother and his hostility toward his father, and gets him on track toward manhood. While there is some evidence to support the notions of castration anxiety in the research literature, American parents in the 1980s are not the same as the Austrian parents Freud was accustomed to when he was forming these views. It is less probable today that the kinds of feedback that would lead a child to formulate this fantasy would occur with today's enlightened parents. In addition, the occurrence of mother-led, single-parent homes in the 1980s is substantial. Development in this different milieu would seem to require at least a significant modification of the classic Oedipal triangle. If castration anxiety and resultant repression remain building blocks of the theory of gender-identity development, they seem to be no longer part of the weight-bearing walls.

Identification, however, as modified by Sullivan, still carries a lot of weight in the formation of gender identity. Sullivan's concept of consensual validation as an ongoing process of identification with chums and later with same-sex colleagues seems to have few if any detractors among researchers. The process has been extended well into adult life; Levinson et al. speak of the need for "mentors" to aid in adult development, and Erikson refers to the attainment of generativity in adult men as a *sine qua non* for growth. Vaillant sees identification as one of the keys to growth and speaks of the rediscovery of the internalized parents during midlife as a source of strength.

Stress on early life experiences continues as a bulwark of developmental theory. Mahler exposed interaction in the mother–child dyad to close scrutiny and discovered very predictable sequenced patterns of behavior. She also hypothesized that certain abrogations of these patterns on the part of the caretaker would lead to severe deficits in personality formation. She points out a number of the short-term effects of these. It remains for longitudinal studies to uphold or discard the case for long-term effects. Other experimentation related to the hypothesis of a critical period for bonding between mother and child (or father and child) may also be a line of investigation that will provide further evidence of long-term effects of very early life experiences. On the other hand, looking retrospectively, Vaillant found little evidence to suggest that early life experiences were powerful influences on his subjects who were watched carefully for 35 years.

Present developments in the field of contemporary particle physics have reawakened interest in the idea of Jung and the Eastern mystics on whose ideas he developed many of his own.[36,37] Zukav[37] reveals that some see the study of physics as synonomous with the study of consciousness itself; that science has come full circle back from the objective study of objects to the study of ourselves in the process of actualization. These comments about contemporary physics are made by way of introduction to thoughts that it is increasingly difficult to dismiss Jung's anima and animus as non-empirically-verifiable and, therefore, of little validity. The collective unconscious, the anima, the animus and the other archteypes that Jung speaks of are as viable propositions today as they ever were.

The hormonal influence to which Money and Stoller point are obviously of enormous importance. Without the properly timed infusion of the male hormone early in the gestation period, there is no male anatomy as we know it. Without a second infusion later, there is no masculinization of the brain and thus no peculiarly male ways of thinking. The third burst of hormones during puberty further refines the male frame. But gender identity is not, as Stoller points out, only the biological reality. It is wrought in the exquisite and sometimes fragile interplay of all of the factors the author has discussed. It is ultimately a dynamic psychological process.

Perhaps the most important and relevant finding is a thread that runs through all these writings that has not been emphasized or explored enough. Freud first advanced it in his furtherance of the concept of delineated states of psychosexual growth. The concept was further refined and elaborated: Jung extended it beyond adolescence to midlife; Erikson built it into a lifespan conceptual scheme. Levinson et al. and Vaillant found evidence that strongly upholds the concept; Vaillant speaks of unfolding patterns as if they unfolded from some internal biological plan; Levinson et al. speak of qualitatively different seasons of life, each with its own character, that each developing person lives through. He sees these as probably universal, transcending race and cultural lines.

The building of an identity, and by inference a gender identity, seen in this light, is a continuing process. It cannot be conceptualized as a static entity that is built and then maintained. It is rather a process that is fluid and flows with the time, context, and individual predisposition within which one finds it; it is relevant only when viewed in that frame. Clearly, in our society, for example, each season of a man's life brings with it different expectations for behavior. The adolescent is expected to sow wild oats, to strike out, and experience. The assertion of adolescent sexuality is functionally relevant. On the other hand, this same assertion would be seen by society as out of step at later seasons. The sexually overassertive middle-ager may be labeled obnoxious or "adolescent" and, even, "a dirty old man." Gender identity and relevant gender-role behavior is best conceptualized as an ongoing process. Vaillant and Milofsky[38] find ample evidence to suggest that the concept holds up well even when applied across socioeconomic levels.

Gender identity, seen in the light of all of the foregoing, can in some respects be likened to Luria's concept of a functional system.[39] It is in part an ideational system susceptible to maturational effects. In other respects it is more easily likened to Arieti and Bemporad's "cognitive construct."[40] It is thus capable of alteration throughout life, and at the same time it is a promoter of life events.

The author has attempted to highlight some of the ideas relevant to the development of male gender identity. The evolving process is intricate, and undoubtedly can take on a myriad of forms. In some ways, it would only be limiting to attempt to define the outcome of so fluid a process. The ultimate definition might most advantageously be seen as dependent on individual interpretation and individual value.

ACKNOWLEDGMENT

The author very gratefully acknowledges the contributions and extensive thoughtful provocation of Terry Stein, M.D. in the preparation of this manuscript, as well as the support of the Psychiatry Department of Michigan State University.

REFERENCES

1. Sullivan HS: The Interpersonal Theory of Psychiatry. New York, W. W. Norton and Company, 1953
2. Allport GW: Becoming: Basic Considerations for a Psychology of Personality. New Haven, Yale University Press, 1955

3. Maslow AH: Toward a Psychology of Being. Princeton, New Jersey, Van Nostrand, 1968
4. Stoller RJ: Sex and Gender. Vol II. The Transsexual Experiment. New York, Jason Aronson, 1975
5. Money J, Ehrhardt A: Man and Woman, Boy and Girl. Baltimore, Johns Hopkins, 1972
6. Forisha BL: Sex Roles and Personal Awareness. Morristown, New Jersey, General Learning Press, 1978
7. Guttentag M, Bray H: Undoing Sex Stereotypes. New York, McGraw Hill, 1976
8. Harrison J: Warning: The male sex role may be dangerous to your health. J Soc Issues 34:65–86, 1978
9. Jourard S: Some Lethal Aspects of the Male Role, in The Transparent Self. Edited by Jourard S. New York, Van Nostrand, 1964
10. Balswick JO, Peek CW: The inexpressive male: A tragedy of American society. The Family Coordinator 20:363–368, 1971
11. Freud S: Three essays on sexuality, in the Standard Edition of the Complete Psychological Works of Sigmund Freud. Vol 7. London, Hogarth Press, 1953, pp 130–243
12. Freud S: Some psychical consequences of the anatomical distinction between the sexes, in the Standard Edition of the Complete Psychological Works of Sigmund Freud. Vol 19. London, Hogarth Press, 1961, pp 248–258.
13. Freud S: The Ego and the Id. London, Hogarth Press, 1927
14. Stoller RJ: Sex and Gender. Vol I. The Development of Masculinity and Femininity. New York, Jason Aronson, 1968
15. Freud S: Three Essays on the Theory of Sexuality. (trans. by J. Strachey), New York, Basic Books, 1967
16. Horney K: New Ways in Psychoanalysis. New York, Norton, 1939
17. Fast I: Developments in gender identity: The original matrix. Int Rev Psychoanal 5:265–273, 1978
18. Chodorow N: The Reproduction of Mothering: Psychoanalysis and the Sociology of Gender. Berkeley, University of California Press, 1978
19. Jung CG: The development of personality, in Collected Works, Vol 17. Princeton, New Jersey, Princeton University Press, 1954
20. Jung CG: The structure and dynamics of the psyche. In Collected Works, Vol 8. Princeton, New Jersey, Princeton University Press, 1960
21. Jung CG: Concerning the archetypes, with special reference to the anima concept. In Collected Works, Vol 9, Part 1. Princeton, Princeton University Press, 1950
22. Jung CG: The psychology of the unconscious. In Collected Works, Vol 7. Princeton, Princeton University Press, 1953
23. Sullivan HS: Personal Psychopathology. Washington D.C., William Alanson White Psychiatric Foundation, 1965 (unpublished), cited in Mullahy P: Psychoanalysis and Interpersonal Psychiatry. New York, Science House, 1970
24. Mahler M: On Human Symbiosis and the Vicissitudes of Individuation, Vol 1, Infantile Psychosis. New York, International Universities Press, 1968
25. Mahler M: The Psychological Birth of the Human Infant. New York, Basic Books, 1968
26. Piaget J: The Origins of Intelligence in Children. New York, W. W. Norton and Company, 1936
27. Erikson E: Identity and the Life Cycle. New York, W. W. Norton and Company, 1980
28. Erikson E: Childhood and Society. New York, W. W. Norton and Company, 1950
29. Sawyer J: On male liberation. Liberation 15:32–33, 1970
30. Pleck J: The male sex role: Definition, problems, and sources of change. J Soc Issues 32:155–164, 1976
31. Farrell W: The Liberated Man. New York, Random House, 1974
32. Levinson DJ, Darrow CN, Klein EB, et al.: The Seasons of a Man's Life. New York, Knopf, 1978
33. Vaillant GE: Adaptation to life. Boston, Little, Brown, 1977
34. Freud A: Ego and the Mechanisms of Defense. London, Hogarth Press, 1937
35. Imperato-McGinley J, Guerrero L, Gautier T, and Peterson RE: Steroid 5 deficiency in man: An inherited form of male pseudohermaphroditism. Science 186:1213–1215, 1974
36. Capra F: The Tao of Physics. New York, Bantam Books, 1977
37. Zukav G: The Dancing Wu Li Masters. New York, William Morrow and Company, 1979

38. Vaillant GE, Milofsky E: Natural history of male psychological health: IX, Empirical evidence for Erickson's model of the life cycle. Am J Psychiatry 137:11, 1980
39. Luria AR: Higher Cortical Functions in Man. New York, Basic Books, 1966
40. Arieti S, Bemporad J: Severe and Mild Depression. New York, Basic Books, 1978

Chapter 4

Androgyny

Jacqueline Boles and Charlotte Tatro

Introduction

What distinguishes man from woman? Are the differences blurring? What are the characteristics of a healthy PERSON? The answers to these and similar questions concern us all, and we can no longer assume the answers. Our assumptions about the psychosocial nature of man and woman are undergoing transformation and few definitions are advanced for androgyny, the new dualism, or sex role transcendance. Currently, the term "androgyny," i.e., an equal number of male and female characteristics in the personality, is in vogue. There are several scales which measure it, and numerous studies which examine it. Androgyny has been positively related to other attributes, e.g., creativity and self-esteem. Many people seek to become androgynous; in fact, androgyny may become the est of the 1980s. Yet, the idea of androgyny is more than a fad. The scales which measure it are based on a view of the relationship between masculinity and femininity quite different from the perspective that was employed in creating the familiar scales which measure masculinity and femininity in the past, e.g., the Adjective Check List.

Further, androgyny, as an "idea in the mind" has freed many people to accept behaviors and feelings in themselves which they would have previously denied. Thus, a man can acknowledge both his masculine and feminine qualities, as can a woman. The "total woman" viewed from this perspective is radically different from her sister as portrayed by Marabel Morgan[1] in her classic fantasy.

This chapter surveys some research related to the development of gender identity and androgyny. New theories on gender-identity formation clarify the relationship between personality and temperamental traits which are biologically predisposed and those which are culturally transmitted and idiosyncratically learned. Specifically, in this chapter the authors (1) review theories of gender-identity and sex-role acquisition, (2) describe and evaluate the major

Jacqueline Boles • Department of Sociology, Georgia State University, Atlanta, Georgia 30303
Charlotte Tatro • Institute for Women, Miami, Florida

scales which measure androgyny, and (3) survey the studies which link androgyny to a variety of social, temperamental, and cognitive attributes.

ANDROGYNY: AN OLD IDEA IN A NEW DRESS

Male and masculinity; female and femininity; no cultures fail to distinguish between the two. Temperament, duties and responsibilities, jobs, personality characteristics, as well as a variety of behavioral attributes all distinguish men from women and maleness from femaleness. However, maleness has not always been conceived of as in opposition to femaleness; rather, some world views consider these two as just aspects of a greater whole. For example, in Chinese thought the male (Yang) and the female (Yin) principles are but two parts of a larger, integrated whole.[2]

Many creation stories recount the division of a whole being into halves (e.g., Hebrew, Greek, Hindu myths). The two sexes, thus created, attempt to reunite; sexual intercourse is often used as a metaphor for the psychic reunion of these two separated halves so that, ideally, the two become "one flesh."

Freud and Jung also recognized the duality of human beings. Freud[3] stated that human beings were constitutionally bisexual; each sex retains certain basic anatomical features of the other. He also argued that bisexual tendencies are present in each person on the psychological level as well.

Jung used many of the insights found in religious cosmologies in his theory of the personality. He saw the anima and animus, the female and male principle, respectively, as universal archetypes that contain large elements of emotion and are stored in the collective unconscious. The anima relates to interpersonal connections, whereas the animus, the paternal Logos, focuses on mind and cognition.[4] Because each of us incorporates the opposite sex archetype, we (1) can manifest characteristics of the opposite sex and (2) can understand and empathize with members of the opposite sex. Thus, because of the presence of the anima in men and the animus in women, we can, indeed, understand each other's needs, passions, and desires. Jung viewed the healthy personality as the integration of the male and female characteristics into one individual personality and argued that humans try to achieve wholeness which presupposes this integration.

Jung recognized that societies attempt, and frequently succeed, in repressing the anima and animus in their citizens, and he warned that the attainment of selfhood (Buddha and Jesus representing two archetypal examples) is not possible until both male and female attributes are fully integrated into the total personality.

Jung's theories and core concepts have been severely neglected by most contemporary behaviorists as they are difficult to operationalize. Most scales which attempt to measure masculinity and femininity are not derived from a theoretical perspective but are merely artifacts of statistical techniques which identify items which differentiate male from female responses. For example, one standard scale uses an item about fear of fire as opposed to fear of earthquakes because men tend to be afraid of one and women the other. This methodological approach precludes the conception of masculinity and femininity as orthogonal; rather, masculinity must be the opposite of femininity (one must not fear both or neither fire or earthquakes).

New theoretical and methodologic developments have pointed the way backwards; in a sense, we are coming full circle back to the idea that masculinity and femininity are just concepts which we use to identify clusters of characteristics. The individual person can contain both male and female aspects in his/her personality, and, as Jung has suggested, the androgynous person may have certain adaptive advantages over those who are strongly sex-typed. The research on androgyny is just beginning; though this chapter will summarize the major developments to date, behavioral scientists are just at the threshold of new discoveries in this important area.

The term "androgyny" comes from the Greek *andro* (male) and *gyne* (female), meaning an individual who possessed both male and female characteristics. Currently, an androgynous person (male or female) subscribes to a self definition which includes both masculine and feminine traits. How much option does the individual have in defining the part of the self-concept which includes gender identity and sex role? How much of what we consider masculinity and femininity is innate and how much is learned and can therefore be unlearned? If those trait clusters which we label masculinity and femininity are biologically produced, then androgyny is impossible. In the next section we review the major theories of gender-identity formation with a view toward separating those gender-related components which are biologic in origin from those which are not.

GENDER-IDENTITY FORMATION

The processes by which embryos become male and female and infants grow up to act in culturally defined masculine and feminine ways are being investigated by researchers in various academic disciplines. Topsy's response, "I just growed," is no longer sufficient. We want to understand the complex steps by which sex differentiation, gender-identity formation, and sex-role acquisition take place.

Sex differentiation occurs during the "critical period" around the sixth week after conception. Normally, if there is a Y chromosome present, the embryonic gonadal tissues will begin to differentiate into testes. If not, the development will continue as before and the gonadal tissue will become ovaries. Money and Ehrhardt[5] have documented many of the problems that can occur between conception and birth which result in sexual differentiation problems; however, for the majority, the process of sex differentiation proceeds normally.

Gender identity is the individual's personal and private experience of his/her gender: the concept of self as either male or female. "I am a female" is a statement about gender identity. It is the most fundamental part of the self and determines most other aspects of the self-concept. Once formed, the gender identity is almost impossible to change.

Though there are several competing theories about the formation of gender identity, it is generally agreed that it is complete for most children between the ages of three to five. Children at this age can make firm statements about their gender, and they tend to choose toys and activities that are deemed appropriate for their gender.

However, authorities disagree over the timing of the development of gender identity. Money's[6] research at Johns Hopkins suggests that between 18 months and two years the child does have an awareness of being one sex and not the other and attaches some meaning to that difference. Kohlberg[7] argues that gender identity does not appear until age three, constant gender labeling until four, and gender constancy until age six.[8]

These arguments about timing involve (1) theoretical issues, (2) problems associated with using preverbal infants in many studies, and (3) semantic issues. Kohlberg's theoretical approach derives from Piaget's cognitive theory which identifies a cognitive shift around age five that allows the child to conceptualize in terms of stable physical categories. Thus, Kohlberg sees gender constancy as most apt to occur at the time when the child's cognitive development will allow it to think in terms of stable characteristics.

Studies using preverbal children force researchers to make assumptions about gender identity based upon indirect evidence like toy preference or picture recognition. Further, the discrepancy between Kohlberg's views and the research of those who have found evidence of some recognition of gender identity in infants (Table I) may be the result of semantic confusion. The child may not comprehend that its gender is permanent, but the child probably "knows" at least for the moment, that "it" is a male or a female. Kohlberg acknowledges that the child's knowledge of his or her own gender is an important step toward the development of a stable gender identity. Could it be that this primitive but critical step must be followed by further cognitive development before gender identity becomes elaborated into stable gender identity?[9]

Research on gender identity (Table I) indicates that it is a gradual process beginning soon after birth when the child first notices differences between mother and father and interacts with each differently. As the infant matures it begins to identify the two sexes by certain cues, e.g., size, height, voice tone, hair length or style. Children also learn to recognize themselves and other same-sex children.

The period between 18 months and two years is a crucial period for the development of gender identity because, in part, a child's vocabulary expands dramatically during this period. Money and his associates[10] demonstrate that children until the age of two can be reassigned to another gender with emotional difficulties, but after two, reassigned children experience severe psychological disturbance.

However, two- and three-year-old children do not conceive of gender as permanent. The presence or absence of cues can lead a child to believe that a person has changed gender. For example, a child may view father, dressing up in mother's clothes, as having changed into a woman because women's clothes are the primary cue by which this child separates male from female. Generally, gender constancy does not occur until the child is between five and seven. Then

Table I. Gender–Identity Formation in Infancy: Related Studies

Behavior	Age	Ref.	Sources
Ability to discriminate between men and women: use of behavioral markers.	9 to 36 months	88	Conn and Kanner
		89	Rabban
		90	Brooks-Gunn and Lewis
		91	Morgan and Ricciuti
		92	Scarr and Salapatek
		93	Culp
Difference in reaction patterns of infants to mother and father	Few weeks +	94	Brazelton, Youngman, and Tronick
Child using genitalia distinguishes between the sexes	3 to 4 years	95	Brooks-Gunn and Lewis
		96	Katcher
		15	Thompson and Bentler
Attention given to same-sex persons	16 months +	97	Slaby and Frey
		98	Lewis and Brooks
		99	Lewis and Brooks-Gunn
Verbal identification: "I am a boy/girl."	18 months to 3 years	100	Gessell et al.
		95	Brooks-Gunn and Lewis
Some knowledge of sex-role stereotypes	2 years	101	Weinraub and Leite
Sex reassignment leads to emotional difficulties	18 months to 2 years	10	Money, Hampson, and Hampson
		102	Hampson and Hampson

the process of gender identity formation is complete. The child knows to which gender category he/she belongs and prefers to remain in that category thereafter. The child must now acquire the complement of temperamental and behavioral attributes which society has defined as appropriate to his/her gender.

SEX-ROLE ACQUISITION

A sex role is "a constellation of qualities an individual understands to characterize males and females in his or her culture."[11] Put another way, a sex role provides a script for playing the roles of male and female in a society. As in a play the characters must know enough of the other's lines to interact successfully. Both men and women must be aware of both role scripts so that they can (1) judge the appropriateness of others' behavior and (2) respond properly to their opposite's lead. For example, for a woman to interact appropriately with a man she must have some fairly specific idea of what he is thinking so that she can respond in a fitting manner.

Acquisition of sex-role scripts begins in infancy as the child starts interacting with its parents and continues on till death. After all, we must learn to be old men and women too.

There are several competing theories of sex-role acquisition, and each major new theoretical development has, in a sense, grown out of the previous one. The five major theoretical perspectives are briefly reviewed in the next section.

IDENTIFICATION THEORIES. Psychoanalytic views of sex-role acquisition rely on the concept of identification. Freud said that fear motivates the child to identify with the same-sex parent: fear of loss of love (anaclitic) or retaliation (defensive).[12] Both male and female infants fear loss of love of the mother. The mother supplies most or all of the child's needs and the child fears that its mother will no longer love and thus continue to provide those "goods and services" which the child requires.

However, around age four the process changes for boys; they discover their genitals. Boys' love for their mothers takes on sexual overtones, and father becomes a threat—a danger. The boy wishes to eliminate his father, but later comes to identify with father as a way of resolving his love–hate–fear feelings. The transition from identification with his mother, his first love object, to his father marks the beginning of the boy's active acquisition of masculinity; he begins to want to learn how to become a man.

The girl keeps the mother as primary love object, but she too experiences difficulties with the relationship as she discovers her genitals or rather apparent lack of them. She blames her mother and gradually turns to her father. She learns to replace her desires for a penis with a substitute—a baby. She realizes that in order to get a baby, she must be like her mother. She identifies with her mother and begins the process of learning femininity.

Identification theory has not been generally supported by the data. Pleck[13] outlines five areas in which this paradigm has not received empirical support: parental identification, effects of father absence, adjustment, cross-sex identity, and Black male identity. Further, available research suggests that external genitalia are not primarily sex-differentiating cues for young children.[14,15] Specifically, Katcher[16] found that 88% of 3 year olds, 69% of 4 year olds, 49% of five year-olds, and 30% of 6 year olds could not distinguish between male and female external genitalia. Also there is little empirical support for penis envy. Sherman's[17] review concludes: "there is little evidence of castration anxiety in women or widespread anatomical envy."

Sex-role acquisition through the process of identification has been reconceptualized by some psychologists who have tied identification to learning and modeling. For example, Sears[18] finds that the child identifies with the mother because she is a secondary reinforcer, having provided the child with both food and nuturance/love. However, the mother cannot be the good-natured provider all the time nor can she gratify the child's every whim. The child must find a way of replacing its mother when she is absent. The child achieves this through identification; by internalizing the mother, the child can have its mother ever present and perfect. Identification with the father is achieved through essentially the same process. The boy loves and therefore wishes to be like his father; he is not driven by fear of castration.[18]

Lynn[19] includes both psychological and cultural factors in his theory of sex role acquisition. He admits identification is the basic mechanism but emphasizes imitation and reinforcement of cultural stereotypes as important parts of the process.

> Typically, in this culture, the girl has the same-sex parental model for identification (the mother) with her more hours than the boy has his same-sex model (the father) with him. The boy seldom if ever is with the father as he engages in his daily vocational

> activities. Consequently, the father as a model for the boy is analogous to a man showing the major outline but lacking most details; whereas, the mother, as a model for the girl, might be thought of as a detailed map.[19]

According to Lynn, male models which reflect the stereotypic male role, e.g., TV and film heroes, sports stars, etc., are important substitutes for the father in providing models for young males. Through a process of gradual "behavior modification" (rewarding masculine and punishing feminine behavior), young boys learn to imitate—not their fathers, whom they rarely see—but the stereotypic male role. Girls continue to model themselves after their mothers.

Kagan[20] suggests that identification may be caused by envy as well as love or fear. The youth may envy the prerogatives of the parents, and thus attempt to identify with and incorporate the parents' attributes so as to achieve parental perks, e.g., freedom, power, money.

Hundreds of studies have generally failed to provide a basis for predicting a relationship between parental and childrens' personality attributes as would be predicted by the "identification theory:"

> Girls and boys are more similar to their mothers than to their fathers, and sometimes are not more similar to a parent than to another adult. Clearly, evidence that children are more similar to the same-sex than to the opposite sex parent does not exist.[21]

SOCIAL LEARNING THEORY. Theories of sex-role acquisition based upon identification presuppose an intense relationship between parents and children; these relationships, though common in Western societies, are not universal. There are cultures in which children do not experience the close, perhaps overheated, emotional ties with parents that are typical in the United States. Further, many investigators find that the concept of identification is difficult to operationalize and measure.

Rather than seeking the cause of sex-role acquisition in internal states, social learning theorists focus on the environment. They seek to identify factors external to the individual's psychic state which influence him/her to model him/herself after parents or other adults.

The three crucial mechanisms which are said to account for sex-role acquisition are observation, imitation, and reinforcement. First, children observe, watch, listen, and learn. They watch parents and significant others, mass media personalities and other public figures, and other children. They learn appropriate behavior for their gender through observation and test with trial and error imitation.

Children observe behavior from a wide variety of sources; most of this they do not attempt to imitate. Why do not more children attempt to fly through the air like Superman, swim under water like Submariner, or simply run away to the circus? Four factors appear to be the major predictors of children's likelihood of choosing adult role models.

The more available the adult the more apt he/she is to be chosen as a role model. The more powerful the adult the more apt a child is to model its behavior on this person. Children are likely to model themselves after adults whom they see as having qualities similar to themselves. Finally, children tend to choose nurturant adults as models.[22]

Though little research supports the modeling theory[23] its adherents maintain that children may learn behaviors they will practice only when they become adults. For example, a young boy may learn how to flirt with girls by observing his elders; however, he may not actually practice flirtation until puberty. In other words, current behaviors do not necessarily indicate what the child knows. Both motivation and level of competence explain which previously learned behaviors will be enacted.

Generally, those investigators with a modeling perspective believe that children learn a behavior complex, i.e., a set of scripts for a wide variety of situations. Occupation, courtship, friendship, and even death and dying: children practice complicated sets of behaviors associated with these life contingencies. Playing house and doctor are but two examples. Small boys and girls may spend hours playing cowboys and Indians or astronauts and aliens. While playing, children run, hide, shoot, help their compatriots, and get shot. When they are shot, they frequently "die." The child clutches his chest, spins dramatically, and falls lifeless to the ground; like a Hemingway hero the child dies with grace and style. When the child becomes an adult and is called upon to fight in the real world, what will be the effect of his/her years of practice? As most researchers point out, we do not yet know.

Whereas modeling theorists deal with complex behaviors, some behavioral psychologists interested in reinforcement study individual behaviors, e.g., sweeping, playing a musical instrument, whittling. The general principles influencing reinforcement are as follows: (1) Positive rewards following a given response increase the likelihood that the response will persist (behavior is conditioned by its effects). (2) Negative reinforcement tends to extinguish the sanctioned behavior. (3) Through the mechanism of stimulus generalization, behaviors related to the one being rewarded or sanctioned will be affected. For example, if a girl is rewarded for vacuuming the floors, she may not only continue to vacuum but also to sweep and mop.

Maccoby and Jacklin,[23] in discussing the role of reinforcement in sex-role acquisition, suggest four hypotheses around which this perspective is organized: parents behave differently toward male and female children; innate differences between the sexes precipitate a set of different responses to each sex from the parent; the behavior of parents is molded by their expectations of what their male as compared with female children can be expected to do; and the behavior of parent to the child is mediated by whether or not the parent and the child are the same or the opposite sex.

This approach assumes that parents have one set of expectations for boys and another for girls and that parents reinforce expectations consistently. Neither of these assumptions is borne out strongly in research. According to Maccoby and Jacklin,[23] "the reinforcement contingencies for the two sexes are not as different as might be expected if parents were socializing children for stereotyped adult roles."

The assumption that parents routinely reward aggression, studying math, and climbing trees for boys and reward girls for reading, sewing, and behaving dependently is unsupported. The situation in which the behavior occurs, the timing, and the mood of the parents affect the decision to reward, punish, or ignore a specific behavior. Only in laboratories are subjects—children or mice—treated consistently.

Studies show that child-rearing patterns, including sex-role socialization, vary with social class, ethnicity, religion, and national origin.[24] Parental values differ widely in America; some parents value independence and achievement while others reward obedience and passivity. The larger society as represented by churches, schools, and the mass media also affect the reinforcement patterns for each child. No wonder psychologists cannot demonstrate either consistent goals of sex-role socialization or patterns of reinforcement.

However, research shows that boys are more rigidly socialized to conform to sex-typed behavior than girls and are more likely to be ridiculed, ostracized, or physically punished for exhibiting cross-sex-typed behavior. For a girl, tomboy behavior is acceptable and often rewarded. Girls who can do "boy things" often have more prestige than their more feminine-acting counterparts. On the other hand, the boy cannot act like a sissy, and parents express more concern about deviations from the norm in the young male than in the female. In sum, girls are allowed to act more androgynously than boys.

Behavioral psychologists, with respect to the effects of imitation and reinforcement on behavior, have examined play groups and games. However, few have been concerned with the interaction that occurs during these activities nor the meanings they have for the participants. A boy may receive praise or gain status as a leader while playing a game with friends; yet, it is the meaning that the child assigns to the activity which may determine whether or not the activity becomes part of his repertoire of behaviors.

SYMBOLIC INTERACTION: MEASUREMENT OF MEANING. Symbolic interactionists (largely sociologists and social psychologists) as well as learning theorists look to the environment, i.e., to factors external to the individual for an understanding of social behavior (that behavior that takes the other individuals into account). The newborn interacts with its environment and begins to learn about cause and effect (crying brings relief from hunger); yet, the infant does not differentiate itself from the external world. The child has no sense of self; it has feelings, emotions, and reactions, but no sense of "me," separate and distinct from others. An infant explores itself, touching and feeling the various parts of its body. Eventually the child discovers its toes and examines them one by one. Then it makes an interesting discovery; watching the child's face, you can see the moment when the child first realizes that it "ends" there, but something else begins. This represents the beginnings of the sense of self.

Gradually, as the child develops, it learns to form images which are associated with objects or people in the environment; the bottle is connected to the mother, who is, in turn, connected to food and surcease from hunger. The child begins to develop significant symbols, i.e., objects that have symbolic meaning which it shares with others. For example, dressing a child in a coat means "going out" for both parents and child; thus, both parents and child share a significant symbol. Language is the most powerful significant symbol and through it the child's repetoire of shared meanings increases exponentially. "All gone," "bye-bye," and "no" communicate to child, parents, and significant others; the child begins to develop a mind and a sense of self.

The primary stages lead to full self-conscious awareness: imitation, play, and game. At first, infants and small children (0–2 years) mimic those around them; most of this behavior has little or no meaning for the child. During the play stage (2–6 years), the child "takes the role of the other," playing the nurse, mommy, fireman, bank robber, or alien. Little girls and boys play house, and some of them at times reverse roles: boys play mother and girls play father. The children practice these roles and begin to understand some of the meanings attached by adults to these behaviors. Matthews[25] observed the unstructured fantasy play of same-sex pairs of children. Some of the four-year-old boys spent time playing "mommy" and "wife." A candid photo of mother taken from these boys' play show "her" cooking, sweeping, telephoning, dropping things for daddy to pick up, and watching the baby. On the other hand, daddy takes photographs, tells mother which car to take, has a large coffee cup with his name on it, and takes control in an emergency situation. Daddies, in contrast to mothers, never panic in a crisis. As children play, they learn to take the role of the other, and because they share a set of significant symbols, they learn to judge the effects of what they say and do on others. The little boy, playing mother, will experience how it feels when a girl, playing daddy, says, 'Stop doing that; you're so clumsy."

As children mature they start participating in organized games, simple in elementary school and complex, highly organized ones, in high school. The child playing in a game must play his/her role (pitcher, tight end) in relation to the roles of others; the player must take these other players into account in order to successfully play his/her role. The pitcher must anticipate what the other players will do in order to act the role well. Through playing in games young people learn to evaluate themselves from the point of view of another (the generalized other).[26] A boy learns he is a "good guy," "team player," or perhaps, "stud." Girls may be seen and come to see themselves as "brain," or "real nice girl." These understandings become incorporated into the self-concept and are part of the way in which we grow to define ourselves as male and female.

> The symbolic interactionist perspective accords primacy to interaction between individuals for the development of the biological infant into a human being capable of intelligent thought. From such interaction, individuals learn attitudes, behavior, and meaning. However, within this view, the individual is more than a passive receiver in the learning process. With the development of mind and self, the individual actively participates in the construction of meaning and so affects the social environment.[27]

Symbolic interaction primarily provides a framework from which to study behavior such as fantasy play of children; it tends to describe rather than prove. The symbolic interaction approach focuses on the way individuals in interaction construct reality; the person is an active participant, not merely the recipient of some others' actions as in social learning theory. Recent theories of sex-role acquisition also concentrate on the active involvement of the person.

COGNITIVE DEVELOPMENT THEORY: THE MIND AS MESSAGE. Many psychologists consider the mind a black box hiding what goes on inside of it from view. The processes taking place in consciousness which intervene between stimulus and response are not readily observable and so are frequently ignored. Kohlberg[28] and his students have been primarily concerned with how thought is structured and have sought to determine the developmental stages that children pass through as they become mature adults.

Kohlberg's theory developed out of the work of Piaget, who studied the development of cognition in children. Children of four think differently from eight year olds; it is not just that eight year olds know more—they think differently from younger children. Kohlberg studied the sex role perception of children as they grew, and he has formulated a series of maturational stages.

Children begin to structure their world through a process of categorization: hot–cold, wet–dry, good tasting–bad tasting, and incidently, male–female. Every person must be one or the other. The child first establishes its gender identity; then the process of acquiring behaviors associated with that gender begins.

The child, having established its gender, proceeds to value those attributes, behaviors, and attitudes associated with his/her gender. "I am a boy; I like boy things." Those attributes which boys come to value are competence, strength, power, and instrumental achievement. The boy values these and wishes to obtain them because they will help him conform to his sense of gender identity. From the point of view of learning theorists,

> sex typed behavior and attitudes are acquired through social rewards that follow sex-appropriate responses made by the child or by a relevant model. The social learning syllogism is: "I want rewards, I am rewarded for doing boy things, therefore, I want to be a boy." In contrast, a cognitive theory assumes this sequence: "I am a boy, therefore I want to do boy things, therefore the opportunity to do boy things is rewarding."[28]

The child comes to identify with the same-sex parent, but identification is the outcome of gender identity and sex role learning rather than its antecedent.

Kohlberg postulates that gender-identity formation begins around age two and is not established until between ages 5 to 7. Much of the criticism of Kohlberg's work focuses on the issue of age at which these events occur (see previous discussion of gender-identity formation), but disregarding the issue of age, some research supports his general theory. Young children show much more rigorous and clear-cut sex-role stereotypes than do adults. In fantasy play children very carefully ensure that fathers do not do mothers' work and vice versa. A child will switch genders (a boy will play mother) if the child wants to do opposite-gender activities. A 4½-year-old girl observed by the authors wanted to drive a car, but the father (played by a four-year-old male) said that she could not because "daddies do that." She promptly said, "Okay, I'll be the daddy now." She became daddy and drove the car around the living room.

The fact that children hold more rigid sex stereotypes than adults may account for some of the difficulty many parents and teachers have in trying to raise children androgynously. These adults have worked unstintingly to provide a gender-free environment for their children and are confounded when these young people conform to sex stereotypes which they have not encountered in the home or school. Usually "society" or "the mass media" are blamed even though, in most cases, the children seem too young to be affected by either.

A teacher in a private school that prides itself on maintaining a gender-free program says,

> during free time our children are encouraged to use their imaginations constructively; yet, most of their play is surprisingly conformist and sexist. A few days ago a little girl was lying on the floor grunting. I rushed over and asked her, "What's the matter?" She said, matter-of-factly, "I'm having a baby; Eric's the daddy." I said, "All girls don't have to have babies; we can do other things if we want to." Her reply was, "Mommies have babies and daddies go to the office."

In further support of the cognitive theory, Kohlberg and Zigler[29] found that intellectually advanced children demonstrate sex-role learning significantly earlier than their less advanced peers. Also, a number of investigators have supported Kohlberg's contention that children are more interested in and more attentive to same-sex children and adults than in cross-sex children.[30,31]

Kohlberg's theory has succeeded in redirecting interest among behavioral science researchers to cognitive processes and the rules by which children acquire, label, and assimilate experiences. Two of the new theories derive from developments in the study of language acquisition and suggest that sex-role acquisition may, too, be innate to human beings.

RULES AND REGULATIONS: RULE AND SYMBOL LEARNING. Some branches of psychology and sociology describe the newborn infant as a *tabula rasa* on which society imprints its values, norms, mores, and customs. Parents, as well as major institutions like schools and churches, socialize children to conform to societal expectations. Children passively receive adult instruction; parents and teachers "mold young minds." New findings in several disciplines call into question this view; ethology and linguistics are but two examples. Research in ethology, sociobiology, and linguistics suggest the importance of innate characteristics which predispose humans to act in certain ways. Two new theoretical perspectives particularly apply to the views of Pleck and Constantinople, the primary researchers to pursue this new approach to sex-role acquisition.

Chomsky[32] pioneered the radical view that the ability to acquire language is an innate characteristic of humans as a species. We have the ability to understand and duplicate grammar and syntax. This competency is content-free in that it is the ability to learn any grammar, not a particular one. Children develop distinct grammatical constructions which they have not learned from adults. For example, small children use "all gone" before a noun as in "All gone mommy," ("-cookies, -grandma, -ice cream.") For Chomsky language is not simply memorized by rote; the human brain actively participates in language acquisition.

Levi-Strauss[33] developed a new approach to the understanding of culture. Structural anthropology seeks to identify and interpret the codes by which societies "mediate and constrain social transactions in complex ways."[34] To order and thus demystify the structure of culture, one must understand the structure of the mind because that which is produced by the mind, e.g., culture, must be organized similarly to the mind itself:

> The structure of the mind is not, however, given to immediate observation. It must be inferred from empirical observations, and the best place to begin to look for this structure, or so Levi-Strauss argues, is in language. Linguistic behavior is thus the behavior par excellence which is governed by rules and structures which are unknown to the actors.[34]

Levi-Strauss believes that the brain is organized rather like a computer, that is, binary opposition. Thus, both language and culture are similarly structured. Hot–cold, good–bad, raw–cooked (which is the title of one of Levi-Strauss' most famous books) and, of course, male–female.

According to Levi-Strauss and other structuralists, the child first begins categorizing in terms of opposites. "The binary opposition is a child's first logical operation."[34] Consequently, structuralist theory predicts that children will (1) identify the oppositional categories male and female and (2) develop rules which would limit behaviors and attitudes to one or the other category.

Chomsky and Levi-Strauss have both contributed to our understanding of the relationship between the mind and its products, and each, in his way, has provided a theoretical basis for new developments in the study of sex role acquisition.

Pleck[35] suggests that a "sex role learning apparatus" similar to the language learning apparatus postulated by Chomsky may act as a processor of sex role images and linkages which are visible to the child. In other words, Pleck argues that the brain may have an area which is predisposed toward categorizing in terms of gender. Pleck's position does not, however, imply that ideas-in-the-mind about gender, once fixed, are immutable. As language usage among not only individuals but also among cultures evolves over time, so sex-role attitudes, beliefs, and behaviors are modifiable, both for the individual and for the society.

Constantinople[9] suggests a "rule-learning" approach to sex-role acquisition, in which attention is focused on the cues children use to categorize by gender. Initially parents primarily supply labels which distinguish between the sexes: boy–girl, mommy–daddy (binary opposites). Soon the child adds cues which categorize male and female, e.g., hair styles, clothing, verbal intonations.

> The major mechanism in the acquisition of distinctive features would seem to be a combination of straight observational learning and direct tutelage, with linguistic tags serving an organizing function. Positive and negative reinforcement would serve both to focus the child's attention on relevant stimuli and to endow sex-role related behaviors with positive and negative affect.[9]

These tags are then used to activate different expectancies in the child. She/he would use them to screen its own and others' behavior for sex role appropriateness in terms of the categories and rules previously developed. Consequently, the young child will hold rigid beliefs about gender-appropriate behavior and will bend the behavior it observes to fit its preconceived models. As the child matures, rules will become less rigid so that more androgynous behavior will be acceptable.

SEX-ROLE ACQUISITION AND THE POSSIBILITY OF ANDROGYNY

This review has traced the evolving history of sex-role acquisition paradigms, beginning with Freud and Jung and ending, at least for the present, with Pleck and Constantinople. In a broad sense, the major theories have focused on three processes: identification, reinforcement and imitation, and cognition.

The rule-learning paradigm offers several advantages as a research model. First, there is extensive research in several disciplines which focus on the relationship between the structure of the brain and behavioral characteristics. Second, a rule-learning approach will explain a variety of findings such as sex-role drift, i.e., individuals become less sex stereotyped as they mature.[9] Rule content and rates of learning vary among individuals and families; thus, this approach offers an explanation of the range of behaviors, attitudes and images associated with gender differences around the world.

The emphasis on cognitive development and/or rule-learning processes for the understanding of sex-role acquisition has an important implication for androgyny. Androgynous behavior may well represent the end point in the sex-role acquisition process. This is the point of view expressed by Block[11] in a seminal article which has influenced much current research on androgyny.

Block's theory is closely related to the ideas of Bakan[36] whose book, *The Duality of Human Existence,* has influenced a number of sex-role theorists. According to Bakan, agency and communion are the two fundamental principles common to all life. Agency, the male principle, is characterized by competitiveness, activity, and independence. The female principle, communion, is marked by concern for others, or selflessness. These two principles represent fundamental modes of existence and they must be balanced for any society to exist. The fundamental task of human society is to achieve such a balance. It is also the fundamental task of the individual to achieve an integration of those two modes. Each, left unchecked, is destructive to the individual and the society. Males must learn to temper their drive toward egoistic self-interest with concern for others. Women's central task is to develop a self-concept based on accomplishments related to self as well as service to others.

Block's sex-role acquisition theory is derived from Loevinger's[37] theory of ego development. For Block,[11] the crucial stage for sex-role acquisition is the one in which children attempt to control their impulses by conformity to external rules. Children are obsessed by rules and external appearances and become aggravated when they perceive deviations from rules. It is during this stage that boys are socialized to control affect and girls aggression.

At the next stage rules are internalized as inner feelings, and inner values and ideas moderate one's definition of masculinity and femininity. Feelings of responsibility shape behavior including sex-role-related behavior. Those who reach the next stage, i.e., the autonomous, are concerned with recognizing societal sex-role expectations and reconciling themselves to their own deviations from those norms. The last stage of development is the integrated state in which the masculine (agentic) and feminine (communal) characteristics are totally integrated into the self-concept. The integrated individual is fully androgynous.

Undoubtedly, there are few people in America and elsewhere who achieve this level of integration described by Block. Most persons are at the stages where either they have not recognized the various components of their social selves or they have been unable to bring these components into a harmonious synthesis. The consequences of this failure may be immense. Becker[38] sees the major cause of "historical alienation" as the unsuccessful attempt to "achieve maximum individuality within maximum community." Androgyny as a social movement may point the way toward an era in human history in which men and women become whole persons and agentic and communal drives are not at war with one another.

If we are to study androgyny, it must be operationalized. In the last few years there has been a major effort to define and measure this rather elusive concept. In the following section, the major scales which are used to measure androgyny are discussed with a view toward identifying their strengths and weaknesses, both conceptually and methodologically.

MEASURING ANDROGYNY

Since Bem[39,40] developed the initial measure of androgyny, others have constructed or modified scales which purport to measure this concept. Currently, there are four scales widely in use: Bem Sex Role Inventory (BSRI), Personal Attributes Questionnaire (PAQ), PRF ANDRO, and Adjective Check List (ACL).[41] In this section we will discuss some common measurement and definitional problems and then compare the four scales in terms of validity, reliability, and usefulness.

PROBLEMS OF DEFINITION AND MEASUREMENT. Problems of operationalization usually derive from inadequate theory. Frequently, scales are constructed with little concern for the concept being measured. Comparisons between the four scales show that they define androgyny differently as subjects classified as androgynous in one may be masculine or feminine in another.[42,43]

Further, the scale developers do not clearly state at what level of generality their scale is applicable: a global self-assessment, behavioral predisposition, or a general mind set. Thus, it is not clear what behaviors can be predicted from subjects identified as androgynous as compared with masculine or feminine.

These scales rely primarily on lists of personality traits, e.g., nurturing, self-sufficient, etc., which individuals apply to themselves. The "trait theory" has been under attack by a growing number of psychologists as the assumption that people have personality traits which they express over a wide variety of situations has received little empirical support. The labeling of individuals as extroverts or exhibitionists has fallen from favor as research demonstrates that people tend to behave in terms of situations in which they find themselves. Mischel[44] found that there is only a .30 correlation between behaviors across situations, rather low if one is attempting to predict behavior on that basis. Since androgyny scales are essentially based on lists of personality/temperamental traits, the utility of these scales in predicting behavior is questioned. Lenny[41] summarizes the problems associated with the measurement of androgyny at the present time:

> Further, the various scales were each developed in a different manner, selected items for inclusion differently, have been validated according to different criteria, have different contents, etc. Again, these methodological differences imply that each scale is assessing a somewhat different concept of androgyny.

FOUR MEASURES OF ANDROGYNY. For reference and comparison purposes Table II summarizes some of the important features of the four scales under review. The first scale developed to measure androgyny and undoubtedly the one most in use, is the Bem Sex Role Inventory (BSRI).

Bem Sex Role Inventory. The 60 items (20 masculine, 20 feminine, and 20 neutral) were selected by a panel of judges from a pool of 400 personality characteristics. Sample items are "Acts as a leader" (masculine) and "affectionate" (feminine). The masculinity score is the mean of the self-ratings on the 20 masculine items; similarly for the feminine.

As originally conceived, the BSRI identified three types: Masculine, feminine, and androgynous. Those identified as androgynous achieved a balanced score, i.e., the difference between the masculine and feminine items was nearly zero. However, Spence, Helmreich, and Stapp[45] showed that the balance method of scoring equated two very different types of individuals; a person who saw himself/herself as having an equal number of positive masculine and feminine characteristics was labeled androgynous. Likewise, an individual who thought of him/herself as equally lacking positive masculine and feminine traits was also classified as androgynous. Spence, Helmreich, and Stapp[45] recommended the use of the median split method (discussed below in the section on the Personal Attributes Questionnaire) to distinguish between these two types. Bem now favors the median split method for calculating the scores derived from her scale.

Factor analysis of the BSRI has identified several components in addition to masculinity and femininity, including social immaturity and self-sufficiency. Further, scores on the BSRI have been related to a wide variety of variables such as self-actualization, manifest anxiety, and even the ability to match musical selections with paintings. Over 80 articles based on this scale have been published, and it continues in wide use.

Personal Attitudes Questionnaire. The Personal Attributes Questionnaire (PAQ) originally consisted of 55 items and is a self-report instrument based on a number of trait descriptions each set up a bipolar basis. These items were drawn from a pool of 130 items which distinguish male from female responses. The scale consists of three subscales; masculine (M), feminine (F), and masculine–feminine (M–F).[46]

Masculine items were defined as characteristics socially desirable in both sexes but believed to occur to a greater degree in males.[46] Similarly, feminine items are socially desirable in all but found more in women. The M–F traits are desirable in one sex but not in the other (example: very home oriented–very worldly). In most research using this scale, the short form consisting of 24 items is used. There is a .90 correlation between the two forms.[46]

Spence and Helmrich recommend the median split (or absolute) method for calculating scores. The median score for normative group forms the basis for classifying subjects into one of four groups: masculine, feminine, androgynous,

Table II. Comparisons between Bem Sex-Role Inventory, Personal Attributes Questionnaire, Adjective Check List, and the PRF Andro Scale

	BSRI	PAQ	ACL	ANDRO
Type of Instrument	Adjective rating scale	Adjective rating scale	Adjective rating scale	true–false
Description	60 adjectives 7-point Likert scale; ask if desirable for man or woman	55 items; 5-point semantic differential; describe self; short form, 24 items	34 items; check those like self	56 statements; describe self
Appropriate for	6 and older	12 and older	14 and older	14 and older
Administration	Self	Self	Self	Self
Variables	Masculinity; femininity; androgyny and social desirability	Masculinity; femininity; androgyny; undifferentiated	Masculinity; femininity; androgyny	Masculinity; femininity; androgyny
Reliability	Test/retest between .89 and .90	Test/retest between .90 and .91	Few data	Test/retest .81
Validity	Evidence for construct validity, especially in regard to masculinity and femininity items	Evidence of construct validity	Probably least reliable of the four	Evidence of construct validity

and undifferentiated. Those who score above the median on both masculine and feminine subscales are identified as androgynous and those who score below the median on both subscales are labeled undifferentiated.

In their recent article, Spence and Helmreich [47] compare the balance (Bem's original method), absolute, and the new hybrid difference median method (which is a combination of the first two) and conclude

> that the manner in which M and F combine is not uniform but varies from one type of dependent variable to another. The absolute method of categorizing subjects does not presuppose a particular type of mathematical combination and is capable of revealing a number of possibilities. The balance method, by assuming a specific *a priori* model (that M and F contribute equally and in opposite direction) is likely to misrepresent many data sets. The difference/median model shares this deficiency.

PRF ANDRO. Berzins, Welling, and Wetter[48] developed a true–false instrument (PRF ANDRO) consisting of 56 statements measuring masculinity and femininity. Derived from Murray's need theory, the masculine items reflect social and intellectual ascendancy, autonomy, and orientation toward risk. The feminine items reflect nurturance, affiliative–expressive concerns, and self-subordination. These two subscales are part of the Personality Research Form, which consists of 400 items.

Subjects check statements they believe apply to themselves. (Example: "When someone opposes me on an issue, I usually find myself taking an even stronger stand than I did at first.") Scoring is based on the median split method, and those who score above the median on both masculine and feminine subscales are labeled androgynous. Berzins, Welling, and Wetter[48] provide norms for researchers interested in using the scale.

Internal consistency coefficients generally range between .67 and .79 and test/retest reliability is .81 for both masculine and feminine subscales. Berzins, Welling, and Wetter summarize,[48]

> The results suggest that the Masculinity and Femininity subscales of the PFR ANDRO scale are independent, reliable, minimally related to socially desirable responding, substantially related to their respective counterparts in the BSRI, convergent with major personality dimensions, and capable of meaningfully differentiating samples varying in age, socio-economic status, and psychopathology.

Adjective Check List. Gough and Heibrun's Adjective Check List (ACL) consists of 300 adjectives, 54 of which are related to sex-role differentiation, at least among college students. As the sex components of the ACL were originally devised, masculinity was opposite of femininity. Even though the ACL may now be scored so as to create a measure of androgyny, this scale is probably the least reliable of the four reviewed here.[43]

The problems associated with the use of the ACL illustrate the difficulties of modifying a scale based upon one conception of the relationship between masculinity and femininity to another model. The ACL sex-role subscales were constructed from the perspective that masculinity and femininity are bipolar opposites; indeed both psychological and physical differences between the sexes were considered in developing the scale.[49] It is less than satisfactory to adopt a scale based upon a conception of a bipolar relationship between masculinity and femininity to measure a concept on the assumption of an orthogonal relationship between these two sex-role variables. Beere's[50] statement about the MMPI explains the difficulties of modifying scales created from one theoretical assumption to measure concepts based on another.

> This instrument has been one of the most frequently used measures of masculinity and femininity. However, recently, researchers have become more critical of it because its development was based on empirical procedures (that is, items that differentiated between males and females comprise the masculinity–femininity subscale), and a respondent cannot score high on both masculinity and femininity (that is, one cannot be androgynous).

Masculinity and femininity: bipolar or orthogonal? Most, if not all of the pre-Bem scales were based on the bipolar view of the relationship between masculinity and femininity. In brief, the view that masculine and feminine attributes are essentially bipolar opposites has dominated the writings of social and behavioral scientists until recently.[46] Based on this view, scales identify four groups: high-masculine vs. high-feminine and low-masculine vs. low-feminine. A subject could not score high in both masculine or feminine components, and many of the scales had built-in "lie detectors" so that inconsistent (androgynous) responses could be controlled.

Today, masculinity and femininity are no longer viewed as opposite ends of a continuum. Masculinity implies one set of attributes and femininity another; thus, it is perfectly possible for one individual to have many masculine *and* feminine attributes as part of his/her self-concept. Now, based on the view that the relationship between masculinity and femininity may be orthogonal, sex role scales such as those discussed in this section can identify four distinct types: high-masculine, high-feminine, androgynous, and undifferentiated (low masculine and feminine). In the following section we will briefly identify the temperamental and behavioral attributes associated with each of these labels.

SUGAR AND SPICE AND PUPPY DOG TAILS: THE COMPONENTS OF MASCULINITY AND FEMININITY

Every culture in the world differentiates between male and female. Indeed, some cultures designate more than two genders; yet universally men are distinguished from women and some separate roles are assigned to each. Cross-culturally, in general men make war, hunt, and do the heavy manual labor. They also direct the major activities of the culture. Women gather food, cook, tend the garden and residence, and rear the children.

Are the differences between what men and women do and the way they act due to biological or social factors? This question is still to be debated. Also, behavioral scientists expend considerable energy, not to say ingenuity, trying to distill the essence of maleness and femaleness. Erikson[51] for example, argued that women concern themselves with inner space, whereas, men thrust themselves into outer space, the external environment. Parsons and Bales[52] suggested that women are expressive while men are primarily instrumental. Witkin[53] characterizes women as field dependent and men as field independent.

These theories, as well as Bakan's which was discussed in a previous section, are attempts to conceptualize a fundamental difference between men and women. Further, most of the scales which measure sex-role orientation, including those measuring androgyny assume a central core for both masculinity and femininity around which traditional attributes associated with maleness and femininity revolve. Bakan's core concepts of agency and communion are useful in describing the attributes of maleness and femaleness as these concepts have been traditionally treated in research and theory.

HIGH MASCULINITY: AGENCY. Only in the last five years has there been much interest in research on the male sex role. However, a significant increase in research which focuses on the male sex role has occurred, and in 1979, Grady, Brannon, and Pleck[54] published an annotated bibliography of over 250 articles and books on the male sex role.

Several writers have attempted to define the core characteristics of maleness.[54,35,55–59] These writers show a remarkable consensus on the core attributes, as illustrated in Table III. There is strong agreement that aggression/violence and success/achievement are central attributes associated with maleness. Aggression is almost certainly related to male hormones, and cross-culturally, men act more aggressively than women.

> Dozens of studies show males of all ages engage in more physical aggression, fantasy aggression, verbal aggression, and play aggression than females do. The differences show up as soon as children begin to play with each other, at the age of two or three and last into adulthood.[60]

Willy Loman, the quintessential fictional salesman, said, "A man can't go out the way he came in, Ben; a man has got to add up to something."[61] The need to achieve appears to be part of maleness cross-culturally. Generally, men strive to achieve in the world of affairs, whether on a tribal, national, or international level. Using a variety of terms to tap this dimension, e.g., ambitious, adven-

Table III. Core Attributes of the Male Sex Role[a]

	Aggression/ violence	Physical action	Dominance	Self confidence	Promasculine antifeminine	Success/ achievement
David and Brannon	×			×	×	×
Pleck	×	×		×		×
Turner	×		×	×	×	×
Boles and Tatro	×	×	×	×		×
Cicone and Ruble	×	×	×			×
Heilbrun	×		×	×		×
Jenkins and Vroegh	×	×				×

[a]Not all characteristics mentioned.

turous, enterprising, and goal-oriented, researchers find that both men and women view men as more achievement-oriented than women.

Physical activity is also a core attribute of masculinity, and considerable research supports the view that men are more physically active than women.[23] Some writers see modern alienation as partly attributable to the fact that men in industrialized societies no longer use their bodies extensively in their work. Man's body as the primary tool in shaping the world is nearly obsolete and the distinctions between men that were created on the basis of it have lost their validity.[62] Both sports and popular culture, e.g., action fantasy films starring Burt Reynolds and Clint Eastwood, reflect men's need for physical activity away from the executive suite or the assembly line.

Anthropologists have never verified the existence of even one matriarchy, i.e., a society dominated by women. Legends of Amazons ruling over men are apparently only fantasies. All known societies are patriarchies, and those which are the most egalitarian are the hunting and gathering ones, which are now nearly extinct.

Some researchers argue that men naturally form dominance hierarchies or pecking orders, whereas women form networks of status equals.[63] In developing the BSRI, Bem found that the two words which best identified masculinity are dominant and assertive.

One of the more enduring mythic images found in American popular culture is the Marlboro Man (Gary Cooper at High Noon). The Marlboro Man, strong and silent, is self-reliant. He is in control but not expressive. The Marlboro Man does not fall apart in crises, and he can, like Daniel Boone, live alone and take care of himself.

Two of the writers (Table III) reviewed here suggest that one keystone of maleness is antifemaleness. If little girls cry, boys don't. Girls play with dolls, so boys must not. Masculine attributes are valued and feminine ones are devalued and shunned.

These six attributes which have been viewed as primary components of maleness are closely related to Bakan's concept of agency. The male acts upon the external environment. He is an active doer.

HIGH FEMININITY: COMMUNION. Investigators generally agree that the essence of femininity involves nurturance and selflessness. For example, Chafetz[64] identified the following as feminine traits: maternal, emotional, compassionate, responsive, and noncompetitive. Stasz-Stoll[65] suggests that for women in American society the following behaviors are prescribed: obedience, nurturance, sociability, and responsibility in the home. Further, Stasz-Stoll points out that for women succorance, self-reliance, and dominance are strongly proscribed. Atkinson, Boles, and Cassidy's[66] study of the self-concept of a sample of Southern "ladies" showed that these women attempt to emulate the behaviors and temperamental attributes of the ideal antebellum female. Adjectives which describe the Southern lady are: simple, good, passive, submissive, humble, sympathetic, kind, hospitable and calm. One respondent, a middle-aged Southern gentlewoman, drew a vivid portrait of the Southern lady, a portrait which might well represent the essence of femaleness:

> A true Southern lady never complains, she meets adversity with dignity and grace. She never discusses money or the cost of anything, and she is infinitely polite to servants and those less fortunate. She puts everyone at ease. She never belittles, ridicules, or criticizes. She greets friends and relatives alike with a hug and a kiss, male and female. She uses no profanity. She always stands for older people when she is young through middle age. She has excellent table manners, often carves with excellence. She keeps her ailments, allergies, and idiosyncracies to herself. She eats with pleasure anything served her no matter what. She believes in putting herself out for company and family, and she is very polite to her husband and children, and it is always clearly understood her husband is the head of the family.

Scales measuring femininity illustrate the consensus among researchers about the core of femaleness. For example, Spence and Helmreich[46] associate the following items with femininity: very helpful to others, very kind, very understanding of others, and very warm in relations with others. Heilbrun[67] includes the following adjectives in the feminine subscale of the ACL: emotional, sensitive, sympathetic, and warm. Compassion and tenderness were found to be the best markers of femininity by Bem.

The essence of femaleness as presently conceived is communion, the concern for others at the expense of self-development. Popular culture provides many examples of this model; one example here will suffice. In a recent film entitled *Marooned,* three astronauts were stranded in space. Back on Earth their wives, via NASA communications, give them encouragement and emotional support as they endure in space while their hopes for rescue are dashed. The wives criticize NASA neither for the mission's failure nor their husbands for undertaking such a perilous assignment. They provide emotional support to the husbands, and not incidentally, to the NASA staff who are attempting to launch a rescue effort. The wives offer emotional support while the men act upon the external world.

ANDROGYNY: THE MIDDLE WAY. An androgynous person possesses a constellation of traits characteristic of both the high masculine and feminine. He/she can be both nurturant and in need of emotional support, depending upon the situation. An androgynous individual may be dominant in one situation and submissive in another, as the person sees him/herself possessing both these traits and is accepting of them. Agency and communion are integrated into the self-concept so that the person is free to utilize whichever traits are appropriate to a given situation.

The median split method labels all the subjects who score above the median in both masculinity and femininity as androgynous. Depending on the scale and the sample composition, between one-third and half of the respondents surveyed since Bem's[39] initial investigation are classed as androgynous. A variety of variables, including age, education, social class, sexual orientation, and ideology account for differences in the percentage of respondents in a given sample who are androgynous. In general, those respondents who are androgynous are middle aged, from the middle or upper class, and college educated. Women, especially educated women who are strongly involved with the Women's Liberation movement, are slightly more apt to view themselves as androgynous than are men.

THE UNDIFFERENTIATED. Those scoring below the median on both masculine and feminine subscales are classed as undifferentiated. Those labeled undifferentiated generally have lower self-esteem scores than subjects in the other three groups.[46,68] Also, undifferentiated women in one study[68] were found to be less adjusted to their life situations than either androgynous or feminine women. They also displayed the most external locus of control of any of the other groups. Showing the highest rates of introversion and neuroticism, the undifferentiated women in this particular study presented a picture of rather poor life adjustment. This may be typical of individuals classified as undifferentiated, but there has been very little research attention paid to this group.

This section contains a brief discussion of the characteristics of the four groups identified in scales currently used to measure androgyny. In the next section, we will discuss the advantages and disadvantages of androgyny for individual adjustment.

ANDROGYNY: BOON OR BANE?

Kaplan[69] defines the major theoretical components of androgyny as situational appropriateness, flexibility, effectiveness, and integration. Bem adds psychological health. In general, research has supported the view that the behavior of the androgynous individual is flexible, situationally appropriate, and effective,[40] and there is some evidence that psychological health is associated with androgyny.[70]

Specifically, Worrell's[71] review shows that androgyny has been compared to sex-typed behavior in regard to the following: "(a) adaptive, flexible and effective interpersonal behavior; (b) self-esteem or positive self-evaluation; (c) freedom from obvious pathology; and (d) broad life-style coping variables." Bem[39] posits flexibility as the *sine qua non* of androgyny by demonstrating that the traditionally sex-typed person manifests less behavior flexibility than the androgynous. The sex-typed person less willingly engages in stereotypically cross-sex behavior, even when that activity is more appropriate or rewarded. Also, the sex-typed person expresses more discomfort when forced to engage in cross-typed activities than the andorgynous individual. Ideally, this flexibility allows the androgynous person to be more successful in a variety of situations than his/her more rigid counterpart.

However, researchers are not unanimous in support of the thesis that androgyny is correlated with flexibility. Jones, Chernovetz, and Hansson[72] concluded from their sample of 1,404 respondents using the BSRI:

> First, the androgyny-equals-adaptability hypothesis seems not to hold for males. In most instances androgynous males scored in the less adaptive direction than the masculine males. However, the notion that androgynous subjects would yield the most desirable patterns of responses across several situations is directly contradicted by the present data in that sex-typed males and opposite sex-typed females with very few exceptions, showed the most flexible and competent pattern of responses.

Several researchers have found a positive relationship between androgyny and self-esteem. For example, O'Connor, Mann, and Bardwick[73] administered the PAQ and the Texas Social Behavior Inventory, which measures self-esteem to a sample of upper-middle-class men and women. They found that "the androgynous men and women were highest in mean self-esteem, followed within each sex by masculine, feminine and undifferentiated." This is essentially the same pattern of findings as Spence and Helmreich's.[46]

However, the causal relationship between sex-role orientation and self-esteem is not clear. Some others[72,74] argue that masculinity is associated with self-esteem rather than femininity or androgyny:

> Present findings suggest that it would be only among women that increased personal satisfaction would be associated with the androgynous person's increased flexibility to engage in cross-sex behaviors.[74]

Androgyny has been linked to mental health in a variety of ways other than general self-esteem, though research reports show conflicting findings. Silvern and Ryan,[74] using the BSRI, found no significant difference between their androgynous and sex-typed students on perceived mental health. In another study androgynous subjects showed higher self-esteem and lower general maladjustment and psychosis than those who were sex-typed.[70]

Jones, Chernovetz, and Hansson[72] specifically tested the hypothesis that androgyny is related to mental health. They predicted that androgynous individuals would show (a) less neurosis, (b) more extroversion, (c) an internal locus of control, (d) higher self-esteem, and (e) fewer alcohol-related problems. They were unable to confirm their hypotheses. In general, masculine sex-role identity for both men and women was associated with positive mental health.

Positive coping strategies are also believed to be correlated with androgyny. Allgeier, Przybyla, and Ruth[75] found that androgynous men and women scored higher than those who were sex-typed in self-actualization, self-regard, and synergy. Berzins, Welling, and Wetter[48] showed that androgynous subjects have greater interpersonal competence and transsituational adaptability than those who were sex-typed. Spence and Helmreich[46] found that the androgynous high school students in their sample had higher achievement motivation than their sex-typed counterparts.

In sum, though a few studies have shown a positive relationship between androgyny and some positive life outcomes, the evidence is at this point inconclusive. The data are confounded by a myriad of methodologic and sample problems; nevertheless, the most serious question is reflected in the title of Silvern and Ryan's paper "Self-rated Adjustment and Sex-typing on the Bem Sex-Role Inventory: Is Masculinity the Primary Predictor of Adjustment?"[74]

There is, at least in Western society, an identification of feminine traits with mental illness. Passivity, dependency, submissiveness, and selflessness are not positively evaluated in our culture. Thus, people who see themselves as dependent and selfless will tend to have low-esteem even if they are women. Highly feminine women suffer a double burden; they have low self-esteem because they possess traits which are negatively evaluated, and they are incapable of functioning well in other than a sheltered environment.

On the other hand, male traits are generally highly valued. Competitiveness, independence, self-reliance, and a certain amount of aggressiveness are admired characteristics and also rewarded. Belote[76] has charged that most clinicians' view of a normal female closely parallels the description of a hysterical personality, whereas the characteristics of a normal male are those of the ideal mature adult. Perhaps de Beauvoir said it best: "Man is defined as a human being and women as a female; whenever she behaves as a human being she is said to imitate a male."[77]

Thus, some investigators argue that androgyny is associated with positive mental health for women because they are "taking on" highly valued male attributes:

> Androgyny vs. traditional sex typing was associated with superior adjustment only among women and only insofar as androgyny was associated with high masculinity. Present findings suggest that it would be only among women that increased personal satisfaction would be associated with the androgynous person's increased flexibility to engage in cross-sex behavior.[74]

Harrington and Andersen[78] found that their subjects who were highly masculine had much stronger creative self-concepts than either their androgynous or feminine counterparts. The authors refer to this as a "masculine advantage."

This masculine advantage is espeically important in business, where the ideal manager has been sterotypically portrayed as having strongly masculine characteristics—The Marlboro Man in the Boardroom. Sargent,[79] in a recent article, argued the advantages of androgyny for managers. Ideally, the androgynous manager could be both forceful and submissive, outspoken and softspoken, depending on the situation. In a recent study, Powell and Butterfield[80] asked 684 business students to identify the characteristics of a good manager. Not unsurprisingly, the good manager was described in strongly masculine terms. Both the relatively young undergraduates and the older graduate students thought the ideal manager ought to have only masculine traits. The graduate women also thought of themselves as having masculine traits in contrast to the undergraduate female students who saw themselves as having mostly feminine traits. Powell and Butterfield believe that the female graduate students adopt masculine traits because they realize that these attributes are necessary for survival and advancement in business.

Because the scientific study of androgyny is in its adolescence,[41] new research on androgyny's relationship to psychosocial adjustment is both sparse and contradictory. The major problems may be summarized as (1) lack of theoretical foundation, which is reflected in scale construction, (2) sampling limitations, and (3) cross-sectional research designs. A few review articles[41,81,71] focus on the crucial problem of sex-role research—lack of theoretical foundation on which to construct scales which actually measure sex-role orientation:

> A substantial portion of manuscripts on sex-role issues fail to explicate a theoretical foundation for the research. This is especially true when a variety of tests or measures are administered. Frequently, little consideration is given to the constructs being measured and their proposed relationship to any sex role theory. In particular default are studies that take a "one-shot" or a "statistical dragnet" approach.[71]

Because of this lack of theoretical foundation, scale items are drawn from traditional sex-role stereotypes. Consequently, a person classed as androgynous possesses (or more accurately views him/herself as possessing) an equal number of stereotypic masculine and feminine traits.

Money,[82] in his provocative new book, suggests an approach that might lead sex-role investigators out of the cul-de-sac into which they have marched. Money[82] asserts that "It should be self-evident that masculine and feminine should be used as mutually exclusive only as in the saying that it is masculine to impregnate and feminine to menstruate, gestate and lactate." However, Money does say that though men and women share the capacity to perform most behaviors, the thresholds for triggering certain behaviors vary by sex.

Researchers might begin by identifying and classifying "basic phyletic mechanisms," and Money[82] lists nine such behaviors which are sex shared but threshold dimorphic: (1) general kinesis; (2) competition; (3) territory marking; (4) defense against intruders; (5) guarding of the young; (6) nesting; (7) care of the young; (8) sexual mounting vs. spreading; and (9) erotic dependence on visual stimuli vs. tactile stimuli. If these nine behaviors complexes are sex shared but threshold dimorphic, then investigators have a basis for constructing scales which reflect behavior in the real world.

Using this approach, androgyny could have several bases. The threshold needed to elicit masculine and feminine behaviors might be highly similar for the androgynous individual. Also, in spite of threshold levels, the androgynous person may choose to engage in typically masculine and feminine behaviors equally.

On the other hand, androgyny might come to represent the attempts of individuals to live more balanced and harmonious lives. These persons may choose to integrate the Yin and Yang, the Animus and Anima, or Communion and Agency. By integrating these disparate congeries of attitudes, values, and behaviors, androgynous persons may lead the vanguard into a new society as envisioned by Jung, Bakan, and others. The available options are the subject of the concluding section.

ALTERNATIVE FUTURES

As mentioned in the beginning of this chapter, androgyny has become something of a movement. Lenny[41] sees some investigators' ideological commitment to the concept and associated lifestyles as a danger to scientific research on the subject as some researchers are so determined to find androgyny beneficial that they allow their biases to prejudice their research designs.

In this section the authors will briefly sketch a few possible alternative futures. Too many factors impinge on social reality to make firm predictions. Social class, region, ethnicity, and religion all independently affect sex-role expectations and behavior. For example, using time budget data, Boles and Tatro[83] showed that in contrast to a national sample of men, their sample of Southern blue collar workers spent fewer hours per week performing household tasks traditionally viewed as female, such as, sweeping and child care. The Southern factory workers were also less liberal than the national sample in their view of women's role in contemporary society.

Not only do demographic and socioeconomic variables make predictions difficult, but events such as depressions and wars affect our sex-role expectations. Within our large-range heterogeneous society, there are those who are experimenting with new lifestyles and equal numbers who long for a return to the "good old days when men were men."

ANDROGYNY: PRESCRIPTION FOR LIVING. Some individuals are already adopting androgyny as a foundation for lifestyle innovations. Many have made the conscious effort to become androgynous, but they have been acting either alone or with one person with whom they are living. One 35-year-old marketing executive described his and his wife's "experiment":

> We had been doing the typical thing—you know—"I'm the man; you're the woman." We started reading, Jung for one. We both made a commitment to try to become androgynous. Though both of us have learned to do new things (my wife took a course in auto repair), we have concentrated on new ways of thinking. I'm trying to get away from old mind-sets: "I must be strong; I must control the situation, etc." It's hard. I backslide often, but my wife and I are committed to this. We feel more of a wholeness and sharing now. Neither of us would go back to what we were before.

Though this couple has shared their goals with a few friends, they are not interested in joining a group or being part of a movement. Yet, springing up around the country are movements organized around androgyny. Probably the best known is the Androgyny Center in San Diego. This center publishes a magazine and sponsored an international symposium.[84] The organization's views of androgyny are broader than that of most sex-role researchers. A list of symposium workshop titles give a picture of the issues considered part of the androgyny movement: left/right brain functioning, androgyny's effect on relationships, child-raising, sexuality, internal energy balancing, physical androgyny (rolfing, etc.), and experiencing the Anima/Animus. We would expect to see the formation of more organizations which seek to merge androgyny with a variety of innovative therapies and "new age" beliefs and rituals.

SEX ROLE TRANSCENDANCE: BEYOND MASCULINITY AND FEMININITY. There is a story told by Pearl Buck. While in New York City, she went out one day and left one of her adopted children at home. When she returned, she asked if anyone had come while she was gone. Her daughter replied, "yes, one person." Pearl Buck said, "Was the person Chinese?" The child replied, "I didn't notice." This is an example of race transcendence.

Are we ready for sex-role transcendence? This construct was first introduced by Hefner, Rebecca, and Oleshensky.[85] They point out (as has been discussed in this chapter) that androgyny postulates the organization of the personality in terms of masculine and feminine stereotypes. Sex role can be transcended and the personality built around other attributes.

Rebecca, Hefner, and Oleshensky[86] suggest the concept "sex role salience" to mean the extent to which individuals do or do not think of certain behaviors in terms of masculinity or femininity. For example, a woman or man might think of him or herself as nurturant or assertive—not feminine or masculine, but nurturant or assertive. The trait descriptors, e.g., strong, emotional, loving, etc., which we traditionally "code" as connoting either masculinity or femininity would no longer carry that meaning. Garnets and Pleck[87] clarify the meaning of this important concept:

> The second kind of change is illustrated by individuals no longer psychologically linking—even positively linking—emotional expressiveness and achievement (or any other psychological characteristics) with males and females by virtue of their sex. It is the difference between saying "it is alright and even desirable for men to be able to cry" and saying "crying (and all other behaviors as well) have nothing to do with whether or not a male is a man."

We are obviously a long way from sex-role transcendence. It would take the imagination of a Ray Bradbury to envisage a society in which sex-role transcendence was the norm. Yet, if we become more androgynous, we may move toward a transcendent society in which the two halves of the personality are reunited so that all of us can create a world in which agency and communion can coexist in each of us without our fearing that we are not after all *really* adequate men and women. The androgynous stage may be a stop on the path to "higher ground."

REFERENCES

1. Morgan M: The Total Woman. Old Tappan, New Jersey, Revell, 1973
2. Bazin NT, Freeman A: The androgynous vision. Women's Studies 2:185–215, 1974
3. Freud S: A General Introduction to Psycho-Analysis. New York, Pocket Books, 1970
4. Jung CG: Two essays on analytical psychology, in Collected Works, Vol. 7. New York, Pantheon Press, 1953
5. Money J, Ehrhardt A: Man and Woman, Boy and Girl. Baltimore, Johns Hopkins University Press, 1972
6. Hampson JL: Psychosexual determinants of differentiation, in Sex and Behavior. Edited by Beach FA. New York, Robert E. Drieger Publishing Company, 1974, pp 108–132
7. Kolhberg L: A Cognitive–developmental analysis of children's sex-role concepts and attitudes, in The Development of Sex Differences. Edited by Maccoby E. Stanford: Stanford University Press, 1966, pp 82–173
8. Emmerich W, Goldman KS, Sharabany R: Evidence for a transitional phase in the development of gender constancy. Child Dev 48:930–936, 1977
9. Constantinople A: Sex role acquisition: In search of the elephant. Sex Roles 5:121–133, 1979
10. Money J, Hampson J, Hampson J: Imprinting and the establishing of gender role. Arch Neurol Psychiatry 72:333–336, 1957
11. Block J: Conceptions of sex role: Some cross-cultural and longitudinal perspectives. Am Psychol 28:512–526, 1973
12. Freud S: A General Introduction to Psycho-Analysis. New York, Pocket Books, 1970
13. Pleck J: Masculinity–femininity: Current and alternative paradigms. Sex Roles 1:161–178, 1975
14. Brooks-Gunn J, Lewis M: Early social knowledge: Development of the knowledge about others, in Childhood Social Development. Edited by McGurk H. London, McThuen, 1978, pp 79–106
15. Thompson SK, Bentler PM: The priority of cues in sex discrimination by children and adults. Dev Psychol 5:181–185, 1971
16. Katcher A: The child's differential perception of parental attributes. Genetic Psychol 87:131–143, 1955
17. Sherman J: On the Psychology of Women: A Survey of Empirical Studies. Springfield, Charles C Thomas, 1971

18. Sears RR, Rau I, Alpert R: Identification and Child Rearing. Stanford, Stanford University Press, 1965
19. Lynn D: The process of learning parental and sex-role identification. J Marriage Fam 28:466–470, 1966
20. Kagan J: Acquisition and significance of sex typing and sex role identity, in Review of Child Development, Vol. I. Edited by Hoffman MM, Hoffman L. New York, Russell, 1964, pp 137–168
21. Brooks-Gunn J, Matthews WS: He and She: How Children Develop Their Sex-Role Identity. Englewood Cliffs, Prentice-Hall, 1979
22. Bandura A: Principles of Behavior Modification. New York, Holt, Reinhart, 1969
23. Maccoby E, Jacklin C: The Psychology of Sex Differences. Stanford, Stanford University Press, 1974
24. Davidson L, Gordon L: The Sociology of Gender. Chicago, Rand McNally, 1979
25. Matthews W: Sex-role perception, portrayal and preference in the fantasy play of young children. Resources in Education, Document No. ED 136949, U.S. Department of Education
26. Lever J: Sex differences in games children play. Social Problems 23:478–487, 1976
27. Chappel N: Work, Commitment to Work, and Self-Identity among Women. Unpublished Ph.D. dissertation. Hamilton, McMaster University, 1978
28. Kohlberg L: A cognitive–developmental analysis of children's sex-role concepts and attitudes, in The Development of Sex Differences. Edited by Maccoby E. Stanford, Stanford University Press, 1966, pp 82–173
29. Kohlberg L, Zigler E: The impact of cognitive maturity on the development of sex-role attitudes in the years 4 to 8. Genetic Psychol Monographs 75:89–165, 1967
30. Slaby RG, Frey KS: Development of gender constancy and selective attention to same sex models. Child Dev 46:849–856, 1975
31. Thompson SK, Bentler PM: The priority of cues in sex discrimination by children and adults. Dev Psychol 5:181–185, 1971
32. Chomsky N: Aspect of the Theory of Syntax. Cambridge, MIT Press, 1965
33. Levi-Strauss C: The Raw and the Cooked. Trans. by Weightmen J. New York, Harper and Row, 1969
34. Scheffler H: Structuralism in anthropology, in Structuralism. Edited by Ehrmann J. Garden City, New York, Doubleday, 1970, pp 56–79
35. Pleck J: The male sex role: Definitions, problems, and sources of change. J Soc Issues 32:155–164, 1976
36. Bakan D: The Duality of Human Existence. Chicago, Rand McNally, 1966
37. Loevinger J: The meaning and measurement of ego development. Am Psychol 21:195–206, 1966
38. Becker E: The Structure of Evil: As Essay on the Unification of the Science of Man. New York, Free Press, 1976
39. Bem SL: The measurement of psychological androgyny. J Consult Clin Psychol 42:155–162, 1974
40. Bem SL, Lenny E: Sex-typing and the avoidance of cross-sex behavior. J Personality Soc Psychol 33:48–54, 1976
41. Lenny E: Androgyny: Some audacious assertions towards its coming of age. Sex Roles 5:703–719, 1979
42. Kelly J, Furman W, Young V: Problems associated with the typological measurement of sex roles and androgyny. J Consult Clin Psychol 46:1574–1576, 1978
43. O'Grady K, Freda J, Mikulka P: A Comparison of the Adjective Check List, Bem Sex Role Inventory and the PAQ, Masculine and Feminine subscales. Multivariate Behav Res 14:215–255, 1979
44. Mischel W: Personality and Assessment. New York, Wiley, 1968
45. Spence J, Helmreich R, Stapp J: Ratings of self and peers on sex role attributes and their relation to self-esteem and conceptions of masculinity and femininity. J Personality Soc Psychol 32:29–39, 1975
46. Spence J, Helmreich R: Masculinity and Femininity: Their Psychological Dimensions, Correlates, and Antecedents. Austin, University of Texas Press, 1978

47. Spence J, Helmreich R: On assessing "androygyny." Sex Roles 5:721–738, 1979
48. Berzins J, Welling M, Wetter R: A new measure of psychological androgyny based on the personality research form. J Consult Clin Psychol 46:126–128, 1978
49. Heilbrun A: Measurement of masculine and feminine sex role identities as independent dimensions. J Consult Clin Psychol 44:183–190, 1976
50. Beere C: Women and Women's Issues: A Handbook of Tests and Measures. San Francisco, Jossey-Bass, 1979
51. Erikson E: Inner and outer space: Reflection on womanhood. Daedaulus 93:1–25, 1964
52. Parsons T, Bales R: Family, Socialization and Interaction Process. New York, Free Press, 1955
53. Witkin HA: Social conformity and psychological differentiation. Int Psychol 9:11–29, 1974
54. Grady K, Brannon, R, Pleck J: The Male Sex Role: A Selected and Annotated Bibliography. Rockville, Maryland, National Institute of Mental Health, 1979
55. David DS, Brannon R: The male sex role: Our culture's blueprint of manhood, and what it's done for us lately, in The Forty-Nine Percent Majority. Edited by David DS, Brannon R. Reading, Mass., Addison-Wesley, 1976, pp 1–48
56. Boles J, Tatro C: The new male model: Traditional or androgynous? Psychoanal 40(3):227–237, 1980
57. Cicone M, Ruble D: Beliefs about males. J Soc Issues 34:5–16, 1978
58. Turner R: Strains of Masculinity. Family Interaction. New York, Wiley, 1970
59. Jenkins N, Vroegh K: Contemporary concepts of masculinity and femininity. Psychol Rep 25:679–697, 1969
60. Tavris C, Offir C: The Longest War: Sex Differences in Perspective. New York, Harcourt Brace Jovanovich, 1977
61. Miller A: Death of a Salesman, Private Conversations in Two Acts and a Requiem. New York, Viking, 1949
62. Ganon J: Physical strength, once of significance, in The Forty-Nine Percent Majority: The Male Sex Roles. Edited by David DS, Brannon R. Reading, Massachusetts, Addison-Wesley, 1976, pp 169–178
63. Boulding E: Women in the Twentieth Century World. New York, Wiley, 1977
64. Chaftez J: Masculine, Feminine or Human? An Overview of the Sociology of Gender Roles, 2nd ed. Itasca, Illinois, Peacock, 1978
65. Stasz-Stoll C: Female and Male: Socialization, Social Roles and Social Structure, 2nd ed. Dubuque, Brown, 1978
66. Atkinson M, Boles J, Cassidy M: Ladies: South by northwest. Paper presented at the Mid-South Sociological Association Meetings, Memphis, Tennessee, 1979
67. Heilburn A: Measurement of masculine and feminine sex role identities as independent dimensions. J Consult Clin Psychol 44:183–190, 1976
68. Hoffman D, Fidell L: Characteristics of androgynous, undifferentiated, masculine and feminine middle-class women. Sex Roles 5:765–781, 1979
69. Kaplan AG: Clarifying the concept of androgyny: Implications for therapy. Paper presented at the Annual Meeting of the American Psychological Association, Washington, 1976
70. Nevill D: Sex-roles and personality correlates. Human Relations 30:751–759, 1977
71. Worrell J: Sex roles and psychological well-being: Perspectives on Methodology. Consult Clin Psychol 44:777–791, 1978
72. Jones WE, Chernovetz OC, Hansson R: The enigma of androgyny: Differential implications for males and females. J Consult Clin Psychol 46:298–313, 1978
73. O'Connor, Mann D, Bardwick J: Androgyny and self-esteem in the upper-middle class: A replication of Spence. J Consult Clin Psychol 46:1168–1169, 1978
74. Silvern L, Ryan V: Self-rated adjustment and the sex typing on the Bem Sex-Role Inventory: Is masculinity the primary predictor of adjustment? Sex Roles 5:739–763, 1979
75. Allgeier E, Przybyla DP, Ruth R: The relationship of androgyny to several indices of psychological functioning. Paper presented at the American Psychological Association Meetings, New York, September, 1979
76. Belote C: Masochistic syndrome, hysterical personality and the illusion of a healthy woman, in Female Psychology: The Emerging Self. Edited by Cox S. Chicago, Science Research Associates, 1976, pp 335–348

77. de Beauvoir S: The Second Sex. New York, Knopf, 1968
78. Harrington D, Anderson S: Creative self-concept, masculinity, femininity and three models of androgyny. Paper presented at meeting of the American Psychological Association, New York, September, 1979
79. Sargent A: The androgynous blend: Best of both worlds. Management Rev 67:60–68, 1978
80. Powell G. Butterfield DA: The "good manager": Masculine or androgynous? Acad Management 22:395–403, 1979
81. Kenworthy JA: Androgyny in psychotherapy: But will it sell in Peoria? Psychol Women Quart 3:321–340, 1979
82. Money J: Love and Love Sickness: The Science of Sex, Gender Difference, and Pair-Bonding. Baltimore, Johns Hopkins University Press, 1980
83. Boles J, Tatro C: The male sex role: Continuity and change. Paper read at the Annual Meeting of the American Psychiatric Association, Chicago, 1980
84. Schonbrook JA: Androgyny Review, Vol. I, 1979
85. Hefner RM, Rebecca M, Oleshansky B: Development of sex role transcendence. Human Dev 18:143–156, 1975
86. Rebecca M, Hefner R, Oleshansky B: A model of sex-role transcendance. J Soc Issues 32:197–206, 1976
87. Garnets L, Pleck J: Sex role identity, androgyny, and sex role transcendance: A sex role strain analysis. Psychol Women Quart 3:270–283, 1979
88. Conn JH, Kanner L: Children's awareness of sex differences. Child Psychiat 1:3–57, 1947
89. Rabban M: Sex role identification in young children in two diverse social groups. Genetic Psychol Monographs 42:81–158, 1950
90. Brooks-Gunn J, Lewis M: Why mama and papa? The development of social labels. Child Dev 50(4):1203–1206, 1979
91. Morgan GA, Ricciuti HN: Infants' responses to strangers during the first year, in Determinants of Infant Behavior, Vol. 4. Edited by Foss BM. London, Methuen, 1969, pp 253–272
92. Scarr S, Salapatek P: Patterns of fear development during infancy. Merrill-Palmer Quart 16:53–90, 1970
93. Culp RE: Visual fixation and the effect of male versus female voice quality. Paper presented at the Society for Research on Child Development meetings, New Orleans, Louisiana, March, 1977
94. Brazelton TB, Koslowski BL, Main M: The origins of reciprocity: The early mother–infant interaction: The effect of the infant on its caregiver. New York, Wiley-Interscience, 1974, pp 49–76
95. Brooks-Gunn J, Lewis M: Early social knowledge, in Childhood Social Development. Edited by McGurk H. London, McThuen, 1979, pp 79–106
96. Katcher A: The child's differential perception of parental attributes. J Genetic Psychol 87:131–143, 1955
97. Slaby RG, Frey KS: Development of gender constancy and selective attention to same sex models. Child Dev 46:849–856, 1975
98. Lewis M, Brooks G: Infant's social perception: A constructivist's view, in Infant Perception: From Sensation to Cognition, Vol. 2. Edited by Cohen LB, Salapatek P. New York, Academic Press, 1975, pp 101–143
99. Lewis M, Brooks-Gunn J: Social Cognition and the Acquisition of Self. New York, Plenum, 1979
100. Gesell A, Halverson HM, Ilg FL, et al.: The First Five Years of Life: A Guide to the Study of Preschool Child. New York, Harper, 1940
101. Weinraub M, Leite J: Sex typed toy preference and knowledge of sex role stereotypes and two year old children. Paper presented at the Annual Meetings of Eastern Psychological Association, Boston, Apr 1977
102. Hampson JL, Hampson JG: The ontogenesis of sexual behavior in man, in Sex and Internal Secretions. Edited by Young WC. Baltimore, Wilkins and Wilkins, 1961, pp 1401–1432
103. Carr A: Forced attention to specific applicant qualifications: Impact of on physical attractiveness and sex-of-applicant biases. Personnel Psychol 34(1):65–75, 1981

Chapter 5

Male Inexpressiveness

Psychological and Social Aspects

JACK O. BALSWICK

> Another thing I learned—if *you* cry, the audience won't. A man can cry for his horse, for his dog, for another man, but he cannot cry for a woman. A strange thing. He can cry at the death of a friend or a pet. But where he's supposed to be boss, with his child or wife, something like that, he better hold 'em back and let *them* cry.
>
> John Wayne[1]

INTRODUCTION

Manhood has traditionally been defined not only in terms of what "real" men should do, but also in terms of what a real man would *not* be caught doing. Inexpressiveness is one of the characteristics of males which has traditionally been defined in negative terms. An expressive male is simply one who has feelings and verbally expresses them. An inexpressive male is one who does not verbally express his feelings, either because he has no feelings or because he has been socialized not to. Another way to think of inexpressiveness is as the lack of affective self-disclosure (see Chapter 16, by Dosser).

In developing the concept of male inexpressiveness the author has developed a typology of inexpressive male roles. Given the temptation to use typologies as excuses to stereotype persons, the author presents this typology as types of inexpressive male *roles* and not as types of inexpressive males. As can be seen in Table I, male inexpressiveness can be categorized on the basis of three criteria: (1) in terms of whether or not feelings are present; (2) in terms of whether or not there is an attempt to pretend to express feelings; and (3) whether the potential object of expressiveness is a female or a male. Three clusters of inexpressive male roles can be identified, each containing two inexpressive roles. The expressive male roles are contained in the upper left-hand

JACK O. BALSWICK • Department of Pastoral and Family Ministries, Fuller Theological Seminary, Pasadena, California

Table I. Types of Inexpressive Males' Roles

		Feeling	Nonfeeling
Verbal	Towards females	Expressive male (Parlor-room boy)	Playboy
	Towards males	Expressive male (Locker-room boy)	Con boy
Nonverbal	Towards females	Cowboy	Locker-room boy (as seen by females)
	Towards males	Good ol' boy	Parlor-room boy (as seen by males)

cell of Table I. In the lower left-hand cell are contained the feeling, nonverbal inexpressive male roles, in the upper right-hand cell are contained the nonfeeling, verbal inexpressive male roles; and in the lower right-hand cell are the nonfeeling nonverbal inexpressive male roles. Since descriptions of each of the inexpressive male roles are given in detail elsewhere,[2] I shall only bother to briefly summarize each role here.

A male who has feelings and verbally expresses those feelings towards both females and males can be considered a totally expressive male. However, some males are expressive towards males and not expressive towards females (locker-room boys), while others are expressive towards females and not expressive towards males (parlor-room boys). As seen by females, some men are locker-room boys because although they may be expressive of their feelings towards other men in the security of the certain "masculine" subcultures, they certainly are not expressive to them. Being dependent upon such masculine subcultures as men's athletic clubs, sports teams, bars, and gaming rooms, masculine identity is secure and the locker-room boy is able to express his more gentle feelings and even physical affection.

After a few beers at the neighborhood tavern, men who have spent the day working in a factory will begin to share their feelings and concerns with each other in a way which does not take place between them and their wives.[3–6] In the locker room athletes will enthusiastically embrace and hug each other following a victory, or openly weep following a defeat. Following the final defeat in the 1976 World Series baseball games, Billy Martin, then the fiery manager of the New York Yankees, announced to the media that he *loved* his ball players. The next year, after the Yankees had just won the world series, Billy Martin and Reggie Jackson (who had been feuding all year) sat before the cameras of national television with their arms around each other proclaiming their affection for each other for the world to hear. Since the athlete's masculinity has been established through his physical prowess, he is free to *be* expressive of his feelings without himself or the spectators questioning his masculinity. The locker-room boy is both more comfortable and also more able to share his feelings with certain other men in sufficiently "masculine" environments.

The parlor-room boy feels more comfortable in expressing feelings towards females than towards males. Research would suggest that a male's greater ability to relate to females may originate in the home, as fathers have been found to be less expressive toward their male children than towards their female children.[7–9] Johnson[9] has noted that while mothers have an expressive attitude to male and female children indiscriminantly, fathers are expressive with their daughters and instrumental with their sons. There is also much within the male subculture which can encourage a male to take on the parlor-room boy role—competitiveness, power grabbing, aggressiveness, and general striving towards one-upmanship. The male who comes to have a fear and distrust of other males or who takes on an insufficient quantity of these "masculine" traits may find himself more comfortable in relating to females than to males. The author's research and classroom conversation with students would suggest that many college coeds function in a "sisterly" relationship with males on campus, and become the "confidant" of men needing to share disappointments over broken romances, discouragements with school, or concerns which are thought too sensitive to share with another male. There is less fear in "spilling one's guts" to a female. The fear that another male cannot be trusted with intimate revelations in a nonexploitive way leads to the use of the parlor-room boy role.

Represented in the lower left-hand side of Table I are two less complicated types of inexpressive male roles. Feeling, nonverbal males learn to play the role of a cowboy towards females and the role of the good ol' boy towards males. Perhaps the best portrayal of the cowboy can be seen in any one of the typecast strong, silent, rugged he-man roles as played by John Wayne. Around women Wayne appeared to be uncomfortable, often unable to speak, especially if he really cared for the woman. Wayne appeared to be more comfortable around his horse than around "his woman." Instead of a forthright pronouncement of "I really love you, darling," any display of affection was likely to be disguised. It should be stressed that the cowboy has strong emotional feelings of affection towards women, children, and even other men, *but* they are never expressed directly.

Although the term "good ol' boy" is primarily a Southern expression, the mass media's portrait of President Carter's brother, Billy, sitting in his service station drinking beer and swapping stories with his male friends has done much to popularize the term. Good ol' boy relationships typically must be cultivated during childhood and nurtured through the trials and triumphs of growing up into manhood. The good ol' boy is completely loyal to the other good ol' boys, who together form a strong in-group or primary group which makes it hard for an outsider to enter. A good ol' boy is one who can be counted on during a time of trouble. He is one who will stick with you "through thick and through thin," and would give you the "shirt off his back" if you were in need.

While conversation may take up much of the good ol' boys' time together, talk usually centers around such topics as the weather, sports, politics, or women, and rarely involves communication of personal feelings to each other. If asked why he did not talk about his feelings the good ol' boy is likely to reply that it is not necessary, that if you have to say it, then it must not be there, or that the expression of feelings is a "womanly" trait. Good ol' boys are men of *action;* they show their love and affection for each other in their enduring friendship. The man who is overly verbally expressive of his feelings is likely to be joked about as one who is "sissy" or "feminine," or as one who lacks "manliness."

Good ol' boy roles are both fostered *by* and the perpetrators *of* a male subculture. This subculture is a storehouse of folk philosophy, humor, wisdom, stereotypes, etc. which is transmitted to small boys as they begin to learn the good ol' boy role. Not only does this common storehouse of memory make it unnecessary for good ol' boys to cement their relationships through expressing verbal affection, but it also renders it nearly impossible for a woman, or even a male outsider, to become a part of this good ol' boy subculture.

A glance at the top right-hand corner of Table I will reveal the names of the two remaining inexpressive male roles. The playboy, in relating to females, and the con boy in relating to males, is void of feelings for the person he is relating to, and thus becomes skilled at pretending to express "feelings." As reflected in the philosophy of his namesake, Playboy magazine, a playboy is a skilled manipulator of women, knowing when to turn the lights down, which drinks to serve, what music to play on the stereo, what topics of conversation to engage in, all calculated to get the woman to bed, and emerge free from any emotional investment in the relationship. In relating to women the playboy may be comparable to Fromm's description of a marketing-oriented personality[10] in which a person comes to see himself and others as persons to be manipulated and exploited. The playboy reduces sexuality to a packageable consumption item which he can handle because it demands no responsibility.

A film version of the playboy would be James Bond. As Bond interacts with women it is with a cool air of detachment, where the women fall passionately in love with Bond, but he remains above it all. A clinical interpretation of James Bond's behavior might even go so far as to question the security of the masculine identity of a man who seems to have a quest to sexually conquer every woman he encounters.

In relationships with other men the con boy role is used to describe the types of manipulative behavior we associate with that of the "con man," "con artist," or "wheeler-dealer" in our society. The con boy becomes a skilled manipulator of other males by means of his ability to convince them that he really likes and cares for them. In the competitive structure of much of the work-a-day world, males learn both that the "techniques" of selling involve flattering and building up the ego of a would-be client, and to be on guard against such manipulative behavior on the part of other males.

Con boys are even able to ethically justify their behavior through membership in male subcultures which rationalize about the manipulation of other men by coming to believe that the "sucker" or naive "mark" deserves to be taken advantage of. The skilled con boy may even achieve status in such a subculture because of his reputation as a skilled manipulator of others. The ethics and philosophy behind the con boy role is that of a modified type of rugged frontier individualist who makes it to the top on his own. The con boy models his behavior after the equally hard working folk hero who had to scheme, connive, and sometimes "claw" his way to the top. The fact that many men report that they feel suspicious of and have a hard time trusting other men may be indicative of the extent to which the con boy role is utilized by males in our society.

EVIDENCE OF EXPRESSIVE DIFFERENCES BETWEEN GENDERS

At this point the reader may be thinking, well, this is all very interesting, but why make so much of inexpressiveness among males, for after all, this appears to be a universal human characteristic? In attempting to answer this question it is necessary to look at some of the accumulated evidence which is suggestive of less emotional expressiveness among males.

The issue is not so much whether there are differences in emotional expressiveness between the sexes, but rather what the nature of these differences is and when they emerge. The literature on sex differences among children leads to the conclusion that young girls and boys are not greatly different in their emotional expressiveness. In their exhaustive search of the literature on the nature of psychological differences between females and males, Maccoby and Jacklin[11] leave the question of the greater emotional expressiveness on the part of girls as inconclusive and open to question. Meador[12] has recently attempted to assess the nature of expressiveness differences between 7–8-year-old girls and boys, utilizing a revision of the Expression of Emotion Scale. She found that girls and boys do not differ significantly in the expression of love, hate, happiness, or sadness.

Studies indicate, however, that by the time children reach high school age, females and males are significantly different in the expression of feelings. Based upon a sample of 1190 high-school-age students, Balkwell, Balswick, and Balkwell[13] found that females score higher than males in the expression of fondness, pleasure, and sadness, whereas males are more expressive than females in verbalizing antipathy. Based upon a sample of 523 college aged students, Balswick and Avertt[14] found that while females are more expressive than males of love, happiness, and sadness, there was not a significant difference between the sexes in the expression of hate. Based upon experimental research utilizing college students as subjects, Allen and Haccoun[15] found that women were consistently more expressive of their feelings than were men. Jourard and his associates have consistently found that men reveal less personal information about themselves than do women.[16–19] Studying the disclosure of feelings in marriage, Levinger and Senn[20] found that wives disclose a greater proportion of feelings than their husbands. Other studies which have focused on affective self-disclosure have also found that females express more feelings than males.[21,22] In attempting to ascertain the effect of situational factors upon gender differences in expressing feelings, Highlen and Gillis[23] and Highlen and Johnston[24] report that females disclosed more feelings than males to best male and female friends regardless of the acquaintance intimacy level.

The evidence seems to be consistent that there are differences in emotional expressiveness by gender which closely correspond to the sex-role stereotyping literature. Females are stereotyped as being more expressive of "feminine" feelings like love, tenderness, happiness, joy, and sadness, and males are stereotyped as being more expressive of such masculine feelings as anger, rage, hate, and resentment. The emerging literature on actual expressiveness suggests that each sex is behaving according to its sex-role stereotype.

EXPLANATIONS OF MALE INEXPRESSIVENESS

To ascertain differences in expressiveness between the sexes is one thing, to explain why there are differences is quite another. Given the limited amount of attention which has been given to gender differences in expressiveness, explanatory theories are still to be developed. What follows are brief statements of representative perspectives which might prove to be fruitful theories of male inexpressiveness.

ROLE THEORY.[25] As a theoretical offspring of symbolic interactionism, role theory is more of an organizing framework or theoretical orientation than it is substantive theory of behavior. Although the concept "role" has been utilized in various sociological and social psychological approaches, the symbolic interactionist's use of "role" places a more dynamic and evolving emphasis on the concept than do other theories. Turner[26] for example, suggested that the idea of "role-taking" shifts emphasis away from the simple process of enacting a prescribed role to devising a performance on the basis of an imputed other role. Interpretation, then, is a key variable, and as Blumer[27] pointed out, should not be regarded as a mere automatic application of established meanings but, rather, as a formative process in which meanings are used and revised as instruments for the guidance or formation of action.

Turner[28] has proposed three essential principles of role theory, which are paraphrased as follows: (a) that clusters of activities are assigned to a given role and once an individual assumes that role he should not dabble in the activities of another person's role; (b) that once a system of roles is developed, social interaction proceeds haltingly unless people play their perspective roles; and (c) that persons take the role of others in order to determine what role to play themselves and how to play it.

In our society, the male role has been imbued with activities which call for task achievement skills rather than emotional skills. As traditionally defined, the adult female role usually includes activities centered in the home and involves the emotional skills of caring for children, whereas the adult male role carries an expectation to earn a living by working outside of the home in occupations which require rational decision making and nonemotional involvement with others.[29] The adult female's dominant role carries with it expressive expectations, while the adult male's role carries with it inexpressive expectations.

This is not to suggest, however, that male inexpressiveness appears only when a male reaches adulthood. Male inexpressiveness is based upon a lifelong institutionally based socialization process which begins in infancy when girls are taught to act "feminine" and to desire "feminine" objects, and boys are taught how to be "manly." In learning to be a man, the boy in our society comes to value expressions of masculinity and devalue expressions of femininity. Masculinity is expressed largely through physical courage, toughness, competitiveness, and aggressiveness; whereas femininity is, by contrast, expressed largely through gentleness, expressiveness, and responsiveness. The male child learns that expressing emotions is not a part of the male role.

Nearly 20 years ago, Hartley[30] and others [31–33] demonstrated that families press these demands early in childhood and frequently enforce them harshly, so that by the time male children reach kindergarten, many feel "virtual panic at being caught doing anything traditionally defined as feminine, as in hostility toward anything even hinting at 'femininity,' including females themselves."[30]

As the male child moves out from under the family umbrella and into the sphere of male peer groups, the taboo against expressing feelings characteristic of females is reinforced. According to studies of the male subculture in schools,[34,35] street corner male groups,[36–38] and delinquent gangs,[39–42] to be affectionate, gentle, and compassionate toward others is not to be "one of the boys." It is to misplay the male role. The mass media seem to convey a similar message. From comics and cartoons through the more "adult" fare, the image of the male role does not usually include affectionate, gentle, tender, or soft-hearted behavior.

Confronted with the image projected by this powerful triumvirate of the family, peer group, and mass media, most young males quickly learn that whatever masculine behavior is, it is not an expression of gentleness, tenderness, verbal affection or similar emotions. Not expressing these types of emotions fits in with other traits of the male role by helping the male avoid "sissylike" displays of behavior, while correspondingly permitting open displays of anger, hostility, resentment, or rage—which are seen as distinctly "masculine." Such selective avoidance of emotional expressiveness is built into the male role which males begin to learn early in life, but which is also reinforced by numerous socializing agents in situations throughout life.

This is to suggest that inexpressiveness is not merely the result of personality traits, but also of life situations, of the roles one is taught to play in society. But again, inexpressiveness is not only a result of the situation, for a male is also influenced by his own view of himself in terms of his role and role performance. Male inexpressiveness is best understood in terms of a male's conception of himself, his perception of the role of the potential target person, and his perception of the potential target person's expectation of him.

FUNCTIONAL-CONFLICT THEORY.[43] As a response to the author's earlier writings, Sattel[43] has suggested that male inexpressiveness might better be understood in terms of sexual politics. What Sattel means by sexual politics is, in actuality, a functional-conflict theory in which male inexpressiveness results from the "instrumental requisites of the male power role."[43] Sattel argues that to wield power effectively, one must convince others that one's decisions are based upon reason and not emotion. Within such a system, the most powerful male is the one who can most soundly convince himself and others that he has divested himself, or the role he plays, of any vestiges of emotion.

Sattell[43] succinctly summarized his explanation within three propositions.

His first proposition (Proposition A) states that "*Inexpressiveness* in a role is determined by the corresponding *power* (actual or potential) of that role." The more powerful the role, the more one will resort to an appearance of rationality and efficiency, as opposed to emotionality, as an attempt to convince others that one's decisions are right. Thus, when an army general or a president of a large corporation announces an important decision, it will be done with an air of emotional detachment. Boys are socialized to be inexpressive because, later as men, they will be expected to be decision makers and wielders of power. The implication contained within Sattel's first proposition is that "inexpressiveness is not just learned as an end in itself; rather it is learned as a means to be implemented later in men assuming and maintaining positions of power."

Sattel's second proposition (Proposition B) states that "Male *expressiveness* in a sexist culture empirically emerges as an effort on the part of the male to *control* a situation (once again, on his terms) and to maintain his position." In this proposition, Sattel is reacting to the suggestion that inexpressive males may learn to become expressive to their wives within the intimacy demands of marriage.[44] Picking up on the suggestion that males might only be situationally inexpressive, rather than totally inexpressive, Sattel described situations of male expressiveness as attempts at controlling the situation. Male expressiveness may be

> a way of "coming on" with a woman—a relaxation of usual standards of inexpressiveness as a calculated move to establish a sexual relationship. Skill at dissembling in this situation may have less to do with handing a woman a "line" than showing one's weaknesses and frailties as clues intended to be read by her as signs of authentic male interest.

Thus, even those instances of male expressiveness which may appear on the surface to be authentic can actually be attempts by the male to control the situation.

Sattel's third proposition (Proposition C) states that "male *inexpressiveness* empirically emerges as an intentional manipulation of situations when threats to the male position occur." Males are not inexpressive because they are unable to express their feelings, but because they *choose* to be inexpressive. The motivating force behind being inexpressive is to be secure and maintain power.

Perhaps as a reaction to what he felt to be a needed corrective to the author's explanations of male inexpressiveness, Sattel has stressed: (a) the harm which male inexpressiveness does to the female rather than to the male; and (b) the intentional rather than the unintentional aspects of male expressiveness (Proposition B) and that the motivation behind inexpressive behavior is desire for power (Proposition C).

COMPLEMENTARY THEORY. As a reaction to the author's role theory L'Abate[45] has argued that male inexpressiveness can best be understood as a complementary reaction to women's overexpressiveness. In failing to find sex differences in research on conflict resolution methods, L'Abate[45] concludes that males and females do not differ in emotional expressiveness. Besides, he argues, his clinical experience would suggest that in 20%–30% of the couples it is the male rather than the female who is more expressive. Very simply put, L'Abate believes that an overexpressive female results in an inexpressive male; presumably when one partner is overexpressive, the other partner will correspondingly be less expressive. In reality, L'Abate's complementary theory suggests that expressiveness must be understood in the context of the dyadic relationship in which behavior occurs.

THE REPRODUCTION OF MOTHERING. In her book, *The Reproduction of Mothering: Psychoanalysis and the Sociology of Gender,* Chodorow[46] manages to present a point of view from a Freudian theoretical perspective which is, at the same time, consistent with feminist thinking. Although Chodorow does not directly present a theory of male inexpressiveness, such a theory is implied in her writing. Chodorow believes that women, rather than men, do most of the parenting as a result of social-structurally induced psychological mechanisms, rather than as an unmediated product of physiology. While women come to mother because they have been mothered by women, the fact that men are mothered by women reduces their parenting capacities. This also results in a different process of maturation in boys than in girls. While both boys and girls begin their lives with an emotional attachment to their mother, boys must learn to identify with their father by denying attachment to their mother. On the other hand girls can continue both their identity with and attachment to their mother.

The nature of a girl's relationship to her mother and the nature of a boy's relationship to his father are significantly different. While the girl is likely to be involved in a personal face-to-face relationship with her mother in the home, the fact that the father is likely to be absent from the home for periods of time means that the boy must derive notions about masculinity from his mother and the culture at large in the absence of an ongoing personal relationship with his father. This results in girls having more of an interactional orientation to the family, while boys receive more of an external orientation from the family.

The close ties which girls have with their mothers will mean that they will most likely desire to be nurturing mothers. Since boys are not closely tied to their fathers, and they deny their attachment to their mother for the sake of their own masculinity, their resulting behavior as fathers will be characterized by emotional distance between themselves and their children. Since fathers are the primary masculine role models for their boys, this emotional distancing behavior will be emulated by their sons. This is to suggest that the same process that produces mothering in girls, produces distancing and inexpressiveness in boys.

Male inexpressiveness is further reinforced by the fact that mothers often turn to their children as potential sources of unfulfilled emotional and erotic desires. As Chodorow[46] states, "Sons may become substitutes for husbands, and must engage in defensive assertion of ego boundaries and repression of emotional needs." Chodorow also believes that, "the very fact of being mothered by a woman generates in men conflicts over masculinity, a psychology of male dominance, and a need to be superior to women."

Although this brief attempt to "abstract" a theory of male inexpressiveness out of Chodorow's insightful writing does not do justice to the richness of her explanations, it does demonstrate how male inexpressiveness might be explained within a psychoanalytic perspective. Although this suggestion is subject to debate, it might be that if Freud were asked to explain male inexpressiveness, he would give a little more credit to the influences of genetically acquired differences between the sexes than does Chodorow.

CONSEQUENCES OF MALE INEXPRESSIVENESS

It is possible to take a functionalist approach and argue that male inexpressiveness is indeed functional to existing societal and familial patterns of relationships. It is the author's contention, however, that male inexpressiveness nearly always presents an obstacle to persons attempting to develop intimate, meaningful relationships to the greatest extent possible. This is not to deny that there may be some positive consequences which are a result of male inexpressiveness, given the existing societal and cultural normative patterns. However, the author is committed to the position that, in the best of all possible worlds, both sexes benefit from the ability to freely and verbally express their feelings.

MALES THEMSELVES. Perhaps the greatest toll of emotional inexpressiveness is upon the inexpressive males themselves, because they are robbed of potentially rich emotional experiences. The personal tragedy in emotional inexpressiveness was illustrated clearly to the author one Saturday afternoon while his wife and he were attending a film version of Shakespeare's *Romeo and Juliet.* The roles of Romeo and Juliet were being played by sixteen-year-old youths; thus, the matinee performance was crowded with high school students. At the very tragic and serious death scene, when his wife and he had lumps in their throats and tears in their eyes, they were surprised to hear the sniffs of most females accompanied by loud guffaws from the adolescent boys. Obviously, the emotional impact was being sidetracked and expressed in a reactional manner to cover up the sad and tender emotions which were not "cool" for adolescent males to express.

It can be physically and psychologically unhealthy for a person to not release and express emotions. Physically, the inability to cry and express emotions is thought to be related to the development of various physical symptoms. Psychologically, the holding in of emotions can result in a person's not being in touch with his or her feelings, which leads to not being in touch with oneself. Articulating feelings helps us become aware of the emotions so that we can learn how to best deal with them. When we do not articulate what we feel, there is an uncertainty about the feelings. Just as talking over a problem with someone is a way to get a better understanding of that problem, so articulating emotions forces us to conceptualize what is being felt.

MALE FRIENDS. Men are less able than women to relate in an open, verbally expressive way to the same sex. There are two aspects of male inexpressiveness which may contribute to this, homophobia and competition. Homophobia is the fear of being close to a person of the same sex. American males show many signs of their fear of being branded homosexual or of having homosexual tendencies. Generally, the more secure a man is in his sexuality the more open he can be in relating to a member of the same sex. The man who is secure in his own masculinity can put his arms around another man or verbally express his affection to him. Although most males would probably deny that they are "skin hungry," they often have needs to be physically stroked and held. James Kirkwood, in his play, *P.S., Your Cat Is Dead!* captures the essence of this in an interchange between two male characters in his play:

> One evening about three months into our friendship, after we'd taken our dates home, we stopped by a bar for a nightcap. We ended up having three or four and when we left and were walking down the street, Pete suddenly slipped his arm around my shoulder. He surprised me; there was extreme warmth and intimacy about the gesture. When I looked over at him, he grinned and said, "That bother you?" "No . . ." I shrugged in return. He then gave my shoulder a squeeze. "Ever since I've known you, you got me pretending I don't have arms."[47]

Compared to other cultures of the world, American males are very undemonstrative and inhibited about showing love to someone of the same sex.

Competition can also be a barrier to the expression of love between male friends. From the time boys are born, they are indirectly taught to compete against other boys. If girls learn to compete for boys, boys learn to compete not only for girls, but also for status and the need to be respected. Although the more traditional symbols of status are such things as achievement in sports, occupation, education, and the amount of money earned, men can compete at almost anything, and will do so in order to gain status. In his book, *Male Chauvinism: How it Works,* Korda[48] relates how illicit sex becomes a status symbol in the corporate business world. In the seemingly sedate atmosphere of the university, men often compete fiercely for status with such things as the number and quality of professional publications, or the number of lectureships one is invited to give. Some professors will not share important scientific information with their colleagues, for fear that someone else will beat them in publishing the information. Even in a prison, where all standards of status are stripped away, status may depend on being the best at playing cards or eating the most food. Homophobia and competition are concomitant factors of inexpressiveness which hinder the ability of males to establish close intimate sharing relationships with each other.

MARRIAGE.[49] With the difficulties that the inexpressive male has in relating as a single person to women, he may come to view marriage as an increasingly attractive alternative. As a husband, he can reduce the pressure to express such emotions by presenting the marriage itself as evidence of this affection ("Would I have married you if I didn't love you?"). Further, his wife may not require him to continually demonstrate the degree of affection and tenderness toward her that a single woman would, because she too can rationalize the existence of such emotions from the marriage relationship. ("He must love me or he never would have married me.") Finally, when the expression of verbal affection, tenderness, and gentleness toward a woman is necessary, it can be done with much less effort and awkwardness by the man who is her husband than by one who is her date. Most couples, if together long enough, develop a set of shorthand symbols through which they express certain emotions and desires, such as a playful pat on the derriere, a certain look, or an arm around the shoulder. These symbols may connote the emotions which the male is inept at expressing and thus require reasonably little "gut-spilling" on his part. They clearly develop in nonmarital as well as marital relationships. But because marital relationships usually endure longer, they present more ample opportunity for the development of a whole array of symbols which will facilitate the expression of "soft" and "feminine" emotions in the least painful way possible for the male.

While marriage may have useful consequences for the inexpressive male, the wife may not define the situation as a solution. Although the wife may resign herself to being married to a person who can communicate his feelings only through nonverbal symbols, she may still hold to the ideal of a verbally expressive husband. Such a marriage situation may not be too different from the highly incommunicative marriage which Cuber and Harroff[50] describes as the *passive* marriage. The consequences of continued inexpressiveness on the part of the male toward his wife may then be dysfunctional to their marriage relationship.

Burgess and Locke[51] made the initial suggestion that the present-day American marriage is more oriented toward companionship and thus carries a much heavier load than in the past. More recently, Blood and Wolfe[52] have concluded that "companionship has emerged as the most valued aspect of marriage today." Male inexpressiveness within modern affectively oriented marriage relationships, then, would likely decrease the chances of a marriage surviving by decreasing the wife's satisfaction with it and thus giving her fewer stakes in its continuance.

Many males who were initially very inexpressive toward all women may learn to increase their level of expressiveness toward women with whom they become seriously involved because such relationships permit the development of symbols which make it less painful to express these emotions. Heiss[53] investigated emotional expressiveness among casual daters, serious daters with no commitment to marriage, and daters committed to marriage. With increased involvement (that is, from casual to committed daters), males become more expressive; so that while females were clearly more emotionally expressive than males in the couples who were casual daters, among the serious daters committed to marriage, males were just as emotionally expressive as females. Leik[54] conducted an intriguing experiment in which he looked at male–female differences when interacting with the spouse of a stranger and when interacting with their own mates. The male was clearly more instrumental and the female clearly more expressive with strangers, but these differences noticeably diminished when they were their own mates.

Like the child who learns a rule and only begins to understand the exceptions to it through further experience, many American males may pick up the principle of inexpressiveness toward women, discovering exceptions as they become more experienced in the full range of man–woman relationships. As a consequence, they may become more expressive toward their wives while remaining essentially inexpressive toward other women—they learn that the conjugal relationship is one situation which is an exception to the cultural requirement of male inexpressiveness.

On the other hand some inexpressive males may never "unlearn" their inexpressiveness, and many wives may incongruently come to value *and* expect an increased quality of nurturance and expression. Within these marriages, male inexpressiveness is certainly one of the contributing factors to the increased divorce rate, as "liberated" women are not as tolerant of the prospect of living the rest of their lives with a man who is not meeting their needs for emotional intimacy.

FATHERING. Fatherhood may bring with it a whole new complexity of demands for inexpressive males. To begin with, women who are now mothers may have increased needs for emotional support and expressiveness from their husbands. While the mother is the primary source of gratification for the infant's rather taxing emotional requirements, the infant is not able to direct positive emotions toward her in return. It can be expected that she will turn to her husband for greater emotional input as a means of encouragement for continuing to meet the infant's emotional demands until she can replenish her own spent emotional resources. As a new mother she will also probably be insecure in handling her new tasks of infant care and need reassurance from her husband in the form of emotional expressiveness. Having just gone through the physically altering state of pregnancy and finding that infant care leaves her much less time and energy to devote to personal beautification, she may strongly desire reassurances that she is still attractive and loved. The emotionally inexpressive male, whose main impact as a father during early infancy may be more determined by his interaction with the mother than the child,[55] may be unable to provide for her emotional needs.

Given the current redefinition of sex roles, greater expectations are being placed upon fathers to provide for the nurturant needs of their children starting from the time they are born. Benson[56] suggests that "the modern father has more intensive nestling and comfort-giving relations with the infant than the peasant father in preindustrial societies." As the infant grows into a child, these expressive tasks expand to include activities such as providing bodily comfort to the child, exhibiting love and encouragement towards him/her, and playing with him/her.

If the inexpressive male has male children, these demands may be especially acute in the early years of his association with them. During their early years, sons can be as desirous of tenderness, gentleness, and verbal affection as girls. Inexpressive fathers may be afraid that their sons will not grow into "men" if they treat them in a tender and gentle manner.

Fatherhood then requires a sudden increase in demands made upon the inexpressive male to produce emotions of tenderness, gentleness, and verbal affection. Although his emotional capacities may have been augmented through practice at expressing such feelings towards his wife, they can still be rather limited. Marriage may serve as a lull between the turmoil of the single inexpressive male and the turbulence of fatherhood. If the inexpressive male continues at his same level of expressiveness or even slightly increases it, he will not be able to perform properly the role of father, and familial relationships may suffer as a consequence.

SOCIETY. In discussing the consequences of male inexpressiveness, thus far, the author has concentrated on its effects upon interpersonal relationships. It may be helpful to consider the possible consequences of male inexpressiveness upon society as a whole. This is a very difficult task to accomplish without falling into circular reasoning, for the author has previously argued that the inexpressive male is a result of societal norms and social structures.

The fact that males are inexpressive allows for the continued justification that because they are that way, they are ill suited for roles which call for a high degree of nurturant caring. Inversely, given the fact that success in the business world often demands that one act rationally and repudiate any emotions or feelings of affection towards other people as a basis for making decisions, it can be argued that men rather than women are best suited to continue in such roles. The same argument might be used to justify political leadership by men rather than women.

The author believes, however, that there will be no women's liberation without man's liberation. While the feminine role will be liberated when it is expanded to include opportunities for achievement, the masculine role will be liberated when it is expanded to include expressiveness of emotions and feelings as acceptable behavior. If men are insecure in their own masculinity and position in society, they will probably be intolerant of increased freedom for women. As women begin to assume new roles, a sense of uncertainty and insecurity will likely occur among males who may very well feel threatened by such new role behavior. This insecurity, however, is not necessary, residing as it does in arbitrary social stereotypes. "If a man is real," writes Brenton,[57]

> Women do not threaten him; nor does he need to confirm his masculinity at their expense . . . if he's secure, he can live his equalitarian life in an equalitarian marriage without fear of having his sexual identity shattered because roles merge or overlap. The secure man is warm, expressive, tender, and creative, yet quite capable of showing a sufficient amount of assertiveness when assertiveness is called for. The secure man can wash a dish, diaper a baby, and throw the dirty clothes into the washing machine . . . without thinking twice about it. (p. 188)

STRATEGIES FOR CHANGE

The strategies which can be utilized to increase male expressiveness are not that different from the strategies which can be employed to change any other type of human behavior. The author has argued that male inexpressiveness can best be understood in terms of both internal factors (personality traits or dispositions) and external factors (the situation itself). In contrast to a strict medical model which conceptualizes the problem of inexpressiveness as being internal to the individual, the role theory model which the author has employed conceptualizes inexpressiveness as behavior exhibited by the individual as he resides within the system. The strategies for change shall include individual therapy, which is a reflection of the medical model, and move towards a systems model as we consider marriage and family therapy, group therapy, cognitive-behavioral training programs, and, finally, social structural change.

INDIVIDUAL THERAPY. When working with an inexpressive male from an individual therapeutic model, some effort will be made to investigate family background and past experiences which may have contributed to the difficulty in expressing emotions. This exploration may uncover specific events which have triggered the blocking of emotional expression. Working through some of these painful experiences and recognizing dysfunctional interactional patterns will hopefully provide incentive for change. Reality testing can assist in discerning inappropriate affective expression. Once an awareness is established, and the desire to change behavior is the individual's goal, various modes of treatment may be appropriate. For example, behavioral procedures such as desensitization and rehearsal, Gestalt techniques such as role playing and empty chair confrontations, rational–emotive approaches such as restructuring belief systems, and relational approaches such as role modeling and improving communication skills, are all treatment strategies which may be useful in helping an individual change inexpressive patterns (see Chapter 13, 15, 16, and 17 in this book).

MARRIAGE AND FAMILY THERAPY. Conjoint therapy with a couple or family is an approach which emphasizes a systems theory framework. The obvious advantage which this approach has over individual therapy is that the therapist has first-hand experience in observing communication among family members and can, therefore, detect dysfunctional patterns. The interactional material which emerges "in session" sets the stage for pointing out ways to improve family interaction. When a cyclical response between an overexpressive wife and inexpressive husband occurs, each can begin to recognize their part in the pattern and can be encouraged to concentrate on specific ways of breaking the established pattern.

In conjoint family sessions, each member becomes aware of the negative effects of inexpressiveness, since it leads to erroneous assumptions and conclusions by other members. The more verbally expressive members, on the other-hand, often err in the direction of not listening, interrupting, and speaking for others. Conjoint therapy provides a real-life situation in which each member can recognize how he/she contributes to the breakdown of the whole system. It becomes a dramatic way of experiencing the interconnectedness of interactional patterns and the recognition of how important it is for all members to participate in the change process. It takes cooperative efforts to ensure permanent changes that will benefit the entire system.

The therapist's role becomes an important factor in the change process as well. Self-disclosure, willingness to be vulnerable, not being afraid of emotions, and dealing openly with anger and sadness are all role modeling examples which demonstrate expressiveness to family members. This creates an atmosphere for similar expressive exchanges between family members during therapy.

Social psychological research indicates that it is much easier to bring about attitudinal change by changing behavior than it is to cause behavioral change by changing attitudes. In a similar vein, the most effective way to change inexpressive males may not be to attempt to change their attitudes toward expressiveness directly, but rather, to change their role commitments. Or put another way, the most effective way to reduce male inexpressiveness may be by changing the social structures which encourage inexpressiveness in males rather than by attempting to change the personalities of males.

In 1974, the author wrote an article for *Woman's Day* entitled, "Why Husbands Can't Say 'I Love You'."[58] This article was primarily directed to wives, suggesting ways in which they might attempt to draw an inexpressive husband out of his shell. The author believes that there is a place for such an emphasis, for some males are better able to become expressive by means of an understanding wife. In a well-taken criticism of the *Woman's Day* article, Sattel[43] points out the danger in burdening the wife with this additional "emotional work" at a time in history when she is probably struggling to define who she is. If the author were to write another article to wives on this subject (the editor strongly suggested that few husbands would actually read the article), he would emphasize the need for a change in the amounts of time spent in certain roles. He would suggest to wives that they encourage their husbands to assume more of the childrearing responsibilities in the home, which may be induced only if they themselves become more involved in activity outside of the home.

GROUP THERAPY. Two types of group therapy appear to be potentially useful in increasing inexpressive males' ability to express feelings—cognitive–behavioral and consciousness raising. Taking a cognitive–behavioral approach, Dosser has proposed an 8-week training program to include techniques utilized in assertiveness training, communication skill cultivation, lecture, discussion, behavioral rehearsal, role playing, modeling, and assignments in real-life expressive behavior (see Chapter 16 in this book).

A neglected impetus for change involves making men aware of the potential gains which changed role relationships can bring. One way of heightening this awareness has been through men's consciousness raising groups. Such groups, where males are able to open up to each other and exchange experiences related to their masculine identities, are undoubtedly enabling males to become more expressive. There is some evidence that such groups are effective in providing the needed impetus for change long after involvement in such a group has ceased. However, a selective factor may be involved in the formation of such groups. The males who are most aware of the stifling effects of our culture's "masculine" emphasis are most likely to be the ones to join such groups. Thus, those men who could benefit most from consciousness raising group involvement are the ones who may never be a part of such a group (see Chapter 14 in this book).

SOCIAL STRUCTURAL CHANGE. There are two types of social structural constraints which need to be changed in order to increase male expressiveness. Systemic linkage between the family and the economy is one area of needed change, and the legal system is another. The fact that the father is usually the main link between the family and the economy means first that he is not around the home very much because his job generally is performed elsewhere. Hence, he has much less opportunity to be expressive towards his children even if he so desires because his job greatly reduces the time he can spend with them. He must usually crowd any attempts at expressiveness into a few hours at the end of a work day, when his emotional resources for doing so are probably lowest, or into increasingly busy weekends. He may thus attempt to telescope his emotional expressiveness into these limited time periods by inventing and improvising shorthand symbols of it, such as purchasing gifts, taking the family on a brief excursion for milkshakes after dinner, playing quick-ending games, making jokes, and telling bedtime stories. Benson[56,57,59,60] suggests that "he runs the risk of becoming little more than a stunt man in the process." The father's being the main link between the family and the economy also means that for approximately eight hours a day, he will likely be exposed through his job to an environment which, by stressing rationality and emotional control rather than emotional expression,[61] will reinforce his initial tendencies not to be expressive. Finally, societal norms regulating ties between the family and the economy take cognizance of the father as the main position that ties the family into the economy by stressing the priority of his work role even when it involves hardships for the family (hence, making it more difficult for him to leave and thus remove a basic link between the family and the economy). If the family can possibly do without the income, a mother is expected to give up her job should it interfere with her relationship to her children; but the father is expected to give priority to his job over his role as a parent.

The legal system provides further discouragement to the father's development of expressive relations with his children by playing down the father–child relationship. Fatherhood *per se,* and thus the father–child relationship, is not a legally acceptable reason for being deferred from the military draft. Divorce laws have traditionally expressed preference for the mother–child relationship at the expense of the father–child relationship by usually giving the mother custody of the children and relegating the father to the position of having to seek legal permission to visit his own children. Fathers can be brought into court for not financially supporting their children; unless physical harm results to the child, as in the cases of battered or neglected children, the laws say little about the absence of emotional support from fathers. The legal system is changing in response to the recognized importance of the father's role. An increase in male expressiveness will follow such structural change, an expectation which one film writer has already attempted to illustrate in the film *Kramer vs. Kramer.*

What is most needed is a change in the amount of time which males are asked to devote to emotion-laden roles. If fathers committed as much of their time to relating to their children as their wives do, it would undoubtedly be reflected in their expressive ability. Part of the needed structural changes has already been initiated by women redefining their role in society; these changes will "force" men to commit greater amounts of their time to roles which carry high expressive expectations.

IMPLICATIONS OF INCREASED MALE EXPRESSIVENESS

Men need to be liberated from the emotional hangups which prevent them from becoming intimate in human relationships. Central to a traditional definition of masculinity has been "the stigma of all stereotyped feminine characteristics and qualities, including openness and vulnerability."[62] Although increased emotional expressiveness is not a panacea for the difficulty men are presently experiencing in trying to work through what it means to be a male in a time of redefinition of sex roles, expressive change can have vast implications for themselves, for the people they know, and for society in general.

The benefits of increased expressiveness for males themselves are both physical and psychological. Physically, release from an inability to cry and express emotions can result in reduction of various medical conditions caused by unreleased stress and holding in emotions. Psychologically, the ability to recognize and get in touch with feelings will provide self-awareness rather than blatant denial and repression. Articulating feelings is one way to get a better understanding of the problem, thus allowing one to go beyond it to do something active and constructive, rather than merely trying to deal with a vague feeling of depression or anxiety.

A second implication of increased male expressiveness has to do with the quality of love relationships. The strong need for nurturance which is characteristic of newborn infants is never outgrown. All of us need to hear and receive overt expressions of love from the time we are born until we die. As we mature from infancy to adulthood, we develop an increasing need for physical expressions of love. Increased male expressiveness will benefit the important people in a man's life—his wife, children, mother, father, and male and female friends.

The quality of the relationships of males who have learned to express their feelings can be expected to vastly improve. A social relationship consists of a bond between two persons who take each other into account. Intimate love relationships are based upon *commitment* and maintained by *communication*. Although the emotions may be involved in love, more than anything else love is a commitment. A commitment involves both rights and responsibilities. From the point of view of the recipient of a commitment, rights are involved. From the point of view of the person giving the commitment, responsibility is involved. True love relationships are always reciprocal and mutual—two-way, not one-way. Each person experiences the relationship as involving both rights and responsibilities.

In the same way that mutual commitment is the *basis* of a love relationship, so mutual communication is the *process* whereby a love relationship is maintained and enhanced. A love relationship does not grow where there is only one-way communication. In a relationship with only one-way communication, only one person is attempting to express personal feelings to the other. At best, one-way communication may keep a love relationship alive; at worst, one-way communication is unable to sustain a love relationship.

The expressive person often makes valiant efforts to sustain the love relationship, while the inexpressive member of the relationship is either unwilling or unable to express his feelings. When an inexpressive person becomes expressive it can have dramatic effects in many areas of his/her life. Instead of the lack of responsiveness serving as a kind of negative reinforcement, the emergence of expressiveness can allow the relationship to grow and deepen. Instead of insecurity resulting from not knowing where one stands in a relationship, the development of expressiveness in the inexpressive person can reduce insecurity and thus the need to resort to devious and most often unproductive types of manipulative behavior designed to evoke some kind of positive response in others. The expression of love is the cement which maintains intimacy in close relationships.

REFERENCES

1. Wayne J: as reported in, A Forum for Changing Men 56:2, 1979
2. Balswick J: Types of inexpressive male roles, in Men In Difficult Times. Edited by Lewis RA. New York, Prentice-Hall, 1980
3. Balswick J: The effect of spouse companionship support on employment success. J Marriage Fam 32:212–215, 1970
4. Hurvitz N: Marital strain in the blue-collar family, in Blue-Collar World. Edited by Shostak A, Gomberg W. Englewood Cliffs, New Jersey, Prentice-Hall, pp 92–109
5. Komarovsky M: Blue-Collar Marriage. New York, Random House, 1962
6. Rainwater L: Family Design: Marital Sexuality, Family Size and Contraception. Chicago, Aldine, 1965
7. Bronfenbrenner U: Some familial antecendents of responsibility and leadership in adolescents, in Leadership and Interpersonal Behavior. Edited by Petrullo L, Bass B. New York, Holt, Rinehart and Winston, 1961, pp 239–271
8. Emmerich W: Parental identification in young children. Genetic Psychol Monographs 60:257–308, 1959
9. Johnson MM: Sex role learning in the nuclear family. Child Dev 34:319–333, 1963
10. Fromm E: Man For Himself: An Inquiry Into the Psychology of Ethics. Greenwich, Fawcett Press, 1947, pp 75–89
11. Maccoby EE, Jacklin CN: The Psychology of Sex Differences. Stanford, Stanford University Press, 1974
12. Meador C: Expressiveness: Self concept and sex differences in children. unpublished paper, 1980
13. Balkwell C, Balswick J, Balkwell J: On black and white family patterns in America: Their impact on the expressive aspect of sex-role socialization. J Marriage Fam 40:743–747, 1978
14. Balswick J, Avertt C: Differences in expressiveness: Gender, interpersonal orientation, and perceived parental expressiveness as contributing factors. J Marriage Fam 38:121–127, 1977
15. Allen J, Haccoun D: Sex differences in emotionality: A multidimensional approach. Human Relations 8:711–722, 1976
16. Jourard SM: Age trends in self-disclosure. Merrill-Palmer Quart 7:191–197, 1961
17. Jourard SM, Landsman MJ: Cognition, catharsis, and the "dyadic effect" in men's self-disclosing literature. Merrill-Palmer Quart 6:178–186, 1960
18. Jourard SM, Lasakow P: Some factors in self-disclosure. J Abnorm Soc Psychol 56:92–98, 1958
19. Jourard SM: The Transparent Self. Princeton, New Jersey, Van Nostrand, 1964
20. Levinger L, Senn P: Disclosure of feelings in marriage. Merrill-Palmer Quart 13:237–249, 1967
21. Fuller FF: Influence of sex of counselor and of client on client expressions of feeling. J Counseling Psychol 10:34–40, 1963
22. Janofsky AI: Affective self-disclosure in telephone versus face to face interviews. J Humanistic Psychol 11:93–103, 1971
23. Highlen PS, Gillis SF: Effects of situational factors, sex, and attitude on affective self-disclosure and anxiety. J Counseling Psychol 25:270–276, 1978
24. Highlen PS, Johnston B: Effects of situational variables on affective self-disclosure with acquaintances. J Counseling Psychol 26:255–258, 1979
25. Balswick J: The inexpressive male: Functional conflict and role theory as contrasting explanations. Fam Relations 28:331–336, 1979
26. Turner RH: Moral judgment: A study in roles. Am Sociol Rev 17:70–77, 1962
27. Blumer H: Symbolic Interactionism: Perspective and Method. Englewood Cliffs, New Jersey, Prentice-Hall, 1969

28. Turner RH: Family Interaction. New York, Wiley, 1970
29. Zelditch MM: Role differentiation in the nuclear family: A comparative study, in Family, Socialization, and Interaction Process, Edited by Parson I, Bales RF. Glencoe, Free Press,1955, pp 307–351
30. Hartley RE: Sex-role pressures and the socialization of the male child. Psychol Rep 5:457–468, 1959
31. Brown DG: Masculinity–femininity development in children. J Counseling Psychol 21:197–203, 1957
32. Gray SW: Masculinity–femininity in relation to anxiety and social acceptance. Child Dev 28:203–214, 1957
33. Hacker HM: The new burdens of masculinity. Marriage Fam Living 19:227–233, 1957
34. Coleman JS: The Adolescent Society. New York, Free Press, 1962
35. Hollingshead AB: Elmstown's Youth. New York, Wiley, 1949
36. Hannarz U: Soulside. New York, Columbia University Press, 1969
37. Leibow E: Tally's Corner. Boston, Little, Brown, 1967
38. Whyte WF: Street Corner Society. Chicago, University of Chicago Press, 1943
39. Kieser RL: The Vice Lords. New York, Holt, 1969
40. Miller B: Lower class culture as a generation milieu of gang delinquency. J Soc Issues 121:5–19, 1958
41. Rosenberg B, Silverstein H: The Varieties of Delinquent Experience. Waltham, Blaisdell, 1969
42. Short JF, Strodtbeck FL: Group Process and Gang Delinquency. Chicago, University of Chicago Press, 1965
43. Sattel JW: The inexpressive male: Tragedy or sexual politics? Soc Problems 23:469–477, 1976
44. Balswick J, Peek C: The inexpressive male: A tragedy of American society. Fam Coordinator 20:363–368, 1971
45. L'Abate L: Inexpressive males or overexpressive females? A reply to Balswick. Fam Relations 29:229–230, 1980
46. Chodorow N: The Reproduction of Mothering. Berkeley, University of California Press, 1978
47. Kirkwood J: P.S. Your Cat Is Dead. New York, Warner, 1973, p 23
48. Korda M: Male Chauvinism: How It Works. New York, Random House, 1973
49. Balswick J, Peek CW: The inexpressive male and family relationships during early adulthood. Soc Symposium 4:1–12, 1970
50. Cuber JF, Harroff PB: The Significant Americans: A Study of Sexual Behavior among the Affluent. New York, Appleton-Century-Crofts, 1965
51. Burgess EW, Locke HJ: The Family. NewYork, American Book, 1955
52. Blood R, Wolfe D: Husbands and Wives: The Dynamics of Married Living. Glencoe, Free Press, 1960
53. Heiss JS: Degree of intimacy and male–female interaction. Sociometry 25:197–208, 1962
54. Leik RK: Instrumentality and emotionality in family interaction. Sociometry 26:131–45, 1963
55. Bartemeier L: The contribution of the father to the mental health of the family. Am J Psychiatry 110:277–280, 1953
56. Benson L: Fatherhood: A Sociological Perspective. New York, Random House, 1968
57. Brenton M: The American Male. New York, Coward-McCann, 1966
58. Balswick J: Why husbands can't say "I Love You." Woman's Day 64:66,67,160, 1974
59. Pleck JH: The male sex role: Definitions, problems, and sources of change. J Soc Issues 32:155–164, 1976
60. Benedict R: Continuities and discontinuities in cultural conditioning. Psychiatry 1:161–167, 1938
61. Guttman D: Women and the concept of ego strength. Merrill-Palmer Quart 11:229–240, 1965
62. David DS, Brannon R: The Forty-Nine Percent Majority: The Male Sex Role. Reading, Massachusetts, Addison-Wesley, 1976

Chapter 6

The Effects of Changing Sex Roles on Male Homosexuals

JOSEPH L. NORTON

INTRODUCTION

Any chapter dealing with male homosexuals' roles needs to begin with the caution that the population studied is anything but clearly defined. For instance, one report[1] indicates that different individuals with similar sexual histories describe themselves variously as heterosexual, bisexual, and homosexual. The male hustler who presents himself as "straight" because he only permits the gay to fellate him, or only inserts in the "fag," is well documented.[2] It is important in counseling to remember that homosexual acts neither cause nor define one's sexual orientation. The simplest definition is "one who has an affectional or sexual preference for a person of the same sex." For some helping professionals, an individual with *no* same-sex experiences but regular fantasies would be called homosexual; for others, only two individuals of the same sex who set as a mutual goal getting each other to climax would be involved in a homosexual act. Enough males respond sexually to pressure on the genitals or other external stimulation that it almost seems as if *intent* should be part of the definition, as Bieber[3] recommended in 1962. Whether one uses the individual's self-definition, or an outsider's count of frequency of the behavior (e.g., the Kinsey[4] data that 10% are primarily homosexual for at least three years in their postadolescent lives), it seems clear that there are vast numbers of American males who see themselves as gay, fear that they may be homosexual, or merely indulge in some same-sex activity as occasion presents itself, without thought of a label. For mental health workers, it is important to recognize that some self-definitions are merely "homosexual panic," but a thorough review of the individual's developing sexuality usually helps. Some adolescents wonder about being homosexual, but the vast majority of gay males "knew" by the time they were in their teens.[5,6]

JOSEPH L. NORTON • Department of Counseling Psychology and Student Development, State University of New York at Albany, New York 12222

CLARIFICATION OF TERMINOLOGY

Gay vs. homosexual. Most gay activists resist the term "homosexual" as too clinical and because it has been used to categorize them and "put them down." Yet some reserve the term "gay" for the self-acceptant, open homosexual, whereas others include all with a same-sex orientation. Some few gays will call themselves "faggot," but resent having non-gays use that term, since it is usually used in a derogatory sense. But the activists resist the famous line in *Boys in the Band,*[7] "Show me a happy homosexual and I'll show you a gay corpse," despite the statement to the contrary in Karlen.[8]

Transvestites. The male transvestite gets sexual (and other) satisfaction from dressing as a woman. While most transvestites are heterosexual, some are homosexual. The gay world often refers to these latter as "drag queens."

Transsexuals. The transsexual males want to be women and feel trapped in the wrong body. Their gender identity is at odds with their biologic development.

Masculinity usually refers to a group of behavior traits and physical attributes characteristic of the male. The macho male struts or rides through "Marlboro country," flexing his muscles and exuding sexuality. This characteristic is made precious to many males; the writer met one young prisoner who killed another male youth who touched the prisoner's crotch. This was an assault on his manhood! (His violent heterosexist reaction might have been tempered had he known the data on gay male athletes.[9]) Yet many masculine men are homosexual and many effiminate men are non-gay. "There is no simple formula for the various degrees and combinations of cross-identification, cross-dressing, effeminacy in men and masculinity in women, homosexuality and transsexualism."[8] It is clinically useful to point out the fundamental differences that distinguish gays from transvestites (desire for same-sex partner vs. sexual satisfaction from cross-dressing) and from transsexuals (desire to be of the opposite sex), and the general public is beginning to understand these differences. Individual cases, however, can include considerable overlap.

Invert. This term was formerly used to refer to those who turned in upon themselves so much that, unable to turn out to the opposite sex, they had sex with their own kind. It is not used extensively anymore, but it is in the title of one of the important works on homosexuality by Marmor.[10]

THE LITERATURE ON MALE HOMOSEXUALITY

Although gays sometimes claim to have been ignored throughout history, facts to some extent belie such accusations. Same-sex activity has been recorded in art over the centuries and has been given attention by hostile legislatures since the early days of this country. Karlen's thorough review[8] gives insight into the ancient days, into the dangers of taking everything written about other cultures' sex lives as fact. He chronicles the early royal involvements and the homosexual house of prostitution run by Mother Clap. One quote: "For at least three thousand years Westerners have been claiming that there is more sex and more homosexuality than in the past" (p. 453). Bieber's classic study,[3] based on 106 male homosexuals in therapy, described them as the products of a weak or absent father and domineering mother. Krafft-Ebing[11] pushed the idea of illness rather than criminality, and homosexuality moved into the Diagnostic and Statistical Manual.[12] Most psychiatrists seemed to agree[8,13] (including those who were themselves same-sex oriented), but voices were raised in protest. Hirschfield[14] and Ellis[15] argued for an anomaly rather than pathology. Lauritson and Thorstad[16] review the early gay liberation movement in Germany, which was brought to a halt by the Hitler regime. But the typical growing American was *not* exposed to the idea of homosexuality as an option; usually the only exposure was to a stereotype of a limp-wristed aesthete. Even in this generation, many a gay male thought he must want to be a woman because he wanted sex with men.

The phenomenon (and subculture) remained very hidden until the Kinsey report,[4] which shocked much of America with its data on same-sex male activity. As Morin points out,[19] Ford and Beach[20] added data showing homosexuality present in almost all species and almost all cultures. Works specifically on homosexuality began to appear,[21] and one publisher even dared publish a book which opened with the sentence, "This is a life-history of a lover of boys."[22] (While pedophilia is a specialization inappropriate for this chapter, it is interesting to note that at least two more-or-less sympathetic books on man–boy love and sex reflect changing attitudes toward sexuality within society.[23,24]) Hoffman's *The Gay World*[2] in 1968 presented a somewhat less grim picture of gay life, and he echoed Krafft-Ebing in pushing for removal of antihomosexual laws.

Immediately after the Stonewall riots in 1969 (when the drag queens and others fought back during one of the routine raids on New York City gay bars), a spate of books began which reflect the development of a willingness to be open, a refusal to apologize, and a beginning of a demand to be recognized as having an alternate form of sexual expression which, for gays, is just as natural as is heterosexuality, in all of its variations, for non-gays.[25–29] More scientific studies and reports also appeared: Weinberg and Williams compared responses from male homosexuals in the United States, Denmark, and the Netherlands, as well as providing an account of the gay subculture in each.[30] Perhaps the best summary of the situation is found in West's 1977 rewrite of his earlier book:[31]

> Paradoxically, further study of the continually increasing volume of publications concerning homosexuality has led to less firm opinions than before. Increasing awareness of the complexities of the subject brings with it the realization that on many issues it would be wise to suspend judgment pending further research.

His two main points in 1977: the omnipresence of homosexuality and the point that a homosexual orientation does not necessarily imply inferiority in other respects. This latter point is continued in two recent works on the topic; Bell and Weinberg[32] describe several types of same-sex orientation, and Masters and Johnson[33] make the point that in general, homosexuals do not differ from heterosexuals in respects other than sexual orientation. Katz' *Gay American History*[34] pulls together hundreds of reports of gay life and gay oppression over the years and brings in the beginnings of the liberation movement. Most recently, two extensive reports on data furnished by thousands of lesbians and gay males have provided extensive data about gay males, their sexuality, and their life-styles.[5,6] While they, like all research, depend on those people willing to complete anonymous questionnaries, the description of their samples makes them the most comprehensive reports about homosexual males yet available.

GAY MALE SEXUALITY

In the middle of the 20th century, gay males who had access to pornography shops could acquire books, usually with pictures, entitled "What Homosexuals Do in Bed." Some gay male activist spokemen, when asked that question, respond "What do heterosexuals do in bed?" But the question is usually a serious inquiry, and Karlen[8] reports that many a person would be startled to discover the error of equating "sodomy" (defined as anal penetration by the penis) with "homosexuality."

Actually, homosexuals do all of the sorts of things that heterosexuals do except penile–vaginal intercourse. Oral–genital sex, mutual masturbation, and general body contact (hugging, kissing, carressing, rubbing) occur regularly. All but 10% in the Spada study enjoy fellatio, while about 75% report enjoying anal intercourse.[5] The Jay and Young data, while presented somewhat differently, do not vary far from such figures.[6] The Bell and Weinberg data[32] are much the same: all reports show performing anal intercourse about 10% more often than receiving it, whereas oral sex seems about equal in the giving and receiving.

Actually, there may be better frequency data about gay males than about heterosexuals in some areas, as the reports indicate that about 10% to 16% of gay males participate in sadomasochistic activities somewhat frequently, and from 6% to 18% in "water sports" (urination). Jay and Young[6] comment that these activities do not seem to be as frequent as the media often seem to indicate.

For the uninitiated, there are better books than the pornography mentioned earlier (although the author can recall one such book as very practical and helpful, teaching about relaxation during anal penetration and giving encouraging advice). Moving beyond others, however, which described exercises to strengthen the hand so it would not tire in masturbating the partner, there are two recent publications that are about comparable, for gays, to Comfort's *Joy of Sex*[35]; they are *The Joy of Gay Sex*[37] and *Men Loving Men*.[36]

In essence, the data from all sources indicate that homosexual sex is varied, varies from person to person, and for the same person, from situation to situation. The range is from celibacy and monogamy to reports of over 1000 partners. Certainly, the stories of compulsive sex, like *Numbers*,[38] are not typical, but not unheard of.[39]

SOME MYTHS DESTROYED BY THE RESEARCH

Gay males and lesbians, with the help of the many non-gay researchers and writers have now "come out" enough to destroy the myths and stereotypes about what it is to be homosexual.[17,25,26,32,33,41,42] And others venture into describing the positive aspects of the gay scene. Among the myths laid to rest are the following:

Homosexuality is a sickness. The American Psychiatric Association in 1974 removed homosexuality per se as an illness from its classification manual. Freedman[45] suggests gays may sometimes be healthier than non-gays.

The cause of homosexuality is known. The one thing that most experts now agree on is that it has not been possible to track down the cause or causes.[8,31,46,47]

Male homosexuals are child molesters. Anita Bryant made so much of this concept that the facts are now clear; homosexual child molestation is proportionately less than heterosexual. Despite a couple of notorious cases (in one of which there is some evidence to indicate the man was actually a homophobe killing the boys for selling their bodies to men), there is no support for any such generalization.[28,48] The related point that being molested is what makes a boy gay is also belied by the Kinsey data,[4] and that of Claiborne,[49] as well as Jay and Young[6] and Spada.[5]

Gay males are limited to hairdressing, interior decorating, and the arts. Jay and Young[6] completely contradict this with their data, as does Spada.[5] Gay lawyers, physicians, counselors and psychologists, as well as teachers, reflect the professions gays enter, as does the gay caucus within the American Psychiatric Association itself. While the Village People may emphasize the stereotypes in their own admirable way, they do reflect the fact that some Indians, construction workers, and policemen are gay.

Gay males play the role of female. Jay and Young[6] indicate that 70% of gay men almost never play a butch or female role; it is clear that most gay men do not play a female role. Spada's data[5] show only seven-tenths of one per cent characterize their relationships with other men as a husband–wife. Five per cent of his men dress in women's clothing, mostly for Halloween; 83% have never so dressed.

Gay males are effeminate, weak, introspective, swishy. With David Kopay as one example,[41] and other studies of gay athletes,[9] there is ample evidence of the falsehood of this generalization.

Being openly gay will destroy your career. With openly gay politicians being elected to office, gay caucuses in many professions, and the National Gay Task Force's published list[50] of companies which publicly state they do not discriminate on the basis of sexual orientation, there is a good deal to contradict this statement. However, this is still true for some in a homophobic society.

Gay men hate women. Many gay/lesbian organizations operate with gender parity; public statements abound to the contrary of this idea.

Open gay role models will persuade young people to be gay. The experts report that sexual orientation seems to be pretty well established by age five, by which time young people have not been exposed to known gays (and the heterosexual role models of the family have not prevented 10% of society from developing into homosexuals).[51,52] A recent study has reported that same-sex oriented households have homosexual children in no appreciably different proportion from non-gays.[53] Riddle's review of the literature[54] on role models leads to the conclusion that children internalize particular traits from a variety of models and that gays are more likely to serve as nontraditional sex-role models than as determiners of same-sex sexual preference.

CHANGES IN GAY MALE SEXUALITY

There is no great evidence that actual changes in types of sexual activity have occurred, although evidence does destroy the ideas held by some that anal intercourse is what is meant when one speaks of male homosexuality. Certainly, coming out has opened up a world of sexual activity to those who had remained inactive (sometimes almost for a lifetime) until freed by the loosening up of attitudes about homosexuality. However, there are some factors worth noting, even if there is no proof they resulted from changing sex roles.

Equality within sadomasochism. While only 10%–20% of gay men report sadomasochistic (S&M) activity, it is a sufficient number to warrant study. Here the stereotype also is belied by the data. The dominance–submission theme is so ingrained in the notion of sadomasochism that the very initials are sometimes used to mean "slave and master." Yet there is some indication that such roles, despite the implication in most S&M pornography, are really often interchanged (and at least, where not interchanged, played within a context of true caring and affection).[6,55] There is actually much love and affection in the S&M scene, which seems to be expressed despite roles. There is also a good deal of security in the S&M scene.[56]

Permission to be nongenital. Whether it is due to changing sex roles or to the increasing awareness–assertiveness–improving-communication movements, some clients report moving to declaring their preference for cuddling, hugging, and body contact over direct oral or anal intercourse. As Litewska[57] points out, concentration of men's sexual feelings in the genitals and the separation of men's sexuality from emotionality have been essential aspects of masculinity. Apparently some gay males are able to move beyond that state.

The aging gay. Although not mentioned previously, the stereotypic old gay was seen as deserted, desolate, depressed and sexless, dreaming of the days of his youth and past successes, yearning for the unattainable beauty. The studies also belie that myth. Many older gay males have a circle of friends, fare as well sexually as at least some of their youngers, and seem pretty well prepared for the vicissitudes of aging.[30,58–60] While most report some decrease in sexual activity from the days of their youth, some who came out late indicate that they have a considerable increase over their almost-celibate days in hiding. The gloomy picture of the ever-wanting old "auntie" is wiped away by reality.

Sexual dysfunction. Virtually nothing has been written about the treatment of sexual dysfunctions of gays. Informal discussion with sex therapists has enlightened the author that some report much the same problems as are found in heterosexual males: mostly impotence, some premature ejaculation problems. As in most heterosexual cases, impotence is related to performance demands or some psychological factor in the situation (for some, with the regular partner; for others, with an unexpected partner).

As for the actual dysfunctions themselves, Bell and Weinberg report that a majority of white homosexual males, but fewer Black, had had troubles with getting or maintaining an erection, lack of orgasm in the partner, being unable to maintain affection for the partner, premature ejaculation, or feelings of sexual inadequacy. Not quite half of both races had had at one time or another, difficulty in achieving orgasm. *The Gay Report*[6] indicates 2% report somewhat frequent or frequent trouble with premature ejaculation, but 62% had not had the problem more than once (51% never). No data are given on impotence, but several (eight from over 4000 questionnaires) anecdotal reports are included, taken from the responses to an open question about hang-ups. But the responses about the importance of erection, both own and partner's, to satisfactory sex, as well as the 53% who said their partner's orgasm is very important to them, reflect that considerable pressure for performance does exist among gay males.

THE DISCOVERY OF HOMOPHOBIA

In 1972, Weinberg wrote about society and the healthy homosexual,[61] and used the phrase "homophobia" to describe the excessive fear of and anger at the homosexually oriented person. Studies have related it to a rigid personality and a narrow view of sex roles as well as to fear of homosexual feelings within the self.[62–64] Currently, attention is being given to ways to alleviate the problem.[65,66] Clinical experience indicates that bibliotherapy can help, using books like Fairchild and Hayward,[46] Silverstein,[67] and Hutchinson.[68] But the best known cure is for the homophobe to get to know several gays, to find that they do not attack or proposition him, and are not monsters. He will find they live pretty much the way he does, including working, paying taxes, even sometimes being a regular church attender. Besides Dignity for Gay Catholics, Integrity for gay Episcopalians, and Affirmation for gay Methodists, the Unitarian–Universalists have an Office of Gay Concerns in denominational headquarters, and the Metropolitan Community Church has over 100 congregations formed primarily for providing church support for gays.

Since the homophobe is most likely to reflect a sexist attitude toward women and to want to remain with his very rigid, narrow definitions of sex roles, the freeing up of gays to be themselves and play their roles as they find them comfortable has allowed them to point out the homophobia in these men.

CHANGES IN LIFESTYLE AND RELATIONSHIPS

A section on changes implies that we know about a situation which no longer exists. Yet the review of the literature has reflected that until very recently, the attitude of disapproval has kept much of the general public in ignorance about homosexuality, although there are early writings that have been found and reported.[8] Most of what was available portrayed the male homosexual as a sinner, a witch, and a sick, deviant pervert. The young man in the 20th century who felt same-sex inclinations met a barrage of swishy comics carressing microphones, by lisping jokes, and limp-wristed gestures. No mention was made of Michelangelo or of same-sex-oriented football players, and only occasional mention of the effete writer. Any research into serious medical writings reflected the aberrant nature of the feelings.

The literature has not provided us with a picture of the typical male homosexual. Some fortunate gays found lovers or at least the subculture. There they felt isolated, but at least supported.[40] Many gays found the gay bar scene by hearing non-gay friends joking about straying into a "queer" bar by accident, and then furtively trying out the place. The role was usually one of being non-gay by day, and hidden at night.[7,18,41] But the recent literature makes clear that a new role is emerging: that of the gay male. Much of the credit for the freedom to develop this role must go to the women's liberation movement (with its emphasis on sex-role stereotypes) and to the Black liberation struggle. It was in 1969 that, with these examples, the drag queens on Christopher Street in New York City fought back during a police raid on a gay bar and the visible role of the gay "out of the closet" began to emerge. This developing role has enabled gay males and lesbians to look at themselves in a new light, to stimulate research, and to come up with a positive self-image.

Documentation of the influence of the women's liberation movement is not extensive in writing, and, in any sense, hard to prove. But attendance at gay liberation rallies over the years, which frequently include speeches by non-gay women, involved hearing time and time again the gratefulness of the gays for the example set by the women and by Blacks.

THE GAY MALE

As emphasized above, recent research emphasizes the variety within the gay subculture. Bell and Weinberg[32] describe their five types: the close-coupled, the open-coupled, the functionals, the dysfunctionals, and the asexuals. Their labels define them fairly well. The close-coupleds look to each other for support, and are closely bound to each other. They are unlikely to regret being homosexual, and have fewest sexual problems, and are less likely to have been arrested. The open-coupleds, on the other hand, are less happy and spend more time seeking satisfactions outside the partnership; they have the widest repertoires of sexual activities. In other respects, however, they are indistinguishable from the homosexual population as a whole. They are the largest group.

The functionals are categorized as matching the "swinging singles" of the heterosexual world. Least likely to regret being homosexual, they more than the others, focused their lives around their sex, were most exuberant, and most active in the gay world. As a group they had had the most arrests, bookings, and convictions for a "homosexual" offense.

The dysfunctionals fit the stereotype of the unhappy, troubled gay; they fit the quote from *Boys in the Band* mentioned earlier (happy homosexual equals gay corpse). They more often regret being homosexual, and have the most sexual problems; they had more problems with the rest of their lives. The asexuals were essentially loners, with less interest in sex as well as less activity with it, with narrower sexual repertoires. They often mentioned not having enough sex, despite their lower interest. Despite their complaints of loneliness, they tend not to seek relationships or to seek gay world activity. Their main difference from the dysfunctionals was in this apathy and disengagement.

Whether or not most gay males can fit themselves into one of these categories, the five again emphasize the differences and range of gay activity (probably here the term "homosexual" would fit better, as most certainly some of these categories do not represent people who are gay in the festive sense). But these data, gathered prior to 1970, do not differ greatly from the two volumes gathered seven or eight years later, in terms of frequency of types of sexual activity, cruising, etc. There seems to be little evidence of actual change of behavior. Yet there is room to discuss changes in the lives and patterns in some areas.

As the role of "open gay" has developed, along with women's changing roles and interest in androgyny, gays' lives have changed. How much credit goes to changing roles, how much to the gay liberation movement, how much to the increase in accurate information about gays (obtained from the healthy ones as well as the unhappy ones in treatment), is hard to say. But there have been some changes for some homosexuals.

Easier to be open. For the gay male, there are now role models; there are numerous books, and even *Time* magazine[69] to reassure him that he is not the only one who feels that way.[17,18,41,70] There are inexpensive pamphlets available to help him "come out."[71–74] There are longer books.[17,18,28,42] He can get three excellent books to give his parents to help them realize they "didn't do anything wrong."[46,67,68]

Two cases indicate the range of clients. One young man, referred by a local counselor when she found he needed gay information, was sure he was gay, had told his mother and his girl friend, but had no ideas of how to go about finding others. A brief discussion of the gay bars and their "protocol," of the local gay community center, of the gay religious groups seemed all he wanted. By the second visit he could report he was making good progress and enjoying himself.

A second took three appointments before he finally reached the office. Violently afraid of being seen coming in, he represented the epitome of the homophobic gay. Much exploration of his sexuality, his background, his hopes, his anxieties about his vocational possibilities if he were gay was needed before he could relax. In fact, relaxation exercises were used, via cassette, to train him to relax. Only after considerable work was he open enough even to consider seeking contact with other gay males.

Avoid the husband–wife, macho–femme roles. How much change there has been is hard to assess. Bell and Weinberg in their 1970 sample[32] say only "Among these coupled, there was generally little evidence of a (masculine/feminine) sex role dichotomy in the performance of household tasks." Jay and Young[6] report that about half of the men have negative attitudes toward role playing, and actually avoid it. However, those authors feel that their respondents do not reveal "any overwhelming commitment to the destruction of role playing." The gay males are interested in the topic and commented on it and on various experiences. Of 2,000 who gave written answers to the longer questionnaire, not one involved in a husband–wife relationship sent in a full description, although some men indicated they were the breadwinner or homemaker. Many men reported they refused to play roles and opposed the consciousness on which it is based. Some men saw the issue as more complex than just getting involved in roles; some reflected ambiguity, with role playing in some circumstances but not in others.

The data reflect that more *do* it than feel positive about it (24% do it sexually, 17% other than sexually, while 20% feel somewhat positive or very positive about it sexually, 13% other than sexually). The approximately one-third who feel neutral about it may imply it is all right for others, or that it is sometimes all right for the respondent. (One could argue that 42% who never do it, 1% once and 21% very infrequently could be reported as 64% who *avoid* it sexually and 70% other than sexually.)

Pressure to change out of the butch–femme roles. Several therapists report patients presenting problems in this area.[75] Others report never having had such patients.[76] It is logical to assume that the push to avoid sex-role stereotypes could affect those who are deeply involved in them. Perhaps the geographic location is related to this, as the first report comes from the South and the other from California, where it is less difficult to be openly gay and couples are less likely to be isolated. Unfortunately, the Jay and Young[6] data are not broken down regionally to verify greater frequency of the role playing in different parts of the country.

New roles for gay males. The gay periodical press, which is ahead of the real professional publications, report two recent trends which may ultimately bring clients to therapists. The one trend is toward "the Castro Clone." This is the macho look, red plaid shirt open at the neck, tight jeans, and boots. Seen as a counteraction to the past stereotype of queen, this appearance is understandable, but the press reacts to it as a problem.

The second is the trend to "leather drag." Again a direct opposite of the sequined queen is this development of the macho leather male. The visored cap, leather chaps, often adorned with chains and metal studs and worn with no shirt, try for the epitome of the male image. For some this also implies a butch role in bed, and for some others the master sadist role in a master–slave, sadomasochistic relationship. The pressure of such roles, and the fears inspired by them, may well lead to future counseling customers. Yet Lee[56] points out that, in one sense, the situation of S&M sex is more controlled than that of most other casual sex; his research verifies, with a description of the role-play-acting involved, what Townsend[55] wrote of from personal experience earlier.

The gay father. Almost nothing has been written about the gay father, although the author knows of individual cases which range the full gamut of contact with their children. Some gay fathers have been seriously restricted even as to visitation rights; others have been awarded the full custody sought. Others share in agreed-upon proportions of time in the keeping of the child or children. Some few males maintain a gay life on the side with full (or at least partial) knowledge of the wife, although Gochros's[77] report on gay husbands does not report encouraging data for such a plan. Most gay fathers the author has met have good relationships with their grown children, if they are past the custody age. Of Bell and Weinberg's sample,[32] 114 white and 14 Black males had been married, and 50% of the whites and 71% of the Blacks had children. Eighteen of the 57 white males had one or more children who suspected or knew of the father's sexual orientation. The fathers reported the knowledge had not affected their relationships with their children. Jay and Young[6] report 13% of their entire male sample have children, and 73% feel positive towards children.

CHANGING ATTITUDES

It is difficult to discuss *changes* in attitudes of gays, as almost no research on adequate numbers of homosexuals precedes the "gay revolution." However, there are some aspects of the current situation worth discussion.

Able to accept their feminine side. While some gays fought their same-sex sexual orientation because they did not want to imitate women,[17,18,41] others, in accepting their homosexuality, were able to find some of the valuable characteristics that are generally reserved for women and absorb them.[78] The majority of gay men describe themselves as having a mixture of masculine and feminine traits.[6] For some few, "androgynous" is the self-descriptive term.

Changing views of the meaning of manhood. Many coming-out stories, although certainly not all, reflect the pain of having been called "sissy," of being put down for not being competitive and athletic, and the endless "proving I'm a man." Some gay males go to the point of affecting leather and Levis (and some of these are unable to accept the right of other gay males to go in *their* kind of drag). The macho image is popular, along with the phrase "If I wanted a female, I'd get a female." However, most gay males at last accept the fact that being gay does not make them any less a man. As described above, most have learned to accept their feminine qualities (and most learn to cook, if only to survive). A whole part of the emerging gay liberation movement is the improvement of the self-image of gays. Far fewer are the self-hating, guilt-ridden men who populated the early reports and literature about homosexuals.[6,79] It is clear that the changing roles women have taken for themselves have influenced this trend for the better.

Yet many men do not go the full way in recognizing that oppression of gays has been tied in with women's oppression, and those gay men maintain the male supremacy patriarchal society which has so long been socialized into all men. But some are breaking away; Snodgrass[80] reflects the changing attitudes that come to some gay males. Some of them go further than damning our patriarchal society and damn the economic and social system, espousing a socialist or Marxist view. But many others remain a part of the middle class, spending $1,000 a year on clothes and travel. This market is just beginning to draw the attention of merchandizers. So changing sex roles does not always change attitudes, although in combination with various other factors, some gay men's attitudes have been changed from what they were socialized to be.

Some see their own sexism: The reluctant patriarchs. Some gays, according to Snodgrass[80] are becoming aware of their own sexism and domination of women. Some gay groups function well with gender parity in leadership, such as the

National Gay Task Force and Gay Rights National Lobby. Some gays call themselves feminists, although others prefer the term "nonsexist male."

Competition. There is much indication that some gay males have overcome one of the barriers to intimacy between men described by Lewis[81]: competition. Yet, if one observes the striving for the best drag outfit (either female or macho), and the fighting over potential partners in many gay bars, it is clear that not all gay men have overcome their socialized need to compete. But it does seem as if it is less tied to one's manhood than the heterosexual who strives to conquer women, or always win the race, or win out in a business deal. Aggressive achievement motivation is not absent in gay males, but in some it is lessened. Power-hungry gays do exist, and sometimes disrupt gay organizations, but for many the role of power-grabbing is not appealing. A shared equality in sex can educate as to the benefits of shared power in other aspects of life.

Awareness of conflicts between transpeople and feminists. Sometimes a conflict has erupted within the gay liberation movement, one which is obvious but not easy to resolve. The drag queens often emphasize the very aspects of femininity which the feminists want to play down: beauty, make-up, sequins and fancy dress, busts, and "feminine" gestures and walk. Often they want to be treated the very way many feminists and lesbians do *not* want to be treated: put on a pedestal and waited on. Also, some lesbians feel uncomfortable in the presence of "made women," the postoperative transsexual, although one such person on a visit to the author's class spent more time arguing women's rights than discussing transsexualism.

Trying to resolve this situation is difficult. It is easy to understand the needs and feelings of each side, and probably the best move (more likely within the gay movement than within therapy) is to work towards greater openness to difference, to greater acceptance of individual differences, and the right of each person to be him/herself.

CONCLUSION

It is clear that the development of the women's movement and the breaking down of sex-role stereotypes has aided the growth of the gay liberation movement, which in turn has freed up many male homosexuals to be themselves, to develop positive self-image, and to be more open about their lives. Little actual change in sexual practices has been documented; for some, more openness to new experiences has developed. For some, new awareness of sexism in most males and an acceptance of the feminine side of self have developed. Basically, the role of "gay male" has made life easier for many homosexual men, while others were comfortable before or remain distressed with their situation. All in all, things should be more positive in the future.

REFERENCES

1. Blumstein FW, Schwartz P: Bisexuality: Some social psychological issues. J Soc Issues 33:30–45, 1977
2. Hoffman M: The Gay World. New York, Basic Books, 1968

3. Bieber I, Dain HJ, Dince PR, et al.: Homosexuality: a Psychoanalytic Study of Male Homosexuals. New York, Basic Books, 1962
4. Kinsey AC, Pomeroy WB, Martin CE: Sexual Behavior in the Human Male. Philadelphia, Saunders, 1948
5. Spada J: The Spada Report, The Newest Survey of Gay Male Sexuality. New York, New American Library, 1979
6. Jay K, Young A: The Gay Report. New York, Summit Books, 1979
7. Crowley M: Boys in the Band. New York, Farrar, Strauss & Giroux, 1968
8. Karlen A: Sexuality and Homosexuality: A New View. New York, W. W. Norton, 1971
9. Garner B, Smith RW: Are There Really Any Gay Athletes? Paper presented at the Society for the Scientific Study of Sex, San Diego, California, June 1976
10. Marmor J: Sexual Inversion, the Multiple Roots of Homosexuality. New York, Basic Books, 1965
11. Krafft-Ebing R von: Psychopathia Sexualis. Trans by Rebman FJ. New York, Paperback Library, 1965
12. American Psychiatric Association: Diagnostic and Statistical Manual of Mental Disorders, 2nd ed. Washington, American Psychiatric Association, 1968
13. Bergler E: Homosexulaity, Disease or Way of Life? New York, Collier Books, 1956
14. Hirschfeld M: Sexual Anomalies. New York, Emerson Books, 1956
15. Ellis H: Studies in the Psychology of Sex, Vol 2, Part 2. New York, Random House, 1936
16. Lauritson J, Thorstad D: The Early Homosexual Rights Movement. New York, Times Change Press, 1974
17. Brown H: Familiar Faces, Hidden Lives: Ths Story of Homosexual Men in America Today. New York, Harcourt Brace Jovanovich, 1976
18. Reid J (Pseud.): The Best Little Boy in the World. New York, Ballantine, 1977
19. Morin SF: Psychology and the gay community: An overview. J Soc Issues 34:1–5, 1978
20. Ford C, Beach F: Patterns of Sexual Behavior. New York, Harper, 1951
21. West DJ: Homosexuality, 3rd ed. London, Duckworth, 1968
22. Davidson M: The World, the Flesh and Myself. London, David Bruce and Watson, 1973
23. Lloyd R: For Money or Love, Boy Prostitution in America. New York, Vanguard Press, 1976
24. Rossman P: Sexual Experiences between Men and Boys. New York: Association Press, 1976
25. Jay K, Young A: After You're Out, Personal Experiences of Gay Men and Lesbian Women. New York, Links Books, 1975
26. Jay K, Young A: Out of the Closets: Voices of Gay Liberation. New York, Pyramid Books, 1972
27. Teal D: The Gay Militants. New York, Stein and Day, 1971
28. Fisher P: The Gay Mystique: The Myth and Reality of Male Homosexuality. New York, Stein and Day, 1972
29. Altman D: Homosexual Oppression and Liberation. New York, Avon Books, 1971
30. Weinberg MS, Williams CJ: Male Homosexuals, Their Problems and Adaptations. New York, Oxford University Press, 1974
31. West DJ: Homosexuality Re-examined. Minneapolis, University of Minnesota Press, 1977
32. Bell AP, Weinberg MS: Homosexualities, a Study of Diversity among Men and Women. New York, Simon and Schuster, 1978
33. Masters WS, Johnson V: Homosexuality in Perspective. Boston, Little, Brown, 1979
34. Katz J: Gay American History, Lesbians and Gay Men in the USA. New York, Crowell, 1976
35. Comfort A: The Joy of Sex. New York, Simon and Schuster, 1972
36. Walker M: Men Loving Men. San Francisco, Gay Sunshine Press, 1977
37. Silverstein C, White E: The Joy of Gay Sex. New York, Crown Publishers, 1977
38. Reichy J: Numbers. New York, Grove Press, 1967
39. Lee JA: Getting Sex, A New Approach; More Fun, Less Guilt. Don Mills, Ontario, Canada, General Publishing, 1978
40. Adair N, Adair C: Word is Out, Stories of Some of Our Lives. New York, Dell, 1978
41. Kopay D, Young PD: The David Kopay Story. New York, Arbor House, 1977
42. Perry T, Lucas CL: The Lord Is My Sheperd and He Knows I'm Gay. New York, Bantam Books, 1973
43. Jay K, Young A: Lavender Culture. New York, Jove Publications, 1979
44. Berzon B, Leighton R: Posivitely Gay. Millbrae, California, Celestial Arts, 1979

45. Freedman M: Homosexuals may be healthier than straights. Psychol Today 8:28–32, Mar 1975
46. Fairchild B, Hayward N: Now That You Know. New York, Harcourt Brace Jovanovich, 1979
47. Money J: Factors in the genesis of homosexuality, in Determinants of Human Sexual Behavior. Edited by Winokur G. Springfield, Charles C Thomas, 1962
48. Tripp CA: The Homosexual Matrix. New York, McGraw-Hill, 1975
49. Claiborne R: Who's afraid of gays? The New York Times, June 14, 1978, p A25
50. National Gay Task Force: Corporate Survey Results. New York, National Gay Task Force, 1978
51. Green R: Sexual Identity Conflict in Children and Adults. New York, Basic Books, 1974
52. Money J, Ehrhardt A: Man and Woman; Boy and Girl. Baltimore, Johns Hopkins University Press, 1972
53. Green R: Sexual identity of 37 children raised by homosexual or transsexual parents. Am J Psychiatry 135:692–697, 1978
54. Riddle DI: Relating to children: Gays as role models. J Soc Issues, 34:38–58, 1978
55. Townsend L: The Leatherman's Handbook. San Francisco, Le Salon, 1972
56. Lee JA: The social organization of sexual risk. Alternative Lifestyles 2:69–100, 1979
57. Litewska J: The socialized penis, in For Men Against Sexism. Edited by Snodgrass J. Albion, California, Times Change Press, 1977
58. Kelly J: The aging male homosexual, myth and reality. Gerontologist: 17:328–332, 1977
59. Francher S, Henkin J: The menopausal queen: Adjustment to aging and the male homosexual. Am J Orthopsychiatry: 43:640–644, 1973
60. Kleinberg S: Those dying generations: Harry and his friends. Christopher Street 2:6–26, 1977
61. Weinberg G: Society and the Healthy Homosexual. New York, St. Martins Press, 1972
62. Freedman M: Homophobia. Blueboy 5, Apr 1976
63. Smith KT: Homophobia: A tensative personality profile. Psychol Rep 29:1091–1094, 1971
64. Silverstein C: Homophobia, Presented at the Gay Academic Union 1, New York, November 1973
65. Morin S, Garfinkle EM: Male homophobia. J Soc Issues 34:29–47, 1978
66. Hyman R: Working with the gay client: Methods of eliminating counselor homophobia. Paper Presented at the Annual Meeting of the American Personnel and Guidance Association, Atlanta, April 1980
67. Silverstein C: A Family Matter: A Parent's Guide to Homosexuality. New York, McGraw-Hill, 1977
68. Hutchinson B: Now What! Miami, Center for Dialog of Dade County, 1977
69. Time, April 23, 1979, pp 72–78
70. Reich C: The Sorcerer of Bolinas Reef. New York, Random House, 1976
71. DeBaugh A: Coming Out! Washington, Universal Fellowship of Metropolitan Community Churches, 1978
72. Mombello R: To Come Out, An Alternative for the Young Male Homosexual. Laguna Beach, R Mombello, 1977
73. National Gay Task Force: About Coming Out. New York, National Gay Task Force, 1977
74. National Gay Task Force: Twenty Questions. New York, National Gay Task Force 1978
75. Solomon K: Personal communication, 1979
76. McWhirter D: Personal communication, 1979
77. Gochros HL: Counseling gay husbands. J Sex Educ Ther 4:6–10, 1978
78. Young A: No longer the court jesters, in Lavender Culture. Edited by Jay K, Young A, New York, Jove Publications, 1979
79. Hall R: The Well of Loneliness. New York, Covici Friede, 1928
80. Snodgrass J: For Men against Sexism. Albion, Times Change Press, 1977
81. Lewis RA: Emotional intimacy among men. J Soc Issues 34: 108–121, 1978

Chapter 7

Sexual Functioning in Relation to the Changing Roles of Men

ROBERT E. GOULD

The Women's Movement, the "sexual revolution," and the more open sexual climate have combined to produce an ambiguous picture, with confusing results that too often reflect the bias of a particular observer or a limited and skewed population. For example, a great number of men are seeking therapy for sexual problems. This was not the case several years ago. What has happened and what does it mean?

There have been several reports of an outbreak of "new impotence" among American men. This began with a brief scientific article published in the *Archives of General Psychiatry* in 1972.[1] The original report cited four cases, and suggested not only that impotence among men was increasing, but that women, specifically the new, sexually "liberated" women, were to blame.

The media seized on this report, giving it wide publicity, and exploited a rather modestly written article "suggesting" that changing social attitudes might be responsible for "(1) Young men now appearing more frequently with impotence and (2) young women more frequently complaining of initial impotence in their young lovers."

A more recent report by Moulton[2] also emphasizes the reactions of sexual dysfunction, including "premature ejaculation, sexual withdrawal, and indifference to the point where the husband may refuse to attempt intercourse for months, even years . . ." She does note, however, that there are "many men who have responded to the new feminism with a new freedom to acknowledge and express a wider range of emotions" and to feel tender without fearing to appear weak.[2]

The question remains: Is there really more impotence and is the Women's Movement really to blame?

ROBERT E. GOULD, • Departments of Psychiatry and Obstetrics and Gynecology and Family Life Division, New York Medical College, and Metropolitan Hospital Center, New York City, New York 10029.

From the author's observations and research, the answer to both questions is no, but with qualifications. There seems to be little question that the "new woman" and the sexual revolution are indeed having profound effects on male potency, but his conclusions are that they are helping more than hurting it.

How does this conclusion square with the obviously increasing number of men coming to therapy complaining of impotence or premature ejaculation?

First, let us examine some of the reasons for this "increase," reasons quite unrelated to feminism and not indicative of a true increase at all.

(1) The new climate of sexual freedom and permissiveness allows everyone to talk more candidly about sexual problems without embarrassment, feelings of humiliation, or guilt. If the cultural climate now allows men's sexual problems to be discussed, then, very simply, men will finally begin to discuss them.

(2) The Feminist Movement has encouraged women to talk more freely to their male partners about their own sexuality. The result, in many instances, has been a collaborative effort to work out problems in the bedroom. Whereas in the past a woman worried about threatening the "fragile male ego" by calling attention to his inadequacies, she now feels free to talk about them and to complain, if appropriate, for both their sakes.

(3) The growth of the sex therapy industry in the past ten years has led to a veritable population explosion of patients with sexual problems, patients who never before have sought any kind of help. Since 1970, when Masters and Johnson began to publish and teach sex therapy techniques for premature ejaculation and impotence, some 5000 sex therapy clinics, many without substantial credentials (an understatement), have opened across the country. Many medical schools now have human sexuality and sex therapy divisions. Just a few years ago, there were no such places to turn to for help with these problems. Therapy by psychiatrists was too long, too costly, and too often ineffective, to attract many men with potency problems. At best, this older, traditional form of therapy could have served only a small number of all those with severe sexual problems. But with sex therapists now numerous and available, and with the help of enormous media publicity, many men with sex problems who would have kept them secret and lived with them now have simply "come out of the closet." Many colleges also offer sex therapy and counseling programs that were nonexistent before the early 1970s.

(4) Finally, the new permissive climate has encouraged more people to engage in more open sexual activity, starting earlier and ending later. If more people are playing the game, it is reasonable to expect there will be a greater number of "strikeouts" as well as a greater number of "home runs."

In light of this, let us return to the original study that supposedly revealed the "new impotence." It is true that more young men are appearing more frequently with complaints about impotence, but does that prove that there is in fact an increase in their numbers? And is there anything really "new" about the problem other than (1) the therapy, (2) its greater availability, and (3) a freer climate in which the problem of impotence is easier to admit?

In scrutinizing the four cases cited in that first widely reported article, one finds little trace of either the "new woman" or her increased sexual freedom.

One of these cases involved a man in his mid-thirties who had sought consultation for impotence because his wife was "unsatisfied by sexual practices limited to foreplay. The patient felt that his problem resulted from lack of experience." He had had no relationships in college with "good girls," but visited prostitutes whom he regarded as "dirty and diseased." He had them perform fellatio in order to avoid "infection." He married in his thirties because it was expected of him, but he had *never* had intercourse or even attempted it. It was his wife's urgings that finally brought him to a doctor. A woman interested in normal consummation of her marriage hardly seems related to Women's Liberation, or to the "effect of women's increased sexual freedom on male partners." In any event, the wife in this case was not the cause of her husband's impotence. The problem had always been there; he had simply never had to do anything about it until his wife expressed a desire for an ordinary sex life in the marriage.

Despite data that largely refute the view that the Women's Movement *per se* is causing sexual problems for men, it is certainly true that some men are indeed being hurt by the revolution. In a stormy sea of dramatic social change, individuals caught by the strong current may be unable to swim along or to swim back to safety.

A previous paper[3] reported on several men whose sense of worth and manliness were threatened when their wives began earning more money than they did. In some cases this was expressed through sexual impotence. The following are some examples of men the author has seen whose sexual potency was compromised by the pressures exerted by the new woman.

Jack A. came into therapy with the complaint "I don't really understand this whole 'Women's Lib' thing. She picked me up and one thing led to another, but when we went to bed I found I couldn't get it up." Jack had been a Don Juan type who found himself impotent with a woman who played the sexually "aggressive" role he was accustomed to playing. In their bar conversation, she had told him that "I have just as much right to sex as you do," and added that he need not try to seduce her. "If I'm attracted to you," she said, "I'll seduce *you*." When the young woman finally said, "O.K., let's go to my place," Jack went but failed to achieve an erection for the first time in his life.

In therapy it became apparent that sex was an expression of power and dominance, not love, and that without these feelings of superiority and control he was uncomfortable with women. He had always been the initiator in sexual encounters and this was the only time he tried to have sex with a woman who did not wait to be asked. He responded to her "challenge" by withholding what she said she wanted and felt she was entitled to: equal enjoyment in an equal sexual partnership. For him to go along with that demand would have undermined his "masculinity." Analysis further revealed that Jack had never before felt any sexual performance of his was being judged, but this time he worried about it, and felt if he did not measure up, she would let him know about it. His reaction was to back away from the challenge and he suffered from a classic form of "performance anxiety."

There are many men like Jack whose background and early training have led them to deal with women as sex objects rather than equals. Their sense of masculinity is based on some combination of a John Wayne/Gary Cooper/Steve McQueen image of what a man is or should be (tough, cool, laconic, unemotional, fearless, invulnerable, a fighter, and a winner). When a "new woman" ceases to find this to be the ideal in her man, what is he to do? Jack is like many men; his conditioning has been so strong that he can find no other way of relating to a woman. He responds by steering clear of the "new woman" and finds an "old-fashioned" relationship, more on the order of "total woman," the Marabel Morgan[4] creation who is virtually a caricature of the submissive, compliant sexual partner whose joy comes from serving and keeping her man happy, no matter what price she pays in her own growth and development. There were enough "total women" around so that Jack saw no need for therapy.

Bill, a physician, and Jane, who started a new successful career, came in for therapy after Jane discovered Bill's extramarital activities, while he was impotent with her. Bill had become impotent when his wife began making more money than he did. For him making money was still synonymous with "masculinity" and power. The truth was that Bill felt uncomfortable not only about Jane's income, but also because she had absorbing outside interests; he resented the independence that the new job gave her. Without her feeling dependent on him as before, he felt threatened and afraid of abandonment. He started sexually withdrawing out of anger and resentment at Jane's changing status. The resulting shaky sense of his own masculine power resulted in impotence.

Although Bill started an affair with a laboratory technician who worked for him, "just to see if anything was wrong with me sexually," the more compelling reason was to vent his anger at Jane (he made it easy for her to find out about the affair) and to reaffirm his sense of masculinity with someone in a clearly dependent position.

This case is by no means unusual, but the outcome of such a marital crisis is dependent on many factors. Bill had enough going both for him and for the marriage. After several months of psychotherapy, he was able finally to accept Jane's achieving and equal position in the marriage. He was further able to see this not as a threat, but an advantage to him. Bill had enough motivation to want to make his marriage work and enough ego strength to permit uncovering his anxiety about losing Jane if she followed an independent career and relationships that did not involve him. Working through his status and image problems and the symbolic values he placed on money, he was relieved of the need to maintain a macho image. He began doing more research, which he enjoyed, though he earned even less money than before. At the same time, he became sexually freer and less inhibited.

In assessing problems like Bill's or Jack's, it is essential not to confuse the new-style assertive woman with the male nightmare image of an aggressive woman. Clearly there are, and have always been, "castrating" women who hate men or need to cut them down. Men have always had trouble relating sexually to such women—but neither the Women's Movement nor the Sexual Revolution can be blamed for that. On the other hand, there are now large numbers of women who are increasingly dissatisfied with their old assigned sexual roles, and their relationships with the opposite sex. These women's changing attitudes and behaviors often present profound new challenges to men. It is a law in physics that when one particle in a field changes, every other particle in that field is also affected and changed. In life, if not in physics, the problem is for all the affected particles in the field to understand how they are affected and in what way changed.

One couple I treated recently offered a good illustration of the "field theory" in action. Jeff's wife Carol had a career as a television producer that she sacrificed because he did not want her to travel. She was also more successful than he in his freelance writing. In many ways, he kept her down and she stayed down to keep the peace (and the marriage). Jeff flirted openly at parties, but flew into jealous rages if a man spoke to Carol alone in a corner. Jeff had never been a good lover, but Carol had dutifully faked orgasms and pretended to be satisfied in order to protect Jeff's self-esteem and shaky sense of his "masculinity." Then Carol joined a women's group and also began therapy. Gradually she began showing her anger and resentment. When she confronted Jeff with them, he responded with premature ejaculation. occasional impotence, and finally, total sexual withdrawal.

In conjoint therapy, Carol told Jeff about her faking orgasms and why sex had not been good for her. Jeff began to work through his feelings of inadequacy, which he had always covered up by trying to dominate Carol. For the first time, there was honest communication between them about sexual desires and dissatisfactions. It turned out that part of Jeff's difficulty in lovemaking stemmed from his suspicion that Carol was not so gratified as she put on; he was never really sure if he was satisfying her. The result was chronic "performance anxiety" which adversely affected both of them every time they had sex. In therapy Jeff was faced with having to develop a sense of worth and self-esteem, without using the neurotic crutch of putting Carol down.

In this case, an emerging "new woman" did indeed cause more sexual dysfunction in the man, but the trouble was transitory, and the end result was a better sex life and a better marriage.

The problems faced by Jeff and Carol, Bill and Jane, and Jack, all reflect reactions to the new sexuality by people in their late twenties and thirties. But perhaps the most dramatic changes are now showing up among college youth who are not so locked into rigid role patterns left over from previous, less liberated eras. The story of Harvey, the reluctant college virgin, emerged in a workshop I conducted during a three-day study of male sexuality at a midwestern college.

Harvey might seem at first glance to be a less predictable kind of casualty. Coming of age in a time of heightened sexual freedom and activity, he suffered acutely from being inexperienced, and, even after falling in love, kept postponing the "moment of truth" because he feared the girl would make invidious comparisons with her previous lovers. With the added anxiety over not knowing what to do in lovemaking, Harvey became a premature ejaculator and finally found himself impotent. That was when he sought help from the college sex counselor. The counselor encouraged him to tell his girlfriend the whole story. She chided him for not being honest in the first place, and then took the lead in teaching him to do what, regardless of the song, does not really come "naturally." Under patient tutelage and with her support, Harvey finally became sexually functional.

There were, of course, many Harveys before the sexual revolution—young men who, lacking experience and confidence or inhibited for a variety of reasons, invariably have found sexual opportunity an anxiety-provoking situation. The Harveys among us have always wondered, "Can I do it right?" "How much is expected of me?" "Will I fail?"

It seems paradoxical that male college students who so often boast about sexual conquests when they are not pursuing them should find that they, of all people, can go "limp" or premature when faced with easier, freer, more available sexual partners. But Harvey, like many of today's college men, went through early adolescence at a time when the "nice girls" he knew were still playing by the old rules—passive, coy, and innocent. He expected girls in college to be as inexperienced as he was. Anxiety struck when he met a "nice girl" who had a healthy and candid interest in sex. Revolution or no, Harvey was not prepared. In counseling, Harvey said he was worried about the girl "throwing him over" for a more experienced lover. But on a deeper level it turned out he still felt that good girls had to be practically raped before they would "give in" sexually. His confusion kept showing up in bed.

The fact is that today's college students, male and female, are caught between the old sexual rules that they learned in high school and the new notions about equality and freedom that are now sweeping the campus, especially among young women moving eagerly toward liberation. The result is often a painful period of sexual dysfunction, especially for the men. Nevertheless, the author has encountered a fair number of male college students who are apparently having a much easier time of it. For varying reasons, these young men grew up with greater awareness of changing mores, and their sex lives seem far better and more rewarding than what their fathers had when they were in their early twenties.

The enlightened young men are benefiting from today's freer sexual climate, not because there is more available sex, but because they are able to share feelings and thoughts about sex with their female peers. Being able to talk about sex with the opposite sex is a heady new experience; helping each other learn how to love seems to free young people from many misunderstandings, deceptions, guilts, and mutual distrusts—in short, all the elements that used to ruin sex for everyone.

Even in Harvey's sexuality workshop, there were other young men who reported discovering this kind of new, improved sex life. Most of them credited it to partners who were freer and had different sexual expectations—not only of men, but of themselves. They helped free the men in their lives from the macho role and they helped them enjoy that freedom. Tom talked about how much more "human" his sexual experiences were now that he did not have to pretend to be something he was not. He *liked* being tender and passive; he was comfortable with a woman who could be assertive without making him feel inadequate. Marshall said, "I really never knew quite what to do with the clitoris or how long to caress a breast before moving on." He was happy to have partners who would tell him what they wanted; far from feeling more "pressured" to perform, he felt "relieved of pressure."

In the lively interchange of this workshop, the young participants also learned a lot about women: that they differed enormously, one from another, in what kinds of sexual caressing they liked, and how, and for how long. The macho myth that a man becomes a good lover by instinct, or that any one "technique" could work for all women, was effectively demolished.

At another college meeting the author attended, male and female students met together to discuss sexuality. The women students were questioned about how much importance they put on male "performance," and the consensus was that it ranked far below closeness, intimacy, mutual respect, and caring.

In a co-ed sexuality workshop, the students talked freely about sexual "turn-ons" and "turn-offs." When some women expressed disenchantment with the traditional he-man type, there was invariably great excitement, lively discussion, and delighted sighs of relief on the part of many men.

In these workshop sessions, men also made discoveries about each other, such as the fact that nobody really knows what to do without at least some help from his partner. They traded secrets about how to encourage a woman to tell, either verbally or nonverbally, what she likes and how she likes it.

The author's experience with these males' sexuality college workshops has led him to subsequently set up similar groups for adult men and women—married, unmarried, and strangers. The object was the same; an ongoing workshop for problems in sexuality and in changing relationships between the sexes. Each session is an informal mix of group therapy, sex therapy, and consciousness raising. The combination seems to work. Women who come (there have been 18 so far) are "semiliberated," engaged in the difficult process of changing into "new women." The men are examining their own sexual attitudes and hangups, each hoping to relate better to the "new woman," and to find the "new man" in themselves. No one who comes to such groups is satisfied with his/her sex life. But their complaints about sex differ sharply from those registered by patients ten or even five years ago, and so do the solutions.

George was married once and had many affairs. He had never asked a woman what she wanted to do in bed; he thought he should know. Also he was only comfortable in certain positions. He never would let the woman be on top; it meant that he would be in the woman's ("inferior") position. When George began to relate to the women in the group as people, not sex objects, he became fascinated by their discussions of *their* sexual needs. Gradually, he began to give up some of his notions about how a man "ought" to behave in bed. George is now beginning to enjoy the "feminine" part of his personality.

Carl has found that allowing himself to cry and to show his emotional side in other ways now makes him feel more comfortable and closer to women. Once he found, through group discussions, that women did not regard this as a failing, but rather as a human trait that they could relate to, he no longer had to keep up a macho front.

Mike used to think the sexual exuberance and openness of his partner were somehow deviant; her uninhibited responses embarrassed him. Now he realizes they are simply a full, healthy sexual expression, and he finds that they turn him on.

One man in the group was disturbed by the idea that women were capable of multiple orgasms. He felt this as a demand to perform better. A woman in the group reassured him that "we aren't interested in performance." As Gilda put it; "I don't care how good you are in bed tonight, or how many orgasms I have per any unit of time. First things first. I want you to respect me, be concerned for me as an equal. I want intimacy, closeness as friends, not only as lovers. After all that, we can worry about orgasms. *If* we still need to."

Ann objected to this as "too easy on men, too much like the old days, when women's orgasms didn't count at all. Remember when they told us it didn't matter if we ever had them, that only men needed sexual release? Now you're saying the same thing: 'Just love me and never mind about my sexual needs.' Well, not me. I want *my* orgasm tonight."

Carl shook his head. "That's how a guy can get performance anxiety! You want it now, or else. What if he doesn't come through?" Ann shrugged. "If a guy wants sex, and a girl doesn't 'come though,' he gets another girl who will. Right?" George sighed, "True, but not right. Aren't we trying to do it differently, not just use each other for orgasms? Sport sex is just for kids, isn't it?"

What becomes apparent in these group sessions is how much both sexes have been missing in life, and how much more they are reaching for. Many of the men still find it hard to renounce their Superman images, to show emotion, tenderness, passivity, dependency. As for the women, many of whom have spent a lifetime playing a submissive role, they often need the support of such a group in order to move onto new, and for them, dangerously independent ground. Both sexes are often testy in relating to each other, especially in admitting inadequacies. But they are making progress. Some even report a richer and more vivid sex life, having learned to emphasize two new things in bed: more touching and more talking. They have begun to know their sexual selves in richer detail. They are less inhibited about learning different roles, to be passive and receptive men, active and assertive women.

The casualties in these groups, like those the author mentioned earlier, are inevitable. No course of treatment works magic, even during a revolution. Drastic change is simply not possible for everyone. Sometimes there are deep neuroses or other personality limitations. Sometimes age is a factor, since it occasionally increases rigidity in personality. And in all forms of psychotherapy, change and movement are marked by pain and a sense of loss which not everyone can weather. With luck, when one gets to the other side, it all proves to have been worth the trip.

A man can only find a new sexual self by sloughing off the old one to which he was assigned by yesterday's culture. Women, now seeking their own true sexual selves, also want to help men find theirs. So if today's new woman seems to be the "cause" of man's sexual problems, she may also be the "cure." Sigmund Freud wanted to know "What does a woman want?" She is now, at last, ready to answer the question. All a man has to do is listen.

REFERENCES

1. Ginsberg, G, Frosch W, Shapiro, T: The new impotence. Arch Gen Psychiatry 26:218–222,1972
2. Moulton, R: Some effects of the new feminism. Am J Psychiatry 134:1–6, January 1977
3. Gould R: Measuring masculinity by the size of a paycheck, in Men and Masculinity. Edited by Pleck J, Sawyer J. Englewood Cliffs, New Jersey, Prentice Hall, 1973, pp 96–100
4. Morgan M: The Total Woman. Tappan, New York, Fleming, and Kavell Co., 1976

Chapter 8

Dual Careers and Changing Male Roles

THEODORE NADELSON AND CAROL NADELSON

INTRODUCTION

That which was first dealt with mockingly in the Women's Movement as the peccadillo of some aberrant radicals has become a part of our laws, lives, and attitudes. There is and will be a continuing struggle, but from now on the issues addressed will be presented to public awareness as serious legal or moral questions. Despite attempts from some quarters to combat the change by designating it only as a transient deviation from the more natural order of male–female relationships, it is safe to predict that its effect will continue to be felt profoundly in the way men and women interact socially, sexually, and at work. Couples engaged in dual careers will be seen as less of a novelty than previously; yet they will encounter problems different from those inherent in the traditional relationships of man-at-work/woman-at-home. For men, raised by fathers and mothers to see their maleness as inseparable from work habits and traditional attitudes, there will be necessary innovation in relationships with their partners and children. Such shifts will contain the potential for discovery along with the risks attendant on shifts from entrenched styles of interaction.

The shift in male role models, certainly those confronted in dual-career families, reflect change on all levels, both in action and in attitudes. Certainly the roles of men and women exert mutual reciprocal influences. The changing relationships in dual-career families will continue generationally, since the attitudes of the partners toward each other and in relation to their roles is pivotal, and will be manifested in child-rearing practices and education for living. Some men will discover the pleasures of domestic life in the newly discovered company of their children.

THEODORE NADELSON • Boston Veterans Administration Medical Center and Department of Psychiatry, Tufts University School of Medicine, Boston, Massachusetts 02111. CAROL NADELSON • Department of Psychiatry, Tufts-New England Medical Center, Boston, Massachusetts 02111.

THE CURRENT SITUATION

There is still, however, inertia to be noted in the fact that children are assigned a place in the social hierarchy corresponding to their father's income, occupation, and education without reference to their mother. The occupation of the "Head of the Household" until 1980 has automatically been reported as that of the husband unless he is no longer present in the home; yet half the women in this country are in the paid labor force, including 46% of those with children.[1,2] Many women have worked for pay in the past; the perceived "deviant" nature of this role is now more difficult to maintain in the face of a continued increase in the number of working women. Yet, even in some communities in which working women constitute the mode, there may be a prevalent view that a working woman is unusual.[3]

We all change slowly, then, and fact is often not as persuasive as ancient myths. Men's fantasies regarding women often have little to do with reality. What has previously been presented as factual history, the house kept bright and warm by the ever-cheerful woman, happy only to do just that, was made up more of individual male wishes rather than woman's needs. It seems now, on review, to be a reconstruction of the male child's ideal. Women may have resented being used as a projective screen for male fantasy but they never have been as consistently public about it until the past decade. The annihilation of the fantasy has been met with varying degrees of discontent by men. In a traditional setting boys learn dependency on their mothers, and as they attempt to develop their male role there is repudiation of that which is female. The relationship with women often shows such continued ambivalence throughout their life.

A successful male executive came to treatment partly at the insistence of his wife when his transient impotence of many years become constant. He loved his wife, and she seemed to share similar feelings toward him. They had met while both were in college. He played football on a major team. After college he joined a number of his classmates who enlisted in the Navy during the Vietnam War. While in combat he sustained a massive wound, leaving a scar on his body. He had related his impotence to shame regarding his scar. His wife loathed it, he said. (She confirmed that belief.) Yet in the course of seeing them in couples therapy it became clear that other sources of dissatisfaction existed, predating the war wound. The husband's mother had been doting and extremely caring. Up until the time he left the home and even when he visited, his mother gave him a great deal of physical care. For example, she had always laid out his clothes, even when he was an adult. She catered to his eating tastes with focused intensity. His wife was in many ways different from his mother; his wife was fair of complexion, and of different ethnic extraction. She was certainly less involved in family relationships. He loved his wife initially because of her distance, and her "coolness." Yet he discovered, subsequently, that her manner also diminished his sexual interest. He attributed his difficulty to an "Oedipal problem." He perceived his mother as a feminine woman (warm, giving), who controlled both father and the household. His father seemed weaker than the way he wished him to be. His mother was always the source of strength and the exclusive repository of need satisfaction.

He had to reject being similar to her in order to be a "man" in the conventional way. His football playing and his military experience was partly a search for manhood. His war injury, which nearly took his life, collapsed the search precipitiously. His wife's rejection of him because of the wound did in his sexual potency with her. Her relative "coolness" was attractive because it defined her as dissimilar to his mother, and so allowed sexual interest. His sexual interest and arousability was dependent on a generally complex and ambivalent view of women. He was forced to repudiate identification with his mother's warmth because that would make him unmanly.

In his choice of a "cooler" woman he sought an identification with those attributes more generally and traditionally acceptable as characteristics to be sought in himself ("cooler," and of "proper" ethnic background). His confusion led to sexual dysfunction as he felt forced to repress his own warmth as too "feminine" and too "ethnic."

SOME WOMEN CAN . . .

Some women can mend clothes, bake bread, wipe noses, sweep the hearth, make love. Some women can write briefs, practice medicine, fly airplanes, direct advertising agencies. There are no women, just as there are no men, who can engage, at the same time, in all with equal facility and feeling. At the beginning of the Women's Movement, which was catapulating some women into positions of executive authority, many men, in an excess of self-righteousness and virtue, "allowed" their wives to make sojourns outside of the home. The assumption perhaps was that husbands might share some of the responsibilities of the household, but more often women were to continue basically in charge of all domestic duties. Taking it as a shared responsibility was, for many men, a service to be performed and paraded in front of others. It established the man as the stronger because he was so "flexible." Professional men particularly have been cared for by women. Many of them, starting with their mothers, have had many of their needs met by women who were concerned with giving to them because that is what women were expected to do—as a sacrifice to the man's higher mission. The man could then be excused from the workaday world of dirty dishes and laundry.

The commonplace chores of domestic life challenge the "liberated" husband's nominal commitment to an egalitarian marriage. Even those who accept household task sharing as the norm usually view their role as accepting assignments, with more or less cheer, but expect domestic executive responsibility to be carried by the wife. Being scrupulous about doing half the physical work, much of it mindless, is not the same as doing half the real work. Worrying about what needs doing and planning ahead for it exacts important costs.

Family executive functions, in our clinical experience, demand a sizable reverberating neuronal circuit, thus preempting major pathways and consuming inordinate amounts of metabolic energy. How else can one explain the common complaint of the married woman physician, that she falls asleep evenings over journals and books when her husband still seems wide awake? The double load of family responsibility and professional responsibility results in wildcat strikes by overworked cortical neurons. As one woman professor said to her equally distinguished husband, "How often do you suddenly think, in the midst of lecturing to a class, 'My God, we have no toilet paper! I'd better stop on the way home and pick some up'." That couple decided, not without some anguish, to contract on alternate months for one and then the other to take full responsibility for the household, including shopping and cooking meals for guests. At follow-up, three years later, the plan is working remarkably well; the husband now boasts, to the considerable discomfort of his male colleagues, of his success in his new role.

After a national meeting a number of years ago (at the beginning of the Women's Movement) a fellow professional had a rude encounter with his own feelings. He had been almost completely ignored by a gathering of women who were all very interested in speaking with his wife. She stayed too long, he thought, and afterward, during a discussion of where to go for dinner, he felt she was too demanding. His response was anger, barely contained. Unable to control himself, he suddenly burst forth, castigating her character as controlling. Subsequently, he realized the source of his feeling in competitiveness and jealousy. Magnanimously (or so he thought) he gave her the gift of saying that he realized he had been acting out anger related to wounded pride and self-esteem. She said, "Yes, I know."

He had expected, he said, that she would soothe his feelings and (consonant with the model of behavior for men and women) give him support for the strength he displayed in admitting that he was jealous. She would say, in the expected scenario, that, after all, "You are strong and I was wrong." That had been demonstrated by his understanding of the angry feelings that he had renounced by identifying them. When she only acknowledged that he was obviously jealous, giving him no reward for his *tour de force* of insight, his anger redoubled. In later years he realized that moment to be a turning point (with no turning back) in the relationship with his wife. Her position was not that of being a wife, mother, and guardian of the hearth merely acting "as if" she were a professional like him. His anger had been continuous because he felt a challenge; and it crystallized at that very moment. She only reiterated that he was, in fact, angry, and she would not remove the reasons for it by reassuring him of his dominance and her submission. The change in him subsequently occurred slowly, reluctantly, and creakingly. Now, he regards his life as a rich one; in fact, he reports that it is hard for him to imagine what it would be like to have a resolutely domestic wife.

Many males in professional couples come only slowly to the understanding that their wives really "mean it," i.e., truly consider professional activities the major endeavor in their lives. Often women arrive at this position with the help of other women; it is our impression that they arrive at it less often as a result of help from their husbands.

Some men indicate that there are times when they feel annoyance or anger engendered by a wife whose professional duties bend the household out of shape. Even those husbands who are beyond expecting a well-run, tidy household often are irritated, e.g., when clothes are not available for their children for a special event. There is often an expectation that the wife should control all aspects of such events, as illustrated by the following incident reported by one of our subjects (after assurance of confidentiality):

> When I made a trip to the cleaners because I remembered that my son was to take his first look at a new school and had no clean clothes, I felt very virtuous and I wore my virtue as an indictment against my wife. It is only in retrospect that I realized that she had set up the appointment for him at the school and that really, logically, we shared the responsibility for the clean clothes equally. Happily, I realize it now without her reminding me, that's too embarrassing. Maybe my encounter with such embarrassment in the past helps to extinguish my annoyance.

However, such reactions extinguish slowly because of long-standing reinforced attitudes regarding women's and men's roles.

WHAT DO WOMEN WANT?

It is a fact that women who choose to have a family are more bound to it than are men. The woman carries the child in pregnancy (a limiting factor in many job situations), and the infant in its earliest years may place limits on activity. The woman has an earlier attachment than her partner to the infant. This attachment is more strongly supported by mandates from society; the child usually is awarded to the mother when custody is questioned. Many women have given up potential careers or delayed them because of their responsibility to their children.

Human striving may be conceptually divided into *species* and *individual* needs, and the woman is biologically deeded as the manifest carrier of species needs. Yet women have as much in the way of individual strivings as do men. Their recognition of such needs predates the more public expression of their wish to such options. The other biological fact is that of the plasticity of the organization of human behavior, whether viewed within the neurological or psychosocial framework. *Some* women (not all) want an equal chance to work and to explore other creative strivings outside of home and children. The men they choose (or who choose them) also must be aware of the importance of that factor in the relationship. Such wishes are not simply reduceable to a basic envy of the body parts assigned to the male gender. That really overtaxes a pale metaphor.

. . . AND MEN . . .

Men do much for love of women. Poets have celebrated that fact. Some male attitudes criticized as inexpressive, violent, or just plain brutal may have their origins in the competition surrounding the seeking of a female partner. Yet many men will state that they have been waiting for women to liberate them from stereotyping appropriate to tribes of hunter–gatherers species engaged only in species survival. The possibility that many women would prefer as a choice a gentle, nurturant man has been a long time in coming.

The Women's Movement has made it possible for women to present that possibility to potential male partners as they have presented the possibility to themselves. Androgyny as a male option has become a discovery for some men. It is occasionally a dramatic shift, but more often men are growing into receptive, warm relationships with their spouses and children. They do it slowly, as such change becomes accepted, or more obviously highly esteemed by their partners. Said in this way, "usual" masculine striving activity is to be seen, at least in part, as a way to please women. To attain women's love, given human plasticity, some men have shifted toward androgyny without any particular sacrifice of their sense of masculinity. That shift also recognizes the capacity in women for what was once seen as a purely masculine prerogative for striving and aggression. In couples where it works there is a pleasing interplay, a duet of rapidly fluxing interaction.

STRUGGLING TOWARD ANDROGYNY

The concept of *androgyny* grew out of the Women's Movement's focus on sex role stereotypes as an unnecessary limit for women. Stereotypes are exaggerations of the observed; the rough averaging of male and female behavior has led to a broadly drawn cartoon of allowable behaviors for each sex. Such generalizations are supposed to contain at least some truth. Yet whatever the small truth, it is far outweighed by actual individual divergence.

Androgyny represents a merger of the usual masculine (analytic, forceful, self-sufficient) and the feminine (gentle, affectionate, tender) traits as revealed by acceptance of such traits as their own by men and women. Androgyny, in a person who merges masculine and feminine traits (rather than an undifferentiated person who endorses neither), is seen as possessing the most positive aspects of humankind:[4,5]

> . . . for fully effective and healthy human functioning, both masculinity and feminity must be tempered by the other, and the two must be integrated into a more fully human, a truly androgynous personality. An androgynous personality would thus represent the very best of what masculinity and femininity have come to represent, and the more negative exaggerations of masculinity and femininity would tend to be cancelled out.[6]

Androgyny, then, is a further extension of flexibility, adaptation, and coping behavior *despite* the imposed sex-role stereotypes usually accepted by both men and women. Those men and women who can, with facility, appropriately employ those traits "assigned" exclusively to the opposite sex move toward a broader spectrum of interactions with each other and their children. Communication, concern, and pleasure can be heightened. For those who are threatened by the concept it should be emphasized that all traits are not demonstrated at all times; that there is a time to be tough and a time to be gentle (and one can be both alternately). Toughness or nurturance are not the characteristics of either sex alone. (Still another source of concern and anger from men is the felt implication that it is only up to them to change; that they are at fault—mostly for their coldness. Change will occur only reciprocally. It is not safe for a man to shift greater emphasis to his potential for nurturance and gentleness if his partner maintains a "helpless female" attitude.)

For men, the Women's Movement exerted a powerful force, most potently for individual men in the direction of what their individual female partners redefined for them as good, engaging, or sexually attractive. The image of a man as necessarily muscular, directed, aggressive, and uncommunicative was probably more quickly broken down on a personal level by a woman partner's personal rejection of such time-worn posturing than by all the persuasive statements coming out of the Women's Movement.

Androgyny can be achieved by some and not by others. For many people in lower socioeconomic situations it still would make male and female relationships unrecognizable. (It is more difficult to achieve such balance in a blue collar class where deviations in the direction of androgyny from traditional male–female divisions are heavily penalized by explicit social stigma.) The effect of the Women's Movement, however, is being felt in every social class in this country, and what was acceptable and usual is being tested by individuals in a way not seen before. The shift is often not noticeable. At times, as a mass phenomenon, movement is glacial. It is more obvious among individual couples, usually with those who have taken on dual careers—even those taken on because of economic necessity. (Also, the war in Vietnam, because it was a "bad" war, influenced many American men on all socioeconomic levels who saw in its political failure a similar failure of the male myth they tried to emulate.)

The Professional Couple

Many professional males in a dual-career marriage are emotionally and intellectually committed to equality. It goes along with their general world view which is antithetical to traditionalism. They have, after all, spent much of their lives in the luxury of intellectual "play"; they often feel like adolescents at times caught in the dissonance between calendar time and their perception of personal aging. They have little trouble with the "expressivity" seen in those of less educational achievement. They really cannot do otherwise; many are wedded to attitudes of "rising above" the conventional and principles of logical necessity regarding equality (or at least they are publicly). Many of their colleagues are increasingly women.

Yet at times what is said privately, to a friend or psychotherapist by a professional man whose wife works, is not dissimilar from the statements of blue collar workers.[8] The issue between men and women has shifted, but not dissolved. Most professional couples the authors know (those in their third or usually fourth decade) take years to reach a semblance of egalitarianism of household management. Many try a rough kind of accounting during the transition; "I take out the trash, you cook the dinner; I clear the table, the cars are your job; the dishwasher is mine." Yet, in this system, future planning is still left to the wife. The spouse who really is in charge, who in truth administers home and children is easily operationally defined by the direction in which heads turn when a child says, "There is no milk; what camp are we going to this summer; I need a new jacket for a school interview." Although there may be a division of labor, the center pivot is held by the wife.

Careers follow parallel paths and usually the husband's is groved deeper. His career may have a longer history to it; he may appear more serious about it, or others may view it as such. Women may drop out for children and start work again later. There is also an expectation, supported by family, usually on both sides, that the husband will follow his career choice and there must be sacrifices by the wife and children. An architect, at work in his own firm for five years, was forced to work longer hours when his partner left him. His mother-in-law suggested to her working daughter (a psychologist) that his upcoming short vacation was "very important" and that she (daughter) should "do all she could" to remove any family worries from his mind. There was no concern expressed about her daughter's career and long hours of work. It was, she said, "all too familiar:"

> She (mother) never regards my job as important—it is a caprice, an unnecessary aspect of my life viewed against the functioning of the family. Despite the effort she knows I make, she sees it as an indulgence.

The wife also knows that in the parallel career paths, her husband (who is working hard) cannot always give her the necessary support either. Sometimes there is desperation. He says

> At least we talk about it—I wish sometimes that she would stay home so I don't have to do double duty . . . but I cannot really expect her to do it. I know—when I think twice—that her career is important also. The trouble is you cannot turn away from the kids. But I cannot turn away from my clients either.

Sometimes, when he "has" to work, he wishes she would take care of the children. Who "capitulates" to the children's demands first? Who blinks? Usually it is the wife. She feels a pull in the direction of giving care and giving up her own needs. She has not been taught another way to be which is acceptable and rewarded as female. She risks not only displeasure of important others, but a sense of failure as a female and as a woman if she feels or behaves otherwise. The traditional path for a woman, with regard to occupational goal, may be quite as deeply grooved as her husband's specific occupational path. The early attitude stays with many women longer, but all seem to struggle with it. Those who must struggle harder against such internalized restraints are often envious and even angry at those women who can give up such a role easily (and write about it) as if it requires no more than extending the right arm.

Yet there are some families in which the woman has, by continued assertion of her prerogative, refused to be drawn into the position of the ultimate domestic resource. That position is usually won over time; it is not always present in the beginning of a relationship. When asked about whether there was milk (bread, eggs, etc.) by their latency age children, one female professional would invariably reply, "I don't know." She was, resolutely, a nonhousewife when asked to be one. She did, however, plan for the children's school, camp, and doctors appointments. Her husband has evolved into the marketer and does more of the casual meal planning. Dinners (with guests) are usually prepared for by both of them. They say that it has been a natural evolution, with no phase of "I'll do this, if you do that." Whoever is home first starts the evening cooking and the children help. At its best it is pleasant; when rushed it is frantic. Despite the availability of a housekeeper they have refrained from asking her to prepare any part of the meal that requires more than placing food in the oven. They all enjoy the warmth and activity of mealtime preparation.

Parents who are members of dual-career couples are often surprised at the amount of actual time the husband spends in domestic duties. They are amazed at the intensity of his interest; and he is surprised, himself, at the discovery of aspects of change:

> The kids need me. Sometimes they say I can be more fun than their mother. I secretly like that; I really am more fun-loving. I can go with the flow, be more indulgent than she can. I think I really am much less practical and so play better with them. I confess that the part of me that is competitive with her takes some pride in the fact that they tell me they like being with me even more than with her. Of course, they probably tell her the opposite, perhaps for different reasons. There is some other part of me that knows the score, however. Of course, the realization of her ambitions was harder won. She went against parents, family, and even more a social tradition that curtailed her ambitions in a real way. If she gives up she is lost. I love her for her efforts too—she is remarkable; I am in awe of her energy and ability and that, also, turns me on. It is not the total woman defined by others that I see; she is often preoccupied—but she has enough for me, she supports me and I support her. She knows I give. We don't count the ways any more. My taking care of the groceries is an act of love. Somewhere in her head and heart she is noticing it. We don't have to tote it up in a double entry bookkeeping system. We feel it together, in a look, a glance, in bed. I never expected I would be this way in a marriage. I wasn't raised to see such mutuality. The kids have always been mine also. I was there when they were born and I changed my share of diapers. It's been good, and it gets better, to my surprise. (An advertising executive whose wife runs a travel agency.)

TROUBLE

It has been observed that marriage, as a system of interactions, can be conceptually separated into two marriages—his and hers.[9] The husband's marriage, despite men's traditional complaint about it and comedians' routines about it, turns out to be unequivocally good for men. They live longer, function better, and thrive in every way better than their unmarried counterparts. That inveterate misogynist, George Bernard Shaw, constructs, like an early sociobiologist, the underpinnings of marriage as a biological mandate; he proposed, in 1903 that woman was "nature's contrivance" for carrying out its highest achievement. Further "sexually, Man is Woman's contrivance to carry out nature's best in the most economical way." Man was invented by woman for this purpose—and he is allowed all his follies, ideals, and heroisms, "provided that the key stone of them all is the worship of Woman . . . of motherhood, of the family . . ."[10] This may be the other side of Shaw's misogyny; his awe and mistrust of women's power.

On the other hand, despite the general need and wish women seem to have for marriage, they paradoxically fare far worse in the marital state than do their husbands. The contrivance which she sets, according to Shaw, then, seems to serve her poorly. Bernard[9] points to the fact that women are required to make more and greater adjustments to change than are their husbands. For the housewife, in a "dead-end job" with little to share with her husband about her world, life can be stultifying. The housewife, then, seems to give up much for the marriage and much for her husband.

The woman in the dual role has seemed to place her position second to that of her husband.[11] Women do this, perhaps, because they are socialized toward the conviction that the family comes first. There is, also, the related strong internalization of the traditional role for women, that of taking less initiative.[12] Home is their arena and husband's needs are primary. Margaret Mead was quoted as issuing the dire warning in 1970 that women in the early wave of the Women's Liberation Movement might be driving their husbands crazy.[9] A supporting finding comes from Burke and Weir,[13] who found that while employed women seemed to be in better physical and mental health with more positive attitudes toward marriage than housewives, the husbands of employed women were in poorer health and expressed more discontent with their marriages. This study indicated that the price to be paid in marriage for women's personal growth and fulfillment is found in their husband's stress and physical debility. A veiw in refutation is entered by Booth.[14] He found methodologic failings in the Burke and Weir paper. In a replication of that study it was found that husbands of employed wives had no greater evidence for marital discord and stress than did husbands of housewives. It is clear, however, that such studies are subject to social and political value systems. There is a lack of clarity about what constitutes contentment or how it is related to social change.

Certainly strongly held social values impinge on both members of the couple. Change in attitude has, however, been rapid within the last eight years. It is parallel with the growing strength and acceptance of the Women's Movement. A 1972 study[9] indicated that "despite cries from radical feminists for emancipation," most married professional women still were basically satisfied with life that includes family first. A recent work suggests a repeat of such a study with the obvious inference that the conclusions in the earlier study would not be found.[15]

Yet, today, although there is more equality "in the air," there is, probably, for many couples, an important leftover derivative of the woman as weaker, less competent, and more dependent than the man. With new-found parity between the sexes, other problems arise for some couples. Equality, when male "superiority" remains the template against which judgments have been made, is often seen as male weakness.[16] This situation holds for the perspectives of men and women, and may lead to sexual dysfunction when both partners register male equality as male weakness. Such difficulties may increase in a couple in which the woman has recently achieved actually greater status than the man. When there is a failure of the defensive perception of "it is all a political manipulation, she gets a lot just by being a woman," many men find themselves angry, feeling misunderstood, and often ready to leave the relationship. At such time there is, for some, a wish for the traditional wife.[15]

Some men discover late in marriage that they cannot endure the privations of a dual-career marriage; they are too directed toward the comforts that traditional wives can provide. They continue to expect that the wife will suddenly find her place in the kitchen or laundry. When the realization occurs that she really means it, that she wants a career, cares less for a tidy house, clean children, and providing creature comforts for husband, the light may go out in his eyes. He may then seek another woman who is more "understanding."

The numbers of extramarital affairs among dual-career couples has not been presented by any study. Writers on the subject of professional couples occasionally mention it, not because there are data, but because one would expect that couples who can break with traditional social interaction can also break with more usual sexual interactions. Such affairs, at least in the authors' experience as therapists, presage marital separation. They may not be the cause of the dissolution of a relationship but rather a sign of it. It is probably still relatively rare in this country (or in the authors' part of it) for there to be either a continuing extramarital affair(s) during which a marriage endures or even rarer that an "open marriage" can flourish. It is more usual (although not generally common) for there to exist occasional sexual interactions with different sexual partners—usually trustworthy friends or colleagues in relationships in which there is little risk of compromising the stable and important ongoing marriage. Such relationships can be friendly, romantic, attended by humor and openness about the necessity for secrecy. If the relationship becomes "serious" it becomes difficult to maintain against the established background of marriage and work. The choice, then, often is for discontinuing the extramarital relationship by both participants.

For the dual-career marriage to work well there must be more in the relationship than the traditional comforts to be provided for, by the wife, as a sacrifice to the husband's needs. A dual career is, still, a social experiment.

Can It Work Better?

Yet, dual-career couples may not always feel that they are involved in a social experiment, certainly not a controlled one. There is often a sense of lack of control, of tumbling through the days, willy-nilly. There are times when, even in the best marriage, the man, of course, wishes that the marriage (or wife) could be traditional and thus make it easier. It often seems, at least for the man, that a double sacrifice is made; he has to give less to his job in order to give more to the family (since she is not doing the whole job) and he gets less time, attention, and comfort from her. In other words many, if not most men in a dual-career marriage still do not perceive that a part of their "job" is at home. Employing a housekeeper is a possible resolution of the problem for those who can afford it and feel that hiring household help is philosophically compatible with their values. Some couples have moved toward more novel arrangements.

An interesting shift from traditional roles of man-at-work/woman-at-home or men and women in dual careers is that of sharing work and family responsibility. Thus, each member of the couple works in a part-time commitment. The part-time work movement has been encouraged by a President, and entered into by those who cannot (for reasons of health) have full-time employment, do not wish to, or are committed ideologically to a "more meaningful life based on a reduced or flexible work (schedule)."[17] This had been tried earlier in Norway.[18]

Equal status is implied for both members of the team, with equal division of labor. The economic difficulty is sizable (income is usually reduced) but such couples often report increased intimacy and sharing. The promise of greater cohesion for families in such a "shared work, shared love" arrangement will be sorely tried during a period of an economic downturn. It also may not be a feasible solution in certain occupational areas.

There are many ways in which dual-career couples may live. The social experiment is not totally contained within a form defined for them (such as, for example, "shared work and love," or "open marriage.") The modes or styles of the relationship are always shifting, and if it lasts, it is dependent on factors relating to the aging and changing personal world of the individuals. The growth of children, social and economic shifts, and a reciprocal wish to keep the relationship going are similarly important. The ability of the man to risk, to shift from his previous position of assumed strength and leadership is important in this. Differences between women and men, assigned as "state" differences, "biologically based," and supported by social and even moral/religious imperatives are challenged within a reciprocal relationship. Interestingly, for the couple "doing it," it becomes commonplace and not worth comment. For those who ask, for example, "How does it feel for your wife to earn more money than you do?," there is sometimes only surprise at the question. It often does not matter at all. For some men, however, it can be a constant source of irritation.

The "limited repertoire" of adult roles, as characterized by a life-cycle model, has also been criticized. A suggested alternative view, more in keeping with human plasticity, is the life-spiral model, with many alternative roles as possible.[19] Some husbands who maintain a "traditional" dual-career family are taking a second look at their priorities, and putting much greater emphasis on family and children than did their own fathers. Support from their wives helps in this; the pleasure derived from exercise of this role becomes for some an important experience. A surgeon in his late forties, married to a nurse, says:

> I started out totally dedicated to surgery. For years I spent day and night at the hospital. I don't want it anymore; maybe I don't need it. I think I lost one of my children because of it. The children want me—I want to be at home, to play music. Do you have to kill yourself and your family to be a good doctor?

The sense of equity in sharing a difficult load, allows a man to view his wife differently. Presenting her with tea or coffee, for example, while she is working, is an extension not only of affection and concern but regard. Emerging from this new interaction is a suffusion of romantic and sexual feelings with respect for a coequal.

CHILDREN . . . AND TIME

We are, as humans, as wedded to time as to each other. We are aware of ourselves today, tomorrow, and yesterday. We view our personal development and the historical evolution of our group, culture, and humankind with varying degrees of interest—but as sentient humans we are conscious of the effect of such changes on our lives. We are aware of aging and the growth of our children who view their world differently from the way in which we saw ours.

We all change. Even those who started a marriage with the idea that change was inherent within us are still surprised by the constancy of change. Many of us, the writers of this chapter included, find that some issues, important at the outset, have become unimportant now. Who does the marketing, or the cooking, or the planning for vacations is not a subject of contention or conversation. (It has the potential for rising to the surface only when the going gets tough and other issues intervene.) For younger dual-career couples, viewing those of us who have been at it for a longer amount of time (and who have, usually, concomitantly fewer tasks and sacrifice directed toward very young children), there is envy and concern. They wonder if we always functioned with less strain than they presently do. They wonder if they can achieve what seems like easy accord. In fact, what matters so much at the outset, an equitable division of labor, given the insistent simultaneous needs of infants and budding career, lessens on those two general scores, as a consequence of time. Other issues become more important, for example, sharing concerns, and an ability to do that in the midst of insistent demands of professional life and interaction.

Change started by relatively few women in the past decade captured the imagination and spirit of others of their sex and quickly entrained men as well. The sense of urgent necessity for a shift in social values toward equity on the part of leaders fired others with the energy to demand change. The movement has evolved as the leaders have aged. Those adults who were adolescents a decade ago have grown to young adulthood in the midst of questioning the traditional lives led by (most) of their parents. The lifestyle they set for themselves and their children may differ greatly from that of their parents. The continuing Women's Movement has supported the possibility of such an option.

There is reciprocity between parent and child as seen early in the child's discriminating development. It is based on a feedback gauged to fulfillment of individual needs.[20] Observed first in mother–infant pairs it is now clear that by three or four weeks of age father–infant interactions, although grossly different from that of mother and child, show the same "reciprocal affective control."[21]

The male child may now grow up with a different perspective regarding maleness. Certainly if father-at-work/mother-at-home has shifted so that father is more present at home, less distant, and more expressive, the boy will grow up holding a different view of maleness and manhood than his predecessors. He may see more of men's potential nurturance and expressiveness and perceive that as an area to be developed.

From another context, the evolution of the Oedipal complex and its manifestations will shift also. Father traditionally has been a distant figure, going in the mornings, returning at night; with mother as the source of ongoing warmth and support. Femininity is then absolutely set aside from male striving within this framework. Women are giving, warm, wished for objects simultaneously to be rejected as models for behavior. Male behavior and activity involves only rough and tumble of the world outside of the home and the pleasure of male company is set aside from that of the company of women.

New generations of boys growing up as men may be able to express a portion of the innate male matrix of behavior previously ridiculed, derogated, or condemned. An optimistic scenario would include the effect of such change on relationships between sexes in play and work, and interpersonal and international violence. We know of course that the changes are not broadly sweeping; they are affected by class lines, geographic and ethnic factors, and history. Yet, the position has been registered and changes in society for men and women are measured against it. The struggle is not entirely women's against men's resistance. Many males see the movement as an opportunity to drop a burdensome stereotypic role.

A time-related phenomenon, particularly among older professional couples, occurs toward midlife. Often the wife, having taken care of domestic duties primarily, is held back from full commitment to professional duties because of the demands attendant on starting a family. As children's requirements for constant attention decrease with time, there is more possibility for women to pursue their own careers. Prompted in part by the encouragement of the Women's Movement (and attendant laws for opportunity) some women have equaled or bettered their partner's positions in terms of money and position.

There is another related phenomenon related to time and aging. Women between forty and fifty, after a later start, are moving ahead in career development, with increasing vigor, as they approach later middle age while their husbands, generally older, have peaked and plateaued.[22] Men often feel burned out, disenchanted with the need for achievement, while their wives are getting a "second wind." For a generation raised in a traditional pattern of man as the leader and mover, and woman as the follower, depression may be exacerbated. Among the consequences of such a "midlife crisis" is the sadly familiar pattern of disengagement from family and remarriage to a younger woman. The attempt to restitute a sense of forward movement and strength by recreating a second family is perilous and not often successful, even with an initially conscientious and willing partner. For a generation raised in a mode which does not emphasize male striving or women's acceptance of "work" solely as the man's prerogative, an alternative, easier, and noncompetitive bargain may be struck at midlife. The view of men, generally as tough and inexpressive, is challenged directly by those who explicitly speak for such social change; and, even, more recently by popular media—television and film. Heroes are often men who can be receptive, understanding, tender, and nurturant toward children. That is seen as worthy of a woman's love, now. It is more "manly" than the "old-grapefruit-in-the-face."

Many women who have achieved their own separate careers feel the pull exerted by the children in the household to a greater degree than do their partners.[20] Professional couples are, by their nature and the nature of their work, demanding. They strongly control their portion of their environment or try to more than do others. This often extends, naturally, to their children. They want their children to develop well, or better than others, and to be happy. That is not dissimilar from other parents but professional couples often feel greater responsibility for mishaps; they tend to see troubles which may be transient as casting a longer shadow. The wife often must worry about it. One wife says

> When something goes wrong—he (husband) notices it. Oh, Tom isn't doing well in math—but he registers it as a complaint as if he is at the garage talking to the mechanic who services the car. I'm supposed to fix what he notices is wrong.

Career women are often susceptible to the feeling that they have not done enough; that they have sacrificed their children's needs for their own careers. Although it is not total, there can be a trade-off of children's needs against the needs of career. Professional women, particularly, in reading the literature on the subject, want to believe that it is quality rather than the quantity of care which matters exclusively. Quality of care, however, is only interchangeable within limits. Forty minutes of "high-quality" care does not equal "being there." A greater amount of time is necessary and flexibility may be necessary for both husband and wife. Child care should not necessarily extinguish either career.

Children are also masters at sensing a mother's guilt and using it as a weapon to get back when feeling that there is not enough (of whatever there is) for them. Larry asked his mother to come to his school's Christmas play in which he was to be one of the Wise Men. None of her careful explanations of why she could not come during her office hours (his father was going to be out of town) consoled him. Later that night, she became so uncomfortable at the vision of her poor son as the only child without a parent present that she cancelled her appointments for the following morning. When she came to school, she found herself the only parent present.[23]

If a father also feels dependent needs are not being met there can be a collusion in which father and child can keep a susceptible mother in a chronic state of doubt. One of the basic issues in the successful maintenance of a dual-career household is the abdication of that kind of interaction. Some mothers may be able to pull it off without help, to repudiate guilt despite the attempt of spouse (and children) to trap her in it. Such women are rare; men earn the love of their spouse by avoiding such dirty tactics and demanding, if necessary, that their children do the same. The whole family may then learn that tasks and pleasures are equally shared. That institutes a potential generational change for the children; a natural acceptance of a woman's right to define her own work priorities. Male role definitions for future generations will change as the result of the exercise of such options, but also, and perhaps more importantly, as they learn, for themselves, the previously little-explored pleasures of parenting and reciprocal equal exchange with their women partners.

REFERENCES

1. Kahne H: Economic perspectives on roles of women in the American economy. J Econ Lit 13:1249–1292, 1975
2. U.S. Department of Commerce Bureau of the Census: A Statistical Portrait of Women in the U.S. Current Population Reports. Special Studies Series Number 58, 1976, p 23
3. Szali A: The Use of Time: Daily Activities of Urban and Suburban Populations in Twelve Countries. The Hague, Morton Publishing, 1971
4. O'Leary V: Toward Understanding Women. Monterey, Brooks/Cole Publishing, 1977, p 108
5. Bem SL: The measurement of psychological androgyny. J Consult Clin Psychol 42:155–162, 1974

6. Bem SL: Beyond androgyny: Some prescriptions for a liberated sexual identity, in Family in Transition, 2nd ed. Edited by Skolnick A, Skolnick T. Boston, Little Brown, 1977
7. Bardwick J: Effect of spouse companionship support on employeemnt success. J Marriage Fam 32:212–215, 1970
8. LeMasters EF: Battle of the sexes, in Family in Transition, 2nd ed. Edited by Skolnick A, Skolnick T. Boston, Little Brown, 1977
9. Bernard J: The Future of Marriage. New York, Bantam Books, 1973
10. Shaw GB: Man and Superman. Middlesex, Penguin Books, 1976, p 147
11. Heckman NA, Bryson R, Bryson JB: Problems of professional couples: A content analysis. J Marriage Fam 39:323:330, 1977
12. Horner M: Toward an understanding of achievement related conflicts in women. J Soc Issues 28:157–175, 1972
13. Burke R, Weir T: Relationships of wives' employment status to husband, wife and pair satisfaction and performance. J Marriage Fam 38:279–287, 1976
14. Booth A: Wife's employment and husband's stress: A replication and refutation. J Marriage Fam 39:645–650, 1977
15. Rice DG: Dual Career Marriages. New York, The Free Press, 1979, p 67
16. Berman E, Sacks S, Lief H: The two profession marriage: A new conflict syndrome. J Sex Marital Ther 1:242–253, 1975
17. Arkin W, Dobrofsky LR: Shared labor and love: Job sharing couples in academia. Alternative Lifestyles 1:492–512, 1978
18. Gronseth E: Worksharing families: Adaptations of pioneering families with husband and wife in part-time employment. Acta Sociologica 18:202–221, 1975
19. Etzkowitz H, Stein P: The life spiral: Human needs and adult roles. Alternative Lifestyles 1:434–464, 1978
20. Brazelton TB: The early mother–infant adjustment. Pediatrics 32:931–938, 1963
21. Brazelton TB, Keefer CH: The early mother–child relationship: A developmental view of woman as mother, in The Woman Patient, Vol II. Edited by Nadelson C, Notman M. New York, Plenum Press, 1982
22. Rappoport R: Dual Career Families. New York, Penguin Books, 1971
23. Nadelson T, Eisenberg L: The successful professional woman: On being married to one. Am J Psychiatry 134:1071–1076, 1977

Chapter 9

The "Abandoned Husband"

When Wives Leave

ELLEN HALLE

INTRODUCTION

Women's changing social roles and social expectations pose new problems for men. One of the troubling issues some men are forced to face is that of adapting to rapidly changing marital relationships when women choose to discard traditional wifely roles.[1] Much has been written about the pain of separation and divorce from the viewpoint of women, but little has been reported on the problems of the "abandoned" male. This paper will describe twenty-six men seen at a mental health clinic at a time of marital turmoil, men who had married in their early twenties, who had been reared in traditional homes, and who had traditional expectations of their wives. The focus of the paper will be on their responses to separation and divorce in their thirties, separations initiated in each instance by the wife.

Though all the men had been rejected by their wives, their characterologic types and response patterns appeared clinically to fall into three categories. Men in Group I had had the longest marriages (and consequently were somewhat older) and were the most successful professionally. The wives of these perfectionistic and demanding husbands felt totally controlled and diminished within the marriage to the point of personal nonexistence. These husbands reacted to their wives' often precipitous departure with outrage and then despair.

The men in Group II were younger, primarily involved in teaching and social work, and saw themselves as nurturing and responsive partners who had been adequate for their wives' needs in the early years of marriage. The shift of their wives' orientation from child-rearing to careers was experienced as disruptive. The wives complained that their husbands were anxious, dependent, unsatisfactory as sexual partners, and inadequate as providers. The men re-

ELLEN HALLE • Department of Psychiatry and Behavioral Sciences, Johns Hopkins University School of Medicine, Baltimore, Maryland 21205

sponded to their wives' withdrawal from the marriage with depression and passivity. Over half assumed primary child care.

Group III were men who were employed in the fields of engineering and computer technology. Their wives described them as distant husbands, emotionally and physically unavailable, overinvolved with their own work, and almost totally unable to communicate feelings. When the wives decided to leave the marriage, the men in this group were angry, but only briefly, and permitted the marriage to end without further fuss.

Three profiles, based on the synthesis of clinical observations, have been developed to describe what seemed to the author to be important differences in behavior, differences which have implications for understanding the nature of the marital conflict and for providing effective therapeutic intervention when consultation is sought. Despite the distinct differences which will be emphasized in this paper, what all these men had in common was the stress of new demands and expectations from their wives, expectations that seemed clearly to have been a consequence of the women's movement of the 1960s and 1970s. Those in clinical practice can expect to see many such problems during this time of transition from one marriage style to another. It is important to recognize not only the intrapsychic elements in each of the partners but also the cultural influences that contribute to masculine "vulnerability"—or at least the vulnerability of males whose sense of self is dependent upon a reciprocal relationship with a woman in the traditional subservient role.

Sample

The material herein reported was gathered from the practice of psychotherapy in a suburban community catering to middle and upper class patients in their early thirties. All of the patients were seen in consultation and treatment by the author. Three were treated in a men's group run by two male therapists as well as being seen on an individual basis by the writer. These patients were seen in the late 1960s to the mid 1970s.

Clinical Findings

Group I will be referred to as the *Angry Grievers*. There were six men in this group; their average length of marriage had been 15 years, and their average age was 37. All were professionals who held well-paid positions, among them a physician, a banker, a research scientist, and a successful business executive. Their predominant character style was obsessional and until the current "emergency" they had felt in control of their lives—and their wives. They functioned well professionally and saw themselves as competent heads of families. All but one had children and all were satisfied with their very traditional marriages. Only one wife had held a job; the others were active in community volunteer work.

Each Angry Griever had come to the clinic with the chief complaint: "My wife is leaving me." Typically, he was in a highly agitated state, with copious crying, and wringing of hands, and complaints of sleeplessness, inability to function at work, and feelings of depression. His wife's departure was regarded as shameful and humiliating, an event that threatened his self-image, a bit of information to be hidden from fellow employees and friends at all costs. Several men spoke of the wife's departure as "like death"; three reported suicidal ideation.

There was much self-blame and regret about not having come to the clinic sooner. In earlier years, each wife had asked her husband to join her in seeking counseling for child-rearing problems and marital dissatisfactions. These men had refused; they regarded consulting a psychiatrist as an acknowledgment of weakness and a reflection of inability to cope. Moreover, they viewed the problems as their wives' problems. They were simply too busy to participate. If the wife was troubled, it was up to her to clear it up.

Now, in the moment of crisis over his wife, the husband spent most of his first treatment session mourning his loss, remembering positive aspects of the marriage, refusing to believe that it was over, and regretting he had not been more responsive.

These men were in acute pain, which their wives were unable to acknowledge directly, presumably because of their massive rage. The wives refused to agree to conjoint meetings and took the position (as reported to the author) that their husbands would want to reassert dominance over them. However, in rare cases where the husband managed to persuade his wife to come to a joint meeting, meetings were disasters; the husbands became domineering and didactic; the wives felt enraged and taken advantage of. None of these men were able to see their wives as individuals until the wives had left.

After some weeks of intense mourning, the intensity of the depression diminished; they returned to work, began to spend more time with their children, and to show an interest in them that most had not displayed earlier. In general, their wives were supportive of their new interest in the children.

Initially all the Angry Grievers experienced brief intense feelings of helplessness and dependency on the therapist. They arrived early for appointments; wished to be seen several times weekly. Though all husbands expressed painful feelings openly during our sessions, when two were evaluated by male psychiatrists for medication, they pulled themselves together feeling they could not let a male see them in such distress. It was "unmanly." After several months, as the reality of their wives' departure was accepted, feelings of rage which had been submerged became the focus of treatment. Wishes for revenge preoccupied these men, especially those whose wives had affairs which they revealed only at the point of separation. Recognizing that they had always felt uneasy in talking about sexual feelings within the marriages, most Angry Grievers found it painful to discuss possible sexual dissatisfactions of their wives. Rage about their wives' infidelity and adandonment helped ward off feelings of depression, and anger was turned on their wives. The wives were seen as cold, calculating, ungrateful, and not worth pursuing. At about this point in therapy, half of the men reported beginning to socialize again and three began dating new partners who were accommodating, admiring, and able to offer needed reinforcement and solace.

Their "new and better partners" did a good deal to fill empty hours and to assuage the narcissistic wound of abandonment. When their self-esteem returned, depression lifted and three men discontinued therapy. The remainder who continued treatment for a longer time had alternating periods of feeling good and periods of feeling worthless, depressed, and self-blaming. Though they were vocationally quite functional, they were not as obsessed with their careers as they had been previously. It was a time for reviewing family histories and personal reflection. Most had had parenting with their mothers playing a shadowy subordinate role to a dominant and often unreasonable father whose son felt unappreciated, competitive, and incompetent in his father's eyes.

When these men began to date again, they were very sought after as desirable bachelors. Although they made real efforts to treat women more sensitively, respond to the new social demands for emotional and sexual "openness," be more playful and less rigid, they were aware of their discomfort and a lack of ease with this new mode. Since all men in Group I left therapy before remarrying, it is not known what their current marital patterns are.

Group II, here called the *Devoted Clingers,* were the largest group, numbering 14 men. Their average length of marriage was seven years and their average age 32. Younger and less affluent than Group I, they held jobs as teachers, social workers, librarians, and government employees. Two-thirds arrived at the clinic at their wives' request. One-third were referred by the Urology Department of the clinic after going there with complaints of secondary impotence. The predominant character style of these men was passive-dependent and passive-aggressive. All couples were seen conjointly. The chief complaint of wives in these partnerships was long-term marital dissatisfaction, specifically emphasizing their lack of sexual interest in their husbands, dissatisfaction with them as providers, complaints that they were poor communicators, and resentment for still being expected to play the traditional female role and yet be strong for their passive mates.

When the husbands were asked to voice their complaints and dissatisfactions, for the most part they were reticent and vague, except to express anxiety and fearfulness about change in their wives' personalities and the possibility of their wives leaving the marriage. Historically, the husbands reported that in the first few years of marriage they had seen themselves as competent, needed, and nurturing to their more childlike wives. An almost symbiotically fulfilling union was pictured by most husbands as they offered help with child care, and empathized with their wives' feelings of depression and isolation.

The wives were regretful for having married too young, having been excessively dependent, generally compliant, sexually inexperienced, and professionally untrained. However, as their children grew older, feelings of depression and restlessness grew and there developed a strong need in these women to change their lives. At least half sought some type of psychotherapy for themselves. The wives began to spend more time and energy in completing educations or going to work. This group was heavily involved in Womens' Movement-type activities: consciousness-raising groups, self-actualization, couples' labs, and assertiveness training. Child care was taken on by husbands, babysitters, or day care. These wives had a high incidence of extramarital affairs, often with their husbands' knowledge. Five couples experimented with open marriage. Wives who had been perceived originally as helpless and naive became, in their husbands' views, aggressive, unreasonable, insatiable women. In return, the wives viewed their husbands as emotionally dependent, personally immature, sexually unexciting, and professionally unambitious.

In conjoint therapy sessions, the husbands minimized problems and placated as their wives demanded that they be different, more competent professionally, more effective personally, and more emotionally expressive. Husbands unable to meet these unrealistic expectations and faced with their wives' desire to leave became extremely anxious, depressed, and pressed more intensely for "closeness," often articulated in requests for sexual contact. Wives were extremely upset over conflicts regarding traditional female responsibilities and the fulfillment of their own "needs." When these wives finally decided to end the marriage, almost half decided to leave children primarily in care of husbands, often saying, "he's a better mother than I am." Husbands responded eagerly to child-rearing responsibilities.

All men in Group II had some individual psychiatric care after wives left. Half were in short-term treatment which focused on need for immediate support, treating anxiety, depression, and in some, worries about sexual dysfunction. In all but one case, dysfunction was reversed, as reported with new partners. After short-term treatment ceased, there was an "open door" policy and these husbands felt free to come as needed for personal crises with children and wives or new partners. The remainder were in long-term treatment at least a year, using a combination of individual therapy and all-male groups run by male therapists.

In all the men in this group feelings of sadness, loneliness, and failure were initially immobilizing. Their wives' leaving brought out their passivity and hopelessness. Some husbands' interests in their wives' new lives were intense as they tried to prolong the attachment through helpfulness, e.g., babysitting, carpentry, running errands. They had difficulty seeing that their helpfulness disguised covert clinging. It was difficult to mobilize their repressed/denied anger and rage and help them to get in touch with aggressive feelings so they could function in a more mature, autonomous manner. Fearful of rejection and sexual failure, these men often were reluctant to make new contacts, but when they did, they felt positive and accepted. Long-term work was often an opportunity to understand that behind the marital struggle was usually an intensely ambivalent relationship with a strong controlling mother. In these men good identification with fathers was usually absent. Ongoing treatment helped these patients deal with separation both intrapsychically on a developmental level and practically with everyday issues. As separation was worked through, they became less compliant. More emotional assertiveness in dealing with wives, bosses, and new partners was usually felt to be gratifying. Therapists who see these men will be dealing directly with dependency issues and must avoid "taking charge" as wives once did. All-male groups run by male therapists are reported to be useful for support, role modeling, self-observation, and helping the patients to take active responsibility.

I will refer to Group III as the *Detached Avoiders.* There were 6 men in this group. Their average length of marriage was 6 years and average age was 31. The husbands' occupations were in the fields of engineering, architecture, computer programming, and real estate. From brief observation, their predominant character style was somewhat narcissistic with obsessive features. These men had looked at married life much in terms of routinized compromise with each spouse filling traditional roles. There was little or no sharing of tasks and feelings. All these men were seen briefly at the clinic at their wives' request just prior to marital breakup. The wives had all been previously treated for the chief complaint of depression and marital maladjustment, reporting that their husbands were not interested in coming in for treatment. Not much is known directly about these men. These wives described their husbands as never having been involved emotionally in the relationship, and as unexpressive, except sexually, where the husbands performed extremely well. These husbands were physically absent much of the time, occupying themselves with work, hobbies, and sports. Many wives suspected husbands' fidelity but were silent. The husbands were seen as pleasant and gregarious by neighbors and friends, but their wives reported them personally as distant and cold.

Wives of Detached Avoiders had been generally uninvolved directly in the Women's Movement. They sought therapy for depression, expressed as loneliness in marriage, fear of getting older and less attractive, and the realization that they wanted more from a relationship than economic security. In these marriages, as long as the wives did not make emotional demands, things went fairly smoothly. Husbands reported being generally satisfied with the marriage, though they admitted they often felt detached and aloof from their wives, children, and people in general. When the husbands were finally forced to come to the clinic, they seemed uncomfortable being in a psychiatric setting and mystified by the intensity of their wives' misery. Willing to be seen with their wives, these men had little interest in exploring personal issues or marital failures. When the wives decided to leave the marriages, their husbands did not protest.

Discussion

As marital patterns are in transition, how can we, as clinicians, be helpful to both men and women? We are seeing more men who are bewildered, hurt, and angry, perceiving women's efforts toward individuation as being directed against them. There is a confusion of role and tasks as couples struggle with change.[2] It is unclear to me as yet what therapeutic approaches are most helpful. A variety were used to meet specific situations. To learn more of what worked therapeutically and what changes, if any, in partners and lifestyles these men and women have made, there must be systematic follow-up of such cases. It is important to note that almost no husbands made the initial psychiatric contact. However, it has been pointed out that in our society, it is women who have been more accepting of the role of the psychiatric patient.[3] Further investigation is necessary to help therapists treat current marital dysfunction more promptly and effectively, as well as to enable men to feel more comfortable or even interested in seeking psychiatric help.

REFERENCES

1. Epstein J: Divorce in America, Marriage in an Age of Possibility. New York, Dutton, 1974, p 76
2. Moulton R: Some Effects of The New Feminism. Am J Psychiat 134:1–6, 1977
3. Chessler P: Women and Madness, New York, Avon, 1972, p 114

Chapter 10

Postparental Fathers in Distress

ROBERT A. LEWIS AND CRAIG L. ROBERTS

INTRODUCTION

According to a number of the authors' colleagues, one group which is finding its way into psychiatric offices in increasing numbers is composed of middle-aged fathers whose children have recently left home. Many of these postparental fathers are experiencing what social scientists have called "the empty nest syndrome."

The terms "empty nest" and "postparental couples" are negative terms in themselves and are symbolic of the ways in which both social scientists and lay people have long viewed that period of family life which stretches from the departure of the last child from the home until parents' retirement. In fact, until rather recently, the transition to the postparental years was seen for most parents as a period of crisis and major discontinuity,[1] since it marked the "desertion" of children from the home or their "abandonment" of their parents. A number of studies have suggested, for instance, that children's leaving home produces many marital conflicts and results for many parents in a loss of roles which are still highly valued in society. One study[2] found that mothers in the postparental years reported lower satisfaction with both spousal love and companionship than did mothers in any of the 15 earlier years of married life. Rollins and Feldman[3] discovered that parents who were launching their children reported the least satisfying family life of all.

Mothers have been thought to experience more crisis and loss than fathers after children depart from the home, primarily since mothers have depended more upon their roles and position as a parent for a major source of their satisfaction and self-identity.[4–7] Journals frequently run advertisements about antidepressants for women who are experiencing the "empty nest syndrome." One study of first admissions to mental hospitals[8] found that 63% of mothers in

---

ROBERT A. LEWIS • Department of Child Development and Family Studies, Purdue University, West Lafayette, Indiana 47907. CRAIG L. ROBERTS • Department of Sociology, University of Minnesota, Minneapolis, Minnesota 44414

the empty nest years had high rates of depression, and 82% of those who had been overinvolved and overprotective of their child were depressed.

A Time of Relief?

Earlier research about the postparental years, however, has been replaced by less pessimistic studies. For instance, most of the studies of postparental couples done since 1960 have found that the majority of mothers and fathers do not experience crisis, but rather view the postparental years as a "time of relief" or even a "second honeymoon."[7,9–17] Moreover, some recent studies suggest that when postparental mothers do experience crisis and great unhappiness, it is usually in the context of poor timing, e.g., an unanticipated life event[14,18] or reorganizations of family relationships which are not successfully completed.[7]

Fathers Can Be Unhappy, Too

Postparental fathers, in contrast to mothers, rarely have been studied. Only four other studies have interviewed the fathers at all.[1,12,16,17] Our own studies of postparental fathers[15] suggest that just as many fathers as mothers report unhappiness following the departure of the last child from the home. For instance, 22% of postparental fathers and 23% of postparental mothers in a random sample of 118 parents in a northeast Georgia county reported feeling unhappy over their last child leaving home. It is important to note that most of the postparental fathers reported feeling somewhat or very happy (42%) or neutral (35%). However, the postparental transition is still problematic if it is a cause of distress for nearly a fourth of fathers.

A description of the 22% of fathers who reported being somewhat to very unhappy is very revealing. These men tended to have had fewer children. They were also somewhat older men and perceived themselves to be more nurturing persons. Additionally, these fathers were also more apt to feel neglected by their wives, to receive the least understanding from them, to be the most lonely and least enthusiastic about their wives' companionship, and to have the least empathic wives.

Most Interest: Most to Lose

One explanation for the unhappiness of these fathers seems to lie in the "Principle of *Most* Interest." Waller[19] suggested many years ago that the person with the least interest in a relationship was the one who has the greatest potential for exploiting the other and, therefore, the greatest power, since he/she would feel the least loss if the relationship terminated. On the other hand, the person with the most interest has the most to lose upon the dissolution of a relationship and therefore is the most vulnerable and should have the most difficult time in adjusting to a separation.

A description of the situation of unhappy fathers is compatible with the Principle of Most Interest, since the unhappy fathers had the fewest children and therefore stood to lose the most with the departure of the last child. They tended to be older fathers who may perceive fewer years remaining in their lives and thus fewer opportunities to be with their children. They perceived themselves to be nurturing and caring men, who should therefore feel more loss with the shrinking of their care-giving, fatherly roles. Finally, and most importantly, since these fathers seemed to have the least satisfying marriages in many respects, they probably had more to lose with their last child's leaving home.

The implications for the mental health of these postparental fathers are serious and problematic. Typical couples can currently expect 16 to 18 years of married life together after their last child leaves home. In fact, the average married couple now spends more years in the postparental period than in any other stage of the family life cycle. One can expect high rates of marital dissolution and psychiatric illness among these unhappy postparental fathers if individual psychotherapy and marriage enrichment are not available to them.

GROWING MALE NURTURANCE

The outlook for men who will become postparental fathers in the future is even more chilling, if it is true, as some suggest, that more young men are becoming nurturant fathers.[21,22] Although there are data which suggest that most fathers of young children indicate some interest in child-care activities and some fathers even arrange their work schedules to be with their young children,[21,23] the actual hours spent in child care by most fathers and the quality of their child care are not well documented.

Research in adult development and aging, however, suggests that men generally become more nurturant during the middle and later years—at a time when women are altering their sex-role behavior in the opposite direction.[24] Neugarten and Gutmann[25] suggest that as men age they become much more receptive to affiliative and nurturant promptings, while women during these years become more responsive toward, and less guilty about, aggression. Lowenthal and Chiriboga[16] found that the personality changes of some wives greatly affected their husbands. The midlife female changes for these women were outward, away from dependency on the husband, and away from support and nurturance of them. The husbands felt that their wives became more precious to them at the same time as these changes threatened the withdrawal of the wives' recognition, affection, and valuing of them. Thus, it may be that the needs of men and women during the middle years often become less complementary.

CASE I

The refusal to acknowledge that a relationship changes when children depart is one manifestation of postparental-father distress. Mr. G., aged 72 and retired for four years, requested treatment at the urging of his only son, aged 34. Mr. G. was obsessed with his son's finances, to the extent of inquiring almost daily into the son's expenditures and keeping a detailed account of them.

Upon learning of her husband's obsession, Mrs. G., aged 64, was openly hostile. Actively involved in running a real estate office, she was home on an irregular schedule but became aware of his frequent calls. She had never been very supportive of Mr. G. and had criticized him throughout their marriage.

The obsessive behavior became the focus of the therapy. The son had lived with his parents through his college years. He married following graduation and moved out of state to attend law school. Mr. G. continued to support his son during law school as he had during the undergraduate years. Each month Mr. G. would make an hour-long phone call to determine his son's needs and then would send him a generous check. It was at this time that he began to keep a ledger of his son's finances.

After the son passed the bar, he joined a law firm in another state. Mr. G. continued to make calls and write checks, but the son now returned the checks. Mr. G. became more anxious, calling more frequently and pressing for more detailed information. By the time the father retired, he was calling weekly. At the beginning of treatment he was making almost daily calls to the son's office.

Treatment was first directed toward overcoming patient resistance. As resistance decreased, Mr. G. focused on his relationship with his own father who had died ten years prior to treatment. Mr. G. had become a businessman against the grandfather's wishes. The grandfather openly chastised Mr. G., who then moved to another city in the same state to reduce contact. The grandfather continued his criticism of Mr. G. until his death. Mr. G. recognized that his own father never changed the manner in which he regarded Mr. G., giving Mr. G. no opportunity to assert his independence. Mr. G. had not experienced his father's "letting go" and thus had no role model for "letting go" himself.

Mr. G. recognized that his obsession was an expression of his need to be valued by both his son and his wife. Because he felt powerless and unneeded in his marriage, the obsession was directed entirely toward his son. This insight enabled him to express his desire for recognition much more directly to both his son and his wife. However, he could not be dislodged from his belief that the son was financially unstable; later he was able to recognize that he could help protect his son's children by creating a trust fund for their education. In time Mr. G. was freed to explore matters such as intimacy and the balance of power in his marriage.

CASE II

Mr. W., aged 52, referred himself for treatment of his depression and alcohol dependency. He contacted the therapist after a business associate refused to ride home with him following a friendly evening of food and spirits.

Mr. W.'s depression was traced back two years to the three-month period in which his two daughters, now aged 21 and 25, were married. His compulsive drinking had begun shortly after his second daughter's marriage.

Mr. W. had very little to say in his description of Mrs. W., aged 49. In contrast to him, she was not a very active person and rarely left the home. Mr.

W. had difficulty describing her reaction to their daughters' marriages. They apparently had not discussed their own reactions to the daughter's leaving.

Mr. W. had always been very close to his daughters, having long discussions with them and taking them to many school and social activities. He played a good deal with them when they were young and took them to parks and camping trips every summer. When the daughters began to date, they often sought their father's counsel.

Mr. W. realized in therapy that his daughters were still very important to him and that he missed seeing them on a daily basis. He was a loving father to them and received a great shock when they left almost stimultaneously. It was hard for him to admit that he must share them now with their husbands.

The loss of his daughters was compounded by the realization that his marriage was less than meaningful. He had made few friends in spite of the many organizations in which he had worked. In actuality, he had no one at the beginning of therapy with whom he could share his life. With the aid of his therapist, Mr. W. began to explore possibilities for enriching his marriage and developing new friendships among male acquaintances.

CONCLUSIONS

These two case studies represent only a few permutations of those recurring themes which we found in our study of postparental fathers. Among the more frequent of these themes were: fathers become more nurturing at the same time that their wives and children have less need to be nurtured; fathers who have spent their early lives working to support their children and wives discover that the other family members now have less need of their support; and fathers discover that their marriages and friendships have become empty shells rather than fulfilling relationships.

In summary, the authors' studies of postparental fathers suggest that about as many fathers as mothers (nearly one-fourth) do exhibit some symptoms of distress when their children leave home. Clinical reports and observations corroborate some survey data which suggest that, owing to cultural changes in both men's and women's sex roles, to developmental changes which appear for most men and women in these middle years, and to the resultant lack of role reciprocity for postparental couples, the numbers of distressed fathers at this stage of the family life cycle may indeed be growing.

REFERENCES

1. Axelson L: Personal adjustment in the postparental period. Marriage Fam Living 22:66–68, 1960
2. Bart P: Depression in middle-aged women, in Women in Sexist Society. Edited by Gornick V, Moran B. New York, Basic Books, 1971
3. Blood R, Wolfe D: Husbands and Wives: The Dynamics of Married Living. New York, Free Press, 1960
4. Burr W: Satisfaction with various aspects of marriage over the life cycle. J Marriage Fam 21:29–37, 1970

5. Cavan R: Family tensions between the old and the middle-aged. Marriage Fam Living 18:323–327, 1956
6. Deutscher I: The quality of postparental life: Definitions of the situation. J Marriage Fam 26:52–59, 1964
7. Deutscher I: From parental to post-parental life. Sociol Symp 3:47–60, 1969
8. Dizard J: Social Change in the Family. Chicago, University of Chicago, 1968
9. Duvall E: Marriage and Family Development. Philadelphia, Lippincott, 1977
10. Fein R: Men's Experiences before and after the Birth of the First Child: Dependence, Marital Sharing and Anxiety. Doctoral dissertation, Harvard University, 1974
11. Fein R: Men's entrance to parenthood. Fam Coordinator 25:341–347, 1976
12. Glenn N: Psychological well-being in the post-parental stage: Some evidence from national surveys. J Marriage Fam 37:105–110, 1975
13. Harkins E: Effects of empty nest transition on self-report of psychological and physical well-being. J Marriage Fam 27:549–556, 1978
14. Levine J: Who Will Raise the Children? New Options for Fathers and Mothers. New York, Lippincott, 1976
15. Lewis R, Freneau P, Roberts C: Fathers and the postparental transition. Fam Coordinator 28:514–20, 1979
16. Lewis R, Casto R, Aquilino W, et al.: Developmental transitions in male sexuality. Counseling Psychol 7:15–19, 1978
17. Lowenthal M, Chiriboga D: Transition to the empty nest. Arch Gen Psychiatry 26:8–14, 1972
18. Neugarten B: Adaptation and the life cycle. J Geriatric Psychiatry 4:71–100, 1970
19. Neugarten B, Gutmann D: Age–sex roles and personality in middle age: A thematic apperception study. Psychol Monographs 72:32–33, 1958
20. Peck R: Psychological developments in the second half of life, in Psychological developments in the second half of life, in Psychological Aspects of Aging: Proceedings of a Conference on Planning Research. Edited by Anderson J. Bethesda, Maryland, Apr 1955
21. Pineo P: Disenchantment in the later years of marriage. Marriage Fam Living 23:3–11, 1961
22. Rollins B, Feldman H: Marital satisfaction over the family life cycle. J Marriage Fam 26:20–28, 1970
23. Rose A: Factors associated with the life-satisfaction of middle-class, middle-aged persons. J Marriage Fam 17:15–19, 1955
24. Saunders L: Empathy, communication, and the definition of life satisfaction in the postparental period. Fam Perspective 8:21–35, 1974
25. Spence D, Lonner T: The empty nest: A transition within motherhood. Fam Coordinator 20:369–375, 1971
26. Waller W: The rating and dating complex. Am Sociol Rev 2:727–734, 1937

Chapter 11

The Older Man

KENNETH SOLOMON

INTRODUCTION

In recent years, the plight of the elderly in American society has received increasing attention from practitioners of social policy and health care, applied researchers in the field of gerontology, and the public at large. It has included cross-sectional examinations of the biologic, psychologic, and sociologic differences between the aged and young as well as investigations of aging as a longitudinal process. The elderly were first considered a homogeneous group of individuals, defined by age, with similar needs, attributes, and problems. Over time, however, it has become clear that the elderly are quite a heterogenous lot, and are comprised of many different groups with their own special characteristics. The Black elderly have different problems from the White elderly, the poor from the rich, the young-old from the old-old,[1] and women from men. Over the last five to ten years in particular, attention has been accorded the special problems of older women, especially widows, and their adaptation.

There has also been a popularization of the developmental problems of pregeriatric individuals, the so-called "midlife crisis." Several investigators, notably Gutmann and co-workers[2,3] and Neugarten and Datan[4,5] have begun to research these midlife issues. Popular books, including those of Levinson et al.,[6] Gould,[7] and Sheehy,[8] have helped to further stimulate these investigations.

However, there has been only the most minimal of examinations of the special characteristics, problems, and needs of older men. These issues range from factors that have a direct effect on the life expectancy of men to a multitude of diseases and psychosocial factors that influence the welfare of the older man in American society. These issues include retirement, health, widowerhood, dependency, and other problems that will be examined in this chapter. Stress and coping in the elderly, with a particular emphasis on the older man, will be a major focus of this chapter. The chapter will also discuss clinical issues for the

---

KENNETH SOLOMON • Levindale Hebrew Geriatric Center and Hospital, Baltimore, Maryland 21215

therapist when he/she is working with an older man who has difficulty adapting to some of the special problems of aging men.

CHARACTERISTICS OF THE OLDER MAN

Who is the older man? It almost seems to be a cliche to say that it depends upon who is defining the person as old and who is being defined. There is no definition of "old" or "aging" that is satisfactory for this purpose. One common definition is based on chronological age. A person is old when he/she has reached the age of 55 (e.g., for membership in the American Association of Retired Persons or many senior citizens centers), 60 (for certain economic benefits of early retirement), 62 (for partial pension benefits), 65 (for Social Security, Medicare, and Older Americans Act benefits), or 70 (e.g., for mandatory retirement) years of age. Being old may be defined subjectively; a person is as old as he/she feels, acts or looks. This has wide variance in any individual from day to day. Another means of labeling a person old is when he/she displays the physical or social concomitants of aging, such as gray hair, wrinkles, slower reaction time, widowhood, or retirement. Unfortunately for this definition, people and organ systems age at different rates. That there is a great disparity in the age at which people define others as old has been clearly demonstrated by Tuckman and Lorge,[9] Powers and Grubbs,[10] and Harris.[11] Indeed, Powers and Grubbs[10] suggest that the concept of "old" may be a false sociologic construct, based on their data that the elderly cannot define what they mean by old. Because of these operational problems, the author will arbitrarily define an older man as a man who has reached his 60th birthday for purposes of this chapter.

Little is known about this population group, for as mentioned above, they have not been the subject of rigorous study. Much of what is known about older men has been researched by anthropologists, and the data that are available comes from cultures other than the American. Because of this paucity of data, much of what is included in this chapter is based on the author's experience as a gerontologist, researcher, and clinician.

There were approximately 23 million people over the age of 65 in the United States in 1974. Approximately 41% of this group were men.[11] As the population ages, the proportion of men to women diminishes; there are approximately 138 women for every 100 men at age 65 and 156 women for every 100 men at age 85.[12] The life expectancy of white men in 1977 was just under 73 years; for white women, it was over 81 years. For Black men, life expectancy was about 61 years. For Black women, it was about 76 years. For American Indian men and women life expectancy was even less, although a similar differential in years is maintained. Older men are likely to be married but older women are likely to be widowed (Table 1).[11–13] Older men are more likely to be living with a family member than are older women (79% vs. 59%) and less likely to be living alone (17% vs. 37%).[12] Only 5% are employed full-time and another 12% have part-time employment; 41% were involuntarily retired.[11]

It has been hypothesized that this difference in life expectancy is primarily biological, that the male is the constitutionally weaker sex. However, when the

Table I. Marital Status of the Elderly[a]

	Men (1970)	Men (1974)	Women (1970)	Women (1974)
Single	7.8	4.0	7.7	5.0
Married, spouse present	68.4	78.0	33.7	39.0
Widowed	18.0	15.0	54.6	53.0
Divorced	5.8[b]	2.0	4.0[b]	2.0
Separated		1.0		1.0

[a]1970 data from Brotman (Ref. 12); 1974 data from Harris (Ref. 11). [b]Includes Divorced and Separated.

causes of death of men are examined, it is clear that most of them are mediated by psychosocial factors and a lifestyle that shortens the lives of men at all stages of adult life. This has been discussed in more depth in the chapter by Solomon describing the masculine role and elsewhere,[14,15] but will be summarized here.

Men are twice as prone to the development of severe cardiovascular disease, especially myocardial infarction, than are women.[14–16] Myocardial infarction is a stress-related disease and tends to occur in people who have the Type A personality.[17] These men are very success-oriented and status-oriented, extremely active, aggressive individuals who are quite tense and inexpressive. They are impatient and have a continuous sense of urgency about time. They are controlling, hostile individuals. They are workaholics and deny their dependency needs. They view themselves as invulnerable. They are, in many ways, only a slight caricature of the traditional masculine role. Other stress-related diseases that affect men more frequently than women include peptic ulcer disease and hypertension (with its resultant renal disease and stroke).[14,16] The stress that men experience frequently manifests itself in self-medication with drugs, particularly nicotine and caffeine. Caffeine intake has been hypothesized to be related to an increased risk of cardiovascular disease. Nicotine intake and cigarette smoking cause lung, throat, and laryngeal cancers (all of which occur three to four times more frequently in men than in women) and is another major factor in the development of cardiac disease. Nathanson[16] has shown that men are less likely than women to perform routine preventive health and dental behaviors, such as being immunized, brushing teeth, and getting adequate sleep. Thus, the masculine role leads to specific behavior patterns that can undermine the health of men.

Self-medication for men commonly involves alcohol. Men are four times more likely to be alcoholics than are women,[18] and are twice as likely to suffer from cirrhosis of the liver, the major cause of death associated with alcoholism.[14,16] Alcoholism is also a major contributor to automobile-related deaths, occupational death and injury, laryngeal malignancies, malnutrition, psychiatric disorders, homicide, and suicide.[19] Illegal drugs are also primarily abused by men, with subsequent morbidity and mortality. In addition, men are frequently killed by virtue of the violence of the masculine role. Most obviously, men serve as combat soldiers. In spite of the fact that modern global warfare wreaks havoc on civilian populations, it is still military personnel on the front lines who are most likely to be killed or seriously injured. Risk-taking behavior manifests itself in repeated accidents and injuries at the workplace or in an automobile. Men tend to kill other men when homicide occurs.

Finally, men have a higher suicide rate than woman. This is a cause of death that increases in frequency with the age of the population.[19] Men are more likely to see themselves as failures and become severely depressed when they are unable to live up to their rigidly defined social role; this leads to increased risks of successful suicide. The means men use to commit suicide are reflections of their masculine role. Men are more likely to kill themselves using violent methods such as weaponry, hanging, or jumping off a building than they are to use more passive methods such as pill-taking or asphyxiation in a gas oven.

It has been frequently stated that the older American man becomes either more androgynous or more feminized over time. It has been suggested by Gutmann and co-workers[2,3,20] and Keith and Brubaker[21] that masculine roles dedifferentiate as men age. However, there are few data to support this hypothesis. Nor are there many data to support the corollary contention that men remain unchangingly masculinized throughout the life cycle.

Some of the data that men become more androgynous were reported by Keith and Brubaker,[21] who reported that the outward behaviors of retired men include an increased amount of time spent around the house helping with traditional feminine tasks, such as putting away clothing, clearing the table, cleaning, and doing the laundry. Similar findings were noted by Hubbard et al.[22] However, these outward behaviors may be only an attempt to utilize additional free time rather than representing any actual change in the person's self-concept or chosen role.

In a Rorschach study, Ames[23] noted that older men were more likely to see women in response to Cards III and VII than were younger men or women. This response is hypothesized to be indicative of a feminine identification in the respondent, and thus, may be evidence supporting the hypothesis that men become more feminized as they age. Other studies,[24–28] using the Thematic Apperception Test (TAT), found that men shifted toward perceived submissiveness and passive mastery over the environment. Problems with these studies are numerous. The research designs were cross-sectional, which means that the data may simply be a cohort effect, rather than the longitudinal effect of aging. The author believes, along with Zubin,[29] that neither the Rorschach nor the TAT have been validated for use with the elderly, although others believe the opposite.[30] These are projective tests, the interpretations of which are subject to a large degree of experimenter bias. Finally, issues of subject fatigue and motivation and sensory limitations were not discussed in the published papers and may have affected the results obtained from these studies.

In several other cross-sectional studies, older men were noted to change in a direction toward femininity. Strong[31] noted an increase in traditionally feminine vocational interests (this study was done in the 1940s). Douglas and Arenburg[32] and Barrons and Zuckerman[33] noted an increase in feminine interests and attitudes. Lowenthal et al.[34] noted that older men were less aggressive, hostile, and ambitious.

In another study, Foley and Murphy[35] found that older men saw themselves as more warm and expressive than younger men, but otherwise adhered to a self-perception of the traditional masculine role. They noted that older men were less concerned, however, about maintaining the appearances of masculinity, a finding supported by Costa and McRae.[36] Jackson[37] found that older men felt that they had lost many of the trappings of the masculine role, such as physical prowess, and work and breadwinner roles, but without a concomitant gain in adoption of feminine roles; however, her sample consisted of residents of adult "rest homes," who may have been deprived of a chance to adopt more feminine roles. Zaks et al.[38] noted, in a cross-sectional study, that there was no change in self-perceived masculinity in men at different ages. They used the Bem Sex Role Inventory and an interview schedule. They did note that masculinity was associated with marital status and parenthood and grandparenthood status, findings that need further elucidation. These studies suffer from problems of test validity and sampling.

There are data that support the hypothesis that men do not become more androgynous or feminized, at least in other cultures. In many West African tribes, or in the People's Republic of China, behaviors expected of younger men tend not to change as men age and new behaviors, further reinforcing the masculine role, may be added. Goody notes that in nonindustrialized societies, over 40% of men do not retire.[39] Mandatory retirement does not exist in China, as noted by Treas,[40] and older men who do retire are given other important and active social roles. In some societies, such as the Gonja of Ghana, many of the men who retire move into other powerful and societally meaningful roles such as chieftainships or judgeships. Simmons noted that chieftainship was only held by old men in the 71 tribes he examined.[41] Thus, male gerontocracy is extremely common form of governance in nonindustrial societies.

Akin to these roles are priestly roles which may also be reserved for elderly men. Sorcery is a particularly potent power invested in older men in the Samburu of Africa, Groote Ejlandt of Australia, and Kikuyu of Kenya. The older Comanche man has powers as the "Peace Chief," to compensate for his lack of physical power. In other preindustrial societies, older men retain rights of polygamy or veto power over the marriages of children, thus assuring older men important roles in maintaining patrifocal family ties and the smooth and continuous functioning of society. Thus, older men frequently remain the "power brokers" in these societies.

On the other hand, Gutmann points out that in many societies, men become more passive.[20] Older Chinese men are expected to be relaxed, meditative, and "noble." In Burmese and Thai societies, older men are likely to pursue religious activities; although these are passive activities, they are also of major importance to society. A similar expectation occurs in the Hindu life cycle, in which the final state, *sanyasa,* involves a renunciation of worldly goods and embracing a relationship with the Godhead; this is also seen in the Druze in the Middle East. Some increased feminization is noted in other societies. Older Fijian men become more outwardly affective and less involved with affairs of men. Older Hopi and Ponro Indian men frequently involve themselves with tasks usually associated with women.

More research is needed to elucidate any changes in gender role behavior in the aging man in American and other societies. There have been several hypotheses proposed to explain these disparate findings. Sinnott,[42] Gould,[7] Levinson et al.,[6] and Guttman and co-workers,[2,3,20] suggest that men, as they age, allow themselves to express a previously repressed part of their personality. Another hypothesis is that increased femininity in older men may be part of the societal stereotype of the elderly. This hypothesis gains support from a study by Silverman,[43] who found that college students were likely to rate men over 65 as feminine on the Masculine–Feminine Stereotype Scale developed by Broverman et al.[44]

The author's hypothesis is that gender-role behavior does not change throughout life unless a conscious effort is made to do so, and that older men are as masculine in their self-concept as they were when they were younger.[45] Some of their outward behaviors may change but for reasons other than a change in gender roles. Rather, they represent a shift from institutionalized roles to informal, or occasionally tenuous roles[46] (first chapter by Solomon). This maintains the interpersonal strategies and comfortable patterns of interaction with individuals with whom the men are intimate and society at large. This maintains the older person's status within his immediate community and family, and protects against rolelessness, anomie, alienation, boredom, and psychopathology. For other men, these same factors, as well as depression, lead to outward changes in the direction of lesser ambition, activity, and aggressiveness. Rather than representing a change in the traditional masculine role, they represent a pathologic result of the ineffectiveness of the traditional role in aging men.

STRESS AND COPING IN THE ELDERLY

Prior to discussing the specific psychosocial stresses that affect older men, it is important to elucidate the characteristic way that the elderly respond to stress (Figure 1).[46–50] All elderly men and women face sequential and severe stress, of both an acute and chronic nature. Elucidation of this pattern of stress response will serve as a framework for a discussion of the specific stresses that elderly men face as well as some of the difficulties elderly men have in adaptation to stress, because of the limitations of the masculine role.

New psychiatric symptoms in the elderly are always triggered by current stress. Faced with stress, regardless of its biologic, psychologic, or social nature, the older individual experiences a diminished sense of mastery over his/her internal and/or external environment. This diminished mastery is frequently not objectively observable. It is the subjective experience of diminished mastery which is crucial to the development of psychopathologic symptoms.

With diminished mastery, the older person experiences increased feelings of helplessness. Helplessness is manifested by feelings of loss of control and autonomy, difficulty in making decisions, and a pervasive sense of doubt. Concurrently, the older person feels ambivalently dependent upon others for help in responding to the present stress. Further contributing to helplessness is the societal stereotype of the elderly. Health care providers and other care givers who work with the elderly frequently reinforce and may even create a learned

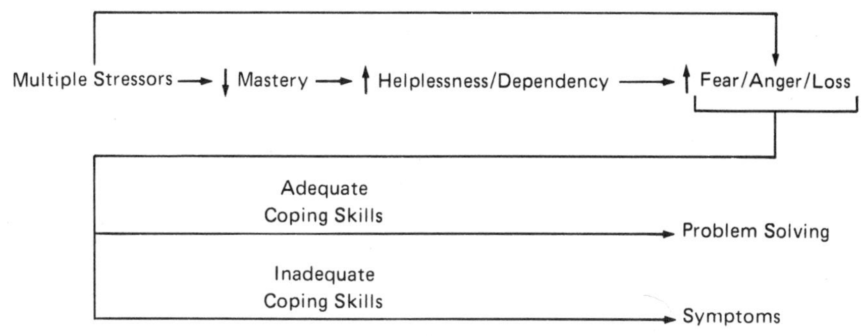

Figure 1. *Stress and coping in the elderly. (Data from Goldfarb, Ref. 48.)*

helplessness in the elderly.[51,52] They do this by accepting the stereotype of the elderly, manifesting the role behaviors and power differential inherent in the sick role,[53,54] and believing that working with the elderly will not be of benefit to the care giver. Feelings of helplessness and dependency lead the older person to experience two possible affects, each biologically mediated by the General Adaptation Syndrome elucidated by Selye.[55] One is fear, as the older person worries about what is to become of him/her as he/she works to resolve the stress. The other affect is anger at self and/or others, and anger over what has happened to the older person as well as anger at experienced powerlessness and loss of mastery. A third affect, that of loss, is also frequently experienced, as the majority of the acute stresses involve the loss of a member of the older person's social support system, social role, or personal attribute.

If the older person has a history of adequate coping skills and is able to utilize them, he/she will begin to problem solve. Any emotional discomfort will be relatively transitory, rarely lasting more than a few days during which he/she may be sad, irritable, anxious, or withdrawn. As the days progress, the older person begins to handle the intensity of his/her affective response to the stressor and attempts to rectify the stressful situation itself. These individuals are rarely seen in clinical practice because they recognize their discomfort as a normal response to stress. As their emotional reactions rarely last more than several days, they feel competent to manage these "problems of daily living" without professional assistance.

However, if the older individual has inadequate coping skills or is unable to utilize previously acquired coping skills, psychopathologic symptoms will develop. The nature of the symptoms will depend upon where the individual's affective responses fall on the fear/anger continuum (Figure 2).[48] They will also be

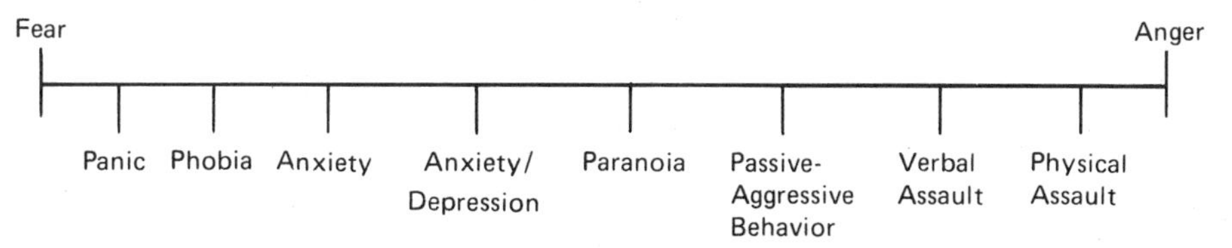

Figure 2. *Psychopathological symptoms in the elderly.*

determined by the intensity of the loss. For example, the older person who experiences fear will evidence symptoms of panic. Less fear and a modicum of anger will lead to symptoms of phobias. On the other extreme, the experience of anger will lead to physical aggression toward others. Less anger and a modicum of fear will modify this to verbal aggression and even more fear will move the individual to display passive–aggressive behavior. The individual with a mixture of anxiety and fear will present to the therapist a picture of mixed anxiety and depression. Adding the affect of loss to this mixture of fear and anger leads to a retarded depression, a clinical presentation more likely to occur if the experience of loss overshadows the intensity of either fear or anger. If the individual is narcissistic and has emotionally overinvested in his/her body, then hypochondriacal and somatic symptoms are likely to develop, regardless of the presence of other symptoms.

There are three groups of older people with inadequate coping skills. One group probably includes the majority of those who develop psychopathology. They have been able to adequately cope with stress throughout life. However, because of severe losses such as the death of a spouse, illness, or retirement, occurring sequentially over a brief period of time, their ego defenses and coping skills may become overwhelmed.

The second group is comprised of elderly who also had adequate coping mechanisms when younger. However, because of brain failure, these individuals are unable to use these coping skills when faced with psychosocial and biologic stress. This leads to psychopathologic symptoms concurrent with the underlying neurologic and/or systemic difficulty.

The third group of older people with inadequate coping skills represents the minority who demand the most time and energy from health care providers and social agencies. This group includes those older people who have never had

Table II. Losses of the Elderly

I. Loss of social support system
   1. Spouse
   2. Siblings
   3. Friends
   4. Parents
   5. Children
   6. Other kin
   7. Neighbors

II. Loss of social role
   1. Occupational role
   2. Shift to tenuous and informal roles
   3. Gender role

III. 1. Health
   2. Independence
   3. Income
   4. Mobility
   5. Adequate housing
   6. Leisure activities

Table III. Role Typology[a]

Role type	Role Expectations/Behaviors	Status
Institutional	Clear	Vague
Tenuous	Vague	Clear
Informal	Clear	Vague
Nonrole	Vague	Vague
Rolelessness	None	None

[a]Data from Rosow (Ref. 46).

adequate coping skills. They include people with chronic schizophrenia and mental retardation, as well as those with unresolved neurotic conflicts and personality disorders that may or may not have been manifested when the individual was younger.

The stresses experienced by the older person may be acute and episodic or chronic and continuous. The events that cause acute, episodic stress may be grouped into three major categories; all are characterized by loss (Table II). One set of losses is in the social support system. The most psychologically devastating of these is the loss of a spouse. Holmes and Rahe note that the death of a spouse is the most difficult and painful stressor that a human being must work through at any age.[56] This is especially true for older women, as 54% of women over the age of 65 are widows, whereas only 17% of men in that age group are widowers.[12] Thus a majority of older women must cope with a change in both their lifestyles and status in society. The spouse may also be lost through severe illness or institutionalization. The plight of the "married widow(er)" has only begun to be recognized as these individuals are accepted neither by the society of widow(er)s nor by that of the married.[57]

Many older individuals experience the death of their even more elderly parents. Siblings, friends, and neighbors who are age peers also die or become seriously ill. And as the population gets older, some older individuals are outliving their elderly children.

Finally, because American society is extremely mobile, kinship networks may be spread from coast to coast. This frequently creates an inadequate social support system for the older individual in distress and may be experienced as a loss almost as devastating as the death of a member of the network.

A second major group of losses concerns social role. Rosow[46] suggests that all social roles have two major dimensions (Table III). One is the clarity of role behaviors and role expectations associated with the role. The other is the clarity of the status of that role in society. Institutional roles are those in which behaviors and expectations are quite clear to all actors involved. Examples are those which make up the bulk of the activities of younger individuals. They include religious, occupational, family, and parental roles. These have been the traditional focus of role analysis.

However, the elderly are more likely to adopt informal or tenuous roles. Tenuous roles are those the status of which is clearly defined; however, the associated behaviors and expectations are unclear. An example is a nominative office such as Chairman Emeritus of the Board, for which the associated status is quite clear and usually high. The expectations of the actor in that role may be unclear or even nonexistent. Other examples of tenuous roles are deviant roles in which status is clear (although low), and behaviors and expectations are vaguely, if at all defined. (Some authors, notably Scheff[58] and Zusman,[59] would disagree with this conceptualization of deviant roles.) Deviant roles include a common role for the elderly, that of mentally ill, and may also include criminal roles and other marginal roles in American society. Rosow[46] suggests that being an old person in society is in itself a tenuous role.

Informal roles are those in which role behaviors and expectations are clear. However, the associated status is unclear and nebulous. These roles have important functions for the maintenance of primary group functioning. Examples, as adopted by the elderly, are the *kibbitzer* at a card game, the neighborhood chauffeur, and a social butterfly at a senior center.

By their very nature, tenuous and informal roles are a source of stress for the elderly. Not only must the elderly grieve over the loss of institutionalized roles, but because of the discrepancy between status and expectations, tenuous and informal roles become a continuous source of psychological dissonance and stress for the older person. As these roles exist at the whim of the primary group or society, their tenuous nature is quite clear to the older person; that, too, becomes a constant source of stress.

The third major set of losses for the elderly are a miscellaneous group that includes loss of health, independence, adequate income, mobility, and adequate housing. These are frequently encountered by primary care physicians and social agencies and are a result of societally determined changes, such as retirement, and chronic diseases that inhibit the functioning of the older person. The major negative effects of these losses are on activities of daily living and may lead to further breakdown of functioning, social loss, and increased stress.

In addition to these acute episodic stressors, there are chronic stressors that the author lables the "victimization" of the elderly.[50] There are four dimensions of this victimization: economic, attitudinal, role, and physical. Like all chronic situations in which the individual is "one-down," the individual feels oppressed, angry, despondent, and helpless, and may turn the anger onto him/herself or explosively outward toward other individuals or society at large.[60,61] Self-victimization, self-blame, and loss of self-esteem go hand in hand with a sense of powerlessness and, at times, apathy. While these phenomena have been relatively well studied in Blacks and other oppressed groups, they have not been studied to any appreciable degree in the elderly, although the author believes that similar dynamic and behavior responses occur.

Economic victimization not only includes illegal "rip-offs" and fraudulent schemes, but also legal and sanctioned policy such as inadequate pensions, the effects of inflation, and business schemes that bilk the elderly consumer of needed funds. One may even consider Medicare a part of this economic victimization; in spite of the presence of Medicare, the elderly person averages \$800–\$1000 per year in out-of-pocket medical expenses.

Attitudinal victimization is the result of the stereotyping of the elderly in society. These beliefs are that[62]

1. The elderly are political conservatives and personally old-fashioned;
2. They have limited activities and interests;
3. They are poor;
4. Physical deterioration is inevitable;
5. They disengage from family and others;
6. They have all positive or all negative personality traits;
7. They are pessimistic;
8. It is the best or worst period of their lives;
9. They are insecure;
10. Senility is inevitable;
11. They are asexual;
12. They interfere in the lives of others; and
13. They are dirty.

As Butler[63] and Solomon and Vickers[64] note, adherence to the stereotype of the elderly leads to the provision of inadequate and/or irrelevant services to the elderly, their individual needs are not identified, and their individuality is lost. This further contributes to the learned helplessness of many older individuals, especially in the health care setting.[51,52]

Role victimization is the shift from institutional to tenuous and informal roles in the elderly. The elderly may then lapse into a state of rolelessness with subsequent alienation, anomie, apathy, and psychopathologic sympotomatology, if they are unable to adopt even tenuous or informal roles.[65]

The last dimension of victimization of the elderly is the physical. This includes the abuse of the older person by his/her children and/or spouse as well as the effects of crime against person and property. It also includes much of the poor treatment that the elderly frequently get from health care givers. This form of physical victimization includes inadequate or inappropriate diagnostic evaluations, overmedication, undermedication, inadequate medication, inappropriate surgery, and inadequate care in custodial institutions.

Given these harsh realities of daily life, it is not surprising that psychopathology in this age group is more common than in any other age group. Nor is it surprising that elderly white men commit suicide more frequently than either men or women in any other group or that elderly women also have extremely high suicide rates.[19] Depression, alcoholism, and psychosis are frequent responses of the elderly to chronic stress and victimization that has no perceived solution and the acute, episodic stresses that severely disrupt the older individual's life.

The loss of traditional gender-role behaviors and the loss of opportunities for the expression of gender-role expectations are particularly stressful for men.[45] Because of retirement, widowerhood, physical illness, rolelessness, and changes in sexuality, men are forced to behave in ways they have avoided for a lifetime. They must adopt some traditionally feminine roles, become expressive, move away from a success orientation to life, take on feminine tasks, and acknowledge their vulnerability. Men who have difficulty adapting to these changes are particularly prone to develop psychopathology. This will be discussed in more depth in the following section.

SPECIAL STRESSES FOR OLDER MEN

RETIREMENT. One of the greatest stresses facing the older man in American society is retirement. The effects of retirement on the older man vary depending upon the nature of his bond to work, the importance of work and breadwinner roles to him, the voluntariness of his retirement, and the degree of his economic and psychological preparation for retirement.[66] Social class also plays a role in choice of and adjustment to retirement, as blue collar workers are more likely to welcome retirement than are white collar workers. In turn, white collar workers are more likely to welcome retirement than are professionals. Indeed, blue collar workers frequently ask for an early retirement as it helps them get away from boring, repetitive work that has been stultifying for years.[67]

Mandatory retirement has been considered a major cause of psychopathology, especially depression and alcoholism, in older men.[45,65] Retirement is less likely to cause psychological difficulties for men who chose retirement and have made adequate provision for their financial, physical, and emotional health during the retirement years. These men have developed interests and activities that are meaningful to them and serve as multivariate sources of pleasure and meaning in their retirement years. Good health and adequate income, important concomitants of life satisfaction,[68] allow these men to enjoy their meaningful realities.

However, men currently entering their sixties and seventies were inculcated with a heavy dose of the American Protestant work ethic in childhood. As noted in the first chapter by Solomon, the work role is the major source of a man's identity, for men define themselves and their status in society by their level and sophistication of productivity. Certain professions, such as medicine, law, and dentistry, are high status professions regardless of how productive the individual is within those professions. Business is a variable status profession, depending upon the size and nature of the business and the person's success within business. As noted in the first chapter by Solomon, the occupational role is intimately associated with the breadwinner role and the man's need to be the sole provider for the financial health and welfare of the family.[69,70] It is also intimately associated with the man's insatiable pursuit of success ("The Big Wheel");[69] this makes the activities of work all the more important.

In addition, many of men's social contacts involve the work arena. Although these contacts have a certain structure that inhibits the development of intimacy between men ("homophobia"), they may be the most supportive and intimate relationships with other men (and perhaps women) that the retiring man has. The retiree loses contact with most of his social network and loses status in the eyes of society (and frequently his peers and family). Under stress, the retiree is no longer associated with a support system that could help him cope. Thus, retirement may directly lead to an aura of uselessness and rolelessness which may be a harbinger of future psychopathology. Diminished income leads to other real problems. And the retired man loses a major, if not the major, source of identity and self-esteem he has.

A 72-year-old man entered therapy for depression. He had coped well with a variety of losses (including widowerhood) and other stresses. The precipitant was loss of his job as a plumber when his employer became bankrupt. He had a reputation as one of the finest plumbers in the city and most of his friends were plumbers. As he said: "I was born a plumber." (His father was of the same occupation.) "What else am I? Who else am I? There's nothing I can do. No one will want to have anything to do with me. I'm useless. There's nothing lower than a plumber who isn't working." (His father died of a heart attack, while working, at age 78.) In a few brief comments, this patient verbalized the loss of role, identity, and social support system that many men experience upon involuntary retirement.

The older man who has given up work roles also confronts issues of intimacy with his spouse in a way that he never had to deal with before. Similar issues develop between the man and his peers, spouse, and children. He is suddenly home with his wife seven days a week, 24 hours a day. He has more time to spend with friends, children, grandchildren, and more frequently in this age of longevity, his parents. If relationships are not to become boring and stultifying, the man must risk intimacy with these people, a risk that involves developing new patterns of interpersonal behavior and a willingness to become vulnerable in the eyes of others. These are changes that are extremely threatening to most men. It is not unusual for couples to report major marital difficulties following retirement. Some of these problems may antedate retirement but are exacerbated by the increased time with and proximity of the partners. Others are new and develop from the ambivalence that the retired man experiences. Humorist Erma Bombeck reportedly stated the problem as follows: "I married him for better and for worse, but not for lunch!"

The use of leisure time also becomes a major issue for the retired man. Appropriate use of leisure time demands the ability to relax, something particularly difficult for a man who has spent a lifetime involved with work and activity. The more emotionally involved with work the individual had become, the more difficult it is to change a behavior pattern that emphasizes activity, aggression, and competition. For example, it is not uncommon for men with the Type A personality to suffer a myocardial infarction following retirement, rather than actually while in the work arena. Even the "leisure" activities of most men are actually disguised work (e.g., mowing the lawn, fixing the car, painting the house). Passive observation of sports may be leisure; however, the emphasis on competition and the associated tension of "rooting" for one's team diminishes the value of this activity as leisure and relaxation.

The loss of role and the inability to find substitute roles that reinforce one's sense of masculinity may lead to a sense of diminished mastery over the environment and a subsequent sense of helplessness, two of the major dynamic factors in the development of depression in the elderly.[47–50,71] The loss of identity is both a narcissistic injury and an existential loss, which also contributes to the development of depression. Many elderly depressed men seen in clinical practice are able to date the onset of their depressive symptomatology to shortly after retirement, as the fantasy of retirement no longer turns out to be as rewarding and promising as the ads for Sun City or Fort Lauderdale.

The stress of retirement frequently exposes neurotic conflicts and symptoms other than depression. A 71-year-old man developed compulsive utterances following retirement at age 64. These symptoms were associated with feelings of anxiety, boredom, and anger. He became asymptomatic following therapy which gave him insight into the dynamic background of his symptoms. Therapy also allowed his interest in travel to reemerge, allowing him meaningful activities to pursue with his wife, thus increasing the intimacy of their relationship of over 40 years.

WIDOWERHOOD. A second major stress for the older man is widowerhood. Widowerhood, being less common than widowhood, has been extremely poorly studied. Widowerhood catapults the older man into a crisis of masculinity, over and above the emotional crisis and narcissistic loss that occurs with the loss of a person with whom he may have been intimate for over 50 years. For example, the widower has been socialized in the dimension of "No Sissy Stuff"[69] (first chapter by Solomon), and now he must adopt new behaviors, all of which are associated with the traditional feminine role: He must do the laundry, cook, shop, and clean the house, roles for which he has been both psychologically and behaviorally ill prepared. The loss of spouse puts an additional demand for affective interchange on the older man, who may now be called upon to cry and grieve, to be expressive, and to share feelings that he may not even know how to label. A 63-year-old man became severely depressed on an anniversary of the death of his first wife. He was unable to label any of his feelings other than to say that when talking about his first wife he felt a tightness in his chest. He was unable to associate that tightness to feelings consistent with the physiologic changes associated with weeping, which he did not do at the funeral. Only once he was able to cry and release his grief, was he able to work through the death of his first wife, repair his relationship with his new wife, reestablish relationships with his friends and family, and become asymptomatic.

Because of the sex differential in survival, the widower may suddenly find himself the object of attention by many other women. This leads to interpersonal strains that he may be ill equipped for, as he may not have related in an intimate way with other women for over 50 years. There may be real sexual demands upon him or he may fear sexual demands which may lead to secondary problems such as social withdrawal or sexual dysfunctions; these may be felt to further reflect negatively upon his masculinity. A 76-year-old attorney (still in practice), once widowed, was invited to dinner (and subsequent sex play) on a nightly basis, by one or another of the many widows in his neighborhood. Only when he developed pneumonia from exhaustion did he realize that he did not have to be a Don Juan to become popular, emotionally intimate, and sexual with the women whose company he truly enjoyed. As men are ambivalently dependent upon a mothering figure, the sudden thrust into a situation without such a person leads to ambivalent expressions of dependency needs, often in the form of psychopathological syndromes such as alcoholism, depression, or hypochondriasis. The overwhelming nature of these various tasks, never before encountered by the man at a time of crisis, coupled with demands that he be "unmasculine," may lead to a prevailing sense of helplessness, another factor in the development of depression in older men.

DISEASE AND DISABILITY. The many diseases that the elderly face and their associated disabilities are a threat to the man's sense of invulnerability. This is the third stress that has special consequences for older men, as the elderly become acutely and chronically ill more frequently than do younger persons. As noted above, these diseases may, in part, be caused by the lifestyles of men and may force men to question their role behaviors, which is in itself extremely difficult. These and other diseases may lead to a chronic loss of functioning and may drastically change a man's lifestyle. For example, the "jock" may no longer be able to play football following his heart attack. Amputation for circulatory difficulties may make a man wheelchair-bound with a subsequent increase in real dependency that may be defended against. The presence of chronic aches and pains may be a constant reminder of a threat to the older man's belief in his invulnerability and may lead to inappropriate expressions of anger or an exaggeration of "macho" behavior. The threat to invulnerability from all diseases may lead to a counterphobic refusal to follow through with medical procedures of either a diagnostic or therapeutic nature.

Two particularly devastating diseases affecting older men are Alzheimer's Disease and multi-infarct dementia. The various dementias effect 2% of the population aged 65 and 20% aged 80;[72] although the snydrome has an equal incidence in both sexes, it is twice as common in men aged 65–70 than in women that age. Its major effect on men is its effect on the man's sense of mastery. The progressive memory loss, disorientation, apraxias, aphasias, agnosias, and inability to function as well as in the premorbid state may be particularly frustrating for the man who sees himself as active, competent, invulnerable, and omnipotent. The difficulty coping with these symptoms becomes manifested in secondary depression or behavioral disturbances. A 77-year-old man with mild Alzheimer's Disease insisted on his active involvement in all aspects of his business. He proceeded to interfere with the work of his employees (to whom he had previously delegated responsibilities) to the degree that his business suffered. This ended when an employee had him declared incompetent by the court.

Older men are less likely to use health facilities than older women. This may not be because they are less ill, but because they are less willing to admit that they may have an illness. This behavior is consistent regardless of the severity of the illness. In part, this is because of the difficulty men have accepting the sick role, as the sick role has several dimensions which are contrary to traditional masculine roles. The sick role means that the man must give up power and control and adopt dependency-inducing behavior.[53,54] The sick role may lead to helplessness and subsequent demoralization.[51,52] The sick role involves passivity and a willingness to express discomfort and pain. As noted in the first chapter by Solomon, all these behaviors are particularly difficult for men to acknowledge as appropriate for themselves.

ROLELESSNESS. A fourth stress is that of rolelessness. As the older man gives up institutionalized roles, he must adopt informal or tenuous roles or lapse into a state of rolelessness. Tenuous roles may be clearly deviant, and although they give some secondary gain to the individual, they do so at major interpersonal cost. Other tenuous roles (e.g., honorific titles such as Chairman Emeritus of the Board), may lead to certain status-associated behaviors in certain arenas, but the true hollowness of such situations is frequently evident to the man who sees himself as truly useless. Informal roles require assent on the part of others in the environment for the individual to take on these roles, for the behaviors are defined by the informal social systems and the primary groups with which the individual interacts. Many informal roles may mean taking on various feminine role behaviors, for they may mean being expressive or being thrust into the company of other men in a way that may force intimacy between them.

However, many fail to adopt meaningful, self-perpetuating informal roles and fall into a state of rolelessness. In other publications, the author has suggested that rolelessness is a major factor in the development of psychopathology through the intervention of stereotyping the older person, the power differential in society at large, a psychological contingency set that leads to helplessness,[51,52] and the development of alienation. For stereotyping to be one of the antecedents of rolelessness in elderly men unfortunately requires that stereotyping and attitudes be translated into behavior—behaviors that maximize the development of learned helplessness. The development of helplessness is the key to translation of societal and personal attitudes into possible psychopathology, as noted in the discussion of stress and coping.

According to Seligman's theory of learned helplessness,[73,74] response–outcome must become independent of the subjective response to stimuli. In some interpersonal situations, a subject's need or a stimulus leads the subject to respond in a way that attempts to satisfy the need. This response is then responded to by a factor in the environment (operant), which leads to appropriate satisfaction of the need and reinforcement of the subject's behavior. In other interpersonal situations, the stimulus forces the subject to seek a response from the operant; if this response satisfies the underlying need, the subject's response is then also reinforced.

However, in either situation, if the subject's response is repeatedly not reinforced by the environment, regardless of its seeming appropriateness, it eventually becomes clear that the subject has no control over response–outcome. Gradually, the subject becomes apathetic, develops the "giving-up–given-up" syndrome of Engel,[75] and learns to be helpless.

By stereotyping the aged person as dependent, "senile," incompetent, and chronically disordered with a poor medical prognosis, individuals do not respond to the older person's behavior and needs but respond only to the older person's custodial or maintenance needs, as perceived by the care-giving individual. These perceptions are frequently different from the old person's own perceptions of his/her needs. The younger person's responses, which are not particularly rewarding or gratifying to him/her, become haphazard, artificially scheduled, or perhaps even nonexistent, thus mirroring the effects of the power differential between generations in society. The older person's individuality and individual needs become lost to the younger.

Some of the major elements of Seligman's theory of learned helpness may now be identified. The older person's responses to his/her own internal needs, whether they be hunger, thirst, pain, discomfort, or growth, not only do not lead to an appropriate response on the part of others, but actually may lead to inappropriate or a total lack of responses. On the other hand, younger persons respond haphazardly and independently of the needs of the older person. Thus, response–outcome becomes uncontrolled by the older person and independent of the older person's response to his/her own needs. This loss of control of response–outcome of his/her behavior eventually leads the older person to give up, with the development of helplessness.

The older man may also come to perceive that all that can be done for him is in the hands of the younger person who maintains control of response–outcome. Once the older person begins to behave in a way consistent with helplessness, the contingencies of his/her environment, e.g., the negative stereotyping of society coupled with any real effects of the older person's social setting and status, only serve to reinforce the helpless behavior. This leads to diminished expectations of the older person and reinforced stereotypes. This further leads to a marked decrease in motivation, more dependency, and more helplessness. Depression, in part related to the loss of control and mastery inherent in the masculine role, complicates this process. The older man may do virtually nothing for himself. In an extreme, the end result is a malodorous room of "senile" old men restrained in geri-chairs, incontinent of urine, not interacting with each other, apathetically staring at a television screen with a rolling picture, and mumbling to themselves.

Thus, stereotypes and ensuing behavior and expectations of individuals in the general population impact both on the contingencies of the environment and on the older person's self-cognition. This directly leads to the older person's learning helplessness.

One contingency that is a reality in the older man's environment is the reality of social loss (Table II). Although some of these losses, such as loss of spouse, lead to a weakening of the older person's social network, many of the social losses could be subsumed under the rubric of role loss. Rosow has noted that the elderly are gradually given increasingly tenuous and informal roles in society.[46] As the author has noted,[76–78] this tends to occur in societies that emphasize industrial production, individualism, and profit. For various reasons, nonproductive, nonconsuming groups are moved to the periphery of society, reinforcing the power differential between the controllers of production and consumption and the majority of social groups in society.

The elderly are only one of these nonproductive, nonconsuming groups in these societies. As the elderly become less profit-producing, their perceived social utility diminishes, they lose power, and they are gradually given increasingly tenuous and informal roles in society (Table III). These roles are generally peripheral to the mainstream of society. Indeed, these roles may be openly devalued. Even in the power elite, age brings questions of competency, as noted in the presidential candidacy of 69-year-old Ronald Reagan. These roles exclude elderly men from meaningful social participation and devalue the elderly as a group. In addition, these peripheral roles further reduce productivity and consumption of goods, so that aged men become progressively more peripheral. However, these peripheral roles remain necessary, as the old person still remains indirectly tied to modes of production and consumption. Along with the changes in roles, however, a more peripheral and diminished status is acquired (or sometimes achieved), and the old person becomes progressively more isolated and powerless, further diminishing perceived social utility. Eventually, if these peripheral, low-status roles cannot be performed because of individual or societal factors (such as illness or grossly inadequate income), the old man lapses into a state of rolelessness. This rolelessness is further reinforced by societal messages of uselessness, such as compulsory retirement or inadequate pensions. These messages of social inutility further divorce the older man from the mainstream of society by alienating him further from modes of production and consumption. Eventually, the old man believes that he is truly no longer a part of society.

This process occurs for men and women in American society. However, there are particular strains for older men that develop from this process. As noted above, men's identity is inseparable from work and productivity. This is taken from the older man and substitutes are not developed. Older women retain household roles; older men enter a state of role limbo. Grandmotherhood in American society has clearer expectations and rewards than does grandfatherhood.

Thus, rolelessness may actually be normative for elderly men in American society. Rolelessness leads to feelings of alienation and anomie, both of which have been associated with depressive symptomatology.[79,80] A loss of self-esteem accompanies the self-blame that occurs with the acceptance of the stereotype.[60,61] Loss of self-esteem has been postulated by several authors to be another important dynamic factor in the development of depressive symptomatology.[81,82] Furthermore, rolelessness directly leads to a sense of helplessness through a loss of control of one's life, which is then further reinforced by the stereotypes that society has for the older individuals. Finally, the loss of social role becomes a major narcissistic injury that stimulates feelings of loss, subsequent mourning, and depression.[83–85]

Older individuals who are not depressed frequently attempt to regain lost roles, albeit sometimes in a caricatured way. Those with personality disorders continue to relate in their life-long maladaptive way. Much of what is clinically diagnosed as behavior problems are attempts by the individual with maladaptive ego functioning to function in a way that had previously been either adaptive or their "habit." However, because of decreased mastery over the environment, these behaviors are exhibited either in a caricatured way, at inappropriate times, or in a way that is potentially dangerous to the individual or the individuals around the patient. Attempts to take away these "quasiroles" may then lead again to a sense of helplessness and dependency, further leading to new psychopathologic symptomatology.

SEXUALITY. The sexuality of older men, the fifth stress, has been studied in depth from the physiologic point of view. Masters and Johnson[86] have noted that sexual potency remains present throughout life and that older men are capable of continued sexual activity. Indeed, approximately 16% of men over age 65 label themselves as "very sexually active"[11] and about 70% of 68-year-old men have regular sexual activity.[87] Because of their small sample size, it is somewhat premature to generalize their findings onto all aged men. Indeed, anecdotal reports suggest that very sexually active elderly men have physiologic function similar to sexually active younger men. According to Masters and Johnson, however, some physiologic changes may occur with age[85]; the penis may not become erect without direct sexual stimulation. It may take longer for the man to achieve an erection and longer for ejaculation to occur. The refractory period may be extended. Erections may not be as hard or as firm as in the younger man. Changes in cardiovascular and pulmonary reserve may lead to fatigue during sexual activity so that the overall amount of time in sexual involvement may diminish. Nipples are less apt to become erect and the sex flush during orgasm is less likely to occur. Testicular steroid levels also diminish (although this is somewhat controversial), leading to changes in the secondary sex characteristics. For example, hair thins out, beard growth slows down, and the voice may become somewhat high-pitched.

Many older men make use of some of the changes in sexual functioning in a positive way. For example, the diminished ejaculatory urge may lead to an increased emphasis on pleasuring the partner as well as the ability to relax and enjoy the sensuality of the sexual encounter. There is less pressure to perform, so impotence and premature ejaculation may reverse themselves. Aging brings a wider variety of sexual experiences so that the older man may be more conversant with multiple positions and techniques necessary for both self-pleasure as well as partner-pleasure.

On the other hand, the older man who has placed heavy emphasis on traditional masculine sexuality may have difficulty adapting to these changes. The older man who is unwilling or unknowledgeable in the changes in his sexuality may become anxious over the loss of an extremely hard erection. This may lead to secondary impotence or premature ejaculation because of an increased need to perform.[88] The physical changes may lead to satyrism or Don Juanism in an attempt to recreate a sexuality stereotypically associated with youth, which also increases performance anxiety and is therefore more likely to lead to further problems with sexual performance.

The older man may also have various physical disorders that may interfere with sexuality. Cardiovascular or pulmonary disease may reduce its ability to sustain performance. Peripheral arteriosclerotic disease may cause Leriche's Syndrome and an associated organic impotence. A similar problem may be secondary to diabetes or hypertension. Many drugs, such as psychopharmacologic agents or antihypertensive drugs, may cause difficulty in sexual performance.[89,90] Prostate or bladder surgery may lead to retrograde ejaculation, which, without proper education of the man, may lead to panic.

Another problem with the sexuality of older men is the belief that once procreation is done, men should not be sexually active, a belief frequently supported by the partner. This belief is further reinforced by the societal stereotype of the older person as asexual.[62] This may lead to ambivalence with subsequent guilt or inappropriate behaviors when sexual urges develop. A 67-year-old widower developed impotence but retained the ability to ejaculate during masturbation, although he could not get an erection. In a somatic way, he was expressing his sexual impulses toward a woman who attracted him, but he felt guilty about "cheating" on his deceased wife, with whom he did not have sex for over ten years prior to her death. He became asymptomatic with therapy.

THERAPEUTIC ISSUES

Androgyny has been reported to be associated with increased adaptability and flexibility in young men and women[91–93] and in old women.[94,95] Although there are neither cross-sectional data for older men nor longitudinal data through the life span of men, it is reasonable to extrapolate from data on older women to hypothesize that the man who has become more androgynous throughout the life span will be able to adapt to the various changes in role as he ages. For example, when faced with retirement, the successfully aging older man will find other meaningful outlets in order to express himself in an active way. As noted above, some of the changes in sexuality noted above may be used in a positive way. Widowerhood may become a time to renew relationships with friends and family and learn, perhaps for the first time, how to become intimate with both men and women. Losses in the social support system may allow the time and energy to make new friends. Aging may also be a time to take on the challenge of new role behaviors. Indeed, any of the changes in old age are a crisis, but crises can be a splendid time for interpersonal and intrapsychic growth.

On the other hand, these various changes in aging may lead to the development of psychopathology. In particular, the older man who has maintained rigid masculine roles throughout life will have marked difficulty adapting to the various changes associated with aging, and this predisposes the man to the development of depression and paraphrenia.[49] These develop following the psychodynamic pattern noted earlier in this chapter.

In addition, the older man frequently experiences depression over the loss of what was and anxiety over the fear of what will or will not be. The repeated losses of love objects become repeated narcissistic injuries to the older person. Narcissistic injuries are experienced as sadness and an existential loss by individuals.[3] The existential loss is colored by the older man's awareness of the limits of his own life span, as noted by LeShan and LeShan[96] and Weinberg.[97] The older man must then question the meaning of his life and what he has done with it. In reviewing his life within a framework of traditional masculine role behavior, he may find himself wanting. He may, like John Wayne, fight on to the end, or he may capitulate into depression. Or he may use the opportunity to grow and change traditional behavior so as to adapt and form a new life with new meaning.

Depressive symptomatology may allow the older man to become dependent and express both dependency and helplessness in a way that is culturally syntonic (i.e., via the sick role).[98] Labeled as sick, he now has permission to express affects of sadness, anger, fear, and loss. He may be able to cry in front of others. Unfortunately, many depressed men cannot express these feelings to others, in part because of lifelong blocks to intimacy and sharing engendered by the masculine role. Rather, they find a way to successfully kill themselves, and suicide rates in this age group is highest of all population groups.[19] Indeed, the fact that men successfully commit suicide more frequently than do women may be evidence that men will carry the socially defined dimension of omnicompetence in the masculine role to the bitter end, as they take their own life.

If however, the older man responds somewhat more ego-syntonically with anger, his symptomatology may be experienced as aggression or paranoia. Paranoia is more likely to occur in the presence of auditory or visual deficits[99] which may be denied by the older man. Another dimension of the development of paranoid symptoms is a lifelong masculine behavior pattern that does not allow intimacy with others, especially men, and reinforces competition and mistrust of others, also especially other men. The development of paranoid symptoms is then ego-syntonic and allows the behavioral expression of much of that which is traditionally masculine, including competition, interpersonal aloofness, and withdrawal, hostility, denial of dependency, grandiosity, and sometimes frank violence.

Several of the personality disorders are partial caricatures of the traditional masculine role. Passive–aggressive, paranoid, narcissitic, and antisocial personality disorders all reflect parts of the traditional masculine role. The expression of hostility, competition, manipulation of others, and shallow relationships that are part of these disorders are exaggerations of similar behaviors in normal men. Faced with the crises of aging, the older man who has a propensity to these maladaptive personality traits is likely to see the maladaptive patterns intensify, frequently with the development of subsequent secondary psychopathology.[49]

The first stage in the intervention with the older man with a psychiatric disorder is what the author broadly calls "crisis intervention."[49,50] Its aim is to reverse the psychodynamic scheme noted above. At first, there is a direct attack on symptomatology. The major modalities utilized in this first step are either pharmacologic or behavioral. For example, if the person has psychotic symptomatology, notably paranoid delusions or hallucinations, antipsychotic medication is indicated. The author recommends that the clinician utilize whatever antipsychotic medication he/she is familiar with and is not contraindicated by concurrent medical problems. The author prefers an intermediate-potency (e.g., mesoridazine, loxapine) or a high-potency e.g., haloperidol,[100] thiothixene, trifluoperazine) drug to minimize possible sedative and anticholinergic side effects of antipsychotic medication. However, one must be aware that Parkinsonian symptoms and toxic psychoses may be even greater problems in many elderly patients than these autonomic side effects.

The presence of a major depressive disorder with vegetative symptoms (Table IV) is an indication for tricyclic antidepressant medication. The author recommends the use of secondary amines (desipramine or nortriptyline) rather than tertiary amines (imipramine or amitriptyline) because of their diminished peripheral anticholinergic,[101] sedative,[102] and cardiovascular effects.[103,104]

If anxiety is a predominant problem, nonpharmacologic techniques may be of greater efficacy than are the pharmacologic. The author's belief that benzodiazepines may not be efficacious ans antianxiety agents[105,106] has led him to explore other modalities for the relief of anxiety in elderly men. He has had good

Table IV. Symptoms of Depression

I. Mood disturbance
II. At least 4 of 8:
  1. Appetite/weight disturbance
  2. Sleep disturbance
  3. Disturbance in activity level
  4. Cognitive disturbance
  5. Disturbance in energy level
  6. Disturbance in usual interests
  7. Disturbance of attention
  8. Suicidal ideation/plans/behavior
III. Duration of at least two weeks
IV. Exclusion criteria: not part of a physical disorder or other major psychiatric disorder
V. Not a normal grief reaction

results in most clients with some of the following techniques. The clients are almost always taught relaxation exercises, either those developed by Jacobson[107] and Wolpe[108] or those used in the Lamaze method of childbirth.[109] This gives the client voluntary control over his symptoms of anxiety. Massage, either done by the client or by another person, is an excellent way of relaxing muscle tension as well as fostering interpersonal communication. Acupressure to the base of the skull just posterior to the mastoid process relieves tension headaches in a matter of minutes for a majority of clients with that problem. A few clients may also benefit from transcendental meditation, Tantric meditation, yoga, or jogging (if the patient's physical condition allows it). Specific symptoms, such as phobias, or compulsions, are quite responsive to behavior modification techniques.[108–110] What is notable is that all these modalities give the responsibility for his own symptom relief and give control of symptoms back to the client, which minimizes helplessness and maximizes the sense of mastery, over and above any specific psychophysiological effects of these techniques. This will be further discussed below.

The therapist then works with the underlying affective responses of fear, anger, or loss. The major therapeutic intervention at this stage is ventilation and the major techniques are clarification of the affect[111] and permission-giving. The older man is actively encouraged to express the affect he is experiencing. It may be necessary to give very clear-cut permission, even going so far as to say, "Its OK to be angry," or "sad," or whatever the affect is. The older man is instructed that not only is it permissible to express affect, but it is an expected part of the therapeutic process that will be constantly encouraged. The therapist may have to actively confront the lack of expression of affect. For some individuals, the therapist may also actively have to label the affect for the patient. With clients with labile personality disorders, limits on the inappropriate expression of affect is necessary.

Anger is relatively easy for the older man to express, as it is a more ego-syntonic affect. Some require limits on and confrontation of the behavioral aspects of the expression of anger, as they may not look or sound angry when acting upon these feelings. The behaviors must be translated into words with the associated affect emoted. It may also be necessary to clarify for the older man that it is frequently considered unmasculine to express his fears or sense of loss, and to cry in the presence of another man (the therapist) or woman. The societal background of the difficulty in ventilation may be explained to the man in the hope that it will then be easier for him to express these feelings. A special problem occurs if the older man suffers from alexithymia, as he may not know how to label his feelings. Techniques dealing with alexithymia are discussed in the chapter on individual psychotherapy by Solomon.

Once the affect has been expressed and labeled, the older man is then given specific behavioral tasks to minimize his experience of helplessness. Emotional, social, and daily living needs are identified and the older person is instructed to respond to those needs with appropriate behavioral responses. Progressively graded and appropriate tasks are given to the older man, tasks in which it can be realistically expected that the older man will be successful. Permission is given to the older man to verbalize and experience his helplessness. Brief psychotherapeutic interventions around issues of dependency and relationships with women and authority figures are frequently appropriate at this stage of therapy. The appropriate use of positive reinforcement to show the older man what he is capable of doing may also diminish his sense of helplessness. Whereas previous phases of therapy tend to utilize the dependency and helplessness inherent in the sick role, these processes are minimized at this stage. This is especially important in institutional settings, such as acute psychiatric hospitals.

Simultaneously, a resurgence of mastery is encouraged, not only by giving behavioral tasks within reach of the patient, but also by emphasizing the person's choice and motivation in seeking therapy. Choice and options in all aspects of life are actively encouraged, in part to move the older person from an external to an internal locus of control, but also to reverse the dynamic process that led to symptoms. The appropriate use of reminiscence as a therapeutic technique[112] will help the older man identify techniques for problem solving and crisis resolution learned in the past; he may again use these same techniques for problem solving in the present.

Olin[113] notes that responsibility for one's own life is a necessary part of the therapy of persons with borderline personality disorders. A humanistic orientation requires that the therapist expand this focus to the therapy of all older people; therefore, it must be made clear to the elderly man that he is responsible for his life and must take that responsibility if therapy is to be successful. The therapist must also help the client create new options to maximize choice and responsibility.

During this stage of therapy, the therapist also makes a direct attack on the particular stressors to which the older man is responding. Biologic stressors are treated with appropriate medical or surgical interventions. With paranoid symptomatology, correction of any hearing or visual deficit may frequently be more valuable than antipsychotic medication. Social losses must be replenished, both through the psychotherapy of grief and narcissistic injury, as well as with concrete ways of helping the older man replenish his losses. Referrals to senior centers, employment agencies, income maintenance, social agencies, or instructions to spend more time with living members of family or friends may be appropriate. New meaning in old and new activities must be developed. Marital therapy and therapy for sexual dysfunctions are as efficacious with older people as with younger patients.[88] Losses in the realm of daily living needs may require that the therapist advocate with and for the patient with various social agencies. The elderly client must be encouraged to experiment with new activities, interests, and relationships, so that he can define and create for himself a new and meaningful social and existential world.

If a major reason why the older person develops symptomatology at this time of life relates to the presence of unresolved neurotic conflicts or a long-standing personality disorder, the second stage of therapy, or the stage of long-term psychotherapy, is begun. In this stage, the therapist attacks the underlying difficulties the individual has with coping as well as his chronic maladaptive responses to stress. Once the person has resolved the triggering crisis, psychotherapy of these underlying dynamic conflicts is absolutely indicated. Older men are appropriate candidates for individual psychotheraphy, which is frequently successful with the population group.[114–116] If the older person has many of the positive ego qualities appropriate for psychoanalytic psychotherapy, that modality should be utilized.[117] Like younger clients, this therapy requires that the older man be motivated for psychotherapy, psychologically minded, and have a modicum of intelligence to be able to work at the abstract level necessary in psychotherapy. The client should have reasonably good ego functioning and impulse control and there should be a relative lack of somatization of symptomatology. As there is nothing that occurs in the process of normal aging that would preclude the development and maintenance of these qualities, psychoanalytic psychotherapy should be considered the modality of choice for treatment of elderly men with neuroses or personality disorders. Indeed, many older people may be treated by psychoanalysis, as noted by Kahana,[118] although the majority will more likely benefit from psychoanalytic psychotherapy.

Some technical modifications may become necessary in working with this age group. If the conflicts have masculine gender-role issues as major component to them, the modifications of psychotherapy developed by Solomon[119] (Chapter 13 in this book) may be particularly helpful. Because some patients may fatigue easily, it may be wise to limit sessions to 30 minutes rather than the traditional 50 minutes for these patients. Sessions should be scheduled at such times as to maximize the older person's alertness and diurnal and other biologic rhythms, as well as special travel needs. Many of the elderly rely on public transportation, limit their driving to daylight hours because of limitations in night vision, or avoid nocturnal excursions into or out of high-crime areas. Taking the history requires longer time because there are more years of experience. History taking should emphasize an assessment of the person's lifelong strengths and how they coped with stress[112] so that these techniques may be utilized and reinforced during psychotherapy. As older men have frequently done many years of self-examination, it may be possible to start psychotherapy at a level of insight that is deeper than with younger clients. In addition, older persons are aware of their limited life span and are more motivated for psychotherapy than are younger persons.[96] Because of this, resistances are diminished, which allows for a more rapid identification and working through of major dynamic issues, followed by the willingness on the part of the older man to put these insights and affective changes into their behavioral repertoire. Interpretations thus may be given earlier in therapy and concentration on resistances may be minimized.

Some older men may not be appropriate candidates for psychoanalytic psychotherapy. If there is more than a minimum of dementia or if the person is unable to work within the transference relationship, supportive psychotherapy is indicated.[120] Supportive psychotherapy should not only emphasize the crisis intervention noted above, but also help the older man devise new ways of coping to minimize the maladaptive effect of the old coping mechanisms on behavior. This is accomplished by an emphasis on the effect of the person's feelings and behaviors on those around him and how that in turn affects the patient in the here and now. It may be necessary to be directive and confrontive to give the patient structured "homework" to attempt to change specific behaviors in a stepwise fashion. Again, the technical modifications noted above and elsewhere[119] (Chapter 13 Solomon on individual psychotherapy), should be integrated into therapy.

Techniques of Gestalt therapy and transactional analysis may be particularly helpful in working with the older man with a personality disorder. If there is a degree of somatization, identification of the emotional concomitants of the somatization may be translated into verbal affective statements. For example, somatic pain may first be concretized so that the older man is asked what his stomach (chest, throat, etc.) is feeling. He is then asked, using a Gestalt technique,[121] to translate that into a statement about what he is feeling. That statement is then used as a bridge to the identification of the underlying affective state. Once that underlying affective state is identified, then the client's maladaptive responses to it can be further identified in a way consistent with either supportive or insight-oriented therapy. Because many older men with unresolved dependency issues behave in a childlike way, various transactional analytic techniques, as well as responses to the individual as an adult and pointing out the childlike ways in which he behaves may be a particular helpful form of interpersonal insight.[122] It is particularly important for the therapist at this stage not to behave in a parental way.

If interpersonal difficulties are a major component of the maladaptive responses, the older man may benefit more from group psychotherapy than individual psychotherapy. Groups of older persons are quite successful in promoting therapeutic changes.[123] They tend to work better when the groups are homogeneous and consist only of older people because many older persons have a reluctance to share in a mixed age group, in which they may be the only older person there, thus allowing younger patients to dominate those groups. However, in a geriatric therapy group, this is generally not so. In addition, because older clients are more likely to be women, there are frequently not enough men in the group to dominate the group, thus allowing for greater intimacy and sharing. The group may be utilized to be supportive, to confront, to suggest specific behavioral modifications, as well as to give insight and feedback on the interpersonal aspects of the individual's personality disorder. Group psychotherapy is particularly helpful in individuals with dependent or passive–aggressive behaviors because the group is frequently unwilling to tolerate the pathologic behavior, thus forcing change in the maladaptive responses to stress with the support and advice of the group. In addition, as there is an element of social isolation in many elderly clients, the group brings to the client a consistent social network that can be expected to be helpful in times of crisis.

Family or couple psychotherapy may be helpful when interpersonal issues within the family are of major importance. It may consist of a very behaviorally oriented approach in which the family is used as behavioral engineers to modify, with classical reinforcement, extinction, or punishment paradigms, the behaviors of the identified patient. Or, a communications, functional, or structural model may be utilized to help clarify the person's needs and to help the family members or spouse behave in a way that maximizes appropriate response–outcome. For the relatively nonverbal individual with interpersonal difficulties living at home, utilizing a family member or a substitute for a family member such as home health aide as an intervenor may be an important element in family or behavioral therapy.

Clients with severe dependency needs or who are schizoid may benefit from day hospitalization or attendance at special social groups for the elderly. These social groups may involve nonthreatening activities and allow for the gradual desensitization of the older withdrawn man to a social network that may be supportive. Day hospitalization may allow the client to structure his life. In the context of nonthreatening recreational activities plus therapeutically oriented groups and individual sessions, there can be moderate success with a severely disturbed older man with a dependent, schizoid, or schizotypal personality disorder. In addition, ancillary social and rehabilitative services that may be necessary and helpful within the context of any of the therapeutic modalities are frequently available. There may be a need to teach budgeting, shopping, or advocacy skills, especially for the chronically dependent or schizoid individual. Assurance that the older man is receiving appropriate and complete social services such as Food Stamps and Medicare may become an important part of developing the therapeutic alliance as well as a way of minimizing some of the social and day-to-day stresses on the client that would interfere with ongoing therapy.

Certain transference reactions may occur with the older man that differ from those of the younger client. One is the parentification of the therapist. While this is no different than the parentification that comprises much of the transference neurosis of psychotherapy with younger individuals, it may be more difficult for the older man to allow these transference interpretations to enter his consciousness. The sense of foolishness at seeing the younger therapist as a mother or father may overwhelm his therapeutic motivation. The parentification may uncover specific and important psychodynamic issues regarding the patient's feelings about his father and the role his father played in this own psychological development. Maternalization of the therapist may uncover difficulties with envy of women, hostility toward women, unresolved Oedipal conflicts, and power needs that underlie some of the development of chauvinistic symptomatology.[124]

Another transference issue is infantilization of the therapist. As the therapist is usually younger and frequently of a different generation than the client, the older man may see his therapist as a child or grandchild, and may relate with him accordingly. One elderly client brought in a deck of cards to teach the therapist how to play gin rummy during a therapy hour. An 86-year-old client called the therapist "Sonny" for the entire first year of therapy. This may be evidence of a positive transference as well as infantilization and it may be utilized by the therapist to allow the older man to experience and express feelings of warmth, intimacy, and trust toward another man. It may also be utilized to help the patient explore his relationships with his children and grandchildren, as well as other intergenerational relationships.

Dependency may become a major problem in therapy with older men. As noted by Menninger,[117] the psychotherapeutic intervention is an unequal relationship. The nature of the relationship is to develop a controlled regression in the client, in part by putting the client into a dependent position. Many men, as noted in the first chapter by Solomon, may run away from this dependent position because it symbolizes an ambivalent relationship with a maternal or paternal figure, or because of the vulnerability that it implies. The experience of sharing feelings in this position may lead to fear of homosexual attack or physical attack by the therapist perceived as father–disciplinarian. This may lead to flight, including absence from a session, silence within a session, intellectualization, and other acting-out behaviors. In group psychotherapy with men, it may be particularly difficult for older men to share, leading to dropping out of the group.[125] Other men try to shift the dependency relationship into another relationship which is more culturally and ego syntonic, the sick role, and thus may present with various hypochondriacal complaints and requests that the therapist examine them, check their blood pressure, or prescribe medications. As the author advocated that the geropsychiatrist accept the role as the patient's primary care physician,[126] and older men are likely to have medical problems, this may be particularly difficult for the therapist to handle without a breakdown of the therapeutic relationship and requires fine tuning of the therapist's clinical skills. Sexualization of the dependency may lead to complaints of prostatic or sexual difficulties.

There are also countertransference issues that develop while doing psychotherapy with older men. Because of the age differential, the younger therapist may see his/her client as a parent or grandparent and may parentify the client. Parentification may inhibit the therapist from working with various clinical issues that arise, depending upon the therapist. Frequently avoided issues are death, sexuality, and marital relationships.

On the other hand, perhaps as a defense against parentification, the client may be infantilized. This frequently is manifested by patronizing statements from the therapist. Infantilization may lead the therapist to bring up issues of dependency and vulnerability when it may be premature for the client to deal with them. Infantilization also leads to a tendency to be inappropriately directive in therapy and to minimize the growth potential of the client.

Stereotyping the older man allows the therapist to see the older man as an ungrowing, conservative, dependent, ill, rigid, sloppy, deteriorating person. Solomon and Vickers[64] have defined a stereotype as "the holding in common by the members of a group of a standardized mental picture representing an oversimplified and uncritical judgment of another group." Given this definition, it can be said that, in general, the acceptance of stereotypes of the elderly by professionals is not any different from that of the general population. The data in support of the opposite idea, that professionals are less willing to accept the stereotype of old people, are limited and nonspecific. For example, Rosencranz and McNevin[127] found that stereotyping was less characteristic of professional and economically advantaged classes; this finding was confirmed by Ivester and King.[128] Thorson, Whatley, and Hancock[129] and Thorson[130] showed that with more years of education, a more realistic set of expectations was held of the aging. In all of these studies, however, professionals were not specifically evaluated.

Most of the published data support the concept that older people are stereotyped as frequently by professionals as by other members of the population. This literature will be briefly reviewed. Although there is a wealth of research on attitudes of other population groups toward the elderly, it will not be reviewed here as it is not specifically germane to the delivery of professional services to the elderly. In general, however, those data are consistent with the studies noted below.

LeShan and LeShan[96] noted that psychotherapists are reluctant to work with clients with a limited life span and were more remote from these clients. Kastenbaum[131] further noted that old people are less likely to receive psychotherapy than younger people. He related this to the status of old people and the fact that psychotherapists rely on unexamined values and stereotypes in determining who is to receive psychotherapy. This has been reiterated by Garfinkel.[132] Dye[133] has suggested that the negative attitudes of care givers facilitates psychological withdrawal in the elderly.

In an early study, Tuckman and Lorge[134] found that professionals who had experiences with the aged via a lecture course accepted stereotypes of old people to the same degree as other students who did not have such a course. Arnhoff and Lorge[135] evaluated 25 fellows in gerontology, all of whom had an M.D. or Ph.D. degree. They found that they accepted many of the stereotypes of old people to a similar degree as other population groups. They also found that this group was more likely to advise palliative therapy rather than a positive growth-oriented therapy for old people.

McGuinness and Knox[136] found that nurses tended to rank psychogeriatric nursing as either their first or last choice of career. Interestingly enough, however, the reasons for first or last choice were similar: more bedside nursing, slow convalescence, and the dependency of the clients. They found that this related in part to stereotypes of old people.

Spence et al.[137] evaluated the acceptance of stereotypes by freshmen and senior medical students and found no difference between the two groups. They also found that in hypothetical life-threatening situations, medical students were more likely to save a young person over an old person, a female over a male, a young female over an old male, a white person over a Black person, but a young Black person over an old white person. They felt that this was response to societal stereotypes as well as a medical training that put an emphasis on chronological age of the client.

Mills[138] found that undergraduate occupational therapy students also held to the stereotype of old people and this prevented them from developing an interest in working with the geriatric population.

Cyrus-Lutz and Gaitz[139] evaluated the attitudes of psychiatrists toward old people and found that although psychiatrists were more aware of many of the positive aspects of the elderly (their humanistic values, their fear of loneliness and isolation, the importance of work, and their wisdom and intelligence), they tended to concentrate on negative aspects, such as memory loss and physical problems, as more relevant to their role as a physician. They found that younger psychiatrists were more out-going and more comfortable with clients over the age of 65 than were older psychiatrists.

York, Fergus, and Calsyn[140] found negative attitudes toward the elderly in nursing staff in nursing homes. These negative attitudes directly correlated with the length of time the nursing personnel worked at the home; in other words, the longer the nurse worked with the elderly, the more negative his/her attitudes were. Similarly, McConnell[141] found negative attitudes toward the elderly among nursing home personnel.

Hickey et al.[142] found that in-service training to a variety of care givers to the elderly did not change their attitudes toward their clients. Younger practitioners, however, tended to become less cynical, to do less stereotyping, and to have less social distance from the aged.

Studies of nursing students by Kayser and Minningerode,[143] Johnson and Wilhite,[144] and Robb[145] showed that nursing students had less positive attitudes toward the elderly than toward other population groups.

Romaniuk, Hoyer, and Romaniuk[146] found negative attitudes among the staff and clients of a psychogeriatic day treatment center. These attitudes were particularly noted in the area of patronizing comments and client self-attitudes and were modified by staff training.

Job satisfaction was correlated with staff attitudes toward the elderly in a study by Montgomery and Wilkinson.[147] They studied staff of health and mental health clinics and nursing homes and generally found negative attitudes toward the elderly.

Brennan and Moravec[148] studied the attitudes toward the elderly of the staff at a Veterans Administration Hospital and found them negative. Following a series of training sessions, attitudes and knowledge improved significantly. Similar findings in a study of medical and dental students were reported by Holtzman and Beck,[149] who also reported an association between the acquisition of knowledge of the elderly and improvement in their attitudes.[150]

Solomon and Vickers[64] studied the acceptance of stereotypes of old people by medical students, housestaff, and geriatric team staff. They found that there were significant differences between these groups of health care professionals and that, in general, medical students and housestaff held to the stereotypes more strongly than geriatric staff. The stereotypes held by these students and housestaff were that older clients have limited activities and interests, were in poor physical condition, were not important to their family, had negative personality traits, were pessimistic toward the future, insecure, and conservative, developed mental and physical deterioration, and were asexual beings.

Beck et al.[151] assessed the attitudes of dental students toward old people. Although somewhat negative to begin with, the attitudes became increasingly negative as the student had more experience with the elderly dental client. The authors attributed this to the students' exposure to a majority of elderly clients with poor oral hygiene remained unchanged. In another study, Ettinger et al.[152] also reported negative attitudes of dental students toward old people.

Farrar and Miller[153] studied the attitudes of social work students, social workers, law students, and attorneys toward older people. Their data supported their hypothesis that the elderly were not preferred clients and that these professionals had negative attitudes toward the elderly.

Psychiatrists were found to hold to many of the stereotypes of the elderly in a study by Ford and Sbordone.[154] Their subjects felt that older clients had a poorer prognosis and that older clients were not suitable candidates for psychotherapy.

Solomon and Vickers[155] examined the adherence to stereotypes of older people of adult protective service workers, most of whom were social workers; the rest were public health nurses. These workers held to most of the common stereotypes of the elderly and viewed older people as conservative, insecure, physically and mentally deteriorated, lonely, meddlesome, and pessimistic persons. The adherence to these stereotypes changed dramatically following intensive training sessions. Similar findings were noted for medical students.

A final blind spot for the therapist is that he/she may use traditional masculine stereotypes as a measure of mental health of the old man. This is in contradistinction to using therapy as an opportunity to change the man's gender-role behavior. The man therapist will frequently find the behavior of the older man ego-syntonic and may be unaware of the lack of affect, avoidance of dependency, and avoidance of intimacy that occurs in the therapeutic setting. However, as noted by Broverman et al.,[44] Kjervik and Palta,[156] and Dreman,[157] women therapists also define masculine mental health according to traditional masculine roles. These blind spots will lead to blocks in therapy, if not the actual failure of therapy. This is discussed in more detail in Chapter 13, on individual psychotherapy by Solomon.

CONCLUSION

Older men have two psychological strikes against them. First is their age, as they suffer many of the losses and crises faced by all older individuals. They respond to these crises in ways that are both idiosyncratic for them as individuals and traditionally masculine. The second strike against them is their masculinity, which may diminish adaptive capabilities. The older man must deal with his own individual issues as well as cope with the stereotyping done of him as old and as a man. It is necessary for therapists to be aware of the special problems of older men, and how to work best with them to enhance the growth and give happiness and meaning to these men in the final stage of the life cycle.

REFERENCES

1. Neugarten BL: Time, age, and the life cycle. Am J Psychiatry 136:887–894, 1979
2. Gutmann D: Individual adaptation in the middle years. Developmental issues in the masculine mid-life crisis. J Geriatr Psychiatry 9:41–77, 1976
3. Gutmann D, Grunes J, Griffin B: The clinical psychology of later life: Developmental paradigms. Presented at the 32nd Annual Meeting of the Gerontological Society, Washington, DC, November 29, 1979
4. Neugarten BL: Adaptation and the life cycle. Counseling Psychol 6:16–20, 1976
5. Neugarten BL, Datan N: The middle years, in American Handbook of Psychiatry, Vol 1, 2nd edition. Edited by Arieti S. New York, Basic Books, 1974, pp 592–608
6. Levinson DJ, Darrow CN, Klein EB, et al: The Seasons of a Man's Life. New York, Alfred A. Knopf, 1978
7. Gould R: Transformations. New York, Simon and Schuster, 1978
8. Sheehey G: Passages. Predictable Crises of Adult Life. New York, Bantam Books, 1977
9. Tuckman J, Lorge I: "When aging begins" and stereotypes about aging. J Gerontol 8:489–492, 1953
10. Powers EA, Grubbs MG: The age identification of older persons: An experience in interviewer-created social reality. Presented at the 32nd Annual Meeting of the Gerontological Society, Washington, DC, Nov 29, 1979
11. Harris L: The Myth and Reality of Aging in America. Washington, National Council on the Aging, 1976
12. Brotman HB: Facts and Figures on Older Americans No. 5. An Overview—1971. Washington, Department of Health, Education and Welfare, 1972
13. Butler RN: Old age, in American Handbook of Psychiatry, Vol 1, 2nd edition. Edited by Arieti S. New York, Basic Books, 1974, pp 646–661
14. Harrison J: Warning: The male sex role may be dangerous to your health. J Soc Issues 34:65–86, 1978
15. Solomon K: The masculine gender role and its implications for the life expectancy of older men. J Am Geriatrics Soc 29:297–301, 1981
16. Nathanson CA: Sex roles as variables in preventive health behavior J Community Health 3:142–155, 1977
17. Kimball CP: Psychological aspects of cardiovascular disease, in American Handbook of Psychiatry, Vol IV, 2nd edition. Edited by Reiser MF, New York, Basic Books, 1975, pp 609–617
18. Chafetz ME, Demone HW Jr: Alcoholism and Society. New York, Oxford University Press, 1972
19. Weiss JAM: Suicide, in American Handbook of Psychiatry, Vol III, 2nd edition. Edited by Arieti S, Brody EB. New York, Basic Books, 1974, pp 743–765
20. Gutmann D: The cross-cultural perspective: Notes toward a comparative psychology of aging, in Handbook of the Psychology of Aging. Edited by Birren JE, Schaie KW. New York, Van Nostrand Reinhold, 1977, pp 302–326
21. Keith PM, Brubaker TH: Male household roles in later life: A look at masculinity and marital relationships. Fam Coordinator 28:497–502, 1979
22. Hubbard RW, Santos JF, Farrow BJ: Age differences in sex role diffusion. A study of middle aged and older adult married couples. Presented at the 32nd Annual Meeting of the Gerontological Society, Washington, DC, Nov 29, 1979
23. Ames LB: Are Rorschach responses influenced by society's change? J Personality Assess 39:439–452, 1975
24. Singer MT: Personality measurements in the aged, in Human Aging: A Biological and Behav-

ioral Study. Edited by Birren JE, Butler RN, Greenhouse SW, et al. Washington, US Government Printing Office, 1963
25. Neugarten BL, Gutmann DL: Age-sex roles and personality in middle age. A thematic apperception study, in Middle Age and Aging. Edited by Neugarten BL. Chicago, University of Chicago Press, 1968, pp 58–71
26. Gutmann D: The country of old men: Cross-cultural studies in the psychology of later life, in Occasional Papers in Gerontology, No. 5. Ann Arbor, Institute of Gerontology, 1969
27. Gutmann DL: Female ego styles and generational conflict, in Feminine Personality and Conflict. Edited by Bardwick JM, Donuvan E, Horner MS, et al. Belmont, Brookes/Cole, 1970
28. Ryff CD, Baltes PB: Value transition and adult development in women: The instrumentality–terminality sequence hypothesis. Dev Psychol 12:567–568, 1976
29. Zubin J: Failures of the Rorschach technique. J Projective Techniques 18:303–315, 1954
30. Kahana B: The use of projective techniques in personality assessment of the aged, in the Clinical Psychology of Aging. Edited by Storandt M, Siegler IC, Elias MF. New York, Plenum, 1978, pp 145–180
31. Strong EK: Vocational Interests of Men and Women. Stanford, Stanford University Press, 1943
32. Douglas K, Arenberg D: Age changes, cohort differences, and cultural change on the Guilford–Zimmerman Temperament Survey. J Gerontol 33:737–747, 1978
33. Barrows G, Zuckerman M: Construct validity of three masculinity–femininity tests. J Counseling Clin Psychol 34:1–7, 1976
34. Lowenthal MF, Thurnher M, Chiraboda D: Four Stages of Life. San Francisco, Jossey-Bass, 1977
35. Foley JM, Murphy DM: Sex role identity in the aged. Presented at the 30th Annual Meeting of the Gerontological Society, San Francisco, California, November 20, 1977
36. Costa PT Jr, McCrae RR: Cross-sectional differences in masculinity–femininity in adult men. Presented at the 30th Annual Meeting of the Gerontological Society, San Francisco, California, November 20, 1977
37. Jackson DW: Advanced aged adults' reflection of middle age. Gerontologist 14:255–257, 1974
38. Zaks PM, Karuza J Jr, Domurath KL, et al: Sex role orientation across the adult life span. Presented at the 32nd Annual Meeting of the Gerontological Society, Washington, DC, November 29, 1979
39. Goody J: Aging in nonindustrial societies, in Handbook of Aging and the Social Sciences. Edited by Binstock RH, Shanas E. New York, Van Nostrand Reinhold, 1976, pp 117–129
40. Treas J: Socialist organization and economic development in China. Latent consequences for the aged. Gerontologist 19:34–43, 1979
41. Simmons L: The Role of the Aged in Primitive Society. New Haven, Yale University Press, 1945
42. Sinnott JD: Sex-role inconstancy, biology, and successful aging. A dialectical model. Gerontologist 17:459–463, 1977
43. Silverman M: The old man as woman: Detecting stereotypes of aged men with a femininity scale. Perceptual Motor Skills 44:336–338, 1977
44. Broverman IK, Broverman DM, Clarkson FE, et al.: Sex-role stereotypes and clinical judgments of mental health. J Consult Clin Psychol 34:1–7, 1970
45. Solomon K: Psychosocial crises of older men. Presented at the 133rd Annual Meeting of the American Psychiatric Association, San Francisco, May 1980
46. Rosow I: Status and role change through the life span, in Handbook of Aging and the Social Sciences. Edited by Binstock RH, Shanas E. New York, Van Nostrand Reinhold, 1976, pp 457–482
47. Goldfarb AI: Clinical perspectives, in Aging in Modern Society. Psychiatric Research Report No. 23. Edited by Simon A, Epstein LJ. Washington, American Psychiatric Association, 1968, pp 170–178
48. Goldfarb AI: Minor maladjustments of the aged, in American Handbook of Psychiatry, Vol III, 2nd edition. Edited by Arieti S, Brody EB. New York, Basic Books, 1974, pp 820–860
49. Solomon K: Personality disorders and the elderly, in Personality Disorders: Diagnosis and Management, 2nd edition. Edited by Lion Jr. Baltimore, Williams and Wilkins, 1981, pp 310–338
50. Solomon K: The elderly patient, in Clinical Medicine. Edited by Spittell JR Jr. Vol XII, Psychiatry. Hagerstown, Harper and Row, 1981

51. Solomon K: Social antecendents of learned helplessness in the health care setting. Gerontologist 22:282–287, 1982
52. Solomon K: Social antecedents of learned helplessness of the elderly in the health care setting, in Sociological Research Symposium Proceedings (IX). Edited by Lewis EP, Nelson LD, Scully DH, et al. Richmond, Virginia Commonwealth University, 1979, pp 188–192
53. Parsons T: The Social System. New York, Free Press, 1951, pp 428–473
54. Wilson RN: The Sociology of Health: An Introduction. New York, Random House, 1970, pp 13–32
55. Selye H: The Physiology and Pathology of Exposure to Stress. Montreal, Acta, 1950
56. Holmes TH, Rahe RH: The social readjustment rating scale. J Psychosom Res 11:213–218, 1967
57. Brandwein C, Postoff R, Steinberg T: The "married widow(er):" A new role. Presented at the 32nd Annual Meeting of the Gerontological Society, Washington, DC, November 28, 1979
58. Scheff TJ: Schizophrenia as ideology. Schizophrenia Bull No 2:15–19, 1970
59. Zusman J: Some explanations of the changing appearance of psychotic patients. Antecedents of the social breakdown syndrome concept. Milbank Mem Fund Quart 44 (Supplement): 363–394, 1966
60. Ryan W: Blaming the Victim, revised edition. New York, Vintage Books, 1976
61. Brody EB: Psychosocial aspects of prejudice, in American Handbook of Psychiatry, Vol II, 2nd edition. Edited by Caplan G. New York, Basic Books, 1974, pp 492–511
62. Tuckman J, Lorge I: Attitudes toward old people. J Soc Psychol 37:249–260, 1953
63. Butler RN: Why Survive? Being Old in America. New York, Harper and Row, 1975, pp 174–259
64. Solomon K, Vickers R: Attitudes of health workers toward old people, J Am Geriatrics Soc 27:186–191, 1979
65. Solomon K: The depressed patient: Social antecedents of psychopathologic changes in the elderly. J Am Geriatrics Soc, 29:14–18, 1981
66. Friedmann EA, Orbach HL: Adjustment to retirement, in American Handbook of Psychiatry, Vol I, 2nd edition. Edited by Arieti S. New York, Basic Books, 1974, pp 609–645
67. Sheppard HL: Work and retirement, in Handbook of Aging and the Social Sciences. Edited by Binstock RM, Shanas E. New York, Van Nostrand Reinhold, 1976, pp 286–309
68. Palmore E: Predictors of successful aging. Gerontologist 19:427–431, 1979
69. David DS, Brannon R: The male sex role: Our culture's blueprint of manhood and what it's done for us lately, in The Forty-Nine Percent Majority: The Male Sex Role. Edited by David DS, Brannon R. Reading, Massachusetts, Addison-Wesley, 1976. pp 1–45
70. Lein L: Male participation in home life: Impact of social supports and breadwinner responsibility on the allocation of tasks. Fam Coordinator 28:489–495, 1979
71. Bibring E: The mechanism of depression, in Affective Disorders. Edited by Greenacre P. New York, International Universities Press, 1965, pp 13–48
72. Kay DWK: The epidemiology and identification of brain deficit in the elderly, in Cognitive and Emotional Disturbance in the Elderly. Edited by Eisdorfer C, Freidel RO. Chicago, Year Book Medical Publishers, 1977, pp 11–26
73. Seligman MEP: Helplessness. San Francisco, WH Freeman, 1975
74. Maier SF, Seligman MEP: Learned helplessness: Theory and evidence. J Exp Psychol: General 105:3–46, 1976
75. Engel GL: A psychological setting of somatic disease: The "giving up-given up" complex. Proc R Soc Med 60:553–555, 1967
76. Solomon K: The development of stereotypes of the elderly: Toward a unified hypothesis. Presented at the 31st Annual Meeting of the Gerontological Society, Dallas, Texas, November 19, 1978
77. Solomon K: The development of stereotypes of the elderly: Toward a unified hypothesis, in Sociological Research Symposium Proceedings (IX). Edited by Lewis EP, Nelson LD, Scully DH, et al. Richmond, Virginia Commonwealth University, 1979, pp 172–177
78. Solomon K: Social antecedents of depression in the elderly: The relationship between societal structure and stereotyping. Presented at the 133rd Annual Meeting of the American Psychiatric Association, San Francisco, California, May 5, 1980
79. Becker E: The Revolution in Psychiatry, London, Free Press of Glencoe, 1964
80. Durkheim E: Suicide (1897). New York, Free Press, 1951

81. Akiskal HS, McKinney WT Jr: Depressive disorders: Toward a unified hypothesis. Science 182:20–29, 1973
82. Akiskal HS, McKinney WT Jr: Overview of recent research in depression. Integration of ten conceptual models into a comprehensive clinical frame. Arch Gen Psychiatry 32:285–305, 1975
83. Abraham K: Notes on the psychoanalytic investigation and treatment of manic-depressive insanity and allied conditions (1911), in Selected Papers on Psychoanalysis. New York, Basic Books, 1960, pp 137–156
84. Freud S: Mourning and melancholia (1917), in Collected Papers, Vol IV. London, Hogarth Press, 1934, pp 152–170
85. Wolff CT: Loss, grief, and mourning in adults, in Understanding Human Behavior in Health and Illness. Edited by Simons RC, Pardes H. Baltimore, Williams and Wilkins, 1977, pp 378–386
86. Masters WH, Johnson VE: Human Sexual Response, Boston, Little Brown, 1966, pp 223–270
87. Pfeiffer E: Sexuality in the aging individual. J Am Geriatrics Soc 22:481–484, 1974
88. Masters WH, Johnson VE: Human Sexual Inadequacy. Boston, Little Brown, 1970, pp 57–60
89. Shader RI: Endocrine, metabolic, and genitourinary effects of psychotropic drugs, in Clinical Handbook of Psychopharmacology. Edited by DiMascio A, Shader RI. New York, Science House, 1970, pp 205–212
90. Kalinowsky LB, Hippius H: Pharmacological, Convulsive and other Somatic Treatments in Psychiatry. New York, Grune and Stratton, 1968, pp 69–70, 136, 149
91. Bem SL: Sex-role adaptability: One consequence of psychological androgyny. J Personality Soc Psychol 31:634–643, 1975
92. Spence JT, Helmreich R, Stapp J: Ratings of self and peers on sex role attributes and their relation to self-esteem and conceptions of masculinity and femininity. J Personality Soc Psychol 32:29–39, 1975
93. O'Connor K, Mann DW, Bardwick JM: Androgyny and self-esteem in the upper middle class: A replication of Spence. J Consult Clin Psychol 46:1168–1169, 1978
94. Gillett N, Levitt M, Antonucci T: The relationship between masculinity, femininity and social competence in three generations of women. Presented at the 30th Annual Meeting of the Gerontological Society, San Francisco, California, November 20, 1977
95. Cherry DL, Zarit SH: Sex-role and age differences in competency, flexibility and affective status of women. Presented at the 31st Annual Meeting of the Gerontological Society, Dallas, Texas, November 18, 1978
96. LeShan L, LeShan E: Psychiatry and the patient with a limited life span. Psychiatry 24:318–323, 1961
97. Weinberg J: Time, age, and timelessness. Am J Psychiatry 135:893–899, 1978
98. Beck AT: The Diagnosis and Management of Depression. Philadelphia, University of Pennsylvania Press, 1973
99. Kay DWK, Cooper AF, Garside RF, et al.: The differentiation of paranoid from affective psychoses by patient's premorbid characteristics. Brit J Psychiatry 129:207–215, 1976
100. Solomon K: Haloperidol and the geriatric patient: Practical considerations, in Haloperidol Update: 1958–1980. Edited by Ayd FJ Jr. Baltimore, Ayd Medical Communications, 1980, pp 155–173
101. Snyder SH, Yamamura HI: Antidepressants and the muscarine acetylcholine receptor. Arch Gen Psychiatry 34:236–239, 1977
102. U'Prichard DC, Greenberg DA, Sheehan PP, et al.: Tricyclic antidepressants: Therapeutic properties and affinity for noradrenergic receptor binding sites in the brain. Science 199:197–198, 1978
103. Jefferson JW: A review of the cardiovascular effects and toxiticy of tricyclic antidepressants. Psychosom Med 37:160–179, 1975
104. Kantor SJ, Glassman AH, Bigger JJ Jr, et al: The cardiac effects of therapeutic plasma concentrations of imipramine. Am J Psychiatry 135:534–538, 1978
105. Solomon K: Benzodiazepines and neurotic anxiety. Critique. NYS J Med 76:2156–2164, 1976
106. Solomon K, Hart R: Pitfalls and prospects in clinical research on antianxiety drugs: Benzodiazepines and placebo. A research review. J Clin Psychiatry 39:823–831, 1978
107. Jacobson E: Progressive Relaxation. Chicago, University of Chicago Press, 1938
108. Wolpe J: The Practice of Behavior Therapy. New York, Pergamon Press, 1969

109. Bing E. Six Practical Lessons for an Easier Childbirth. New York, Bantam, 1969, pp 36–52
110. Shaefer HH, Martin PL: Behavioral Therapy. New York, McGraw-Hill, 1969
111. Bibring E: Psychoanalysis and the dynamic psychotherapies. J Am Psychoanal Assoc 2:745–770, 1954
112. Butler RN: Successful aging and the role of life review. J Am Geriatrics Soc 12:529–532, 1974
113. Olin HS: Psychotherapy of the chronically suicidal patient. Am J Psychother 30:570–575, 1976
114. Verwoerdt A: Clinical Geropsychiatry. Baltimore, Williams and Wilkins, 1976, pp 60–64
115. Sparacino J: Individual psychotherapy with the aged: A selective review. Int J Aging Human Dev 9:197–220, 1978–1979
116. Knight B: Psychotherapy and behavior change with the noninstitutionalized aged. Int J Aging Human Dev 9:221–236, 1978–1979
117. Menninger K: Theory of Psychoanalytic Technique. New York, Harper and Row, 1958
118. Kahana RJ: Psychoanalysis in late life. Discussion. J Geriatric Psychiat 11:37–49, 1978
119. Solomon K: Therapeutic approaches to changing masculine role behavior. Am J Psychoanal 41:31–38, 1981
120. Peck A: Pscyhotherapy of the aged. J Am Geriatrics Soc 14:748–753, 1966
121. Perls F: Gestalt Therapy Verbatim. Lafayette, Real People Press, 1969
122. Maxwell J, Falzett B: OK Childing and Parenting. El Paso, Transactional Institute of El Paso, 1974
123. Goldfarb Al: Group therapy with the old and aged, in Comprehensive Group Therapy. Edited by Kaplan HI, Sadock BJ. Baltimore, Williams and Wilkins, 1971, pp 623–642
124. Woods SM: Some dynamics of male chauvinism. Arch Gen Psychiatry 33:63–65 1976
125. Solomon K: Sex roles and group therapy droupouts. Am J Psychiatry 136:727–728, 1979
126. Solomon K: The geropsychiatrist and the delivery of mental health services in the community. Presented at the 32nd Annual Meeting of the Geronotological Society, Washington, DC, November 26, 1979
127. Rosenkranz HA, McNevin TE: A factor analysis of attitudes toward the aged. Gerontologist 9:55–59, 1969
128. Ivester C, King K: Attitudes of adolescents toward the aged. Gerontologist 17:85–89, 1977
129. Thorson JA, Whatley L, Hancock K: Attitudes toward the aged as a function of age and education. Gerontologist 14:316–318, 1974
130. Thorson JA: Attitudes toward the aged as a fuction of race and social class. Gerontologist 15:343–349, 1975
131. Kastenbaum R: The reluctant therapist. Geriatrics 18:296–301, 1963
132. Garfinkel R: The reluctant therapist 1975. Gerontologist 15:136–137, 1975
133. Dye CA: Attitude change among professionals. Implications for gerontological nursing. J Gerontol Nurs 5:31–35, 1979
134. Tuckman J, Lorge I: Attitude toward aging of individuals with experience with the aged. J Genetic Psychol 92:199–204, 1958
135. Arnhoff FN, Lorge I: Stereotypes about aging and the aged. School Soc 88:70–71, 1960
136. McGuinness AF, Knox SJ: Attitudes to psychogeriatric nursing. Nurs Times 64 (Supplement): 127–128, 1968
137. Spence DJ, Feigenbaum EM, Fitzgerald F, et al.: Medical students attitudes toward the geriatric patient. J Am Geriatrics Soc 16:976–983, 1968
138. Mills J: Attitudes of undergraduate students concerning geriatric patients. Am J Occup Therapy 26:200–203, 1972
139. Cyrus-Lutz C, Gaitz CM: Psychiatrists' attitudes toward the aged and aging. Gerontologist 12:163–167, 1972
140. York J, Fergus E, Calsyn R: The implications of staff attitudes for a nursing home mental health training program. Presented at the 28th Annual Meeing of the Gerontological Society, Louisville, Kentucky, October 28, 1975
141. Mc Connell SR: The effects of organizational context on service providers' attitudes toward old people. Presented at the 30th Annual Meeting of the Gerontological Society, San Francisco, California, November 20, 1977
142. Hickey T, Rakowski W, Hultsch DF, et al: Attitudes toward aging as a function of in-service training and practitioner age. J Gerontol 31:681–686, 1976

143. Kayser JS, Minningerode FA: Increasing nursing students' interest in working with aged patients. Nurs Res 24:23–26, 1975
144. Johnson DM, Wilhite MJ: Changes in nursing students' stereotypic attitudes toward old people. Nurs Res 25:430–432, 1976
145. Robb SS: Attitudes and intentions of baccalaureate nursing students toward the elderly. Nurs Res 28:43–50, 1979
146. Romaniuk M, Hoyer FW, Romaniuk J: Helpless self-attitudes of the elderly. The effect of patronizing statements. Presented at the 30th Annual Meeting of the Gerontological Society, San Francisco, California, November 20, 1977
147. Montgomery D, Wilkinson A: Intervention in the organizational environment: Correcting the mismatch between staff attitudes and agencies' activites. Presented at the 31st Annual Meeting of the Gerontological Society, Dallas, Texas, November 20, 1978
148. Brennan SJ, Moravec JD: Assessing multidisciplinary continuing education as it impacts on knowledge, attitudes and behavior in caring for the elderly. Presented at the 31st Annual Meeting of the Gerontological Society, Dallas, Texas, November 19, 1978
149. Holtzman JM, Beck JD: The impact of medical and dental education on student's attitudes toward the aged. Presented at the 31st Annual Meeting of the Gerontological Society, Dallas, Texas, November 19, 1978
150. Holtzman JM, Beck JD: Palmore's Facts on Aging Quiz: A reappraisal. Gerontologist 19:116–120, 1979
151. Beck JD, Ettinger RL, Glenn RE, et al.: Oral health status: Impact on dental student attitudes toward the aged. Gerontologist 19:580–584, 1979
152. Ettinger RL, Beck J, Kerber P, et al.: Dental student confidence in prosthodontics and attitudes toward the elderly. Presented at the 32nd Annual Meeting of the Gerontological Society, Washington, DC, November 28, 1979
153. Farrar DR, Miller RH: Professional age related attitudinal conflicts of social workers and lawyers. Presented at the 32nd Annual Meeting of the Gerontological Society, Washington, DC, November 28, 1979
154. Ford CV, Sbordone RJ: Attitudes of psychiatrists toward elderly patients. Am J Psychiatry 137:571–575, 1980
155. Solomon K, Vickers R: Stereotyping the elderly: Changing the attitudes of clinicians. Presented at the 33rd Annual Meeting of the Gerontological Society of America, San Diego, California, November 25, 1980
156. Kjervik DK, Palta M: Sex-role stereotyping in assessments of mental health made by psychiatric-mental health nurses. Nurs Res 27:166–171, 1978
157. Dreman SB: Sex-role stereotyping in mental health standards in Israel. J Clin Psychol 34:961–966, 1978

Chapter 12

Where Have All the Heroes Gone?

Another View of Changing Masculine Roles

WOLFGANG LEDERER AND ALEXANDRA BOTWIN

Let us face it: When we are talking today of the changing role of males in society, we are referring to their diminishing role and their diminishing maleness.

It started quite some time ago and it resembles some long drawn out sexual suicide. For it began with the machine and the Industrial Revolution—and the machine was invented by men. It was the machine that deprived men of one of their few natural advantages over women, their greater physical strength. It takes a strong man to clear ground and plow a straight furrow, but a teenage girl can run a tractor. A smith must have muscle, but an assembly worker needs only patience, and women are more patient. When it comes to modern technology with its tiny electronic assemblies, women are not only more patient, they do it better. Even in war, that old proving ground of manhood, now that the fighting is to be done more and more by gadgets and less and less by bodies, women can push buttons and set dials as easily as men.

Industrialization and the corporate world, which treat men as interchangeable parts of a social machine, have not only done away with the glory of sweat, they have also removed the father from the home and thereby diminished him. It may be objected that fathers always left home, sometimes for months and years at a time, in fishing and trading ships, on expeditions of exploration or war, and they were exalted thereby, not diminished. Yes, but there was glory to that, those ventures took courage, they were—to use the key word of our title—heroic. They involved facing a dangerous task for the ultimate benefit of someone else, a man's family, his country, or even humankind. But there is nothing heroic to a job in factory or office and, above all, to "a job any woman can do." Men used to be jealously proud of their purely male jobs. They felt it would be bad luck to have women on ships, in the mines, on a hunting party; now that

---

WOLFGANG LEDERER AND ALEXANDRA BOTWIN • Department of Psychiatry, University of California, San Francisco, California 94118

there are women miners and sailors and even soldiers, men feel a little naked; the mantle of pride and dignity that came from doing a purely male job has been stripped from them.

But a man is not just brawn. Over the millennia men have prided themselves on being more brainy, too. Have men not invented, without any female help, philosophy, mathematics, and all of the sciences? From their bastions of learning, have they not dispensed, without female assistance, all the blessings of social and political theory, of technological practice? Was it not men alone who put technical civilization together and made it run? But now the women assert that men just kept them out; and intruding into traditionally masculine space, they prove themselves quite the equals, and occasionally the betters, in most fields.

What have we left that is specifically male? The question betrays the answer; we have all but forgotten manliness, we account ourselves lucky if we can still prove maleness. "It is no longer in war," writes Diana Trilling, "that men are invited to measure their heroic capacities, but in lovemaking." And she adds, "Certainly it is a kamikaze enterprise in which men engage when they take on the sexual mission assigned to them by an Erika Jong or a Gael Greene."[1] Note the tone of amused, condescending compassion, so fully justified; for it is precisely when we are reduced to maleness, in the sexual sphere, that we are at the worst handicap: Performing the more uncertainly, the more we need to prove ourselves thereby, and competing with a partner who can outperform us, orgasm for orgasm, with one hand behind her back.

This amused condescension has been hounding us for many years, ever since Dagwood appeared in the comic strips and all the endearing, weak, fumbling fathers vied for laughs on television. Many years ago Philip Wylie, in his acidulous *Generation of Vipers*,[2] described how momism corroded the father, how Mom, staying home with her mama's boy, diminished the absent father into insignificance. Mom is no longer staying home, but her move into the man's world has not been counterbalanced by an equivalent resumption of a paternal role by men. The office is no longer a man's world, but the woman still rules the home. She rules the home, and the kindergarten, and the grade school, and she is present as an equal in high school and college, so that, in the eyes of the boy, his father has no special status whatever.

It is precisely for the sons that the derogation of fathers is so calamitous. A son desperately needs his father to be strong and secure, so that he, the son, can hope to grow up to become strong and secure himself. He needs his father to be courageous, to be in some sense a hero, not only to furnish a worthy model but also, on occasion, a worthy adversary.[3]

Let us explain this last point with the aid of mythology. There is no finer, no more radiant figure in all the imaginings of the human mind than the young hero setting out to do battle against the forces of evil. He encounters them—typically—in the shape of a dragon, and he fights the dragon—typically—to save a maiden. His victory—typically—results in his becoming king of a realm previously barren, but now abounding in fertility. In time, as the hero ages and his fertility decreases, he himself becomes a dragon, just as the dragon he slew had, in earlier times, been a hero.[4]

This scheme is of immense importance and wisdom. The young hero is not only the spirit of spring, of the new vegetation that overcomes the barren dragon of winter and drought; he is the spirit of any change and innovation, fighting against an old and established order that has become rigid and sterile. Let us note carefully: He is always fighting, not just to destroy that old order, but to institute a new one; his fight is never for his own glory alone, but always for the betterment of humankind.[5]

So when we ask, what is a man all about, then we can give a very simple answer: A man's task is to try and become a hero. This means that he must go up against the older generation, must challenge them, must unseat them, must take their place, must in turn and in his own way do their job of caring, providing, ordering, and protecting. The motto has always been and will always be: The old king must die, so that the new king may rule.

But what if the father was never king? What if father, in the eyes of the mother and therefore of the son, was a weakling, a nonentity, or altogether absent? Then the chances are that the son, lacking both a shining example and a worthy adversary, perceives no call to heroism, but that he will dally away his youth in idle mischief and purposeless boredom.

This is, in fact, where we are today. Fifty years ago Freud who, like most of his early followers, was steeped in hero lore and constantly drew from it for his psychological metaphors, speculated about the "misery of the masses" in America who, he felt, lived without heroes.[6] Thirty years ago Riesman[7] described other-directedness, the now dominant mode of deriving values, not from ideal standards or examples but, for lack of anything better, from the Joneses, from momentary fashion. Fifteen years ago the senior author suggested the designation "sans-identity" for the aimless young men we saw so many of in our practices.[3] And today we focus on the narcissistic personality[8,9] and the culture of narcissism[10] as the dominant mode and the dominant pathology of the present. We are said to be living in a fatherless society.[10,11] And because, in the absence of strong fathers, we have no reliable vehicle for transmitting positive values, the male superego tends to lack the component we call the ego ideal. It tends to be deficient in its positive, directing, and protective functions. What does persist is the cruel, archaic superego of earliest childhood, and so we deal with patients who not only will not or cannot assume responsibility, make choices, or engage in long-range commitments, but who are so self-defeating that they regularly demolish the dependent relationships they need in order to survive.

It is tragic in the true sense of the word, namely, that the best efforts of the hero are fated to bring about nothing but calamity for him and his world. It is tragic that Freud and all the rest of us after him have helped to bring about the current misery.[12] Just at a time when social conditions undermined the authority and prestige of fatherhood, our therapeutic emphasis has encouraged, first in individual patients, but eventually as a social mass phenomenon, a withdrawal from the urgent but frightening problems of reality into a narrow preoccupation with the self and its needs and aches, into a fascination with the complexities of the unconscious and a retreat from real trouble into mysticism, drug intoxication, and the whole trashbag of all the world's superstitions. Psychology has opened the door to the psychic, ego psychology has led to egocentricity, and among the popularizers,[13] to unabashed advocacy of the most limited selfishness. Finally, the authors doubt not but that the consistent derogation of the superego as harsh, cruel, and oppressive has filtered down to the public as a derogation of conscience, has helped to convert guilt into nothing but guilt feelings, and responsibility into supposedly neurotic feelings of obligation.

But if it is tragic that we have inadvertently contributed to a further loosening of a social fabric already weakened by social change,[14] then there is in it on the other hand the hopeful suggestion that, where we were effectively destructive, we just possibly could be constructive with equal effectiveness. In order to achieve this we must, of course, not just describe what *is* happening—we must find the courage to commit ourselves to what we think *should* be happening. And so, with regard to our particular topic, the question becomes: What *should* be the coming role of males in society?

The authors have already gone out on that limb. Since the beginning of human time, if we go by the oldest records extant, men have been inspired by hero models, have striven to be heroes themselves, and in this pursuit have felt manly and good. Nor do we have to go all that far back. During the very same years which saw the origins of the "me-generation"[15] and its current efflorescence into a "poor-me-generation," history also provided some shining hours. There were many instances of true heroism in recent wars, and there were many instances of true heroism among the war resisters. There were silent heroes of the war on poverty and lonely heroes in the Peace Corps. And of course there were, and still are, heroes, some famous and many more unsung, in the civil rights movement.[16] It seems that, given an occasion, men and women gladly rise to it, and act as heroically as their forebears have ever done. And there seems to be the same old hunger for heroics in our youngsters, even though one could question the credentials of popular figures such as Superman, the characters of "Star Wars" or *The Lord of the Ring*. The good urge is there, but what of the occasion? In what arena can men still strut their stuff?

We are bedeviled here by the circumstance mentioned initially, that women can do anything a man can do, so that it would be hard to find a pursuit in which men only can excel. And yet, that is what it would seem to take to restore to them some of their pride and social function.

The solution, the authors believe, lies in this: That while men and women can be equally heroic, their actions affect them differently. When a man acts like a hero, it makes him feel and look more manly; when a women acts like a heroine, it does not make her more feminine. On the contrary, it shows up what we perceive as a masculine quality in her. Jeanne d'Arc was a heroic female, but she was not exactly feminine. We do not know whether she would ever have become a wife and mother, had she not been burned first. Or let us recall another fighting woman, Brunhilde the Walkyrie, who lived in a circle of flames and not only expected a suitor to penetrate it but, before she would give him a kind word, would require that he best her in armed combat. The moral seems to be that such a strong and combative lady must seek a man even stronger than she so that, through his egregious manliness, he may make even her feel feminine.

Lest this sound a bit fanciful, consider a different sphere of action where the same condition prevails. Intellectual brilliance, too, makes a man more of a man, but a woman of equal brilliance is perceived not as being more womanly, but as formidable in a mannish way. When it comes to finding a mate, such women look for, and apparently need, a man of superior intellect. An attempted union with a lesser man is likely soon to fall apart. Much the same can be said of administrative–executive–political authority: that many a woman is as capable as a man, but the authority is seen to defeminize her, so that in fact the great women politicians of our time entered upon their careers after they had raised their families and, for one reason or another, were without husband. But surely the most common example pertains to the earning of the daily bread. Men can work and hold a job and so can women. But a man must earn money, unless he is devoted to a cause or a creative effort and absolves his obligation to society in that manner. By and large he must earn money in order not to feel and look like a parasite, whereas a woman may very well choose not to earn money without thereby diminishing her femininity by one iota. And again, when a woman does have a job, she is likely to want a mate who earns at least as much as she and preferably more, in order that they shall both feel right about the arrangement.

So there are areas which, while perfectly accessible to women, enhance maleness: Physical strength, intellectual brilliance, financial competence, political leadership; all these make a male more manly. And that women can and do function in the same realms should not make the men feel that they have been relieved and can go off-duty (although this is often the result), but should spur them to that extra margin of performance which both sexes need to feel comfortable with each other.

By the same token, and for the sake of everybody concerned, it is high time that men should make a truly heroic effort to regain some of the importance they have surrendered in their own home. Boys need strong fathers, as mentioned above. Girls need the love of strong fathers to feel lovable as women. And women need husbands they can respect. Therefore a man should stand up and be counted and be counted on, not only on the job. But whenever his understanding and his conscience so dictate, he should stand up to his wife and to his children and to the whole amorphous other-directedness that, by way of the media and his children's friends, threatens to swamp the house.

Such a stand is likely to entail much conflict and aggravation, and together with the uncertainty of having done the right thing, a real fear of having caused harm, so that a man may well feel tempted to shirk the whole business. But in this regard, let the authors recall an episode in the life of that great hero, Ulysses. When on his long and arduous voyage it became inevitable that he would have to sail his ship through a narrow passage between two dreadful dangers, namely the many-headed dragon Scylla on one side and the sucking whirlpool Charybdis on the other, he was advised by Kirke, a sorceress who meant him well, to sail close to the monster rather than risking the vortex.[17] The story is symbolic. The many-headed dragon, Scylla, represents anxiety and fear. The whirlpool sucking down into darkness and death is depression and despair. The arduous voyage is life itself and the ship and its crew the cares and responsibilities to which man is committed. As to Kirke, the wise woman, she counseled Ulysses well, for to cringe before the challenge and to back off from fear means falling victim to depression, means betraying one's charge and risking death, if not of the body, then surely of the spirit.

The authors believe this proposition to be a basic human truth, easily demonstrable in daily life. And it follows that as psychotherapists we must, like Kirke, counsel our patients that rational understanding and emotional expression may be desirable, but never enough. They must, if they are to avoid or to emerge from depression, confront their anxieties, take the risk of making decisions and commitments, and proceed in the face of their fear.[18]

There are some who would think it contrary to our basic credo as therapists to advocate anything. But even Freud, while neutral as to detail, had a basic conviction as to what would be best for his patients. He expressed it in the maxim: "Where id was, there ego shall be." Implied is the more general proposition that any personality growth which is perceived as possible then also becomes a challenge, a categorical imperative that says: Be the best you can be. Psychotherapy must pose this imperative. And as to the changing role of the male, it must demand that he become once more what he very well knows he could be: A hero.

REFERENCES

1. Trilling D: The Liberated Heroine. London Times Literary Supplement, October 13, 1978, pp 1163–1167
2. Wylie P: Generation of Vipers. New York, Rinehart, 1942
3. Lederer W: Dragons, Delinquents and Destiny: An Essay on Positive Superego Functions. Psychological Issues Monograph #15. New York, International Universities Press, 1964
4. Lederer W: Oedipus and the serpent. Psychoanal Rev 51:619–644, 1964–65
5. Lederer W: Historical consequences of father–son hostility. Psychoanal Rev 54:248–276, 1967
6. Freud S: Civilization and its discontents, in Standard Edition of the Works of Sigmund Freud, Vol 21. London, Hogarth Press, 1961, p 115
7. Riesman D: The Lonely Crowd. New Haven, Yale University Press, 1950
8. Kohut H: The Analysis of the Self. New York, International Universities Press, 1971
9. Kernberg O: Borderline Conditions and Pathological Narcissism. New York, Jason Aronson, 1975
10. Lasch C: The Culture of Narcissism. New York, Norton, 1978
11. Mitscherlich A: Society without the Father. New York, Harcourt Brace and World, 1963
12. Erikson EH: Young Man Luther. New York, Norton, 1958
13. Ringer RJ: Looking out for #1. New York, Funk and Wagnalls, 1977
14. Lasch C: Haven in a Heartless World, New York, Basic Books, 1977
15. Wolfe T: The me decade and the third great awakening, in Mauve Gloves and Madmen, Edited by Clutter and Vine. Toronto, Bantam Books, 1976, pp 111–150
16. Beardslee WR: The Way Out Must Lead In: Life Histories in the Civil Rights Movement. Atlanta, Emory University, 1977
17. Homer: The Odyssey, XII, v. 73–110
18. Wheelis A: How People Change. New York, Harper and Row, 1973

Chapter 13

Individual Psychotherapy and Changing Masculine Roles

Dimensions of Gender-Role Psychotherapy

KENNETH SOLOMON

INTRODUCTION

The Feminist Movement has led women to question traditional feminine roles in all areas of life, including marriage, family, career, relationships, and sexuality. These questions have led to discomfort and conflict for many women, usually associated with the crisis affects of anxiety, fear, confusion, and sadness, and their symptomatic counterparts. The discomfort of those women seeking professional help frequently cannot be assuaged by traditional psychotherapeutic approaches. Nor can they frequently be worked out by less traditional therapies, including Gestalt therapy, Transactional Analysis, and those psychotherapeutic approaches that have evolved from the Human Potential and Humanistic Psychology movements. Consciousness-raising and women's support groups have been beneficial for some women, but have limited value for others.

Some women therapists, aware of the limitations of these modalities for working with feminist issues, have begun to develop new therapeutic techniques. As described by Wolman,[1] this therapeutic approach, known as feminist therapy, has its own set of expectations, goals, and techniques and builds upon more traditional psychotherapies while focusing on societal and gender role issues specific for women. These include an examination of the sociocultural antecedents of the feminine role, an egalitarian change in the hierarchical structure of the therapist–client relationship, and the explicit understanding that feminist and other gender-role issues are a primary focus of the therapeutic contract.

As women have changed, men have been forced to respond to these changes. For example, men professionals suddenly find themselves being su-

---

KENNETH SOLOMON • Levindale Hebrew Geriatric Center and Hospital, Baltimore, Maryland 21215

pervised by women. Other men find themselves adapting or failing to adapt to a growing spouse. Or a salesman may discover that "one of the boys" at dinner is a woman, necessitating sudden changes in behavior. As noted by Gould (Chapter 7 in this book) and Moulton, [2,3] women's sexuality has ramifications for the traditional sexuality of men.

Most men have variably adapted to these changed role expectations and new demands on themselves. For some men, the behaviors that constitute male chauvinism have become more intensified. Other men have become more emotionally unresponsive to women or have found themselves unable to respond to women because of a lack of adequate responses in their behavioral repertoire. Other men have come face-to-face with their inexpressiveness, overemphasis on rational problem solving, or competitiveness.

Many men do not want to change traditional gender-role behaviors and would prefer a return to the "good old days" of *kinder, kirche,* and *küche*. They see this as the only appropriate place for women in American society. Other men want to change some of their traditional masculine role behaviors because they feel an obligation to their wife, their girlfriend, or to society. These men believe that specific changes in themselves would be a means of diminishing the intergenderal conflicts they perceive to be swirling, maelstromlike, around them. A third group of men choose change because they feel they have been able to identify many of the negative and positive aspects of the traditional masculine role and are seeking these changes for their own personal growth. Some of these men are motivated by hostility toward women and see themselves as oppressed. Others are motivated by what they perceive to be the advantages of androgyny, both for themselves and for significant other persons in their lives.

Many authors have noted the need to be aware of gender-role issues in clients seeking individual,[1,2,4–17] group,[9,18–23] and marital or family[9,24] therapy. In the context of individual psychotherapy with men, a few authors have noted specific clinical issues within the client;[5,9,16,17] these will be elaborated upon in several sections of this chapter. They have begun to address these as clinical issues because of increasing evidence of gender-role strain and conflict in men requesting psychotherapy coupled with an awareness of the many negative effects of the traditional masculine role on the physical[25–27] and mental health of men[28,29] (Chapter 2 by Solomon; Chapter 1 by O'Neil).

As had happened with women and issues related to feminine gender roles, traditional psychotherapeutic approaches have been found to be lacking in their capabilities for working with men faced with gender-role issues. While traditional psychotherapies and appropriate pharmacotherapy are frequently helpful with some of the more classical neurotic or psychotic symptoms that some of these men also demonstrate, certain of these specific issues have necessitated the development of new psychotherapeutic techniques and the modification of others. It is the collection of these techniques and a specific conceptual approach to psychotherapy that the author calls gender-role psychotherapy.

In this chapter, the author will discuss these techniques and adaptations of individual psychotherapy that he has developed from working with men with problems related to masculine gender roles. He will also discuss special transference and countertransference issues that emerge in psychotherapy with men. Other chapters in this book will discuss behavioral techniques (Chapter 16, by Dosser, Chapter 15, by Goldfried and Friedman), and group psychotherapeutic techniques (Chapter 14, by Stein) that have also been evolving over the last several years. A chapter from the vantage point of a woman therapist will discuss similar issues (Chapter 17, by Bernardez).

GENDER-ROLE PSYCHOTHERAPY DEFINED

Gender-role psychotherapy has its roots in psychoanalytic psychotherapy and utilizes psychoanalytic theory and techniques as its nucleus. In addition, conceptual and technical changes are derived from other forms of psychotherapy, especially Gestalt therapy, Transactional Analysis, radical therapy, client-centered therapy, humanistic psychology, and existential psychotherapy. Major modifications are also derived from feminist therapy.

There are several major conceptual changes that differentiate gender-role psychotherapy from other forms of individual psychotherapy. The most major change is that masculine gender-role issues are explicitly agreed upon as a major focus of therapy. This agreement is an inherent part of the therapeutic contract and leads to other conceptual and technical modifications of traditional psychotherapy.

The therapist conceptualizes masculine behavior in an integrated way, seeking to interdigitate multiple biologic, psychologic, and sociologic inputs into behavior. However, he/she emphasizes the sociocultural inputs and social learning as major epigenetic dimensions in the development of masculine role behavior. Furthermore, the therapist is acutely aware of the sexism in American society and how men contribute to and are affected by it.

In addition, the therapist is sensitive to issues of competition, inexpressiveness, intellectualization, power "games," and homophobia, both within the therapeutic setting and in society at large. There is a heightened awareness of dependency, intimacy, control, and sexual needs of the client. In addition, the therapist is aware of the potential for antifeminism that might develop so as to work with that problem in a therapeutic way.

Technically, the therapist–client relationship is more egalitarian than in traditional psychotherapy. The client is responsible for defining the goals of psychotherapy with the therapist's help. The therapist may serve as a role model for the man client and may share personal experiences to do so. The therapist must be more active in expressing his/her affect within therapeutic sessions. The therapist must also relate to the client in a nurturing, affectively caring way.

Finally, more consistent with humanistic therapies, the bulk of therapeutic work is done in the here and now. Although reference is made to past experiences, including those from childhood, gender-role psychotherapy focuses on the interactions within the therapeutic relationship and in the client's immediate past and future. The major exception to this occurs during examination of the client's relationship with his father.

The primary goal of gender-role psychotherapy is to move the client's role functioning in the direction of psychological and behavioral androgyny. Androgyny is the integration of positive aspects of both masculine and feminine roles within the person's ego so that he/she can flexibly call upon a wide behavioral, affective, and cognitive repertoire to respond as any situation demands. Androgyny represents an important aspect of conflict-free ego functioning, and gives the person the psychological tools necessary to satisfy needs for self-actualization. Several authors[30–34] (Chapter 4, by Boles and Tatro) have noted that androgyny is associated with flexibility, adaptability, ego strength, self-esteem, and problem-solving skills in men and women. Thus, helping the client move into a more androgynous mode of functioning will lead not only to symptom relief, but to personal growth, the ability to handle future changes, and to function alloplastically as he/she ages.

INDICATIONS

As with any intervention of a medical or psychologic nature, the specific intervention must be tailored to the specific problem. Indications and contraindications (relative and absolute) for any intervention must be clearly defined. Thus, like other forms of psychotherapy, it is necessary to delineate the indications for gender-role psychotherapy.

Gender-role psychotherapy may be utilized as the sole therapeutic modality or as an adjunct to other forms of psychotherapy or pharmacotherapy. For the man who enters therapy with specific gender-role problems or issues and who does not manifest psychopathology, a brief psychotherapy of this type may suffice. For a man is interested in personal growth and understanding regarding gender-role issues, a more extensive gender-role psychotherapy would be indicated.

However, some men enter therapy because of neurotic or psychotic problems or because of manifestations of a personality disorder. The classical neurotic and psychotic symptomatology is handled psychotherapeutically in traditional ways. When gender-role issues arise in these therapeutic situations, the techniques of gender-role psychotherapy are important adjuncts to the main psychotherapeutic activities. For example, a man with an underlying compulsive character structure requested therapy. He wanted to change his personality structure because of the overwhelming anxiety it engendered. In therapy, it was also discovered that he found himself unable to relate to some of the role changes his wife was developing. Techniques of psychoanalytic psychotherapy were necessary to uncover and work through issues of unresolved hostility, control, and dependency that were major psychodynamic roots of his underlying character structure. However, it took different therapeutic techniques for the man to understand the changes in his wife and to develop a behavioral repertoire necessary to allow him appropriate and mutually satisfactory interactions between him and his spouse.

The therapeutic techniques of gender-role psychotherapy are indicated for any man facing gender-role issues. The techniques to be described may be used with schizophrenic, neurotic, or relatively intact individuals who are dealing with issues specifically related to masculine gender roles. These gender-role issues include the effects of the affective, cognitive, and behavioral components of the traditional masculine role on the man. They also include any conflicts and strains within this role or caused by adherence or change in the role. These role conflicts may either contribute to or result from the client's presenting symptomatology. These techniques may be integrated into the process of psychoanalytic psychotherapy or other psychotherapies, as they are intended to allow the therapist to work with these specific gender-role issues and not to modify underlying pathological character structures or neurotic or psychotic symptomatology.

THERAPEUTIC ISSUES

There are three groups of men who are apt to complain about gender-role conflicts and strains and who request therapy for these conflicts and their sequelae. One group is comprised of those men who complain about changing roles but who do not want to change. They are the unchanging men in a changing world. The other two groups of men are changing men in a changing world. One group consists of those men who have been forced to change in order to maintain work, marital, or sexual relationships. The other group consists of those men who choose to change role behaviors for political/social reasons or their own personal growth and self-actualization.

The unchanging men in a changing world are upset about the changes in roles of men and women in American society and are having great difficulty adapting to these changes. They consider these changes wrong, perhaps even sacrilegious or immoral. Many are openly contemptuous of "libbers" and see changing roles as a threat to the family, and even the fabric of society itself. These men frequently demonstrate many of the behavioral characteristics of male chauvinism, although these men are not necessarily "macho," John Wayne–Charles Bronson–Clint Eastwood types of individuals. An example is a 54-year-old minister who requested therapy because he was upset about his wife's autonomy following her graduation from social work school and her beginning a new job. This man had not adopted many traditional masculine role behaviors. For example, he was a relatively passive individual who was quite sensitive and caring and was able to express positive and negative emotions freely in the company of both men and women with whom he was intimate. However, he had been inculcated with many traditional masculine values and beliefs about the appropriate roles of men and women in American society and was unable to change these values when faced with changes in his own marriage.

Many of these unchanging men in the changing world complain of anxiety, depression, anger, and sense that they are not in touch with the world around them, all in relation to gender-role conflict and strain. Most of these men are already in therapy for other reasons, such as a personality disorder or a schizophrenic process. This group of men, because of major difficulties in ego functioning, frequently exaggerate many characteristics of the traditional masculine role. It affords them clear ego boundaries and structure and allows them to develop a sense of identity, a consistent interpersonal behavioral repertoire, and the *ur*-delusion that there is an order in the world. These are necessary for maximal ego functioning in these individuals. These men function relatively poorly in most areas of life, including work, interpersonal relationships, and cognitive functioning. The issues of masculine gender roles that they present in therapy are frequently secondary to major intrapsychic and interpersonal conflicts and develop from the same psychodynamic roots. These clients usually require multiple modalities of intervention.

Another group of men also enter therapy with similar symptoms: anger, depression, anxiety, and a sense of being adrift in the world. These men, whom Woods[35] considers to be the true "male chauvinists," have adopted the behaviors and values of the traditional masculine role to an extreme. These men are psychologically and physically aggressive, are work- and success-oriented, are relatively inexpressive, and place a heavy emphasis on rational problem solving. These men have a rigid set of values in which they feel that everyone and everything has its appropriate place in life; these values are particularly resistant to change. This group of men frequently have a submerged but pervasive sense of hostility toward a world they cannot trust. In addition to a suspicious cognitive style, they also cannot trust the world because it is changing in spite of their attempts to control their external environment.

Although these men do not fit the diagnostic criteria for any particular personality disorder, they have many of the behavioral and dynamic characteristics that are essential components of the personalities of obsessive–compulsive, paranoid, antisocial, and passive–aggressive individuals. Although their behavior is frequently impulsive, their cognitive styles are extremely future-oriented and they frequently seem to be living for and in the future. They treat women with "respect," "dignity," and "deference," as long as women respond in a traditional way. These men place an emphasis on external manifestations of traditional intergenderal role behaviors, such as opening doors for women, taking off their hats in the presence of women, or standing up when a woman comes into the room. Intellectually, they may see nothing wrong with women working, but they strongly feel that women should not work instead of bringing up children. They also believe that women should not hold jobs that might diminish the status of their husbands. These men frequently believe that the man should be the primary, if not sole breadwinner for the family, even in times of crisis,[36] and frequently prefer to work at a second job rather than have their wives go out and work. Many of these men frequently meet the criteria of the type A personality[37] and frequently do not enter therapy until they have developed a major physical problem, such as a myocardial infarction or peptic ulcer.

Woods[35] has identified four major areas of intrapsychic difficulty for these men. These are unresolved infantile strivings and regressive wishes, hostile envy of women, Oedipal anxiety, and power and dependency conflicts related to their self-esteem. It should be noted that these are important psychodynamics issues for all men. These conflicts permeate the psychological development of boys and their lack of resolution is reinforced by societally derived behaviors that allow men to repress, deny, or "sublimate" these conflicts in their interactions with women. This is discussed in more detail in Chapter 2, by Solomon.

The Oedipal anxiety frequently manifests itself in a "Madonna–prostitute" complex. By using the primitive defense of splitting, men can idealize women as either "all good" or "all bad." Women are believed to be pure and good and are placed on a pedestal and treated with a deference that should be accorded an archetypal mother. Seeing women, especially women with whom the man is close, in such a positive light dilutes the Oedipal anxiety because the man can then minimize sexual strivings towards the women who now substitute for mother. Sexual impulses toward these women may be sublimated by making them mothers. Other women to whom he feels attracted are seen as entirely bad so that he may project his guilt and libidinal impulses onto an unconscious remnant of mother toward whom he felt attracted. Having a woman like mother, but who is not mother, diminishes the anxiety of competition with the father. Thus, these women can become sexual playthings, and not related to as human beings. These defensive maneuvers only work as long as the gender-role situation remains rigid and stereotyped. Compulsive defenses may be adopted to control the environment to assure this situation as well as to contain guilt and hostility.

The hostile envy of women (which the early feminists clearly identified) maintains itself by an attempt to keep women "in their place." Men rationalize this situation by seeing the women's place as having many advantages. For example, women do not have the pressures of the day-to-day world of work. They have the joys of nurturing children. They gain freedom from many worries by not being financially responsible for the household. They are allowed to be expressive. However, the feminine role is structured is such a way that a traditional woman must be dependent on the man; this is a manifestation of the unconscious hostility toward women men experience. Many of the behaviors which are superficially polite and respectful are subtle messages that tell the woman that she is inferior, incompetent, weak, and a second-class citizen.

The third set of dynamic conflicts are those about power and dependency. Adler[38] felt that men have a will to and a wish for power to minimize their fears, vulnerability, and dependency, especially dependency on women. This not only helps dissipate some of the unresolved Oedipal anxiety by minimizing dependency upon "mother," but it also allows the man to deny that he may need women. This, in turn, bolsters his self-esteem and sense of invulnerability. Power not only diminishes dependency but may also be used to keep women "in their place." Thus, it is used to allow the hostility of women that these men experience to become behaviorally manifest. By keeping roles rigid, regressive wishes of infantile dependency and nurturance can then be satisfied in a way that is highly structured and disguised, allowing a man a means of maintaining his self-esteem while gratifying infantile needs.

A 38-year-old man was referred for psychiatric evaluation by the court. He had a long record of recurrent arrests and prison terms for assault, armed robbery, passing bad checks, selling drugs, and parole violations. He saw physical fighting or competitive interpersonal manipulations as his only means of problem solving. He frequently beat his wife, sisters, mother, and other female relatives and in-laws. "I take out my inadequacies on them," he said. He viewed women as irrational, overemotional, dependent "things" who needed the protection, guidance, and direction of a strong man. He became violent with women whenever he became aware of his dependency needs, to which he responded by exerting power. He developed severe tension headaches whenever he expressed emotions other than anger. His life goal was to "never become vulnerable, especially with a woman." He hated women and manipulated them for whatever he could gain, including housekeeping chores, sex on demand, and money (his wife worked as a prostitute at his insistence). Many of his men "friends" looked up to him as a role model and tried to emulate his behavior, reinforcing his sense of power and control of others. As this example shows, the male chauvinist takes many of the characteristics of the traditional masculine role and exaggerates and adapts them to serve as culturally syntonic as well as ego-syntonic defenses against these underlying unresolved dynamic issues.

If the individual is also schizophrenic, many of these underlying issues are even more intense, frequently leading to the adoption of this male chauvinist stance in an extremely rigid way. According to Searles,[39] many schizophrenics have difficulty resolving or accepting their unresolved dependency needs. When dependency needs are intense and society dictates that the man deny these needs, the seeds of major conflicts are sown. If in the context of other infantile psychodynamic difficulties, double-bind communication, the tenuous ego development of the so-called schizophrenogenic mother, biologic and/or genetic defects, or any combination of the many factors that have been hypothesized to lead to the development of schizophrenia, the issues of unresolved dependency and unresolved infantile wishes may be exacerbated and may be "resolved" by the development of highly rigid, stereotyped, "macho" chauvinistic behavior.

Furthermore, the child who has been unable to master the first two periods of psychosexual and psychosocial development is thrown into a complex and confusing Oedipal situation, not unlike some of the family situations described by Lidz and his co-workers,[40,41] and forced to work through issues for which he is psychologically unprepared. This may lead to a dramatic rise in the normal Oedipal anxiety that is seen in children, which may then remain unresolved. Denial of this conflict is aided by the development of a need for power, as well as chauvinistic behavior. When one complicates this dynamic with problems such as concreteness, difficulty with attention, poor object relations, a diffuse identity, and the presence of psychotic symptoms, the issue of masculine roles becomes both extremely difficult for the patient to handle as well as a major crisis that must be worked with in order to move ahead with other therapeutic work.

To complicate therapeutic work further, schizophrenic patients are particularly prone to have difficulty in defining their own needs and desires and separating these from those of society and their families. Identity and role behaviors and expectations are frequently and mistakenly merged. In this context, further diffusion of ego boundaries may then cause anxiety, depression, and very frequently, an exacerbation of psychotic symptomatology, although the person may be maintained on an adequate dose of antipsychotic medication. In addition, the adherence to very rigid, stereotypic, chauvinistic behavior helps the patient create a clear identity and ego boundaries for himself and thus helps ward off the development of confusion, anxiety, and psychosis. However, this is done at the expense of limiting his adaptive and coping potential and putting himself in many situations which he is unable to resolve because he is either unaware or unwilling to admit the other side, the "feminine" side, of his personality.

Men who are not so rigidly chauvinistic may enter therapy with similar presenting complaints of anxiety, depression, and existential conflict, because of more specific problems in their relationships with changing women. Some of these men have been described by Halle[42] (Chapter 9 in this book), who discussed her work with men whose wives have left them. These men want reassurances that their value systems or behaviors are "OK." They frequently request guidance so that they can treat women the way women want to be treated. At the same time, they want to maintain their own chauvinistic value system and behavioral repertoire. They want to change some of their behavior, but only specific behaviors at specific times, in specific situations. There is a large element of manipulation in this therapeutic request, as they aim to get what they want from women without having to give up any part of what they perceive to be their masculinity. They want to learn how to play a new "game" and not make any significant change in their own role behavior or self-concept. Many of these men come to therapy with a sense of confusion regarding women. They frequently paraphrase Freud's legendary remark: "My God, what do women want?" These men find it extremely uncomfortable when women challenge many of their traditional behaviors. They have difficulty working with women who may be in conventional masculine work roles. They also have difficulty relating to sexually assertive women. A slightly less chauvinistic group of men want reassurances that although they are changing their outward behaviors, their traditional masculine values are still appropriate.

Another group of unchanging men are those men whose major complaints relate to sexuality. They are uncomfortable with sexually assertive women or feel that women are placing excessive demands upon their performance. They cannot accept women who demand sexual behaviors that maximize sensuality rather than genital performance. They believe in the "double standard" of sexuality and feel that sex is a man's prerogative. Even most men in sexually liberated lifestyles, such as swinging, maintain the sexual double standard and are threatened by women asserting their sexuality. These men tend to present with a mixture of the various affects and symptoms noted for the other men noted above. They also frequently request reassurance from the therapist that women are wrong and that the masculine sexual value system and behavioral system is the appropriate one.

Another group of men present with the problem of inexpressiveness. They do not perceive that they are inexpressive, but come to therapy because of secondary manifestations of it, such as depression, psychophysiologic disorders, or a physical disorder such as hypertension or peptic ulcer disease. Another consequence of inexpressiveness that frequently leads to therapy is the inability to express anger and hostility until it becomes explosive. These men are unable to share many of their frustrations with others. Nor are they able to identify the psychological or somatic concomitants of various negative affects until they become so intense that the person explodes, frequently with physical aggression toward another individual.

A 63-year-old man came to therapy with a severe depression. In part, his depressive symptomatology related to an inability to grieve over the loss of his first wife who had died six years previously. At that time, he was unable to cry or express any outward manifestations of grief, anger, guilt, or ambivalence over the loss of a love object. These feelings remained repressed until he remarried. Following the first anniversary of his first wife's death that occurred after his remarriage, these feelings came into consciousness. These affects overwhelmed him and led to the development of a severe depressive episode.

A 38-year-old laborer could not express feelings of anger at his boss or frustration with what he perceived to be a lack of success in his life. He periodically would strike his wife at the slightest provocation, although he was perplexed and guilty over this behavior. When he learned to verbalize the underlying feelings that he displaced onto his wife, his physical abuse of her finally stopped.

Another type of unchanging man who seeks out therapy is the overrational man. This man puts a premium on rational problem solving for all of life's difficulties and is unable to comprehend or relate to the affective distress of others. These men are frequently plagued with doubt, since they see all possible consequences for any particular action. They are able to identify many important reasons for one decision and many other and equally important reasons for the opposite decision. Thus, their cognitive style is similar to the obsessive–compulsive style described by Shapiro.[43] These men frequently seek therapy because of ineffectiveness in the workplace, especially if they have a management position, because of the effects of this doubt. Because of their commitment to being rational, they are unable to relate with other individuals on an affective level; they may also seek out psychotherapeutic intervention for this problem.

The second group of men who seek therapy are those men who feel that they are being forced to change because of a changing world. These men externalize their reasons for therapy to resolve ambivalence about entering therapy. The manifest reason for requesting therapy is their subjective discomfort caused by difficulties adapting to the changing individuals and situations around them. They seek out new ways of relating and behaving, not for personal growth, but to gain symptom relief. The motivation for some of these men includes seeking support from a nurturing individual or ventilation of anger. Many of these men present with secondary interpersonal or marital conflicts, sexual dysfunctions, or work concerns. Halle[42] (Chapter 9 in this book) has identified some of these men who seek therapy after their wives leave them. It is interesting to note that none of the men that Halle discusses had any desire to actually make any major change in their role behaviors, self-concepts, or value systems. These men have conflicts and dynamics similar to those of the men in the first group, but they are not as severe, so that some motivation for therapeutic change is apparent. Whereas the first group of men seek therapy with the intention not to change masculine role behaviors, this group of men want to change only specific masculine role behaviors to ease their own subjective discomfort.

The third group of men are the men who choose to change. One subgroup of these men are men who frequently verbalize a personal and societal responsibility to further the role changes in women. These men, however, frequently have no intrinsic desire to change. Their manifest motivation seems to be purely altruistic, and solely what they perceive to be for the good of women. These women are not only specific women in their lives, such as wives or children, but may be women in general. These men seek help in changing many external role behaviors. For example, many want to learn child-care skills. Others seek support in making a decision to diminish their work hours so that they can be at home with their wife or children. They may seek permission to allow their wives to return to school or pursue a career. They want to be comfortable with their wives' newly developed autonomy or to learn to be more sensual in the bedroom.

These men do not, however, request changes in other aspects of the masculine role. For example, they do not seek to develop skills that allow intimacy with other men. Nor do they seek to change their rational cognitive mode. Nor do they seek to integrate the external behavioral change into their self-concept of themselves as men. Indeed, upon deeper examination, many of these men harbor a deep hostility and envy of women. What is manifested as altruism is an attempt to work through the envy of the feminine role by adopting the outward trappings of the role. These men frequently express hostility toward women with complaints of being "oppressed" by women. They seek to neutralize this hostility by becoming "feminine" in outward behavior. What are complaints of not being allowed the feminine role can be accompanied by identification with the perceived aggressor and adoption of the traditional feminine role. These men display their feminine roles in a competitive way, much to the envy of other men. This is another identification, for other men respond to these men with the same chauvinist dynamic that motivates this group of men to change.

These men usually request short-term therapy and are rarely symptomatic. They request help with solving a specific problem. However, if they remain in therapy once the task is accomplished, they frequently identify and work with other aspects of the masculine role that negatively affect their lives. From that point, psychotherapy of the psychodynamics of chauvinism become feasible.

The other subgroup of this group of men are those men who are motivated by self-actualization needs. These are men who have identified problems, conflicts, and strains in the traditional masculine role, its relationship to their selves and their needs. On the surface, the desired changes in behavior seem to be the same as the previously mentioned group. For example, they may seek support in taking on new child-care responsibilities. However, they are not taking on child-care responsibilities primarily so that their wives can return to work or school or because of an underlying chauvinistic dynamic, but because they want to relate more intimately with their own children. These are men who have identified masculine issues such as dependency, intimacy, and inexpressiveness, as issues that inhibit their own personal growth. These men are actively attempting to redefine their values and behaviors as well as their inner sense of what it means to be a man.

The conflicts and psychodynamic issues dealt with in the context of gender-role psychotherapy are as varied as the individuals seeking therapy. Many of these conflicts are those delineated by Woods[35] and noted above, but are less intense in those individuals who are less severely disturbed. As the individual is more self-motivated for therapeutic growth, the issues worked on in therapy more frequently relate to those particular problems that are part of the negative core of the masculine role, as identified by David and Brannon[44] and in Chapter 2 by Solomon. These will be briefly discussed below.

One major issue that arises in therapy with men is dependency and fears of dependency. As men become aware of their dependency needs they may become anxious about these needs, for these directly challenge their belief that they should be able to "go it alone" ("The Sturdy Oak"). Dependency is also a "feminine" trait, traits which men actively avoid. Thus, men attempt to deny or repress these dependency needs. They may adopt various behaviors, such as an increase in risk-taking or competitive behaviors, to deny dependency needs. Dependency needs are frequently denied within intimate relationships and inhibit the development of intimacy with important persons in the individual's life. As these dependency needs are also manifestations of unresolved pre-Oedipal infantile needs to be emotionally and physically nurtured, men may manipulate others, usually women, to subtly meet these needs. A 69-year-old self-made millionaire and fiercely competitive businessman let his wife choose his daily wardrobe, schedule his social life, and manage household financial affairs because he was "too busy" to pay attention to these "picayune details of life." He became extremely anxious when faced with the necessity of handling these tasks during his wife's extended convalescence from major surgery.

Closely associated with dependency issues are fears of vulnerability. It is particularly difficult for a man to come face to face with his lack of omnipotence. The American man's belief in his omnipotence is so strong that it functions as an *ur*-delusion. Any threat to this omnipotence is a source of anxiety to the man, frequently resulting in panic. Indeed, the act of entering therapy, which is in itself an expression of emotional vulnerability, may be so anxiety-provoking for the man (by challenging his omnipotence) that he may be unwilling to stay in therapy and may drop out after very few sessions.[45] A 55-year-old marathon runner became moderately depressed following a broken ankle. He feared that his body was now weakened and could be unpredictably attacked by aging and disease, which would make him less masculine. He counterphobically began to run before his ankle completely healed, leading to further damage, surgery, a total withdrawal from competitive running, and a severe depressive episode requiring psychiatric hospitalization.

Ambivalence about intimacy with others is another important conflict of men who are seen in psychotherapy. Men tend to seek out intimacy with women but do not know how to be intimate. They fear this intimacy, for they fear engulfment by the psyche and soul of another. Men are frequently unable to separate intimacy needs from sexual needs. They may misidentify sexual impulses as desires for intimacy or vice versa. Sexual relating is also less risky for the ego than relating intimately to another person for sexual behaviors do not require vulnerability through communicating openly to others. A 33-year-old single man consciously sought out a sex partner whenever he felt the need to be close to a woman. When asked why, he replied, "If I told a woman that all I wanted was a hug, she'd think I was either crazy, impotent, or a fag."

The desires for intimacy with other men are also ambivalent. In part, they are due to the individual's identification with a societally defined homophobia. This homophobia can block attempts at intimacy in homosexual as well as heterosexual men, for each has grown up with the same societal prohibitions. The issue of intimacy also has its Oedipal and pre-Oedipal roots in the person's relationship with his own parents, particularly his father. Most men have not had intimate relationships with their fathers because their fathers have been as programmed with the traditional masculine role as have the sons. The time most boys spend with their fathers has traditionally involved activities such as sports and active hobbies, and has not involved the sharing of intimate feelings and experiences. Very few men have seen their fathers cry or experience anxiety and thus have not been able to experience the emotional intimacy with men in their childhood that could serve as a model for intimacy with men in adulthood. A poignant example of this is the relationship between father and son in the play *I Never Sang for My Father*.[46]

A fourth issue frequently worked with in therapy with men is loneliness. This is more existential rather than classically psychodynamic, and is related to the three previously discussed problems. The avoidance of loneliness may be a major drive in the interpersonal life of all people,[47] but men create their own loneliness because of barriers they erect in their interpersonal relationships. In part, these barriers evolve from the difficulty men have in expressiveness and intimacy with others. Many men have identified and are variably comfortable with "unmasculine" needs. Yet, because of masculine role socialization, they are unable to share these needs with women for fear that they will be seen as "unmasculine." The outward manifestations of the masculine role then become overvalued at the expense of the man's inner psychological state, because of the socialized need of men to preserve external appearances at all costs. However, men also cannot share these feelings with other men because of homophobia, and this same need to maintain the outward trappings of the masculine role, the lack of role models, and the absence of anything in a man's behavioral repertoire that would allow the sharing of feelings with other men. A 49-year-old professional man was having many questions about what he wanted from his career. He also was having difficulties in his relationship with his wife. He would frequently call men friends to arrange time to share some of his concerns. But when he met with his friends, their talk was frequently about football, politics, or technical issues related to his work. He finally admitted that he did not know how to talk with other men about the things that really bothered him.

Men's sexuality is another frequent concern that is discussed in psychotherapy. Performance needs and fears are often expressed. Fears of demands by women and anger at women's sexuality are discussed and may be used as a defense against an examination of the man's own sexuality. Confusion of sexuality and intimacy, as noted above, is also a common problem. Ambivalent desires about becoming more sensual may be expressed. Fears of impotence may be expressed by the man as a belief that he is homosexual. Therapeutic roadblocks may occur as men in therapy are also unwilling to express feelings of being "turned-on" by specific women (including the therapist). Sex is frequently discussed in a sexist "locker room" way or in a very intellectualized manner. The client may attempt to conceal any evidence of sexual ignorance or lack of sexual experience for fear that the therapist may see him as less of a man. A 22-year-old man occasionally spoke vaguely of his previous sexual experiences. Only in the third year of therapy did the therapist find out that his client was a virgin.

Aggression may be another common issue worked on during therapy. The expression of anger is one of the few affects allowed to men. Yet, it is the expression of anger that is frequently a source of interpersonal and societal discomfort and may lead to the man's entering therapy. This is because the expression of anger is usually active and behavioral, rather than verbal, causing discomfort in the client and in others. The client may enter therapy to learn how to express anger in a verbal, more interpersonally appropriate, and less destructive way.

Inexpressiveness is another problem that is faced in psychotherapy with men. The inability to express affect and the need to concentrate on rational, cognitive data and modes of functioning may lead to an emphasis on the cognitive aspects of psychotherapy by the client. Rationalization and intellectualization may be the most common defenses used by men in psychotherapy. The client may attempt to deal with affective issues in a cognitive way and defuse the affect. He may be particularly resistant to the expression of affect in his therapy sessions, especially if they are negative affects such as weakness, fear, and sadness. When expressing affect, it is frequently verbalized but with the physical concomitants of the affect absent.

The man may be resistant to changing many aspects of the masculine role because of his fear of feminization. An attack on the masculine role may be viewed as an attack on his own masculinity, rather than a need to change that which is a cause of subjective discomfort. Even the man who is highly motivated to change masculine role behaviors may be reluctant to adopt certain behaviors as an alternative because of his fear of being labeled as feminine, or worse, homosexual.

A final issue that must be continuously faced in gender-role psychotherapy is the response of the client's environment to the changes in his behavior. Grant[48] has noted that for a Colorado rancher, although the macho role may have negative marital consequences, a change to more androgynous role functioning may be equally or more devastating to the man's interpersonal and business relationships. When helping a man change his masculine role behaviors, it must be kept in mind that many of these behaviors are not sanctioned by other men or by society and the man will have to face much discomfort in his interpersonal relationships and with the rest of society. For example, an employer may not take kindly to a man reducing his hours so he can participate in child care. Or a man who seeks intimacy, rather than just sex, with women will no longer find that in a singles bar but may not know of other options to meet women. Spouses, parents, peers, and children may be variably supportive of these changes as they will require and necessitate changes in their own ego-syntonic gender-role behaviors that may also be extremely threatening. In summary, the man becomes deviant and others respond to him in accordance to that role.

TECHNICAL NOTES

As noted earlier in this chapter, the technical framework used in changing masculine role behavior is that based on principles of psychoanalytic psychotherapy, with modifications. This technical framework includes the judicious use of questioning and defining[49] as well as clarification, exploration, and interpretation.[50]

Modifications are necessary, however, because much of the process of psychoanalytic psychotherapy is consistent with maintenance of the traditional masculine role. The cognitive emphasis of psychoanalytic psychotherapy needs techniques for the expression of affect to supplement it. Actively supportive techniques are necessary for the client to have a role model who can be utilized as a sounding board for new behaviors. The sociocultural orientation of much of the technical interventions is supportive, as it links the client with other men and allows for a more comprehensive understanding of individual behavior than does a psychodynamic approach alone.

Questioning is a therapeutic technique that is frequently underutilized in psychoanalytic psychotherapy. An exception to this reluctance should be made when working with masculine roles. Questioning is a precursor of clarification and is particularly useful in helping the man define how he sees the masculine role and its alternatives. Questioning allows the client to examine his own concept of himself as a man. Questions may be used to help the man identify what he sees as the consequences of his changed behavior and to identify examples of behavioral change and consequences within his own life and in the lives of other men he may know. These may serve as both positive and negative examples of various behaviors that he may want to consider. It may also help him clarify his goals for therapy, increasing the chance of collaboration and cooperation and equalizing the therapeutic relationship.

Clarification may be used for feedback of the client's affective responses. As many men are unaware of their affective responses in psychotherapy, both clarification and questioning may be utilized to help the person identify how he is responding. The therapist verbalizes and labels the affect the client is experiencing, but does so as a question, to allow the client the opportunity to integrate the cognitive and affective states. Another clarifying technique, derived from Gestalt therapy, is to have the man express what a body part is doing. This may then be utilized to help him identify his underlying affective state.[51] Clarification and a paraphrased repetition of what the client has said may also help change the conceptual framework of therapy from an individual to a sociocultural one that sets the stage for explanation and interpretation.

Explanation is the educative function of psychotherapy. Many men have not thought about the psychological or societal evolution of their gender-role behavior. Explanations in gender-role psychotherapy should be within a cultural framework. The therapist should explain the nature of specific aspects of the masculine gender role that are disturbing to the client, the positive and negative effects of the masculine role on men in general, and the societal development of these roles. Explanations should be utilized to further develop a sociocultural framework for interpretation. They should always be timed so that the explanations are relevant to the specific role behaviors in question and occur after the client has experienced the affect associated with the behaviors and their consequences. This serves to diminish some of the anxiety that the man experiences when dealing with these issues. Explanations can then be expanded to help the individual understand how his own gender-role behavior has developed. Explanation also serves the political analysis dimension of gender-role psychotherapy, through an examination of societal and personal sexism.

Interpretation is the keystone of psychoanalytic psychotherapy. Interpretation is also the most important technique in changing masculine roles. Like explanations, interpretations should be offered within a cultural framework rather than a psychoanalytic framework. Interpretations serve to link the individual and his psychodynamic and behavioral conflicts with the sociocultural framework that has been developed. Interpretations should be used to show the client how he perpetuates his own gender-role behavior and how he uses these behaviors in his relationships with others. It is utilized to help the client see how he is relating to his therapist as a man (or woman), both within the transference relationship and within the real relationship that coexists in therapy. Another area of transference interpretation that should be emphasized is the client's relationships with his own father and male children, and how that has contributed to the development of masculine role behaviors. Interpretations should be timed so that the client may immediately feel the affective impact of the interpretation as well as be able to make cognitive use of it. If an educative framework has been developed and accepted prior to the interpretative process, the interpretation will be comprehended by the client and will be processed in further therapeutic work.

Supportive techniques are an integral part of the psychotherapy of changing masculine roles. As many of the changed behaviors adopted will be new, uncomfortable, and strange to the client and members of his network, it is necessary for the therapist to actively encourage the ventilation of the discomfort the client experiences in adopting these new behaviors. Clear permission-giving by the therapist is necessary to allow for ventilation. It is extremely important for the therapist to verbalize his empathy when this occurs. The client must be aware that any change in his behavior is a matter of personal choice and responsibility and that the therapist will support the client's choice. It is occasionally appropriate and necessary for the therapist to share some of this own discomforts when he too was undergoing similar behavioral changes. If the therapist is a woman she may share analogous behavioral changes, although this is riskier and may easily intimidate the male client, regardless of how "liberated" he may seem.

Confrontation is an extremely helpful technique with clients in certain specific situations. Because the behaviors that are being changed are ego-syntonic for the man, confrontation must always be supportive and coupled with an explanation of why it is necessary for these behaviors to be changed so rapidly.

One situation that requires confrontation is when the change in gender-role behavior is crucial, as when these behaviors are severe enough to cause conflicts that may lead to an exacerbation of psychotic symptoms. For example, a 29-year-old paranoid schizophrenic man was able to control his symptomatology without medication as long as he was working. Because of seasonal variation and his employer's financial problems, he lost his job and rapidly became anxious, agitated, and paranoid. Financial difficulties forced his wife to get a part-time job, leaving him at home with the roles of babysitter and housekeeper. He found this situation to be intolerable and eventually acted upon his aggressive impulses, destroying most of the furniture in the house and striking his wife and child. Over the course of a tense, protracted session, he began to realize that he was not any less of a man because he was not working. This was accomplished largely through gentle and supportive confrontation of his violent behavior as "pseudomacho," challenging his link between his self-esteem and his work, and confronting him with the results of his behavior. The author interpreted the issue of control of his impulses and control of his environment from a cultural standpoint. Hospitalization was avoided as his anxiety and aggressive impulses diminished over the course of the session. Eventually, he was able to repair the damage in the relationship with his wife with the help of family therapy. After several months he was able to find himself a new job, thus improving his self-esteem.

With certain individuals, such as passive–aggressive and antisocial men, confrontation may be the only therapeutic language they understand. A 26-year-old passive–aggressive man required confrontation in order to change his sociopathic, aggressive, controlling behavior. He had a long history of physical explosions against his wife and friends, and refused to accept limits of any sort (this included escaping from jail on one occasion). All therapeutic work with this man had been a failure until he was confronted with the fact that he was not acting like man, but like a caricature of a man. The author called him a "cartoon," offering to help him change that image. This led to further acting up, but he was also able to start utilizing this information and changed his behavior. His modified behavior became less self-destructive and less stereotypically masculine. He continued to have a major problem with dependency needs, which remained a major issue in individual and group psychotherapy.

When other therapeutic techniques have failed, confrontation may be the only way of breaking through the resistance to changing masculine roles. A 56-year-old depressed man droned on about the same complaints for months. His affect was quite bland and he made no progress. Various therapeutic techniques, both psychotherapeutic and psychopharmacologic, were of no avail. Finally, the author confronted the client with his own anger and boredom and confronted the passive–aggressive nature of the client's behavior. He was told that he was acting in a typically "macho" manner by being inexpressive, controlling, and playing a power "game" with the author. The client broke down in tears and began to move to new material concerning these very issues between him and his wife.

Another important therapeutic technique is touch. Although there is a strict prohibition on touch in traditional psychotherapy, a prohibition that has its historical roots in the disputes between Freud and Ferenczi, the appropriate use of touch has specific uses in gender-role psychotherapy. It may be used to bring out the masculine prohibition against touch as a therapeutic issue. Touch may be used as a supportive technique; touching a hand or forearm may be a concrete expression of empathy, intimacy, and support by the therapist. It may also be utilized to examine these issues as well as the client's homophobia and sexuality. Touch should only be utilized if the therapist is completely comfortable with that modality and as an expression of support and empathy. At first, it should always be accompanied by a verbal expression of the therapist's feelings.

Individual consciousness raising may be utilized with those men who have made some changes in their masculine role behavior and who desire a structured examination of most, or all, aspects of the masculine role and its consequences. The framework developed by Moreland[52] is a useful set of consciousness-raising goals that can be modified to suit each client's needs. The length of time and number of sessions devoted to each topic is determined by the importance of each topic for the client and the amount of work each client is willing and able to expend on each topic. Moreland's framework allows for discussion of many issues faced in therapy in an organized way. Included are issues related to achievement, relationships with men, relationships with women, emotionality, and sexuality and sensuality.

A final therapeutic technique is therapist disclosure. This technique must be judiciously used so that the therapist serves as a role model for the client without stimulating feelings of competition, resignation ("I can't be as 'liberated' as my therapist, so why try"), or submissiveness in the client. There are two types of therapist disclosure used in gender-role psychotherapy. The more common is the expression of the therapist's affective response to the client's behavior or reported behavior. By letting the client know when the therapist is happy, angry, or bored, for example, in response to the client, the client learns the appropriate verbalizations and labels of affects as well as the immediate impact of his behavior on another person. This type of therapist disclosure makes the therapist more "real" to the client, enhancing the collaborative aspects of gender-role psychotherapy.

The second type of therapist disclosure involves the therapist disclosing a life event that is analagous to the client's. This should be used only when the client is stymied either in problem solving or affective response to this own life events. The therapist may then model a response in a supportive way to help create behavioral and affective options for the client.

SPECIAL PROBLEMS

Certain types of clients have special needs or present special problems when changing role behavior. As noted above, schizophrenic clients frequently have more intense conflicts around the issues of dependency and intimacy. Work in the area of changing role behavior with schizophrenic men must be much more supportive, gentler, and proceed at a slower pace. If the schizophrenic man's only identity comes from his stereotyped masculine role behavior, taking away this identity may be more detrimental than helpful. One must develop alternatives to this behavior that are comfortable and syntonic for the individual in order to avoid an exacerbation of psychotic symptomatology.

Narcissistic, passive–aggressive, borderline, or antisocial clients frequently behave in a way that caricatures the traditional masculine role. These "macho" individuals are very reluctant to change their role behavior and may do so only under external duress. Because of this, confrontation during therapy with this kind of client becomes a particularly valuable technique. Indeed, severely narcissistic clients are probably better treated in group psychotherapy to avoid their attempted manipulation of the therapist which helps them avoid changing their pathological role behavior. The role of group psychotherapy is discussed in detail in Chapter 14 by Stein.

Compulsive clients tend to emphasize the cognitive mode of functioning and to be particularly success and activity oriented. In working with compulsive clients it is important that permission-giving for affective responses be extremely clear, especially if these responses involve affects of aggression and hostility, for the compulsive person is particularly defensive of these affects.[53] The therapist should show the compulsive man how affective responses can be utilized in a positive way by modeling them and thus break through the intellectualizing defenses of the compulsive individual.

The specific problems of elderly men have been discussed in Chapter 11 by Solomon. It is important to note that feminine behaviors of older men may not mirror their subjective psychological state and that they usually wish to retain more traditional masculine behavior. Their feminine behaviors may be completely secondary to their changed social situation. The older man also faces many life changes that impact upon the masculine role. Those changes and therapeutic modifications for working with the older man are discussed in the above-mentioned chapter.

Alexithymia is a frequent problem in men. Alexithymia is the inability to identify, label, and experience certain emotional states. Alexithymia can be considered the extreme of inexpressiveness. Men suffering from alexithymia as a symptom are unable to verbally express an affect or its physical concomitants, label the affect, or psychologically experience the affect. It has been hypothesized that alexithymia is a major factor in the somatization process that leads to psychophysiologic and psychosomatic disorders[54,55] and substance abuse.[56]

A technique the author developed to break through alexithymia is derived from Gestalt therapy.[51] When the alexithymic man talks monotonously and inexpressively discusses an emotionally charged issue without the expression of affect, asking questions such as "what are you feeling?" is particularly useless.

The individual usually responds to those questions with "I don't know" or "OK" or a similar nonaffective response. When repeatedly faced with that, the therapist should then move to the somatic sphere. Paying particular attention to the nonverbal aspects of affect, the therapist then focuses on a somatic sensa-tionan is experiencing. For example, he/she may ask, "What does your chest feel like?" or "What are your eyebrows doing?" or the therapist may use a mirror or videotape feedback[57,58] to show the person his facial expression. Once the somatic sensation is acknowledged as present and identified, the patient may then be asked to rephrase the statement, substituting the word "I" for the body part. For example, the client at first might say, "My chest is feeling heavy." Then he would be asked to take ownership of that feeling, by stating "I am feeling heavy." He is then asked to identify what kind of feeling he knows can occur with the body sensation he is experiencing. For example, a "heavy"chest may be associated with fear, sadness, or crying. A frown may be seen as a concomitant of seriousness of purpose or anger. The individual then is asked to identify which of these affects is most related to what he is talking about. Once that is done, the person is then asked to identify the actual affect he is experiencing and take ownership of it. This process is repeated many times throughout therapy before the man is able to start to spontaneously identify the affective content of what he is experiencing and break through the separation of thought and affect.

TRANSFERENCE ISSUES

As in all therapeutic relationships, a transference relationship develops in gender-role psychotherapy. This transference relationship is frequently utilized, as in psychoanalytic psychotherapy, as the core medium for therapeutic change. In changing masculine roles, this transference relationship itself is frequently a take-off point, not only for discussion of the transference relationship itself, but for discussion of the specific role behavior that needs changing, its underlying affects, and its societal framework and etiology.

The act of being in therapy in itself becomes the first major transference issue to develop within therapy. How the client feels about being in therapy and his feelings about the therapist then should be examined very early, sometimes in the first session. It is not uncommon for the author to ask his men clients during his initial evaluation how they feel about being treated by a man, and how they feel about expressing feelings to another man. This immediately sets the stage for an ongoing examination of the transference relationship within the context of a man-to-man framework. Women therapists may utilize a similar process, as exemplified in a case report by Stevens.[5]

The regression that occurs in therapy becomes the second important transference issue to emerge. This regression is responsible for the eventual expression of many of the underlying psychodynamic and role conflicts expressed by clients. This regression occurs in the presence of attempts to maintain a collaborative, egalitarian, nonauthoritarian therapeutic relationship. Indeed, the regression may be an intrinsic part of any healing relationship.[59] Regression is also a source of resistance, for the client attempts to avoid regression and the awareness of painful material that follows. The resistance is examined as it develops and interpreted within the context of masculine role issues. These issues that develop because of the therapeutic regression are handled by the therapeutic techniques discussed earlier in the chapter. As the regression itself leads to feelings of weakness and vulnerability, controlling the regression by the therapist allows for examination of these feelings, rather than panic and flight of the client.

Intimacy with another individual is another major transference issue. This is complicated if the therapist is also a man because of homophobia. Therapy with men frequently slows down after less than ten sessions because of the man's fear of intimacy with the therapist. The men respond to this threat of intimacy by switching from an affective to a cognitive, intellectualized mode of functioning. They may spend many hours discussing irrelevant and detailed facts about their external life rather than the affects, memories, and experiences in their inner emotional life. Dreams are rarely reported during this time. Rather than seeing these facts as therapeutic themes, it is important for the therapist to realize that the true issue is intimacy with the therapist. The therapist should handle this by bringing up references to both the transference and the real relationships of therapy within a context of client conflicts with intimacy. This should be done very supportively and with the appropriate explanations about the difficulties that men have relating to other men (or women).

Closely related to problems in intimacy are issues of trust. Trust implies a sharing of intimacy and vulnerability, and a lack of competition. As a projection of their own fears, men in therapy may angrily accuse their therapist of breaking confidences or questioning their trust. They will frequently act out in an attempt to compete with their therapist. For example, some men will come to a session with many interpretations rolling off their tongue. These men are competitively attempting to show the therapist how much they have been working on their problems. They also show the therapist how they can live without their therapist, which is a subtle display of hostility, mistrust, and flight from intimacy. Like other transference issues that develop early in therapy, issues of trust and intimacy must be confronted.

A major transference issue that develops in therapy with men is that of dependency. As Menninger[59] has pointed out, psychotherapy is an unequal relationship in which one person, the client, is emotionally and physically dependent upon the other person, the therapist. This develops in spite of all attempts to formulate a more equal bond. Once dependency on the therapist is acknowledged by many men, they become anxious, leading to therapeutic examination of this vital and core conflict.

Another transference issue is that of homosexual fantasies for the man therapist. Because of homophobia, this is frequently anxiety provoking but rarely reported unless the therapist specifically asks. These fantasies are frequently disguised in dreams. It is important for the therapist to give the client clear permission to experience these fantasies for these fantasies will become an acknowledgment of the man's inherent bisexuality. They must also be interpreted to show how a block in these fantasies may lead to a block in the development of relationships with other men. To minimize the effects of homophobia, it is important to clarify to heterosexual men that fantasies are not the same as behavior or action, and that feeling attracted to another man or having a fantasy about another man does not make one homosexual or feminine. These fantasies may also be utilized to further examine issues of dependency, vulnerability, trust, and intimacy.

Specific transference responses to the man therapist, although idiosyncratic for the client, may open the door to examination of the client's relationships with important men in his life. Parentification of the therapist mirrors the client's relationship with his own father or other male authority figures, such as grandfathers, teachers, and employers. Infantilization of the therapist will lead the client to examine his relationships with younger, less dominant men in his life, such as his sons, grandsons, students, and employees. In addition, transference reactions may cross general boundaries so that the client may examine his relationship with his mother, wife, daughters, or other significant women in his life.

COUNTERTRANSFERENCE ISSUES

Countertransference issues are extremely important in the gender-role psychotherapy. Most of these countertransference issues can be simply explained by the fact that traditional masculine behavior is ego-syntonic for the great majority of men and, to a lesser degree, women psychotherapists. The relative newness and lack of direction and popularity of the Men's Liberation Movement has not forced therapists to be sensitized to masculine gender-role issues within themselves. As men and women therapists find traditional masculine role behavior ego-syntonic, they may be unaware of how they are reinforcing an inappropriate role behavior. For example, much of psychoanalysis and psychoanalytic psychotherapy is conducted in a cognitive mode. For the man therapist and man client, this is an extremely comfortable mode of functioning and may lead to the therapist being blind to the need for affective expression by either himself or his client.

The most important countertransference issue is the standards psychotherapists use to define the mental health of both men and women. The data of Broverman et al.,[60] Chesler,[61] and others [62–65] support the hypothesis that both men and women therapists retain the commonly accepted stereotypes of the traditional masculine and feminine roles as their respective standards of mental health for each sex. In another study, by Kjervik and Patla,[66] this hypothesis was supported for men clients only. Only Billingsley[67] and Dreman[68] report data that dispute these findings. Dreman's study,[68] however, was done with Israeli psychotherapists (who have a cultural background of greater gender-role egalitarianism) and is thus not comparable to all the other studies, which were completed in the USA.

It is important for the gender-role psychotherapist not to adopt any conceptualization of a standard of mental health that is directly tied to traditional gender roles. For one thing, gender roles are changing, and this immediately invalidates any standard. Secondly, a humanistic perspective provides a therapeutic ideal that individual clients have different and idiosyncratic needs and behaviors that may or may not mesh with traditional gender roles. Moreover, satisfaction of and comfort with these needs, coupled with an ability to adapt, solve problems, and become intimate are more akin to a humanistic conception of mental health than is a rigid set of "liberated" values.

Another important countertransference issue is the therapist's fear of change in his/her own role behaviors and expectations that are ego-syntonic. For example, the therapist may fear intimacy with his/her client or fear a homo/heterosexual fantasy of his/her client. Changing masculine roles for the client may lead the therapist to examine his/her own value system and role behaviors. As traditional masculine roles are ego-syntonic for both men and women, any confrontation of these roles in another person may lead to subjective confrontation within the therapist. The therapist may then either avoid certain role behaviors and conflicts in the client, deal with them in some stereotyped and superficial way, or behave in some nontherapeutic way because of his/her own anxiety.

Difficulty in the expression of empathy may lead to particular problems for men therapists. As noted by Abramowitz et al.[69] and Hoffman,[70] women therapists are more empathic than men therapists. Men therapists are more likely to resort to corrective action rather than sharing the affective experiences of the client. This may lead to an unconscious encouragement of acting out by the client or a blind spot, in which the therapist is unable to see how the client uses action as a resistance to therapy.

Related to this is what Farrell[18,20] calls self-listening. While seemingly listening to his client, the man therapist will be unconsciously working to interpret the clinical data in a preconceived way. Therapeutic interventions are then projections of the therapist's psyche rather than reflections of the client's. This is a subtle form of competition that is also a barrier to intimacy and maintains an unequal and authoritarian therapeutic relationship.

Aside from an overemphasis on cognition and intellectualization, another blind spot that may be ego-syntonic to the therapist is the man patient's need for success. Therapists are socialized to pursue success and status, as are clients. This may be particularly true if the therapist is in an academic setting and is living and working in a similar or analogous corporate structure as the client; he/she is likely to miss subtle problems that the client develops because of his/her own attachment to an analogous bureaucratic system. It is also likely to be true if the therapist places great emphasis on the acquisition of material rewards for his/her work.

Analogous to transference issues of parentification and infantilization, gender-role psychotherapy may uncover unresolved issues between the therapist and his/her father, sons, and other important men in his/her life. It is important to acknowledge these issues as they arise and occasionally appropriate to share them with the client. Should they arise frequently or lead to repeated difficulties conducting therapy, the therapist should consider entering therapy or joining a consciousness-raising or support group to help resolve these issues.

It is easy for therapists who are actively growing and changing from traditional role behaviors to be impatient or angry with clients who prefer traditional roles or who are slow to change. It must be remembered that the internatlization of societally defined roles is strong, having developed over a lifetime. Patience and support is necessary, for change may occur in the most chauvinistic of men. As long as the client is accepted for who he is, his beliefs and values respected, and gender-role issues contractually remain a valid focus of psychotherapy, change is likely to occur. To respond with revolutionary fervor is a therapeutic mistake that may irreparably damage the therapeutic relationship. Should the therapist be unable to keep his/her values from interfering with therapy, referral to another therapist is indicated.

CONCLUSION

With the techniques described in this chapter, it is frequently possible to change masculine role behavior. As with all therapies, the better the person's ego functioning, the easier this job will be and the more sophisticated will be the degree of change. The more the person is truly motivated to change his role behaviors, the easier and more lasting the job will be. With some men, six to eight sessions, primarily aimed at support, clarification, and ventilation, may be all that is necessary. With other men, it may take years of psychodynamic psychotherapy, in which changing masculine behavior is only a part of the process. If these men are extremely disturbed, pharmacotherapy may also be necessary. With individuals with personality disorders, group therapies may also be particularly valuable.

In addition, it is important for the therapist to change. As therapists themselves adopt traditional masculine and feminine roles as their standards for mental health, the author has previously suggested that men therapists join consciousness-raising groups[16] to further their own growth as men. Other men's groups, especially support groups, may be equally helpful. Men and women therapists must examine their biases and eradicate their gender-role blind spots. If men therapists are able to relate intimately to other men therapists (as well as other men and women), they will be able to maximize the changes in their own role functioning. This will allow them to deal with the issues of masculine roles in a nonjudgmental, growth-oriented way that will be of benefit to client and therapist alike.

REFERENCES

1. Wolman CS: Clinical applications of feminist theory. Presented at the 132nd Annual Meeting of the American Psychiatric Association, Chicago, Illinois, May 17, 1978
2. Moulton R: Psychoanalytic reflections on women's liberation. Contemp Psychoanal 8:197–223, 1972
3. Moulton R: The fear of female power—A cause of sexual dysfunction. J Am Acad Psychoanal 5:499–519, 1977
4. Moulton R: Sexual conflicts of contemporary women, in Interpersonal Explorations in Psychoanalysis. Edited by Witenberg EG. New York, Basic Books, 1972, pp 196–217

5. Stevens B: The sexually oppressed male. Psychother: Theory Res Pract 11:16–21, 1974
6. Baruch GK, Barnett RC: Implications and applications of recent research on feminine development. Psychiatry 38:318–327, 1975
7. Pleck JH: Sex role issues in clinical training. Psychother: Theory Res Pract 13:17–19, 1976
8. Seiden AM: Overview: Research on the psychology of women, Vol. II. Women in families, work and psychotherapy. Am J Psychiatry 133:1111–1123, 1976
9. Wong MR, Davey J, Conroe RM: Expanding masculinity: Counseling the male in transition. Counseling Psychol 6:58–61, 1976
10. Marecek J, Kravetz D: Women and mental health: A review of feminist change efforts. Psychiatry 40:323–329, 1977
11. Moulton R: Some effects of the new feminism. Am J Psychiatry 134:1–6, 1977
12. Lerner HE: Adaptive and pathogenic aspects of sex-role stereotypes: Implications for parenting and psychotherapy. Am J Psychiatry 135:48–52, 1978
13. Maffeo PA: Conceptions of sex role development and androgyny: Implications for mental health and for psychotherapy. J Am Med Womens Assoc 33:225–230, 1978
14. Nadelson CC, Notman MT, Bennett MB: Success or failure: Psychotherapeutic considerations for women in conflict. Am J Psychiatry 135:1092–1096, 1978
15. Kaplan AG: Toward an analysis of sex-role related issues in the therapeutic relationship. Psychiatry 42:112–120, 1979
16. Solomon K: Therapeutic approaches to changing masculine role behavior. Am J Psychoanal 41:31–38, 1981
17. Stein TS: The effects of the women's movement on men: A therapist's view. Presented at the 132nd Annual Meeting of the American Psychiatric Association, Chicago, Illinois, May 16, 1979
18. Farrell W: Women's and men's liberation groups, in Women in Politics. Edited by Jaquette J. New York, John Wiley and Sons, 1974, pp 171–199
19. Schonbar RA: Group co-therapists and sex-role identification. Am J Psychother 27:539–547, 1973
20. Farrell W: The Liberated Man. New York, Bantam Books, 1975
21. Wolman CS: Therapy groups for women. Am J Psychiatry 133:272–278, 1976
22. Bernardez-Bonesatti T, Stein TS: Separating the sexes in group therapy: An experiment with men's and women's groups. Int J Grp Psychother 29:493–502, 1979
23. Rounsaville B, Lifton N, Bieber M: The natural history of a psychotherapy group for battered women. Psychiatry 42:63–78, 1979
24. Berger M: Men's new family roles—Some implications for therapists. Fam Coordinator 28:638–646, 1979
25. Nathanson CA: Sex roles as variables in preventive health behavior. J Community Health 3:142–155, 1977
26. Harrison J: Warning: The male sex role may be dangerous to your health. J Soc Issues 34:65–86, 1978
27. Solomon K: The masculine gender role and its implications for the life expectancy of older men. J Am Geriatrics Soc 29:297–301, 1981
28. Solomon K: The depressed patient: Social antecedents of psychopathologic changes in the elderly. J Am Geriatrics Soc 29:14–18, 1981
29. Solomon K: Psychosocial crises of older men. Presented at the 133rd Annual Meeting of the American Psychiatric Association, San Francisco, California, May 7, 1980
30. Bem SL: Sex-role adaptability: One consequence of psychological androgyny. J Personality Soc Psychol 31:634–643, 1975
31. Foley JM, Murphy DM: Sex role identity in the aged. Presented at the 30th Annual Meeting of the Gerontological Society, San Francisco, California, November 20, 1977
32. Gillett N, Levitt M, Antonucci T: The relationship between masculinity, femininity and social competence in three generations of women. Presented at the 30th Annual Meeting of the Gerontological Society, San Francisco, California, November 20, 1977
33. Cherry DL, Zarit SH: Sex-role and age differences in competency, flexibility and affective status of women. Presented at the 31st Annual Meeting of the Gerontological Society, Dallas, Texas, November, 1978

34. O'Connor K, Mann DW, Bardwick JM: Androgyny and self-esteem in the upper-middle class: A replication of Spence. J Consult Clin Psychol 46:1168–1169, 1978
35. Woods SM: Some dynamics of male chauvinism. Arch Gen Psychiatry 33:63–65, 1976
36. Lein L: Male participation in home life: Impact of social supports and breadwinner responsibility on the allocation of tasks. Fam Coordinator 28:489–495, 1979
37. Kimball CP: Psychological aspects of cardiovascular disease, in American Handbook of Psychiatry, 2nd edition, Vol IV. Edited by Reiser MF. New York, Basic Books, 1975, pp 609–617
38. Adler A: Understanding Human Nature (1927). Trans by Wolfe WB. New York, Fawcett, 1965
39. Searles HF: Dependency processes in the psychotherapy of schizophrenia. J Am Psychoanal Assoc 3:19–66, 1955
40. Lidz T, Fleck S, Cornelison AR: Schizophrenia and the Family. New York, International Universities Press, 1974
41. Lidz T: Family studies and a theory of schizophrenia, in Annual Review of the Schizophrenic Syndrome, Vol 3. Edited by Cancro R. New York, Brunner/Mazel, 1974, pp 386–402
42. Halle E: The abandoned husband: When wives leave. Psychiat Opin 16:18–19, 22–23, 1979
43. Shapiro D: Neurotic Styles. New York, Basic Books, 1965, pp 23–53
44. David DS, Brannon R: The male sex role: Our culture's blueprint of manhood and what it's done for us lately, in The Forty-Nine Percent Majority: The Male Sex Role. Edited by David DS, Brannon R. Reading, Massachusetts, Addison-Wesley, 1976, pp 1–45
45. Solomon K: Sex roles and group therapy dropouts. Am J Psychiatry 136:727–728, 1979
46. Anderson R: I Never Sang for My Father. New York, Dramatists Play Service, 1968
47. Mijuskovic B: Loneliness: An interdisciplinary approach. Psychiatry 40:113–132, 1977
48. Grant RL: Discussion [of papers on psychotherapy and the changing roles of men in society]. Presented at the 132nd Annual Meeting of the American Psychiatric Association, Chicago, Illinois, May 15, 1979
49. Olinick SL: Some considerations of the use of questioning as a psychoanalytic technique. J Am Psychoanal Assoc 2:57–66, 1954
50. Bibring E: Psychoanalysis and the dynamic psychotherapies. J Am Psychoanal Assoc 2:745–770, 1954
51. Perls F: Gestalt Therapy Verbatim. Lafayette, Real People Press, 1969
52. Moreland JR: A humanistic approach to facilitating college students learning about sex roles. Counseling Psychol 6:61–64, 1976
53. Salzman L: Treatment of the Obsessive Personality. New York, Jason Aronson, 1980
54. Nemiah JC: Alexithymia. Theoretical considerations. Psychother Psychosom 28:199–206, 1977
55. Flannery JG: Alexithymia. II. The association with unexplained physical distress. Psychother Psychosom 30:193–197, 1978
56. Malinow K: Doc, my meth isn't holding me: An analysis of the narcotic withdrawal syndrome. Presented at a scientific meeting of the Maryland Psychiatric Society, Towson, Maryland, March 6, 1980
57. Berger MM: Multiple image immediate impact video self-confrontation. Presented at a scientific meeting of the Association for the Advancement of Psychoanalysis, New York, October 25, 1972
58. Berger MM: A preliminary report on multi-image immediate impact video self-confrontation. Am J Psychiatry 130:304–306, 1973
59. Menninger K: Theory of Psychoanalytic Technique. New York, Harper and Row, 1964
60. Broverman IK, Broverman DM, Clarkson FE, et al.: Sex-role stereotypes and clinical judgments of mental health. J Consult Clin Psychol 34:1–7, 1970
61. Chesler P: Women and Madness. New York, Doubleday, 1972
62. American Psychological Association: Report of the Task Force on sex bias and sex-role stereotyping in psychotherapeutic practice. Am Psychol 30:1169–1175, 1975
63. Delk JL, Ryan TT: Sex role stereotyping and A-B therapist status: Who is more chauvinistic? J Consult Clin Psychol 43:589, 1975
64. Abramowitz CV, Abramowitz SI, Weitz LJ, et al.: Sex-related effects on clinicians' attributions of parental responsibility for child psychopathology. J Abnorm Child Psychol 4:129–138, 1976
65. Delk JL, Ryan TT: A-B status and sex stereotyping among psychotherapists and patients. Toward a model for maximizing therapeutic potential. J Nerv Ment Dis 164:253–262, 1977

66. Kjervik DK, Palta M: Sex-role stereotyping in assessments of mental health made by psychiatric-mental health nurses. Nurs Res 27:166–171, 1978
67. Billingsley D: Sex bias in psychotherapy: An examination of the effects of client sex, client pathology, and therapist sex on treatment planning. J Consult Clin Psychol 45:250–256, 1977
68. Dreman SB: Sex-role stereotyping in mental health standards in Israel. J Clin Psychol 34:961–966, 1978
69. Abramowitz CV, Abramowitz SJ, Weitz LJ: Are men therapists soft on empathy? Two studies in feminine understanding. J Clin Psychol 32:434–437, 1976
70. Hoffman ML: Sex differences in empathy and related behaviors. Psychol Bull 84:712–722, 1977

Chapter 14

Men's Groups

Terry S. Stein

Introduction

Groups of men have existed throughout history. Men have congregated in all male groups in every society to accomplish a wide variety of political, social, religious, economic, recreational, and personal tasks. Most of these groups, whether large in size, such as an all-male army or religious order, or small, such as a meeting of the male tribal leaders in a primitive society or a gathering of a totally male corporate board of directors in an industrial society, have both reflected and served to maintain cultural definitions of masculine and feminine gender roles. Quite simply, men have met in all-male groups to perform certain functions which have most often been separated from the functions women perform. The purpose of this chapter is to describe a type of men's group which differs from these other exclusively male groups. The specific functions of this type of men's group are to encourage examination of how the masculine gender role is experienced by individual men and to explore new ways of enacting this role.

Two major categories of such men's groups, consciousness-raising groups and psychotherapy groups, are described in this chapter. While the purposes and characteristics of these two categories of men's groups are not always clearly differentiated, either theoretically or in practice, they can be viewed as distinct entities and will be described as such. Throughout the chapter the use of the term "men's group" will refer, unless otherwise specified, to small groups of men who meet on a regular basis and who have identified one of their purposes for meeting to be the examination of the masculine gender role. The manner in which they accomplish this purpose will be shown to vary widely from group to group. All of them, however, have developed as a result of two historical factors: first, the entire biologic and cultural history of differences between men's and women's gender roles, a history which significantly shapes the characteristics of

---

Terry S. Stein • Department of Psychiatry, Colleges of Human Medicine and Osteopathic Medicine, Michigan State University, East Lansing, Michigan 48824

the very men's groups which have been established to alter definitions of the masculine gender role; and second, the contemporary movement to describe and alter traditional definitions of gender roles. This movement was labeled in America in the 1950s and the 1960s as the Women's Movement and is now described by some as part of a larger human potential movement. These two factors—the historical differences between masculine and feminine gender roles and the contemporary movement to alter the definitions of these roles—underlie the development of men's groups in America today and provide a basis for understanding many of the characteristics of men's groups as they presently exist.

Throughout this chapter, the author will present his own experiences with men's groups in order to illustrate certain characteristics and applications of these groups. His experiences have included participation as a member in a year-long leaderless men's consciousness-raising group, as a psychotherapist in four men's psychotherapy groups, and as a leader of numerous men's discussion groups and workshops on men's issues. Each of these experiences has provided him with a rich opportunity for personal and professional growth.

He will also present in this chapter a brief historical background of men's groups in America, develop a rationale for these groups, describe some of the characteristics of men's groups, and discuss possible applications of such groups in the mental health field. Each of these topics will be discussed within the context of the larger topic of this book, the changing male role in American society.

HISTORICAL BACKGROUND OF MEN'S GROUPS

The history of men's groups is short and poorly documented. Nevertheless, understanding this history can help us to identify some of the characteristics of men's groups and to appreciate better many of the issues which can arise in such groups. An early account of a group of men meeting together to examine the experience of being men was written in 1971 and is entitled *Unbecoming Men.*[1] This book is a collection of brief essays written by the members of a men's consciousness-raising group. The title chosen for the book suggests an essential dilemma faced by the participants of any men's group. Men, who by definition reflect at least in part the masculine gender role, come together in these groups to learn how to "unbecome" men. Many of the characteristics attributed to the masculine gender role in American society, such as assertiveness, competitiveness, and independence, may be contradictory to the stated goals of men's groups, which include introspection, self-disclosure, sharing of affective experiences, and diminishing competition and the use of power in oppressive ways. Thus men, who represent masculinity, seek in men's groups to become, according to social definitions, unmasculine. This inherent contradiction in the very concept of men's groups—the contradiction of men seeking to "unbecome" men—provides a significant theme throughout the brief history of men's groups.

The essays in *Unbecoming Men* suggest another important theme which persists today in most men's groups: many of the men in this group describe an awareness that they want to change as men as a result of interactions with women who were a part of the Women's Movement. The relationship between women changing their concept of feminine identity and men changing their concept of masculine identity is complex. The contemporary Women's Movement began in America in the 1950s and by 1971, when a small number of men's groups were beginning to form, women had already articulated many aspects of the roles they wanted as women in society, had offered serious criticism of men's roles, and had begun to meet in a variety of types of women's groups. Thus, women had very clearly been the first to question traditional notions of gender roles, and men were the followers. The reasons for this phenomenon have been examined extensively and usually include issues related to the maintenance by men of power over women. Farrell[2] has suggested that the development of separate Women's and Men's Movements is a distinctly American process and that other countries, such as the Scandinavian ones, have instead developed a Human Liberation Movement. The relevance of this separate history of the Men's and Women's Movements in America is that men frequently enter men's groups with a sense of isolation from the struggles of women, with feelings of self-criticism as men which are in part a response to the real critique of men and the male role presented by feminists and other women, and with an awareness of following women in changing. These themes have become important determinants of the characteristics of some men's groups.

The author's experiences with men's groups also began in the early 1970s, when he was asked to participate as a leader and as a resource person for women's groups in order to assist these groups in examining their reactions to the presence of a man following being together as a group of women. He began to develop an interest in feminist writing at the same time. Many of his female friends and patients were also describing to him the distress they saw in their male partners and friends in reaction to changes which they were undergoing as women. Gradually men began to report directly their concerns in relation to the women they knew who were changing their views of themselves as women. These concerns were presented by a wide range of types of men including some who came to him because of psychiatric disturbances.

Based upon these experiences, he decided to start a men's psychotherapy group which could address both the emotional distress of his male patients and the social issues regarding male–male and male–female interactions. He also realized that being in a men's group himself would be of benefit in understanding better his own experience of being a man. He began to read the few books and articles about men available at that time. He realized that his interest in being in a men's group was not a solitary one when two friends shared with him their similar interest. They each invited other men to participate in such a group. Eventually eight men came together to discuss how they wanted to conduct their group. The experiences in this group will be presented in later sections of this chapter.

Like the group of men in *Unbecoming Men,* most of the other men's groups which have been written about in the professional literature[2,3] can be described as consciousness-raising groups. They tend to be leaderless, exist in nonprofessional settings, and focus on altering the social expectations placed on men. The fact that men in such groups tend to challenge existing social expectations for men has led to an apparent reluctance to form or at least to report about such groups within settings which represent and reflect more traditional social values, such as hospitals or community mental health centers. Those few men's groups which have met within an institutional setting[4,5] have been formed in universities. This may simply reflect the fact that the university is the setting where many professional publications originate. These groups are more structured in format, following either an educational or psychotherapy format, and may utilize examination of issues of masculinity as only one of several approaches to change.

Newspaper and other public media accounts[6] provide the only other descriptions of men's groups. The groups described in these accounts are formed in churches, in men's centers, or outside of any organized setting by groups of men who work together or have some other common interest. The largest number of such groups are probably formed in large urban communities or in university settings. Almost all of these groups seem to follow a consciousness-raising format, although many of them exist primarily as support or discussion groups without an explicit goal of change for the participants or for society. Because of the paucity of reports about men's groups, it is impossible to determine exactly how many men participate in such groups, what the outcomes for the members are, and for what reasons the groups were originally formed. Recently national organizations such as Free Men have been formed with the specific purposes of encouraging communication about gender roles through conferences and of promoting the formation of men's groups. The formation of men's groups does not seem to be a widespread social phenomenon, however. A much larger number of women's groups have been reported about in the professional and popular literature.

Part of the reason that so few men's groups have been described in the literature may also be viewed as a direct result of the very purpose and structures of these groups. The purpose of these groups is to change the way males are required to perform as men in our society. To exist within traditional and male-oriented settings could be counterproductive to the stated goals of such groups of men. To report in a systematic fashion in the professional literature on men's groups also could be viewed as a derivative of the same ways men have always been required to be: systematic observers who often maintain power through a scientific, logical approach to their experiences. Many of the men who enter men's groups are trying hard to alter these expectations for themselves, and to do so many require being outside the mainstream of professional and other social organizations.

This brief history of men's groups in America demonstrates several important issues relevant to these groups. First, while there are several published references to men's groups, actual studies are practically nonexistent. Second, the phenomenon of men's groups came after the start of the Women's Movement and the formation of a large number of women's groups. Third, the history of men's groups reflects some of the problems inherent in all male groups with which such groups have to struggle. These problems include the difficulty for a group of men who themselves represent masculinity to accomplish the task of "unbecoming" men and the related difficulty of developing strategies for groups which are not stereotypically masculine but which will at the same time allow honest expression of the masculinity of the group members. Fourth, men's groups have developed along two lines, those formed outside of professional settings, such as consciousness-raising, political action, and support groups, and a small number formed in traditional professional settings, primarily universities, and which may utilize a combination of consciousness-raising, educational, and psychotherapy approaches.

In subsequent sections of this chapter, the author will demonstrate how these historical issues relevant to men's groups are useful in formulating a rationale for men's groups and for understanding both the problems which arise in such groups and the possible applications of these groups in the mental health field.

RATIONALE

The rationale for men's groups is in the most general sense a belief in the need for men as a group to change their behaviors, belief systems, and affective experiences. A number of authors have discussed the problems for men in these areas.[7–10] In a separate paper[11] the author presented six areas of concern related to gender-role issues which have been identified by men: a generalized difficulty and anxiety in relating to the changing role of women in society, changes in the fathering role, examination of the male role in work and recreation, a wish by men to change affective style, alterations in the nature of adult relationships, and changing patterns of sexual functioning. Small groups of men meeting together to share concerns and to change in these areas may be particularly helpful for some men.

Experiences in the men's consciousness-raising group in which the author participated illustrate how one group of men interacted about their concerns in these areas. The topics discussed in this group included relationships with male and female partners, relationships with parents, the experience of being fathers, feelings about each other, sexuality, careers, and many other aspects of the men's lives. Together they lived through many important life events, including marriage, separation and divorce, graduation from college, the birth of a child, questions of homosexual identity, sickness of parents and other relatives, and stress in personal relationships. They also began to share meaningful events among themselves. Late in the life of the group they took a weekend retreat in a setting on a lake. This and many other shared activities served to expand their conceptions of how they could be together as men.

The nature of the sharing and the content of the discussions in this group were undoubtedly determined to a large extent by certain common characteristics. All of the men were between the ages of 20 and 40, most were students or members of the faculty of a large university, several had careers in psychology or psychiatry, and all shared an interest in the examination of their experiences as men. For the author, this men's group was a valuable resource for support, for learning about himself as a male, for helping to focus his professional interest in the particular concerns of men in contemporary America, and for developing new ways of relating to other men and to women. Today, four years after the ending of this group, several of the men in this group remain among his closest friends. All of the men had an important impact on his life.

His gratitude and respect for the men in this men's consciousness-raising group has continued to this day. In this group the author learned how to care about men as an adult; he learned also how to fight with men in totally new ways; he began, as a result of experiences in the group, to explore more deeply the relationships with his son, his father, his brother, and other important males in his life; and finally, as a result of learning more about himself as a man, he reevaluated his relationships with women and began to establish patterns of intimacy with women which did not involve traditional expressions of sexuality or power. While no political activities were directly undertaken by the group, several of the group members have become involved in other men's activities following being in this group. All of them were deeply affected by the experiences of sharing with each other the personal parts of their lives, parts which most of them had previously tended to share primarily only with women, and of allowing other men to become important to them as close friends.

Being in a men's consciousness-raising group was invaluable in preparing the author to work with men's psychotherapy groups as well. The men's psychotherapy groups with which he subsequently worked have consisted of from six to eight members and have all been conducted on an outpatient basis. The men who composed these groups have ranged in age from 18 to 60, and they have presented with a wide range of psychiatric problems. Some of the men were experiencing only mild symptoms of depression and disturbance in interpersonal relationships when they entered the groups. Others presented with symptoms of severe depression, borderline personality disorder, or character disorder. Several of the men had had extensive previous psychotherapy, had been hospitalized, or had received psychotropic medication. These groups all met weekly and were relatively short-term (six to eight months) with closed membership. Three of the groups were conducted in conjunction with women's groups led by Teresa Bernardez, M.D. The coleaders have reported on several aspects of these groups in a separate publication.[5]

Consistent themes have emerged in each of these groups. Many of these themes are described elsewhere in this chapter. But certain themes may be of particular interest in helping to elucidate further a rationale for men's psychotherapy groups. First, the men in all of these groups have expressed a concern with whether or not they can fully relate to each other in the absence of women. This concern appears different from the common experience of psychotherapy groups which are struggling to define their pattern of interaction as a group and to achieve a degree of cohesiveness. It seems rather to reflect a feeling of lack of interpersonal competence on the part of men.

A second and related concern expressed by all of these men's groups involves the nature of affective or feeling expression within the group. Expression of certain types of feelings directly within the group, especially those feelings perceived to be associated with vulnerability, such as sadness, affection, sexual attraction between men in the group, and feelings of intense anger, is initially inhibited within these groups. Again, this lack of affective expression appears different from experiences of groups in general. While members in any group may require a certain amount of time together before they can begin to express their feelings directly, the members of a men's group seem particularly reluctant to display their feelings. The eventual release of this affective inhibition in these groups tends to disconfirm the idea that men are unable to express feelings directly. It does appear to support the idea that men can learn to express feelings more openly if given the opportunity. The capacity to share feeling experiences varied considerably, of course, among the men in these groups and was to a large extent independent of the factor of gender. The occurrence of an initial affective deadness within these groups, however, seems specifically related to the fact that they were all male in composition.

These examples of one men's consciousness-raising group and four men's psychotherapy groups are presented in order to highlight certain themes and types of interactions which can occur in such groups. From these examples and the descriptions of other men's groups available in the literature, several specific purposes and functions of men's groups can be presented which together form a rationale for such groups. This rationale serves to differentiate men's groups from other types of groups and to describe the unique contributions of men's groups to society in general and to the field of psychotherapy in particular. The specific purposes and functions of men's groups which are not currently accomplished in any other type of group will now be presented.

Membership in a men's group represents in itself a statement of nontraditional masculine values. Men who wish to change themselves as men often begin this process by affiliating with a group of men who have similar values and interests. Since men's groups are a new social development and have arisen in large part as a result of the Women's Movement, a willingness to enter a men's group is an important statement by an individual man that he wants to change. For many men, this may represent the first step in a whole series of life changes related to his experience of being a man.

Men's groups provide an opportunity for men to relate to other men in an interpersonal setting without women. Many men in our society rely on women to perform a wide variety of interpersonal functions, such as caretaking, nurturing, and expressing certain types of feelings more associated with the feminine role.[12] In an all-male group, men are left to accomplish these functions on their own without the support of women. In such a setting, men may learn to perform many of the functions which they previously felt could only be done by women.

Men's groups serve as a means for demonstrating to men how they behave when they are with other men. Competition, striving for success, a wish to dominate, assertiveness, aggressiveness, and intellectualization are characteristics associated with the masculine role.[13] These characteristics can be expected to appear in groups of men meeting together, and in time men in men's groups may learn to express them in new ways. Struggles to win or to dominate other men, when they arise, can be experienced, examined, and altered in men's groups. The manner in which a particular men's group examines and helps to alter stereotyped masculine behaviors will to a large extent determine the success of the group in helping its members to change.

A men's group represents a nontraditional male activity for its members. When men come together in groups they generally do so for a specific purpose or to accomplish a task, both in work and nonwork areas. Although men's groups do have a personal, political, or psychotherapeutic purpose for the members, they will generally not have the same product-oriented or competitive goals as other groups of men. The task of sharing personal feelings, thoughts, and hopes with other men provides an opportunity to behave in nonstereotypically masculine ways, an opportunity which may not be available to many men in any other area of their lives.

The relationships in men's groups can serve to highlight the ways in which members have related to other significant men in their lives. Men's groups, especially those having a heterogeneous composition with respect to age and other characteristics of the members, may provide an opportunity for members to see important aspects of relationships to fathers, male children, authority figures, or male peers. The men may initially interact with other group members in ways which are similar to interactions with significant males in their lives outside of the group. If the group facilitates the experiencing and sharing of these "here and now" relationships, its members may acquire a greater understanding of the ways in which individual men and men as a group are encouraged to interact with other men according to stereotyped masculine patterns. This understanding can lead to important changes in relationships with men outside of the group through the formation of new relationships which are not based on patterns of authority, competition, or other traditional factors in male–male relationships.

A men's group can provide a setting in which to explore special topics which are frequently difficult for men to talk about, such as dependency and homosexuality. Adherence to the masculine gender role prescribes for men a masculine identity which emphasizes independence, lack of noncompetitive physical contact between men, and exclusion of sexual feelings between men. In challenging the traditional masculine role, a men's group can encourage the expression of feelings of dependency, passivity, weakness, and sexual feelings for other men. The open acknowledgment of such feelings within a group of men can serve to diminish the men's concerns about these areas and to reinforce a greater openness in sharing a wider range of other feelings as well.

Men's groups may lead to the greater understanding of special problems for men, such as male diseases, an excessive need to achieve, reactions to divorce, and difficulties in parenting. Certain topics are of interest to men either because they are exclusively male problems, such as men's illnesses, or because they generally involve a particularly masculine experience in American society, such as the frequent separation of men from their children following divorce. The opportunity to hear about other men's experiences in these areas may be especially helpful to men in two ways. First, some stress for individual men in these areas may be alleviated merely by learning that other men experience similar concerns. Second, some men's groups may attempt to alter the male experience in these areas either by supporting individual men in challenging social norms, as when a man is encouraged to obtain custody or joint custody of his children, or by focusing the entire group's activity in a particular area of concern to men. An example of this type of group is one that is specifically organized to alter existing divorce or child custody laws.

Men's groups can serve to alter the nature of adult male–male relationships by promoting caring and friendship between men. Many men primarily relate to other adults in structured settings which preclude the sharing of feelings, concerns, fears, hopes and expectations, and empathy. If such interpersonal sharing takes place at all, it occurs within the family setting, and for many men it fails to occur at home as well. Men's groups can be a mechanism for learning how to develop adult male friendships, either through the establishment of relationships with other men in the group or by applying the learning experience in the group to relating in new ways to men outside of the group.

Men may learn new patterns of relating to women in men's groups. Men who participate in a men's group often have an awareness of changes in the role of women in society and are attempting to change the gender-role expectations and norms for men as well. The relatedness between changes in men and women is a recurrent theme for most men's groups, and relationships with women may be the central focus of some men's groups. Regardless of the extent to which the group explicitly discusses relationships with women, however, these relationships can be expected to be affected because the men are changing their ideas about themselves as men. The nature of specific effects will vary considerably, of course, depending on such factors as the degree of political consciousness of the men in the group regarding gender-role issues, the quality of existing relationships with the women to whom the group members relate, and the motivation of members to experiment with nontraditional patterns in male–female relationships. These patterns can include establishing nonsexual friendships with women and assuring equal power in relationships with women.

Men's groups can serve to increase the social and political awareness of men as a basis for eliminating individual and institutional sexism. Some men's groups are organized for the specific purpose of promoting radical change in existing gender arrangements. All men's groups, by encouraging awareness of gender-role characteristics for both men and women, can help to increase the sensitivity of men to prejudices and injustices in society related to sexism. With such a heightened sensitivity, individual men can become more aware of their own beliefs and behaviors which previously may have served both consciously and unconsciously to oppress women as a group and to restrict their own experiences of becoming more fully human.

Each men's group will vary considerably in the extent to which it addresses these issues. Similarly the outcomes of such groups for individual members will vary depending on many factors, including the stated purpose and interests of a given group, the type of men who compose it, the format of the group, the setting in which it occurs, the presence or absence of a group leader or therapist, and the length of time the group meets. Nevertheless, a group of men which comes together in order to examine concerns about gender-role characteristics can provide an opportunity which is not presently available in any other type of group. Some of the variable factors which determine the specific characteristics of a particular men's group are discussed in the next section.

CHARACTERISTICS OF MEN'S GROUPS

Small groups of men have been shown to have characteristics which are different from the characteristics of women's groups and mixed groups. Aries[14] demonstrated differences in these three types of groups which she believes reflect the sex-role demands of conventional society. She showed that

> . . . men had more personal orientation in a mixed setting, addressed individuals more often, spoke more about themselves and their feelings, while in an all-male setting they were more concerned with the expression of competition and status.

She also demonstrated that over time in a small discussion group men tend to benefit more from a mixed setting and women tend to feel less restricted and benefit more from an all-female setting.

Several other authors have also reported on specific problems in men's groups. Farrell[2] extensively examines some major barriers to successful interaction in men's consciousness-raising groups which derive from the very conception of the masculine role in American society. One such barrier is the tendency of men to intellectualize. Through this process, men may become psychologically insightful or politically aware at an intellectual level without really changing underlying attitudes, beliefs, and behaviors. Another barrier to which Farrell refers is an inability of men to overcome their attachment to a hierarchy of values which places males' values over females' values in a social interaction. A technique which he identifies as reinforcing the male hierarchy of values is "self-listening," which refers to a process of listening to another person only for the purpose of sharing one's own experiences and reactions and not for purposes of genuinely appreciating the speaker's experiences. Farrell believes that men employ this technique of exchange both with other men and with women. He further believes that utilization of this technique and the maintenance of attachment to males' values in group interactions leads to the development of such interactive traits as dominating, interrupting, condescending, showing disrespect, and aggression, traits which can interfere with showing empathy and warmth in interacting with others. Farrell's analysis of male interaction in consciousness-raising groups is consistent with Aries' findings about all-male discussion groups. He believes that these patterns are demonstrated by men in mixed groups with women as well.

Washington[15] identifies several additional problems for men in consciousness-raising groups. He describes the initial decision to participate in such a group and a sustained willingness to continue to attend as the two major problems for such groups. Other problems he identifies for men's groups include anxiety about homosexuality within the group and a tendency for the men to use intellectualization.

Efforts to overcome some of the problems which men may have when interacting in groups have led to several suggestions for how to structure men's groups. Wong[4] outlines a series of activities and possible discussion topics for male self-help groups. Moreland[16] describes a course of seminars for increasing college students' awareness about sex roles. Farrell[2] believes that men's groups need a facilitator initially in order to overcome males' inhibitions to group interaction, but that the facilitator should play a diminishing role over time in the groups.

The factors identified by Aries, Farrell, and others which interfere with communication between men meeting in small groups may significantly determine the characteristics of men's groups. The author's experience shows that for most men's groups these factors, when they are examined and when they are successfully managed within the group, may also provide a stimulus for further personal growth for the individual men in the group. Breaking through barriers to communication which present themselves as masculine patterns of relating to other persons appears to be the most satisfying experience reported by the men who have participated in men's groups. Certain specific features of men's groups, including the nature of the contract, the process, the pattern of leadership, the dynamics, and the presence of conflicts about changes will significantly influence the degree to which a particular men's group will successfully overcome the problems men have in interacting in small groups.

CONTRACT. Any group must have a task and a set of assumptions, guidelines, and rules which will presumably lead to the accomplishment of this task. The task and rules of operation determine the contract for the group. The task of most men's groups is generally stated as a personal one for the members, to increase awareness about men's issues and about alternatives to social prescriptions for male behaviors. Some men's groups also attempt to undertake broader political or social activities related to these issues, but even these groups may still emphasize the individual member's responsibility for gaining awareness and changing.

The rules of operation of men's groups are much more variable. Some groups function according to clearly specified guidelines which establish requirements for attendance, what may be discussed, how long the group will meet, and other rules which determine the structure of the group. Other groups may be loosely organized, meet sporadically, and not decide in advance what will occur during meetings. The degree of organization and adherence to rules may significantly influence what can be accomplished in a given men's group. Style and degree of organization is of particular importance in men's groups because the male role in society tends to emphasize hierarchy and organization. The wish by some men's groups to operate without established rules may promote overcoming traditional male patterns of interaction, but it may also encourage disorganization within the group, leading to nonattendance or lack of shared purpose among the members.

The specific contract for a men's group will vary considerably, of course, depending on whether it is a psychotherapy, a consciousness-raising, or some other type of group. Men in a psychotherapy group may be expected in general to be experiencing a greater degree of emotional distress than men in other types of groups. As a result of their distress they have "contracted" with a therapist in the hope of obtaining relief. Consequently, the factors of identified emotional distress and of working with a therapist will determine certain characteristics of men's psychotherapy groups, such as degree of structure and setting. The contract of a consciousness-raising group may, in contrast, involve only an agreement among the members to increase personal awareness about the experience of being a man. Because of the relationship between the contract of a group and how the group is structured, the nature of the contract can be seen to be an important determinant of how a particular men's group will overcome the barriers to communication among its members.

PROCESS. Most men's groups will at some point directly address issues of communication between members, or in other words, attend to the process by which the group functions as a group. The manner in which a group addresses its process will vary considerably depending on other characteristics of the group. The characteristic of men's groups which seems to be most consistently helpful to the members is simply the opportunity to interact with other males about issues related to being men. Thus, a helpful process in men's groups is one that facilitates interpersonal communication among its members. In the initial phase of the group, some specific structure for demonstrating existing modes of interaction and for eliciting the concerns of the members may be desirable for most groups. By discussing selected topics, reading certain books about men, allocating time for each member to talk about his concerns, designating a group leader or facilitator, or combining these approaches, the group may encourage the development of a sense of cohesiveness and sharing among the members. Later in the group's life, these initial arrangements may yield to a more loosely organized process in which members spontaneously interact regarding certain shared problems or individual concerns. Because of the varied composition, settings, and contracts of men's groups, the process which any given group follows will vary considerably.

An awareness of which areas may be particularly problematic for men in groups and an attention to ways in which the process the group follows can be helpful in addressing these areas will be crucial in determining the success of the group. For example, a group of men who have decided to participate in a consciousness-raising group and who share a concern about expressing feelings with other men may want to avoid a group process which focuses on intellectual topics or reading books. A process which focuses on here and now sharing of feelings between the members or which encourages the revealing of emotionally important concerns may be more relevant for this type of group. In contrast a group of students who want to learn about gender-role issues during a set period of time may benefit more from topic discussions. A flexible combination of various group processes which highlights the concerns men have allows the men to interact about these concerns, facilitates a greater level of awareness, and provides an opportunity to behave in new ways is the ideal process for most men's groups.

PATTERNS OF LEADERSHIP. Leadership is an extremely important variable in men's groups. Participants and observers in these groups agree that competition for dominance is an almost universal phenomenon in groups of men. The dilemma for most men's groups, if they recognize this struggle for dominance, is to establish a balance between leadership, which can provide some consistent direction and facilitation for group exchange, and nonadherence to traditional patterns of leadership, which are often directive, prescriptive, or authoritarian.

The original purpose of the group will influence the pattern of leadership. If the group is formed for purposes of psychotherapy or education, then a therapist or instructor will usually serve as a leader. If the group is constituted specifically for consciousness-raising or political action purposes, then leadership patterns will vary considerably. Some groups may rotate leadership, others may agree that there is no established leader, and yet other groups may utilize a set structure, such as a topic-discussion format, which addresses leadership by selecting a discussion leader. The setting in which the group occurs may also significantly influence the leadership patterns. For example, a group which meets to learn about sex-role issues in a college classroom may benefit from the structure and direction provided by the instructor. A group whose purpose is to significantly alter the life styles of its members may require experimentation with a variety of patterns of leadership.

Style of leadership is also an important issue for a men's group, regardless of how the leadership function is structured in the group. Moreland[16] has emphasized the need for group facilitators in college classes about sex-role issues to be aware themselves about sex-role constructions and to model nontraditional patterns of behavior. It is difficult to imagine the members of a men's group achieving a higher level of awareness about sex-role issues and changing themselves if they were to be led by a person demonstrating only traditional sex-role attitudes or behaviors. Female leaders have apparently not been extensively utilized in men's groups, but this approach may provide an alternative for some men's groups which could both demonstrate that women can be in helpful positions of leadership in relation to men and at the same time provide for men a realistic representation of feminine qualities within an otherwise all-male group. Other groups may benefit from periodic consultations by outside leaders who are requested to assist the group in overcoming specific problems or to offer expertise in an area of particular interest to the group at a given time.

If a group decides to establish itself without a designated leader or facilitator, it may encounter problems which can result in dissolution of the group, stagnation within the group, or, if successfully handled, an enhanced sense of accomplishment by the group. If the group does continue to function, the risks of conducting a men's group without a designated pattern of leadership are that the group members may persist in openly competing for leadership through the life of the group, thereby reinforcing traditional patterns of male–male interaction, or that the members may deny that competition exists at all. The latter outcome may serve to encourage even more unconscious mechanisms for achieving dominance through the use of intellectualization or reaction formation. Groups which can successfully overcome these problems without adhering to traditional forms of leadership may serve as the best laboratories for expanding male consciousness. Leaderless men's groups which cannot overcome these problems can benefit from utilizing alternative strategies for leadership, such as requesting help from outside consultants or temporarily designating a leader from within the group.

DYNAMICS. The dynamics of a group refers to the themes, conflicts, and style which are characteristic of a particular group. Men's groups reflect the dynamics of small groups in general as well as certain dynamics which can be viewed as unique to groups of men. It is these unique dynamics of men in groups which will be discussed in this section.

Many of the dynamics of men in groups reflect the nature of the masculine gender role. Some of the attributes which are associated with the masculine role in American society are assertiveness, aggression, independence, rationality, competitiveness, seeking of power, an action orientation, a tendency not to be introspective, little expression of certain emotions (such as sadness, vulnerability, helplessness, and caring), and being less nutruring than women in relationships. While an individual man may possess these attributes to a greater or lesser extent, groups of men can be expected in general to exhibit these traits more than either groups of women or groups of both men and women together. Thus the dynamics of groups of men highlight many of the same themes, conflicts, and styles which are a product of the masculine gender role itself.

Most men's groups will struggle at some point with how to obtain the proper balance between allowing those masculine traits which help to organize and coalesce the group and discouraging expression of those traits which may tend to dissolve the group and threaten its continued survival. (And often a single trait may be helpful to the group at one point in its existence and may be a hindrance at another point.) This struggle is not an easy one and is reported as occurring in varying ways in virtually every men's group which has been described thus far in the literature. The struggle can be illustrated by examining how a single masculine-linked characteristic, such as competitiveness, may manifest itself in a group. Competitiveness can be an extremely valuable characteristic which may serve to motivate an individual or a group to achieve certain goals; but it may also be experienced as a burden to an individual man and oppressive to others if the competitiveness becomes a requirement in all interactions. Many men experience both these positive and negative aspects of competitiveness and may even enter a men's group with an awareness of their mixed feelings about competitiveness. Within the group itself, however, especially in a group which encourages fairly open-ended interactions, the men may become so competitive, either because of a wish to compete or of a fear of not competing that the group may not be able to establish a climate for helpful communication. The struggle for most groups is neither to curtail completely the expression of this competitiveness, which may be a shared concern of many men in the group, nor to encourage its display to such a degree that the group cannot function. Some groups may structure their meetings so rigidly with agendas or rules that it appears as though competition does not exist among the members, and other groups may spend so much of their time arguing, disagreeing, or debating that they never alter their expression of competitiveness.

The dynamics of men's groups can be viewed in the most general sense as a struggle to achieve the expression of the entire spectrum of human attributes within an all-male setting. This struggle will continue in men's groups until a greater flexibility in the masculine gender role is achieved in American society. Most men who enter men's groups will seek to balance their learned tendencies to be competitive, aggressive, powerful, in control, and rational with newly discovered capacities to be nurturing, supportive, and expressive of feelings. The greatest barrier to achieving this balance appears to be an excessive display of the so-called masculine attributes. In contrast, the most helpful factor in attaining this balance seems to be the motivation on the part of the men who enter men's groups to gain access to the so-called feminine attributes. The helpful integration of these characteristics can be the major accomplishment for a men's group.

CONFLICTS ABOUT CHANGE. Three specific conflicts regarding change often present themselves in men's groups and are a reflection of certain themes with which men in general are concerned today. These conflicts involve struggling with ambivalence about change, establishing a positive image as a man which incorporates both masculine and feminine traits, and resolving guilt associated with being a man. The members of a men's group must arrive at a motivation to change which is stronger than the motivation to maintain the *status quo* of gender-role arrangements. The evidence that men suffer as men in our society is overwhelming. Goldberg[17] has documented many of the negative aspects of being a man in America today, including a shorter life span than women, a higher crime rate, greater victimization as a result of crimes, and a higher incidence of many chronic diseases. But because men in fact continue to be in positions of dominance, continue to possess economic, educational, and political power, and continue to exercise prerogatives not available to women, giving up an association with the traditional masculine gender role is unacceptable to many men. Even if men, as individuals, derive little actual gain from the masculine role, they still have an association with power simply by being men. Women have the clear objective in their struggle to change to obtain certain social rights, privileges, and power which have been denied them. Men, in contrast, will have to yield some of their privileges and power if they are to change. Many men refuse to examine their role as men or, even if they begin such an examination by participating in a men's group, will present an ambivalent motivation to alter their beliefs, attitudes, and behaviors as men. This reluctance to risk a loss of some of the benefits of being a man in our society prevents some men's groups from promoting true change in their members.

A second conflict with which men's groups must struggle in order to allow change is to establish a more integrated sense of masculinity which does not deny traditionally "feminine" traits. Chodorow[18] has stated that the masculine identity is to a large extent the result of a process which encourages boys not to be like their mothers. Many men, as a result, fear becoming like women if they acknowledge certain characteristics, such as the wish to be nurturing, passive, and dependent or the desire to possess other attributes traditionally associated with women. But to learn new ways of being men may be impossible for some men until they have first acknowledged their fears of being like women. The fear may be expressed in groups as anxiety about homosexuality or concern about being a "sissy," but it derives from an underlying devaluation of certain feminine-identified qualities. Miller[19] has described some of the social consequences of this devaluation. As a result of the conflict between the recognition by some men that they no longer want to be like men are supposed to be and the coexisting fear of being like a woman if they do not behave like men, some men's groups may have difficulty in fostering new positive images for their members. The recognition of this conflict and the gradual opportunity to experiment with new attitudes and behaviors may free the men to achieve a more flexible sense of identity as a man, an identity which can incorporate both masculine and feminine attributes.

A third conflict in some men's groups involves the personal guilt which men may tend to assume as a result of criticism of the masculine role. Criticism of the masculine role by some feminists and dissatisfactions with men expressed by individual women can lead to a personal sense of guilt on the part of some men simply because they are men. This guilt, if excessive, may prevent a group of men from freely examining what actual responsibility they have in their lives for oppressing women and ultimately from arriving at new definitions of masculinity which are associated neither with guilt nor with oppression. Resolution of this conflict requires careful exploration (within a nonjudgmental setting) of both the positive and negative aspects of being male. Either self-denigration or excessive criticism by others can inhibit such exploration and interfere with arriving at a new positive image of oneself as a man.

TYPES OF MEN'S GROUPS

Several types of men's groups can be described, based upon the stated purposes and the format of the group. These include support, political action, consciousness-raising, discussion, educational, and psychotherapy groups. All of these types of groups share two characteristics: (1) at some point in their life they are all male in composition and (2) during the course of the group an opportunity is provided to discuss or to take action regarding concerns related to the masculine gender role. Most of the general characteristics of men's groups presented in the preceding section can also be demonstrated to be descriptive of the several types of men's groups. However, the form of expression of these characteristics in a particular men's group will depend to a large extent on how the members define their group. For example, some ambivalence regarding changing the masculine role can be expected in most men's groups. This ambivalence may be explicitly acknowledged in a men's discussion group. In contrast, a political action men's group may never talk about ambivalence regarding change, but may instead express this ambivalence through focusing their activities on greater rights for men and ignoring equal rights for women.

The different types of men's groups may address similar areas of concern even while talking about different content areas and behaving in very different ways. The political action men's group may talk about and try to change social and legal structures which define patterns of interaction between men and women (such as marriage and divorce laws) or between men and their children (such as child custody laws or child support arrangements). The consciousness-raising group, which may be more focused on awareness within the group, could simply talk about the individuals' experiences regarding these concerns. And a men's support group may focus on participating together in certain activities which in our society usually take place between men and women, such as going on outings with children or providing emotional support to one another. This latter group, by focusing on personal activities, may want to restrict the opportunities for intellectualizing or for behaving in traditionally masculine ways as, for example, by becoming involved in politics. The content of these three groups' discussions and their behaviors will be very different, yet each of them is addressing an underlying concern with the nature of male–female and male–male relationships and is attempting to alter the existing patterns of such relationships.

Two types of men's groups, the consciousness-raising group and the psychotherapy group, are particularly relevant to the mental health field because of their potential applications in psychotherapy and because of the different assumptions regarding change underlying these two types of groups. Both men's consciousness-raising and men's psychotherapy groups have a stated goal of change for the members with respect to their beliefs, feelings, and behaviors regarding gender roles. Both types of groups may also utilize a variety of means, including support among members, education, discussion, experimentation with new behaviors and therapeutic interaction, to accomplish change. But the underlying assumptions regarding how change is best accomplished are very different for these two types of groups.

The literature on women's groups provides some clarification of the differentiation between consciousness-raising and psychotherapy groups. Kirsh[20] has outlined two basic theoretical elements of difference between them: (1) the degree of reliance on an hierarchical and unequal patient–therapist relationship in contrast to peer equality, and (2) the amount of emphasis on intrapsychic and individual in contrast to social change. Consciousness-raising groups tend to emphasize peer equality and goals of social change; psychotherapy groups rely more on an unequal patient–therapist relationship and stress individual change. Because psychotherapy is often seen as a conveyer of existing social values, some feminist writers[21] have argued that traditional psychotherapy is not the appropriate mechanism by which women can alter their concepts of themselves as women. To a large extent the factors of hierarchical relationship between patient and therapist and of focus on individual change are contradictory with the goals of change articulated by some women. Thus, Kirsh's differentiation between consciousness-raising groups and psychotherapy groups serves to point out possible problems inherent in changing patterns of social role expectations for women through traditional forms of psychotherapy.

Certain differences between masculine and feminine identities and between the masculine and feminine gender roles suggest additional issues which must be considered in evaluating for men the effectiveness of consciousness-raising or psychotherapy groups. First, the critique of the traditional client–therapist relationship in psychotherapy by feminist writers is based to a large extent on how the greater assumption of power by the therapist generally reinforces the social experience of men in power over women since a larger number of men have been therapists and a larger number of women have been clients. For men, who have not been in the client position as frequently as women, the acceptance of lesser power and the accompanying position of dependency on the therapist (who may be either female or male) may represent a helpful change in their usual social role.

A second difference between men and women relates to the greater focus on introspection and on issues of inner identity in women and the greater focus on activity and outer identity in men. Erikson[22] identified the developmental basis for these differences. Writers such as Hopkins[23] have recently demonstrated changes in the relative importance of issues of inner and outer identity for women. Similar studies of men have not been undertaken. But generally men as a group could still be expected to represent less capacity for introspection than women and greater emphasis on concerns about outer or social identity. This essential difference may suggest that men who wish to alter their expression of the masculine gender role may benefit more than women from participating in more traditional forms of psychotherapy which emphasize introspection and individual change rather than social change. The relevance of these differences between men and women to change in same-sex groups must be tested in further research in this area.

Regardless of these theoretical issues regarding the different types of men's groups, the largest number of men's groups described in the literature follow a consciousness-raising format. These groups have formed over the past decade in America with the primary purpose of bringing men together to discuss experiences with traditional expectations associated with the masculine gender role and to explore alternative ways of being men. While the actual number of men who have participated in such groups cannot be determined, it is clear that they have arisen throughout the country, that men's consciousness-raising groups appear to serve a need for a certain segment of the male population, and that they have been formed primarily outside of psychiatric and other mental health settings. As long as this need continues to exist, men's consciousness-raising groups can be predicted to continue to exist as well. The extent of increase or decrease in the number of men's consciousness raising-groups will depend on at least three factors: the future course of the human potential movement in general in the United States, the evolution of the movement to examine and alter gender-role definitions for men and women, and the effectiveness of men's consciousness-raising groups in providing a forum for accomplishing member's goals.

At the present time there is no evidence to suggest how extensively psychotherapists utilize either men's or women's consciousness-raising groups as a viable alternative resource for their patients. Since men's consciousness-raising groups are usually leaderless and considered nontraditional, this type of men's group will probably continue to exist outside of settings where an organized practice of psychotherapy takes place. Arguments can be raised that to attempt to alter this situation would be beneficial neither to the men who participate in these groups nor to the practitioners of psychotherapy. For the members, any attempt to impose an institutionalized structure on men's consciousness-raising groups would undermine many of the goals and characteristics of the groups as they presently exist. And for many psychotherapists, working within a consciousness-raising format in a men's group would be inconsistent with their current conceptualizations of psychotherapy.

In contrast to the brief history of men's consciousness-raising groups, groups of men have met together in professional settings for psychotherapy and educational purposes since at least the turn of the century. The early history of group psychotherapy[24] consists to a large extent of groups of men who were brought together in wartime and in certain all-male or primarily male settings, such as prisons, military hospitals, and drug treatment centers. But only recently have men's psychotherapy groups which have the stated goal of examining issues of masculinity been formed in professional settings. No precise delineation of how this goal is accomplished or of the extent to which a particular psychotherapy group emphasizes this goal will be attempted. However, all of the men's psychotherapy groups which are referred to in this chapter do share three characteristics: (1) The group has the structure of a psychotherapy group, including at least a designated leader or leaders (psychotherapist), a contract to engage in a psychotherapeutic process, and a regular meeting place and time. (2) There is an explicit acknowledgment by both leader and group members that gender-role concerns are appropriate matters for discussion. (3) The opportunity is provided for concerns related to gender roles to be expressed during the course of the group, either through a direct focus on such material or through examination of these concerns as they relate to other material presented in the group. These three characteristics serve to differentiate men's psychotherapy groups both from other types of men's groups, such as consciousness-raising, political action, or educational groups, and from other all-male psychotherapy groups which do not explicitly examine gender-role issues.

The differentiation between men's psychotherapy groups and psychotherapy groups which are simply all male is an important one which involves assumptions regarding the interplay between specific psychosocial factors such as gender roles and emotional disturbance. While a psychotherapist who believes in the importance of the relationship between social forces and individual emotional distress and specifically between gender-role expectations and emotional disturbance may not apply this belief in the practice of psychotherapy, a person who does not believe in this relationship or who actively opposes it could not be expected to examine it effectively within the context of his or her practice of psychotherapy. Therefore, the requirements that a men's psychotherpy group must by definition explicitly acknowledge the importance of gender-role concerns and must in some manner address these concerns serve to confirm that the psychotherapist at least will bring a particular belief system to the group. He or she may more or less actively attempt to encourage group members to share these beliefs, but this is not a universal or even necessarily a desirable undertaking.

In summary, a necessary condition for a men's psychotherapy group of the type being discussed in this chapter is that at least during part of its life it will be all male. But the quality of being all male is not a sufficient condition for defining this type of men's psychotherapy group. In addition, the all-male psychotherapy group must incorporate a belief system regarding the relationship between gender-role expectations and emotional distrubance and provide an opportunity for expression of conflicts in this area in order to be labeled a men's psychotherapy group.

OUTCOMES

No systematic research has been undertaken to determine the outcomes of the several types of men's groups. Yet those men's groups which have been described are subjectively reported to be positive experiences by the men who have participated in them. Although the characteristics of women's groups and men's groups have been shown to be different in many respects, it may be helpful to examine some of the research about the outcomes of women's groups in order to arrive at a better understanding of outcomes for men's groups.

Most authors who have reported on the outcomes for women's groups have described positive changes for women who have been members of either a women's consciousness-raising or a women's psychotherapy group.[25–27] There is a great variation in the manner of reporting outcomes, but the positive changes for women in women's groups can be grouped into four general areas: (1) women's groups provide an opportunity for increased affiliation with other women and for recognition of women as a distinct social group with specific characteristics; (2) women's groups lead to the acquisition of a more positive internalized sense of identity as a woman; (3) women's groups lead to more egalitarian relationships with men; and (4) women's groups lead to a greater awareness of sexism, promote the expression of anger against sexism, and increase women's determination to change rigid gender-role definitions for themselves and within society in general. These outcomes suggest that women's groups provide a means both for increasing a woman's personal sense of positive identity as a woman and at the same time for promoting change in the social requirements and restrictions regarding how a woman is supposed to behave.

To the extent that men's groups attempt to accomplish outcomes comparable to women's groups, similar positive outcomes could be described as enhancing an individual male's image of himself as a man and promoting for men in general a greater flexibility in their expression of the masculine gender role. The extent to which a particular men's group accomplishes these outcomes will depend on the purposes and characteristics of the group. For example, different specific outcomes can clearly be expected following participation in a men's consciousness-raising group and in a men's psychotherapy group. A group of men meeting together for purposes of personal awareness will share different goals than a group of male psychiatric patients who come together because of emotional distress. Some more specific positive outcomes can be postulated for men's groups in general, however. The effectiveness of a given group in achieving these outcomes can only be determined through the systematic study of actual groups over time. These predicted outcomes for men's groups derive from the rationale presented in a previous section of this chapter and from reports by individual men who have participated in such groups.

First, an increased awareness about the masculine role and about an individual man's experience of being male in American society can be expected. Every type of men's group should at least provide an opportunity for acquiring this awareness even if the members vary in the extent to which they actually do so. For some groups, particularly educational groups, this outcome may be the primary goal of the group. Other types of groups, such as men's consciousness-raising groups, will generally view this as either an early or partial goal during the group's life. A men's psychotherapy group may emphasize this goal to a greater or lesser extent depending on the severity of emotional disturbance and the relevance of this issue to the problems of the individual men in the group.

A second outcome can be a greater sense of personal freedom as a man. This outcome would result from acquiring a greater flexibility in expressing feelings and from engaging in activities which are generally considered unmasculine, such as rearing children and entering traditionally female professions. With the support of other men in a group, men can be freed to experiment with more options in their lives and to make choices based to a greater extent on personal interests and talents and less on social stereotypes for masculine behavior. While this outcome may be an ideal result of any personal growth experience, it has particular relevance with respect to the dimension of masculinity presented in men's groups. A greater sense of personal freedom in other areas of one's life as well can result from the experience of being in a men's group for many men.

A third positive outcome is greater satisfaction in interpersonal relationships. Men, through understanding themselves better as men, may also acquire a greater understanding of women. A recognition of real differences and real similarities between men and women can replace stereotyped impressions of how men and women are or should be. The experience of encountering other men within a men's group can also lead to greater empathy with men in general. Some men's groups may meet periodically during their existence with women's groups to explore new ways of interacting with women. Other men may enter a group of both men and women following participation in a men's group.

A fourth and final outcome for men's groups is a change in relationship to social institutions. Recognition of individual and social sexism directed against both men and women and exploration of nonsexist approaches can encourage personal and political confrontation of discrimination based on gender. For some men this confrontation may take the form of direct political action to change laws and regulations which promote such discrimination. Other men, who do not choose to become politically involved, may still acquire a greater understanding of how they relate to the authority of social institutions and as a result alter their personal patterns of interactions with these institutions. For example, a man who is about to become a father may, following participation in a men's group, challenge established regulations where he works which discriminate against men with respect to paternity leave.

APPLICATIONS OF MEN'S GROUPS IN THE MENTAL HEALTH FIELD

The discussion of the characteristics of men's groups, the different types of men's groups, and some general outcomes of men's groups provides a background for looking at the specific application of men's groups in the field of mental health. In the following section the author will examine the clinical application of men's groups in the practice of psychotherapy.

Men's groups have not been extensively utilized either as an approach to psychotherapy or as a method of educating mental health professionals. Several reasons other than the fact that men's groups are not a widespread phenomenon in American society in general can be suggested for the paucity of experience with men's groups within the mental health field. First, as described in a preceding section, these groups can be difficult to work with because of the problems men present in communicating when in small groups. Some psychotherapists may not work with men's groups as a result of their awareness of these problems and because of a lack of experience in successfully resolving such problems within an all-male setting.

A second reason for the small number of men's groups in the mental health field may derive from the fact that working with such groups can confront the male psychotherapist with the same conflicts with which the men in the group must struggle. These conflicts include ambivalence about changing gender-role arrangements, difficulty in arriving at new expressions of masculinity, and guilt about being a man. In addition, the lack of responsiveness of men in general to issues raised by the Women's Movement can also occur among male psychotherapists and may lead to reluctance or even to inability to examine concerns about gender roles presented by male and female patients. This reluctance may be expressed in a theoretical argument that the proper scope of psychotherapy does not include social issues, or it may be expressed even more directly in the form of actual disapproval of changes in gender-role expressions in patients. Recent efforts to educate men who are hostile or apathetic to changes in women[28] may also be helpful for some of those male psychotherapists who are unwilling to examine their own experiences of being male and of relating to women. Such efforts could promote in these therapists an increased awareness, a greater sensitivity, and an enhanced skill in addressing concerns regarding gender-role experiences which are presented by both male and female patients.

Other reasons for the small number of men's groups in the mental health field include a general unfamiliarity with and lack of information about this approach to working with patients, the smaller number of men as compared with women who enter psychotherapy and who are therefore available for participating in men's groups, and the absence of evidence regarding the effectiveness of men's groups in helping men who are in emotional distress. Utilizing men's groups on a wider basis and in a variety of settings, reporting in the professional literature on such clinical experiences with men's groups, and systematically studying the outcomes of these groups for men who participate in them will provide a basis for determining the actual usefulness of men's groups as an approach to psychotherapy.

The clinical discussion of men's groups presented in this section is based largely on the author's experience as an educator and a psychiatrist who has worked with such groups. Recently he has found among mental health professionals an increasing interest in and enthusiasm about the use of men's groups. He believes that this growing responsiveness to the idea of men's groups is in large part a result of the effectiveness of women's groups in addressing problems with gender-role expectations among women. The extent of further application of two types of men's groups, consciousness-raising and psychotherapy groups, may determine the ability of mental health professionals to work with parallel concerns among men.

THE APPLICATIONS OF MEN'S CONSCIOUSNESS-RAISING GROUPS. Men's consciousness-raising groups can serve to increase the awareness of men about problems arising as a result of enacting rigid, stereotyped gender-role expectations, to offer support for men who are sharing similar concerns in these areas, and to promote change among these men. These groups can be a valuable community resource to which men who present to psychotherapists or other mental health workers with such concerns can be referred in the same manner in which patients are referred to other community "self-help" groups.

Increasingly, no single approach is offered for the treatment and care of patients who present with mental health problems; rather attempts are made to provide medical care, psychological and behavioral treatment, attention to the social support system of the patient and, if necessary, legal intervention. The validity of using men's consciousness-raising groups as part of such a comprehensive treatment program for some men cannot be stated at this time. However, increased belief[29,30] in the need for broad-reaching behavioral and social interventions in the practice of psychotherapy and of medicine in general suggests that social support systems which are perceived to be helpful—as men's consciousness-raising groups are by the men who participate in them—should be made more available to patients. While the actual relationship between beliefs and behaviors associated with the masculine role and the development of disease may never be precisely determined, efforts by men to achieve attitudes and behaviors which appear to be associated with a greater degree of health can nevertheless be supported. The mental health field can contribute to this holistic movement through its practitioners' being informed about the existence of men's consciousness-raising groups and then recommending participation in such groups for those men who might benefit from them. It can also contribute to this movement to promote mental health in men by further studying the relationship between specific diseases and the psychological and social expression of the masculine gender role.

Three examples where a recommendation to participate in men's consciousness-raising group could be viewed as part of a comprehensive treatment and care program for men can be presented. These examples are the substance abuse patient, the cardiac patient, and the patient diagnosed as having one of the broad categories of disturbance classified as reactive or adjustment disorder and associated with depressive symptoms. Patients with each of these categories of disease include large numbers of men, and factors described as being associated with the disease also represent characteristics which are related to the definition of the masculine gender role. Specifically, each of these disorders involves, in addition to many identified and hypothesized biologic factors, particular patterns of reacting to and coping with stress in the environment. The male alcoholic patient who reacts to anxiety by drinking, the compulsive, driven man who develops hypertension or has a heart attack, and the man who reacts to divorce with symptoms of severe depression can all be viewed as men who are in part enacting aspects of the stereotypic masculine role in American society. Through hiding feelings, through behaving in an excessively competitive and aggressive manner, or through viewing the loss of a relationship with a woman as a cause for lowering of self-esteem and helplessness, these men may be enacting pathological extremes of the masculine role.

Selecting men who could be referred to men's consciousness-raising groups will depend on two factors: first, the careful evaluation of the appropriateness of such a group for an individual man and second, the availability of such groups within a particular community. Within the midwestern community in which the author practices, several such groups currently exist. One men's group has met for over five years in a local church. Several of the members of this group have entered psychotherapy following participation in the group, and other men have joined this group as a result of being in psychotherapy. Separate groups have been formed on the initiative of other men who have either been patients or colleagues of the author. These groups have served for some men as a valuable adjunct to psychotherapy for purposes of consciousness raising and support; for others they have provided a setting in which emotional problems which could better be resolved within a more traditional and structured psychotherapy relationship are first recognized.

A second application of men's consciousness-raising groups within the mental health field is their direct use in the training of mental health professionals. Participation in a men's consciousness-raising group could accomplish this goal of increasing the individual male mental health practitioner's self-awareness regarding gender-role issues. The results of a systematic encouragement of men's consciousness-raising groups for these men cannot be predicted at this time. However, it is clear that professional mental health training and continuing education programs have failed to pay attention to gender-related issues and sexism among men. Arguments regarding the proper scope of psychiatry and other mental health disciplines or the relative biological or psychosocial emphasis of a particular training program may be used against the idea of a direct application of men's consciousness-raising groups in mental health education. However, the increasing number of reports of women's groups for female residents and psychiatrists[31,32] suggests that there can be advantages for similar groups of men as well. Within the field of psychiatry, Robertiello[33] is one psychotherapist who has written about his experiences in a men's consciousness-raising group, and participation in such groups by male psychiatrists has now been reported about by a small number of male psychiatrists at recent annual meetings of the American Psychiatric Association.

Opinions about the advantages and value of men's consciousness-raising groups for mental health practitioners will probably continue to vary considerably depending both on perceptions regarding the role of psychiatry and the other mental health professions in general and on the interests and skills of individual professionals. But for some of these men, and potentially a large number, the experience of participating in a men's consciousness-raising group may be an important opportunity to increase self-awareness and to understand better the particular concerns of male and female patients regarding gender-role issues. This opportunity has not yet been realized by mental health professionals on a large scale.

The Applications of Men's Psychotherapy Groups. Evaluation, Selection, and Uses of Men's Psychotherapy Groups. The clinical applications for men's psychotherapy groups discussed in this section remain, at this point, suggestions for use, since there exists little evidence that such groups have actually been utilized within the mental health field. Two principles must be considered if these applications are to become viable therapeutic alternatives. First, the same requirements which exist for evaluating the appropriateness of an individual patient for any psychotherapy group must also be applied in selecting men for participation in a men's psychotherapy group. Consideration is given to the setting and purpose of the group, the degree to which an individual man could benefit from participating in group psychotherapy, and the composition of a particular group. Both the general principles regarding selection of patients for small groups and the specific criteria of the individual practitioner in selecting patients for groups will apply to men's psychotherapy groups as well. A second principle which must be applied is that men's psychotherapy groups must be studied as they are tried so that greater precision can be arrived at in predicting their usefulness for individual men.

Men's psychotherapy groups may be the desired treatment of choice for three types of men who are evaluated to be otherwise appropriate for group psychotherapy. These three types of patients are those with significant disturbance in interpersonal relationships, those with concerns about gender identity, and those men with specific concerns related to gender-role performance. These categories of patients may present with a wide variety of specific diagnoses and individual concerns, but each may benefit from participation in a men's psychotherapy group. Depending on the degree and nature of individual disturbance, a men's psychotherapy group may be the single approach to care or may be used in conjunction with other approaches, such as the use of medication or in combination with individual, marital, or family therapy.

No consistent criteria for selecting those men who could benefit most from men's psychotherapy groups can be presented. The psychotherapist must first be willing to consider this treatment approach for his or her patients and then must attempt to understand how a particular man's concerns could best be worked with within the setting of a men's group. A helpful approach to selecting men for a men's psychotherapy group will involve assessment of the same areas which are evaluated in all patients combined with a particular emphasis on deciding how an all-male setting might be appropriate for an individual patient. For example, in obtaining a developmental history, specific developmental lags which are identified, such as failure to develop a relationship with father or failure to establish meaningful same-sex friendships during latency, may be reflected in current problems in interpersonal relationships. The opportunity to work with these problems within the environment of a men's psychotherapy group may be helpful for some men. Experimentation with a variety of types of groups will help to determine the usefulness of men's psychotherapy groups for different types of patients. For example, a married couples' group may benefit from having separate all-male and all-female sessions during the course of the group. And men who have experienced similar life situations, such as divorce or job difficulties, may find a men's psychotherapy group particularly useful.

Men with a variety of physical diseases may also find a men's psychotherapy group helpful because this type of group would provide an opportunity to discuss those aspects of the disease which are associated with being a male in American society. The masculine gender role could be especially relevant in considering two aspects of physical disease, the hypothesized relationship between the etiology of a variety of diseases, such as hypertension and heart disease, and patterns of coping with stress, and the impact of physical incapacitation on the ability of men to function as males are expected to perform in our society. An excessive requirement for men to achieve and compete may contribute to the development of physical disease in some men. The real or perceived loss of this ability to achieve and compete associated with illness for other men may lead to distress in the area of masculine identity. Thus, both the causes and the effects of physical illness may for some men be related to their experience of the masculine gender role.

The types of groups which would be appropriate for such men would depend on the degree of associated psychopathology. Many men's groups which might be formed in general medical settings would probably not be designated as psychotherapy groups, but rather would be discussion groups which focus on reactions to loss, such as the loss of sexual functioning and of ability to work which result from some illnesses. The important difference between these groups and groups of men which already exist in medical settings would be the focus on issues of gender-role expression and the relevance of these issues to the illness. For example, groups of male cardiac patients who presently meet for purposes of regular exercise and education could also be structured to encourage discussion of losses associated with being men. Men's psychotherapy groups constituted of men with physical illnesses could be appropriate for those patients with seriuos psychopathology which develops in relation to their physical illnesses.

Men's psychotherapy groups may also be useful within those institutions, such as military hospitals and prisons, which are almost exclusively all male. Identified psychiatric populations within these institutions who are also evaluated to be appropriate for group psychotherapy could benefit from participation in a men's psychotherapy groups. The rationale for such groups derives from a belief in the interplay between the particular psychiatric disorder of an individual and his environment. In some all-male institutional settings, such as prisons, there is an increased likelihood that the environment may reinforce the development of particularly destructive expressions of the masculine gender role, including violence and excessive regimentation. Psychiatric patients within these settings may be especially vulnerable and could benefit from examination of their experience of being men within these settings. All male institutions or other settings, such as male wards in mental hospitals, may also foster the development of particular concerns related to the experience of being a man, such as fears of homosexuality, anxiety concerning athletic performance, or performance in other traditionally masculine areas. Men's psychotherapy groups or men's discussion groups may be helpful for men with these concerns as well.

THE THERAPIST IN A MEN'S PSYCHOTHERAPY GROUP. The author's experiences in working with men's psychotherapy groups will serve to illustrate some of the problems the male psychotherapist may encounter in such groups. Generally he conducts psychotherapy groups with a combination of the group-as-a-whole approach described by Bion[34] and approaches utilizing individual interpretation and interpersonal interactions. In working with men's groups, he has sometimes experienced requirements which seem contradictory with his role as leader in these groups. The beliefs he holds as a group psychotherapist and the manner in which he applies these beliefs may tend to reinforce the notion that he, as a male leader, represents aspects of an aloof, nonfeeling, and authoritarian masculine role. His parallel belief in the necessity for the therapist in a men's psychotherapy group to model nontraditional behaviors and attitudes has at times led to a conflict for him in his perception of his role as a psychotherapist. The gradual resolution of this conflict through the integration of these seemingly discrepant views into a single belief system has resulted in a more consistent pattern of leadership, a pattern which provides for a greater flexibility in his role as a therapist not only in men's groups but in all of the groups within which he works.

The pattern of leadership which the author now attempts to follow incorporates some of the same masculine-identified and feminine-identified characteristics which the men in the groups are seeking to integrate as well. One example of his changing belief system has been to view his interpretations, which still derive from an awareness of unconscious and dynamic processes in groups and individuals, as *alternative* insights. Thus, he attempts to listen to his patients without utilizing what Farrell[2] labels as the masculine technique of self-listening. Many psychotherapists may believe that their interpretation of a patient's experience is the only correct interpretation and therefore listen to patients only in order to state their own insights and values about these experiences. While a therapist of any theoretical orientation may arrive at similar conclusions about what is effective in working with patients, the particular belief which the author holds, in part as a result of working with groups of men, is that the process identified as self-listening is a derivative of the masculine gender role. As such, the therapist in a men's psychotherapy group may choose to demonstrate actively that he can simply listen to a patient or that he can admit the inappropriateness of an interpretation following discussion with the patient. Through such choices the male psychotherapist can demonstrate directly that men can be more passive in interactions and can admit errors even while being in positions of perceived authority.

Another example of the author's behavior which has altered because of his changing belief system has been the degree to which he presents intellectual in contrast to affective interventions in men's psychotherapy groups. Because many men have difficulty expressing feelings directly, encouragement of the greater expression of feelings may over time be more helpful to these men even at those times when an intellectual insight appears to be more appropriate or obviously relevant. The author also utilizes self-disclosure regarding his immediate feelings when appropiate in order to model the expression of feelings for men. Through a greater emphasis on showing feelings and a decreased use of intellectualized interpretations, he has attempted to integrate his beliefs about the need for changes in men with his beliefs about the role of the psychotherapist. Unlike other therapists who may demonstrate similar behavior, he has undertaken these changes because of his particular understanding of gender-role characteristics and of the need to provide greater flexibility for both men and women in the expression of these characteristics.

While each male psychotherapist working with a men's group will determine the nature of his role as a function of his belief system, his personality characteristics and the needs of a particular group, all male therapists who work with such groups will be confronted with particular issues which may challenge their conception of their roles as men and as psychotherapists. For the author, issues concerning authority, male silence, expression of feelings, and sexuality recurrently arose during his work as a therapist in men's psychotherapy groups. An important task for each therapist will be to distinguish between those aspects of his individual concerns which arise in reaction to intrapsychic transference and countertransference material and those which arise as a result of interpersonal and social challenges to stereotyped attributes associated with the masculine role. Such challenges will occur for the therapist as well as for the patients in men's psychotherapy groups.

MEN'S PSYCHOTHERAPY GROUPS IN PRACTICE. A clinical example of one men's group with which the author has worked will serve to highlight certain of the characteristics of men's psychotherapy groups, some of the problems in working with these groups, and possible outcomes for the members of men's groups. This group consisted of six men who were highly homogeneous with respect to age and to educational and socioeconomic levels. All of the men were between 20 and 35 years old, had some college or graduate school education, and were either currently employed or in school. Three of the men were married and three were single. This group first met for several sessions in a mixed group with an equal number of women, subsequently met for twelve weekly sessions as a men's group and then returned to the mixed group setting. Teresa Bernardez, M.D. and the author were coleaders for the mixed group.

Videotaped segments of the initial session of this men's group have been shown for purposes of training to several audiences of mental health professionals. This session has consistently stimulated similar observations and reactions in these audiences. The men in the group discuss a wide range of topics of concern to them with particular emphasis on problems of relating both to other men and to women. The pattern and content of the discussion demonstrate a general lack of straightforward affective expression by the men, a high level of intellectualization, a frequent reference to women and to the qualities women possess which seem unavailable to the men, and a virtual absence of direct interaction between the men. The content of the verbalizations does not always seem to flow in a clear manner from speaker to speaker, largely because the men rarely speak directly to each other. In spite of these qualities, the group generally evokes a strong reaction in the audiences who observe it in response to the intensity of the wishes conveyed by the men to be different and the degree of isolation they describe in their interpersonal relations. These factors are directly described by this group of men as a derivative of pressures they feel to behave in stereotypically masculine ways, including denying expression of their feelings, requiring the presence of women for conveying feelings related to intimacy and caring for others, and following certain rules of interaction with other men which emphasize athletic and other forms of competition. Other groups of men with whom the author has worked have described similar experiences but have not always linked these experiences as directly to their perceptions of characteristics associated with the masculine gender role.

One direct exchange does occur in this session between two men and illustrates the fear some men have of being like women if they change their ways of behaving as men. Prior to this exchange, several of the men talked about their dissatisfaction with the feeling that they had to compete with other men or to act in certain ways, such as hiding their feelings when they were upset and showing an interest in athletics, in order to be accepted as men. One man then talks about his wish to be different in how he shows his feelings than most men seem to be. Another man responds to this expressed wish by saying, "That's what I don't like about you sometimes. You seem to want to be like a woman." This derogation of characteristics which appear unmasculine and are identified with women (You will "be like a woman" if you show your feelings differently than other men) seemed to be shared by all of the members of this group. Even the man who had expressed his wish to change how he showed his feelings agreed with the second man's disapproval of his appearing to want to be like a woman. At the time of this exchange, the specific qualities associated with a feminine expression of feelings had not even been identified, and the men seemed to be reacting to a generalized fear simply of being unmasculine or of becoming effeminate. Subsequent development of this theme revealed an underlying fear of loss of potency and effectiveness which is associated with losing a sense of masculine identity. This internal masculine identity may be perceived to be particularly fragile when it is viewed as largely equivalent to characteristics attributed to expression of the masculine gender role.

The pattern of discussion in this group, the nature of the concerns expressed by the men, and their initial attempts to resolve these problems can be viewed within the context of a large number of theoretical frameworks. A group psychotherapist emphasizing the interpersonal dynamics of the members might understand this group session as a demonstration of immature and unsuccessful patterns of relating and seek to encourage different patterns of relating among the men. Such a view would attend to both the process and the content displayed by these men. Another therapist, having a more analytical and intrapsychic orientation, might approach this group with an understanding based upon the distorted or unsuccessfully resolved conflicts regarding dependency and identity conveyed by the men in the group. Both of these views would be accurate and could serve as a basis for helping the men to change, but neither alone incorporates an appreciation of the extent to which social pressures require men to behave in certain masculine-identified ways and prohibit men from demonstrating other feminine-identified traits.

It is this additional level of understanding, one which recognizes the importance of characteristics associated with gender roles in determining thoughts, feelings, and behaviors, that is essential in working with a men's psychotherapy group. As a result of the author's belief in the importance of gender roles in understanding what happened to the group, his interventions during the first session were few in number and were intended primarily to clarify comments by the members and to focus their discussion more on the here and now of the group and between the members. Such interventions would serve both to model for the men a less active and controlling male presence and to encourage a more immediate interpersonal exchange between the men. One of these interventions described the intellectual quality of the discussion about men in society and linked this quality to possible fears about what would happen in the immediate setting of this all male group. The initial reaction to this intervention was denial of fear in the group. One man stated that he felt more comfortable in an all-male setting, and another man stated that he perceived this group as a controlled "laboratory," which would not evoke such fears. After the initial denial of this fear, however, and following the author's listening to their disagreement, one man proceeded to talk about his fears of homosexuality. Soon after this comment, the exchange between the two men regarding men becoming like women occurred. Both of these comments served to move the men to a more direct expression of feelings and to a more immediate interaction with each other.

The eventual outcomes for the members of this short-term men's psychotherapy group were both positive and negative. Several of the men reported a sense of dramatic improvement in their understanding of themselves as men and in their behaviors in interactions with men and women outside of the group. One married couple were in the mixed group together, and participated separately in the two same-sex groups. Their marital relationship, which had been highly stressful for both partners prior to the group, changed significantly following being in the group. Both the man and the women were able to accept the wife's striving for greater independence through returning to school and beginning her own career. The husband, during the course of the group, learned about his reactions to his wife's changes, expressed his own difficulties in accepting his altered role as husband and father, and explored new ways of establishing his independence as a man.

In contrast, another man dropped out of the group following the return to a mixed group setting after the twelve sessions as a men's group. The conscious focus of his dissatisfaction was intense anger at the author. He reported that in contrast to the female therapist the author appeared "unavailable" to him. In addition to presenting his own dynamic and conflictual issues, this man also seemed to represent the views of several other men in the group who had not had well-established relationships with their fathers and who had difficulty establishing adult relationships with male authority figures. The lack of significant relationships with males for individual men may be recapitulated in a men's group through extreme difficulty in establishing meaningful relationships within the group or through the presence of persistent anxiety and ambivalence as aspects of male–male relationships are explored.

This particular men's psychotherapy group may have been especially problematic for this man for two reasons. First, the group was so short in duration that there was not sufficient time for him to work through conflictual material. Second, the experimental structure of this group, which alternated between a mixed and a same-sex composition, may have worked against the resolution of or actually reinforced this man's problems. He had been raised almost exclusively by women, and like several other men in the group, he attributed many expressive and relational capacities almost solely to women. When the men's group met after first meeting together with women, he reported a loss of a sense of being able to relate as openly. And the eventual return to the mixed setting seemed to precipitate his decision to leave the group. This return of women to the group may have represented to him a reminder of feminine attributes which now seemed even more unavailable to him and which he believed to be similarly absent in me. Thus, while several factors worked against the direct resolution of this man's conflicts within this group, a major factor seemed to be the variable structure and composition of the group. His situation suggests the importance of understanding the personality structure and dynamics of each man before recommending psychotherapy in a men's group.

This group was atypical in comparison with the other men's psychotherapy groups with which the author has worked in two respects: first, none of the men in this group demonstrated signs of severe emotional distress and second, the group was the shortest-term men's group the author has conducted. But the eventual outcomes, given the nature of the members' concerns and the length of time the group lasted, were comparable for this and the other groups. Five of the six men reported satisfaction with their experiences in the group and demonstrated significant improvement in their presenting problems, which included moderate depression, anxiety in interpersonal relationships, and significant disturbance in marital relationships. In addition to the positive changes described in these areas, the five men all reported an enhanced self-esteem with respect to their expression of the masculine gender role. While similar changes might be accomplished in other types of groups, the specific focus on feelings, thoughts, and behaviors associated with the masculine gender role seemed to promote a more rapid and significant positive change in interpersonal relationships as well as in the other areas of concern to the members.

These changes were demonstrated within the group itself as well as in descriptions of experiences outside of the group. The fears of becoming like women initially expressed by the men were further clarified in later sessions of the group and served to highlight the irrational and stereotyped nature of responses to expressions and behaviors associated with the masculine and feminine gender roles. None of the men in fact simply lost masculine-associated attributes or acquired feminine-associated attributes. Instead, all of them experimented with demonstrating a greater range of characteristics in their internal representations of themselves as men, in their interactions with other men, and in their relationships with women. This simple acquisition of flexibility in the expression of gender-associated characteristics was the single most positive outcome for most of the men and resulted in a greater ability of the men to express feelings of vulnerability, caring, and dependency and a diminished need to compete, to dominate, and to appear aggressive in relations to others.

All of the men's psychotherapy groups with which the author has worked have led to many valuable outcomes for the men in them. The resolution of the problems with which the men initially presented has appeared to take place as readily as in other types of group settings. And the men in these groups have in addition been able to explore concerns related to the masculine gender role which are problematic for many men today. All of the groups which have met periodically with women's groups as well have reported satisfaction with these experiences and have viewed the opportunity to meet in both same-sex and mixed-sex settings as beneficial to them. In his future work with such groups, the author intends to refine further both the technical aspects of working with men's groups and the description of specific indications and outcomes for these groups.

CONCLUSION

Men's groups have been explored in this chapter as a social phenomenon, as an approach to psychotherapy, and as a part of the author's personal and professional experiences. Their relevance for individual men will depend on many factors including interest, motivation, and capacity to function within a small group setting. Each of these factors must be considered by the clinician in evaluating individuals for participation in men's groups. The greater utilization of men's groups within the field of psychotherapy can provide many men with the opportunity for an enhanced appreciation of themselves as men and for greater satisfaction in their relationships with other men and with women. The wider application of men's groups in the training of male mental health professionals can also lead to an increased awareness about gender-role concerns on the part of psychotherapists. For some men, traditional masculine activities such as athletic events and club or lodge meetings have been supplemented or even replaced by participation in men's consciousness-raising, support, or psychotherapy groups. The purposes of this chapter are both to inform the mental health professional about this occurrence as it relates to a growing number of men's lives and to encourage an increased interest in the direct application of men's groups in psychotherapy. The future of men's groups as an approach to psychotherapy will depend on the careful examination of the benefits such groups provide to the men who participate in them.

References

1. Bradley M, Danchik L, Fager, M, and Wodetzki T: Unbecoming Men. Albion, California, Times Change Press, 1971
2. Farrell WT: Women's and men's liberation groups, in Women in Politics. Edited by Jaquette J. New York, Wiley, 1974, pp 171–199
3. Pleck J, Sawyer J: Men and Masculinity. Englewood Cliffs, New Jersey, Spectrum Books, 1974
4. Wong MR: Males in transition and the self-help group. Counseling Psychol 7:46–50, 1978
5. Bernardez-Bonesatti T, Stein T: Separating the sexes in group therapy: An experiment with men's and women's group. Int J Group Psychother 29:493–502, 1979
6. Amann D: Moving towards men's liberation. Chicago Tribune, Section 12, pp 1, 4, Aug 5, 1979
7. Farrell W: The Liberated Man. New York, Random House, 1974
8. Fasteau MF: The Male Machine. New York, McGraw-Hill, 1974
9. Goldberg H: The Hazards of Being Male. New York, New American Library, 1976
10. Tolson A: The Limits of Masculinity. New York, Harper and Row, 1977
11. Stein T: The effects of the Women's Movement on men: A therapists view. Presented at the Annual Meeting of the American Psychiatric Association, Chicago, Illinois, May 16, 1979
12. Miller JB: The future of female–male relationships. Presented at the Annual Meeting of the American Psychiatric Association, Chicago, Illinois, May 16, 1979
13. Spence J, Helmreich R: Masculinity and Femininity. Austin, University of Texas Press, 1978
14. Aries E: Interaction patterns and themes of male, female and mixed groups. Small Group Behav 7:7–18, 1976
15. Washington C: Men counseling men: Redefining the male machine. Personnel Guidance J 57:462–63, 1979
16. Moreland J: A humanistic approach to facilitating college students learning about sex roles. Counseling Psychol 6:61–64, 1976
17. Goldberg H: The New Male. New York, Morrow, 1979
18. Chodorow N: The Reproduction of Mothering. Berkeley, University of California Press, 1978
19. Miller JB: Anger and aggression in women and men. Presented at the Annual Meeting of the American Academy of Psychoanalysis, New York, December 2, 1979
20. Kirsh B: Consciousness-raising groups as therapy for women, in Women in Therapy. Edited by Frank V, Burtle V. New York, Bruner/Mazel, 1974, pp 326–54
21. Chesler P: Patient and patriarch: Women in the psychotherapeutic relationship, in Women in Sexist Society. Edited by Gornick V, Moran BK. New York Basic Books, 1971, pp 362–392
22. Erikson EH: Childhood and Society. New York Norton, 1963
23. Hopkins LB: Inner space and outer space identity in contemporary females. Psychiatry 43:1–12, 1980
24. Anthony EJ: The history of group psychotherapy, in Comprehensive Psychotherapy. Edited by Kaplan HI, Sadock BJ. Baltimore, Williams and Wilkins, 1971, pp 4–31
25. Bernardez-Bonesatti T: Women's groups: A feminist perspective on the treatment of women, in Changing Approaches to the Psychotherapies. Edited by Grayson H, Loew C. New York, Spectrum Publications, 1978, pp 55–67
26. Brodsky AM: The consciousness-raising group as a model for therapy with women. Psychother: Theory Res Pract 10:24–29, 1973
27. Newton E, Walton S: The personal is political: Consciousness-raising and personal change in the women's liberation movement. Presented to an annual meeting of the American Anthropological Association, 1971
28. Choate RB: Personal communication. May 23, 1979
29. Pelletier KR: Mind as Healer, Mind as Slayer. New York, Dell, 1977
30. Stachnik TJ: Priorities for psychology in medical education and health care delivery. Am Psychol 35:8–15, 1980
31. Benedek EP, Poznanski E: Career choice for the woman psychiatric resident. Am J Psychiatry 137:301–305, 1980
32. Kirkpatrick M: A report on a consciousness-raising group for women psychiatrists. JAMWA 30(5): 1975
33. Robertiello RC: A Man in the Making. New York, Marek, 1979
34. Bion WR: Experiences in Groups. New York, Basic Books, 1961

Chapter 15

Clinical Behavior Therapy and the Male Sex Role

MARVIN R. GOLDFRIED AND JERRY M. FRIEDMAN

INTRODUCTION

Men rarely present themselves for treatment because they have identified problems associated with their roles as men. Yet such problems may often be at the core of the difficulties they do present with: difficulties they are experiencing in their marriages, problems with excessive use of alcohol, sexual dysfunctioning, stress-related problems, as well as the full array of psychological difficulties one is likely to encounter clinically. Behavior therapy, while having relevance to an increasingly more diverse set of clinical phenomena, has had little to say directly about problems centered around men's issues. However, behavior therapy does have a history of flexibility in areas of application, as it provides the clinician with more of a technology than a direction for specific areas of applicability. Behavioral procedures originally developed for one specific purpose have often later been applied to a wide variety of other clinical problems. The newly emerging field of "behavioral medicine" has drawn extensively on behavioral intervention methods for purposes of dealing with various physical disorders. And assertion training, while originally developed with no thought whatsoever as to its utility in dealing with problems associated with the female sex role, has nonetheless been used to help women become more instrumental in their functioning.

While the feminist movement can be credited with highlighting the relevance that assertion training has for women in our society, there has been little discussion of how various therapeutic procedures may be particularly appropriate in working with men clinically. Yet, the knowledge of the behavioral, cognitive, and emotional patterns associated with the male role can be extremely

MARVIN R. GOLDFRIED • Department of Psychology, AND JERRY M. FRIEDMAN • Department of Psychology and Psychiatry, State University of New York, Stony Brook, New York 11794

helpful in sensitizing clinicians to important factors that may be contributing to the presenting problems of male clients. Thus, knowledge that a male alcoholic's drinking behavior provides him with a nonthreatening and socially acceptable social context within which he may relate with other men on an intimate basis can provide therapists with information that can be useful in planning their therapeutic intervention.

The goal of this chapter is to explore some beginning links between the heretofore separate areas of behavior therapy and the male sex role. It begins with a brief overview of what it means to be a "man" in our society, emphasizing the premium placed on emotional inexpressiveness and excessive instrumentality. It then moves on to a consideration of some of the clinical problems that bring men for treatment, particularly marital conflict, sexual dysfunctions, and excessive drinking. Next, it deals with the scope of contemporary behavior therapy, and describes some intervention methods relevant to problems of men, such as relaxation training, cognitive restructuring, communication and negotiation training, sex therapy, and assertion/expressiveness training. The issue of psychological androgyny is considered, and the chapter concludes by returning to a discussion of the larger social system that one needs to attend to in any attempt to change men's functioning.

ON BEING A MAN

Boys learn to be a "psychological" male very early in life. As Bem[1] points out, most children are already behaving in accordance with their assigned sex role by the time they are in nursery school, but can still role play the opposite sex quite accurately. As children grow older, however, sex differences become even more pervasive. Males are motivated towards achievement and power, females toward affiliation and dependency.[2]

From athletics to the military, the masculine role stresses skill, competition, strength, endurance, aggression, and winning, while at the same time discounting emotional intimacy, dependency, and vulnerability. These two characteristics, namely, *male inexpressiveness* and *high instrumentality,* typify what it means to be a man in our society. Knowledge of these two patterns of functioning can be of immeasurable help to the practicing therapist in working with men clinically.

MALE INEXPRESSIVENESS. While all individuals have limitations in their ability to be expressive and open in their relations with others, men are particularly deficient in this aspect of human functioning. The very nature of "manliness" in our society emphasizes that men be objective, striving, tough, goal-oriented, unsentimental, and emotionally inexpressive. Perhaps the most typical emotional response available/permissible for men is that of anger, often resulting from interference with their goal-oriented behavior. The fear is, that if he is tender, if he weeps, if he shows weakness, other people (and he himself) will view him as inadequate and inferior, and certainly less of a "man." Thus, men frequently seem obliged to hide much of their real self, not only from the rest of the world, but from themselves.

Jourard[3] has hypothesized that the inexpressive aspect of the male role may account for the fact that men die sooner than women. Trying to seem manly, according to Jourard, is a kind of "work" that consumes energy and imposes stress. Therefore, manliness carries a chronic burden of energy expenditure and stress that could easily be a factor related to man's shorter life span. Jourard further suggested that if men are trained to ignore their own feelings in order to pursue the instrumental aspects of manliness, they will be less sensitive to internal signals that all is not well. They do not stop work until the destructive consequences of their behavior pattern has progressed to a point of total collapse.

"Manly" men, according to Jourard, are unaccustomed to self-disclosure and are characterized by less insight and less empathy than women. After self-disclosure patterns are developed, they are often maintained by the rewards or punishments in the environment. So even those men who may have the capacity and desire to express feelings may refrain from doing so because of fear of ridicule or rejection. This fear is most likely a realistic one. A study by Derlega and Chaikin[4] found that males who did not disclose information about a personal problem were rated—by women and men alike—as better adjusted than males who did disclose, while the opposite was true for women. Being reluctant to make themselves known to another person, including their spouses, it follows that men are more difficult to love, have more difficulty loving others, and find it especially difficult to love themselves. A number of research findings substantiate the linkage between the traditional male role and men's difficulty in relating to both women and other men, and may be found in a review by Lewis[5] and in Chapter 5, by Balswick, and Chapter 16, by Dosser in this book.

With the strong cultural prohibitions against any demonstration of intimacy between men, many adult males have difficulty having really open, trusting, emotional friendships with other men. As Fasteau[6] has pointed out, it is a bit ironic that many American men report their closest male friendships developing through sports or war, a time when they are bonded together to destroy or overcome others. An absence of role models for intimacy, a socialization towards competition and winning, and an aversion to vulnerability, all form severe barriers to intimacy between men. Several studies have demonstrated the power of the competitiveness between males from childhood to adulthood.[7–9] Clearly it is hard to reach out affectionately to another male if he is viewed as a competitor. If this were not enough, homophobia, the fear of homosexual contact or of appearing to be homosexual to others, exerts a particularly strong force within our culture to keep men from getting to know each other too intimately. Thus, male to male touching, except during contact sports, is something American men in particular seem to avoid. This may be some reflection of the general difficulty among many men in distinguishing between intimacy and sexuality; there appears to be a fear that experiencing one will automatically open the door to the other.

In a book that is aptly titled *The Male Machine,* Fasteau[6] describes not only the nonexpressive aspects of the male sex role, but also its highly instrumental nature. As Fasteau observes:

> The male machine is a special kind of being, different from women, children, and men who don't measure up. He is functional, designed mainly for work. He is programmed to tackle jobs, override obstacles, attack problems, overcome difficulties, and always seize the offensive. He will take on any task that can be presented to him in a competitive framework, and his most important positive reinforcement is victory. He has armor plating which is virtually impregnable. His circuits are never scrambled or overrun by irrelevant personal signals. He dominates and outperforms his fellows, although without excessive flashing of lights or clashing of gears. His relationships with other male machines is one of respect but not intimacy; it is difficult for him to connect his internal circuits with those of others. In fact, his internal circuitry is something of a mystery to him and is maintained primarily by humans of the opposite sex. (Ref. 6, p. 1)

It is evident that what men lack in interpersonal expressiveness, they make up for in their highly instrumental, goal-oriented approach to life.

MALE INSTRUMENTALITY AND THE TYPE-A BEHAVIOR PATTERN. The energy, anxiety, and stress expended on fulfilling the highly instrumental socially prescribed male role has a price. Not only do men miss out on many of the potential pleasures of life, but life itself may be shortened.[3,10] In fact, men do not live as long as women. In 1970, male death rates exceeded those of females by as much as 180% for those under 24, and by 110% for 55–64 year olds.[11] Although this apparent "fact of death" may be due to the genetic superiority of females over males, there is increasing evidence that the instrumental behavior pattern of men may play a significant role in this differential mortality. Of all the causes of death, cardiovascular disease remains the number one health problem in this country, with death rates from heart disease being twice as high for men as for women.[12]

Over the past ten years, research on heart disease has broadened to include the influence of psychological and social factors as well as medical and hereditary ones. In particular, the coronary-prone behavior pattern has been receiving an increasing amount of attention by researchers in the field.[13,14] Based on the work of Rosenman and Friedman, as well as subsequent efforts by others, the highly instrumental Type-A style of functioning has been found to be characterized by some or all of the following: an excessive competitive drive, an intense striving for achievement, a persistent involvement in multiple functions subject to deadlines, easily provoked impatience, time urgency, overcommitment to vocation or profession, abruptness of gesture and speech, an habitual propensity to accelerate the pace of living, an excess of drive and hostility, tenseness of facial musculature, restlessness, hyperalertness, and feelings of being under the pressure of time and challenge of responsibility. Those who show the opposite pattern, that is relaxation, serenity, and lack of time urgency, are known as Type B. Type A persons are often so committed to their vocations or professions that they neglect other aspects of life, such as family and recreation. They are described as active and energetic, and at the same time perfectionistic and unable to relax. It is not surprising that several of the attributes of Type-A behavior are those usually associated with the successful, urban, upwardly mobile, middle-class male. The behaviors that make up the Type-A pattern are, in fact, strongly *encouraged* in our society, and certainly not considered psychopathologic or socially deviant. In fact, ambition, goal-directiveness, and time urgency are precisely those qualities on which our society was built and continues to function.

The introduction of Type-A behavior pattern as a causative factor in coronary heart disease, particularly among men, was met with a great deal of skepticism and reserve by the medical and mental health community. Perhaps the concept was difficult to accept because the Type-A behavior pattern described so many of the professionals in these fields! Nonetheless, evidence has continued to mount, leaving little doubt that such a behavior pattern has a direct causative impact on heart disease.[15] In a major prospective study,[16,17] it was found that Type-A behavior proved to be a significant predictor of heart disease, independent of any associations with the standard risk factors. Even when one controls for the effect of other risk factors, Type-A men are twice as likely to develop or die from heart disease than are Type-B men. Following a first myocardial infarction, the risk of a subsequent one for Type-A men is approximately twice that experienced by Type-B men.

Type-A behavior is clearly more consistent with the traditional male than female role, and in fact, is more common among men than women.[11,18] This sex difference in the prevalence of Type-A behavior possibly contributes to men's higher rate of heart disease and mortality in general. While the sex difference may reflect both inherited factors as well as differential socialization—that is, society's tendency to reward men more than women for such Type-A behaviors as competition, aggressiveness, and ambition—available evidence suggests that the latter is more likely to constitute the determining factor.[19–23] It is particularly noteworthy that sex differences in Type-A behavior decline dramatically when factors of occupation, socioeconomic status, and age are taken into account. Women employed outside the home, particularly those past the age of 25, are more likely to manifest Type-A behavior patterns than are women not employed outside the home[23] and have Type-A scores that are closer to those of men.[22] Hence, the pattern is not so much a male pattern, but actually one that is associated with the traditional male sex role, so that women who assume this role may also be assuming the Type-A behavior pattern.

As suggested above, one of the most salient characteristics of the Type-A behavior pattern is an habitual sense of time urgency, reflected in the attempt to participate in too many events given the amount of time available. Type-A individuals usually behave as if they can successfully cope with anything. In this context, it is of considerable interest to contemplate the reverse of this: To the extent that individuals do *not* believe that they are able to control the forces in their lives, they eventually reach a state of "learned-helplessness"[24] and are typically found to be psychologically depressed. By contrast, Type-A individuals approach almost all tasks with active attempts at controlling the environment, and find it difficult to accept the fact that there may be situations over which they *have* no control.[25] In contrast to depressed individuals, they appear to have adopted an attitude of "learned invulnerability." It is almost as if we are dealing with two ends of a continuum, both of which are maladaptive. At one extreme, we have depressed individuals (typically women) who do not perceive themselves as having much ability to control anything in their lives; at the other end, there are the Type-A individuals (typically men) who believe that they are capable of coping with anything and everything. Both extremes depict the stereotypic definitions of what it means to be a female and male in our society.

WHAT BRINGS MEN INTO THERAPY?

Although an increasing number of men are starting to realize that emotional inexpressiveness and high instrumentality are frequently self-destructive, these male characteristics *per se* do not usually bring men into therapy. More typically, men seek therapy when their lives are not going well, and even then it is the authors' experience that this frequently happens at the insistence of someone else—either wife, girlfriend, physician, or employer. Although mental health professionals might argue that it requires a fair amount of strength to acknowledge personal upset, especially since such acknowledgment often carries with it the anticipation of punishment from others, it is not typically viewed this way by men themselves. In a sense, an individual who is willing to seek out professional help is more likely to be viewed and view himself as behaving in a manner more consistent with the "feminine" than with the "masculine" role.

Some men who enter therapy do so because of problems that may be construed as a less than successful incorporation of the male sex role into their functioning. These might include such problems as unassertiveness, underachieving, or being overly "emotional." Other men seem to have personal difficulties because they have incorporated the male sex role all too well. For example, a man may enter therapy at the insistence of his physician, usually after finding it difficult to make the necessary lifestyle adjustment following a heart attack. With increases in unemployment, more men are entering therapy in a state of crisis following the loss of a job and the associated loss of self-esteem. Although the family may be able to get by financially on the wife's earnings, the man may nevertheless experience great distress and/or depression. Other men enter therapy at the insistence of their employer, because of absenteeism resulting from chronic drinking behavior, or an inability to get along with fellow employees. Sexual difficulties, such as erectile failure, premature ejaculation, or low sexual desire may be other reasons for men seeking therapy, frequently at the insistence of their partner. An ever-increasing number of men are entering marital therapy, albeit reluctantly, with little understanding of what has gone wrong in their relationship. In most of these instances, men have little insight into the causes of their problems, particularly those that may have to do with how their role as a man creates difficulties for them. Some of these issues will be illustrated with three typical problems that men bring into therapy: marital distress, sexual dysfunction, and problems associated with excessive drinking.

MARITAL DISTRESS. The divorce rate in the United States has been estimated to range from 33% to 50%.[26] Moreover, Lederer and Jackson[27] found that 80% of the couples they interviewed reported having considered divorce at some time in their relationship. The very structure of contemporary marriage—or perhaps more approximately, lack of structure—helps foster conflict and marital dissatisfaction. Recent cultural changes certainly may be a large contributing factor to the growing divorce rate. In treating couples that have come for marital therapy in recent years, it is not uncommon to find that distress in the relationship is associated with the changing guidelines on which the marriage is based. This "upsetting of the applecart" is modifying a system that many have seen as a blessing for men at the expense of women.

Clearly defined roles of "husband" and "wife", though not necessarily resulting in happiness, tended to promote stability in the past. It is not unusual to find couples who have been married for a long period of time, but who interact in a very limited manner and never really get to know one another. They go their separate ways and interact not as unique individuals, but in terms of their respective socialized sex roles. These couples often do not show overt signs of distress, and may describe themselves as bored rather than unhappy. It is when people begin to question their marital roles and the rights and responsibilities associated with them, or are faced with a change in their family system, that marital distress can become overt.[28] Within an egalitarian relationship, rights and responsibilities are open to discussion, compromise is necessary, and consensus is required for decision making. As roles within the marriage change to incorporate more independence, jealousy can become a problem. With greater independence, there are more opportunities for the actions of the wife to be viewed as disloyal. For women, career opportunities or friendships outside the marriage, and other environmental factors may compete with her husband for her attention and may be a source of conflict and distress within the relationship. Also, if additional rewards are present in the outside world, more are required within the relationship to maintain it as a reasonable alternative.

When a couple enters marital therapy, it is not unusual to see the wife reaching out, exploring, and growing in a way completely incomprehensible to her husband. She may be working outside the home, going back to school, seeking a career, or in general developing her own individuality. Frequently, husbands are at a loss, and respond with anger, depression, and bewilderment. The implicit marriage contract with which they entered the relationship has been broken. A wife may have been dependent, passive, and helpless early in the marriage, but now has become more self-reliant, less eager to please, and better able to assert herself. She may no longer be the "sweet little thing" he married. It is certainly not surprising that a women may grow discontented with her "wifely" role long before her husband does. Although these changes may have been due to a wife's consciousness having been raised, they can also result from economic circumstances requiring that both partners work outside the home.

Scanzoni[28] presents evidence showing that attempts to transform traditional marital systems into more equal companionship marriages result in inevitable conflict and strife. Part of the problem is that spouses have not learned the skills necessary to help a companionship marriage function smoothly. Problems in communication are particularly devastating in marital relationships where couples are struggling to redefine the rules by which they interact. In fact, one of the most frequently occurring problems reported by couples in distressed relationships is the failure to communicate.[29,30] Just as men are frequently frustrated in their report that they simply "do not know what women want," women are often irritated by their male partners' lack of expressiveness. This lack of expressiveness and conflict over changing roles can have a strong impact on sexual functioning.

SEXUAL DYSFUNCTION. An attitude that has pervaded our culture is that the only problem men experience with their sexual behavior is that there is not enough of it. Although many men do experience sexual difficulties, the prevalence of such difficulties is not easily determined. The male myth that all men should be able to "perform" well at all times[31] makes it especially difficult for men to acknowledge and seek help for any sexual problems they may experience, such as premature ejaculation, erectile dysfunction, inhibited ejaculation, and inhibited sexual desire.

Men have to be "on"—for other men, for women, and for themselves. For men in which the traditional male role is firmly entrenched, there is increased difficulty and stress ahead as women become more successful in standing on an equal footing ("competing") with men. This is most strikingly seen in men's sexual interactions with women, where men often seek nonemotional involvement, as intimacy and dependency with women is "unmasculine." The quest for competence and performance, highly valued male traits, extends into the sexual area, causing a great deal of potential problems for men. Sexually, the man has almost always been viewed as someone who is always ready, able, and willing. This social script is learned early in life, well before the boy actually experiences any sexual feelings *per se*. As a man, he strives to get sex any way he can, reaching orgasm with as little tenderness, communication, and relating as possible. In fact, getting a woman to agree to sex has typically been viewed as full proof of masculine charm and power. In more recent years, many women are not willing to put up with this kind of male response, and require and expect a good deal more.

The recent emphasis on female sexuality and the acknowledgment of women as sexual beings has, for many men, changed the way they interact with their sexual partners. One of the most salient features of the masculine stereotype in our society is that a man, especially when it comes to sex, has no doubts, questions, or confusion. He knows what he has to do to have good sex.[31] To admit ignorance, concern, or a sexual problem is seen as a sign of vulnerability and weakness, and the accompanying risk of being considered something less than a real man by both women and men alike. To the extent that men adopt the stereotypic role for male sexual functioning, they may perceive any feedback as added pressure to "perform" as a good lover and to be responsible for their partner's sexual satisfaction.

The description of the instrumental, nonemotional "male machine"[6] may be somewhat of an exaggeration for many men in our society. Nonetheless, even those men who are somewhat in touch with their feelings and can allow themselves to be somewhat vulnerable, have bought into some part of the male myth. Consequently, when they "fail" sexually, when they are not as "good lovers" as they believe they "should" be, they often react in ways that can make their problem even worse.

There has been a noticeable change in the nature of the sexual difficulties that couples present to sex therapy centers, the incidence of low sexual desire appearing to be on the increase. A review of 39 recently completed cases at the Sex Therapy Center at the State University of New York at Stony Brook shows that 27 included complaints of low sexual desire. Of these, 17 (63%) involved low sexual desire on the part of the male. This higher incidence of low sexual desire among men is similar to the findings at other sex therapy centers,[32] and is especially interesting since low desire was not even identified as a sexual problem by Masters and Johnson[33] or by Kaplan in her earlier work.[34] This increased incidence may merely be a reflection of therapists' recent recognition of these difficulties, or may constitute an actual change in those who present themselves for therapy. It is certainly the case that males presenting with low sexual desire in the absence of any other dysfunction was virtually unknown until the late 1970s, and it has been suggested that this is at least somewhat of a reflection of the changing sex roles in our society.[35]

EXCESSIVE DRINKING. It has been estimated that approximately half of all first admissions to psychiatric hospitals in the United States are the result of problem drinking. Alcoholism has also been linked to the incidence of automobile accidents, various physical diseases, suicide, crime, absenteeism in the work place, and shortened life-span. According to a national survey by Calahan,[36] heavy drinkers tend to be of lower socioeconomic status, have little or no higher education, are single, divorced, or separated, are likely to be residents of large cities and, most relevant to the theme of this chapter, tend to be male. In fact, Calahan has found that the prevalence of drinking-related problems was more than twice as great among men than women (43% as compared to 21%). Men are more likely to become intoxicated, to experience blackouts, to use drinking to cope with feelings of tension and depression, and to have their drinking behavior threaten their marriage. Other surveys have found the prevalence rates for men to be even higher, reporting estimates of five times as many men than women experiencing such difficulties.[37]

The various theories of why people resort to excessive drinking have been dealt with at length by clinicians and researchers (e.g., Marlatt and Nathan[38]). Certainly, many forces within our society directly encourage drinking behavior (e.g., movies, advertisements), with only lip service being paid to some of its more serious consequences. Numerous social pressures from peers to drink exist in various subcultures. Indeed, the bar often functions as a setting in which a good deal of male socialization occurs. Inasmuch as alcohol serves as a central nervous system depressant, drinking also becomes reinforced by virtue of its ability to reduce feelings of tension. In addition, drinking can serve to help men slow down, loosen their inhibitions for social interaction, and become more socially expressive. To the extent that men believe it is inappropriate to have and express such feelings as upset, tenderness, and fear, alcohol can serve as a useful aid in facilitating such feelings without directly acknowledging them. When under the influence of alcohol, greater expressiveness among men carries less of a negative social sanction, as it can be attributed to the intoxicated state of the person and not the person himself.

Although there is still no consensus on any comprehensive theory for the development and maintenance of alcoholism, there is a growing recognition among workers in the field that modeling and other social learning factors can greatly enhance the likelihood that an individual will drink to excess. Inasmuch as the consumption of alcohol is typically conceived of as being a sign of masculinity in our society, the risk factors for the development of excessive dependence on alcohol are hence far greater for men than women. In his work on the possible modeling effects associated with heavy drinking, Marlatt[39] reports that the male heavy drinker has had a history of observing a same-sex model in his life who also drank to excess. Female drinkers, on the other hand, as well as males who were only light drinkers, were less likely to have had such models in their backgrounds. Marlatt further suggests that "It seems likely that many male problem drinkers have been influenced strongly by exposure to peers who drink heavily and by the cultural acceptance of drinking as a 'macho' expression of masculinity" (p. 329). There also exists evidence to indicate that excessive drinking typically occurs in situations where there is a sense of control by external sources, such as when there is evaluation or criticism by others, an unpleasant interpersonal encounter with another individual, a difficult life crisis, and other similar forces.[39]

Although men may voluntarily rely on drinking to reduce their feelings of tension and facilitate social interaction, the physical and psychologically addictive properties of alcohol eventually begin to play an increasingly more significant role. The therapeutic goal becomes that of assisting the individual not only in controlling his drinking behavior, but also to more effectively teach him to deal with those factors that may have contributed to the original need to drink.

BEHAVIORAL INTERVENTIONS

Behavior therapy has evolved over the past twenty years to a point of greater sophistication and breadth. Therefore, before describing some of the behavior therapy methods that may be useful in working with men clinically, it might be appropriate to first describe the characteristics of contemporary behavior therapy.

As a way of appreciating the scope of behavior therapy, one may view the field as comprising three separate but interwoven trends: classical conditioning, operant reinforcement principles, and cognitive psychology. Central to the *classical conditioning* emphasis, which has its roots in Hullian learning theory and Pavlovian conditioning, is the observation that stimuli appearing in temporal/spatial proximity tend to become functionally similar in eliciting various autonomic reactions. The *operant reinforcement* trend in the behavior therapy movement is based on the principle that much of our behavior is maintained by its consequences, and that altering reinforcement contingencies can have some very important effects in changing various problematic patterns of behavior. The third and newest trend in behavior therapy, that of emphasizing *cognitive* processes, is more recent in nature. Recognizing that principles of classical and operant conditioning were inadequate to explain and alter the full range of clinical problems likely to confront a therapist, behavioral clinicians and researchers began to emphasize the role of cognition in behavior maintenance and change. Work in the area of cognitive behavior therapy has developed fairly rapidly, and has been applied to such diverse areas as anxiety, depression, unassertiveness, anger, impulsivity, alcoholism, and eating disturbances.

It is unfortunate that behavior therapy is so often depicted as representing a clearly delineated "school" defined by a given pool of intervention methods. Behavior therapy has gone far beyond systematic desensitization or the contingent delivery of M&Ms, and defining it by such techniques is clearly shortsighted. Indeed, the pool of techniques that are employed by those who call themselves "behavior therapists" is continually changing. In providing a broader conceptualization, Goldfried and Davison[40] indicate

> that behavior therapy is more appropriately construed as reflecting a general orientation to clinical work that aligns itself philosophically with an experimental approach to the study of human behavior. The assumption basic to this particular orientation is that problematic behavior seen within the clinical setting can best be understood in light of those principles derived from a wide variety of psychological experimentation, and that these principles have implications for behavior change within the clinical setting. (pp. 3–4)

Following from this point of view, there are certain characteristics that are typically associated with a behavioral orientation to clinical work. These include the importance of operational definitions, the need for an ongoing behavioral assessment, an ahistorical emphasis, the systematic nature of the intervention, the emphasis on empirical verification, and the view of therapy as training in coping skills.

Operational Definitions. Although behavior therapists use such general terms as "anxiety," "depression," and "unassertiveness," it is recognized that these concepts represent general classes of an individual's response, and consequently must be operationalized in more specific ways. Thus, to say that a given client is "anxious" requires a further delineation of both the kinds of situations in which this reaction occurs (e.g., closed places, social gatherings, heights) and the particular response system associated with this reaction, be it cognitive, physiologic, or motoric.

Behavioral Assessment. Any given client's presenting problems are viewed as dependent variables, and it is up to the clinician to search out those independent variables that are likely to produce change. These may consist either of variables associated with clients themselves, or may entail some change within their current life situation. Thus, in conducting a behavioral analysis, the clinician frequently looks for potential stimulus antecedents of the problem, organismic variables within person (cognitive as well as physiologic), specific aspects of the behavior pattern itself, as well as consequent variables (e.g., the reaction of others) that may serve to reinforce certain behaviors and discourage others.

Ahistorical Emphasis. Because behavior therapy focuses on the here and now, it is sometimes mistakenly believed that it underplays the importance of the individual's past. In actuality, behavior therapists most readily acknowledge the important role of past learning experiences, either in the form of role models that may have been available to clients, or through the different reinforcement patterns to which they have been exposed. Where behavior therapy is ahistorical is in its approach to the intervention process, the essence of which is the facilitation of new learning experiences. This is very much within the spirit of what Alexander and French[41] have described as "corrective emotional experiences," in that insight into the historical origins of one's problems are not seen as being needed in order to bring about a change in the present.

Systematic Approach. Perhaps more than any other orientation, behavior therapy is characterized as being systematic in its approach to clinical problems, specifying (together with the client) the treatment goals as well as the therapeutic steps that will be used in achieving such objectives. In the clinical outcome research carried out in behavior therapy, therapists are frequently guided by treatment manuals that are specially designed for the problems at hand. Within routine clinical practice, clinicians frequently have plans and goals for each therapy session. We would like to emphasize, however, that "systematic" should not be read as "mechanistic." Without a sensitive, caring, and empathic approach to clients, even the most systematic of behavior therapists is apt to fail.

Empiricism. Behavior therapy is characterized by its strong research emphasis, which has been credited with advancing the field of psychotherapy research since the mid-1960s.[42] At the time of this writing, approximately half of the psychotherapy research projects funded by the National Institute of Mental Health are being carried out by behavior therapists. In a recent review of current knowledge about therapy, Frank[43] has concluded that data currently exist to indicate the effectiveness of behavioral procedures with certain clinical problems (e.g., fears, phobias, sexual dysfunctions). In light of Frank's long-standing and almost exclusive emphasis on the nonspecific factors associated with therapeutic change, this acknowledgment is particularly noteworthy.

Coping Skills. Because of its emphasis on a systematic and relatively directive approach to therapy, behavior therapy has often been criticized as fostering dependency and undermining the individual's own autonomy. Starting in the early 1970s, behavior therapists responded to this criticism, and developed procedures by which clients themselves could learn more independent coping skills.[44,45] The coping-skills orientation within behavior therapy carried with it the very clear implication that the therapist is a teacher, supervisor, and consultant, who works with clients in a collaborative effort to teach them behavioral and/or cognitive strategies for functioning more effectively.

Having provided this brief overview of behavior therapy, some of the behavioral interventions that may be relevant in dealing with problems associated with the male sex role will be presented. The behavioral procedures to be considered are relaxation training, cognitive restructuring, communication and negotiation training, sex therapy, and assertion/expressiveness training. It should again be emphasized that even though a series of distinct interventions are to be described, they are not meant to be applied in a mechanistic manner, but rather as part of a comprehensive treatment program tailored to meet the needs of individual clients. Different instances of seemingly similar problems may be a manifestation of very different causal determinants, requiring different intervention procedures for their effective elimination. Moreover, a given problem cannot usually be adequately handled by means of a single therapeutic technique. The complexity of human behavior is such that multifaceted intervention procedures are more often the rule than the exception.

RELAXATION TRAINING. Clinical research using relaxation as an active coping skill has found it to be effective with a variety of different anxiety-related problems[46] Included are such diverse problems as hypertension,[47,48] tension headaches,[49] insomnia,[50,51] speech anxiety,[52,53] test anxiety,[54–56] and interview anxiety.[57] Inasmuch as men all too often fail to tune into their bodies, relaxation training may be particularly helpful in allowing them to become better aware of internal signs of stress before they become extreme. Thus, by training individuals both to recognize and cope with their feelings of tension, the clinician can provide clients with an effective coping skill that can be used in a wide variety of different stressful life situations.

Training procedures for relaxation have been in existence for some time. They were originally outlined by Jacobson[58] and later incorporated by Wolpe[59] into his procedure for systematic desensitization. In the early use of systematic densensitization, it was noted that although the technique was presented as a means of deconditioning specific fears and phobias, many clients often construed the relaxation component in a very different way. By conceptualizing the relaxation training as a skill for coping with a variety of stressful events in their lives, they often were successful in reducing their anxiety reactions by themselves even before systematic desensitization could be applied within the consultation session. It is indeed fortunate that these clients never read the research literature, which at the time indicated that what they were doing was not supposed to work. Eventually, the literature caught up with what was going on clinically and several articles appeared, presenting relaxation training as an active coping skill for combating anxiety.[60–62]

Within this general coping framework, relaxation training is conceived of as fitting a paradigm very much like that associated with biofeedback, whereby clients learn to become more aware of the sensations of tension as they are beginning to build up, and then to respond to such signals by means of the relaxation response. Despite minor variations in relaxation training procedures, most methods involve training clients to alternatively tense and relax various muscle groups, after which a more advanced phase is introduced which involves learning to relax by merely letting go. Eventually, clients learn to become more and more adept with the relaxation response, and then are in a better position to employ it in various life situations when needed.

In regard to problems related to the male role, relaxation training may be used by problem drinkers as an alternative to alcohol for reducing their anxiety, as a means of eliminating the anxiety that may be interfering with a man's ability to experience sexual arousal, and to help men reduce the high levels of stress that often accompany Type A behavior. Suinn[63] has developed an anxiety management training program involving the use of relaxation skills for the treatment of Type A individuals which, like other programs of this sort, is typically carried out in a group treatment format. Ironically enough, group treatment seems to capitalize on those male characteristics that constitute part of the problem in question. As Roskies[64] points out, the group treatment mode provides the individual with an unusually relevant source of motivation, for "no-self-respecting Type-A man, even a reformed one, is going to allow others to benefit from treatment while he does not."[64] Apart from the context in which it is presented, it seems likely that relaxation training, while it can help the Type-A individual to cope with perceived levels of stress, may do little to alter the highly instrumental behavior pattern that is the source of such stress. To accomplish this requires a more basic change in the rules that govern such behavior.

COGNITIVE RESTRUCTURING. The impact that societal role definitions offer for men has profound effects on the way they view themselves and the world around them. These role conceptions are well learned during the course of one's lifetime, and eventually take on the form of various implicit assumptions of how one is to behave. Contemporary work on behavioral approaches to cognitive restructuring can be relevant in uncovering such assumptions, and consequently can function as a form of consciousness raising for men in reevaluating their inexpressiveness, their implicit problematic guidelines for marital interaction, the social-evaluative anxiety that may result in excessive drinking, their homophobic concerns about close relationships with other men, and the unrealistic standards that motivate their excessive and tension-producing instrumental behavior pattern. In this last context, we would maintain that the most effective treatment procedure with Type-A individuals is not so much teaching them how to reduce their levels of stress, but rather having them learn more realistic rules or scripts by which they can approach various life events. Cognitive restructuring has the potential for helping men identify both their realistic and unrealistic expectations of themselves and reevaluate their goals and the methods for achieving them. This clinical impression has received some empirical support in a study by Jenni and Wallersheim,[65] who compared a stress management program with a cognitive intervention program based on rational–emotive therapy. Although both treatments were more effective in reducing self-reported anxiety levels when compared to a no-treatment control, their findings indicated that the cognitive therapy was more effective than the stress management intervention for men who had the highest degree of Type-A characteristics.

A variety of different methods of implementing cognitive restructuring have been proposed by behavior therapists. Beck[66,67] has described procedures by which clients may be taught to become better aware of, and consequently to change, certain illogical thought patterns, such as the tendency to draw arbitrary inferences from instances, to overgeneralize from a given happening, and such "cognitive deficiences" as the failure to attend to or incorporate experiences that occur. Similarly, Lazarus[68] has described various maladaptive thought processes that may be in need of change, such as dichotomously viewing things as being either "good" or "bad" and the assumption that certain mores within our society are logical ways of viewing things rather than conventions. Meichenbaum[69] acknowledges that unrealistic perceptions of events may mediate problematic behavior patterns and emotions, but places greater emphasis on training individuals in more effective ways of coping than on changing misconceptions. Thus, individuals are taught to make use of such coping self-statements as "Take one step at a time," "Relax, you're in control," and "Worry won't help anything." Meichenbaum has developed procedures by which such coping self-statements may be employed together with relaxation skills. Drawing an analogy between an individual's personal problems and the problems dealt with by research scientists, Mahoney[70] suggests that a "personal science" may be achieved by training clients to specify general problems, collect information, identify patterns or causes, examine options, narrow these options and experiment, compare data, and then extend, revise, or replace their options. Each of the methods proposed above involve relatively structured steps for teaching clients more appropriate ways of cognitively appraising situations, and for encouraging the use of such skills in real-life situations.

A procedure that has been found to be particularly useful for helping individuals reevaluate their view of potentially upsetting events consists of systematic rational restructuring,[40,71] a therapeutic technique in which rational–emotive therapy[72] has been fitted into a more structured, social-learning framework. There are four basic steps that are associated with rational restructuring: The *first* step involves helping clients to recognize that self-statements mediate emotional arousal. Here the therapist's goal is to help clients accept the general assumption that their emotional reactions can be directly influenced by labels, expectations, and self-statements. The automatic quality of these expectations and beliefs is emphasized, so that clients understand that although they may not make deliberate self-statements prior to or during emotionally upsetting situations, they nonetheless react *as if* they view the situation in a given way.

The *second* step involves having clients acknowledge the irrational or unrealistic nature of a series of beliefs that individuals typically hold, the most frequent of which are the expectation that it is essential to receive approval and love from others in order to have any feelings of self-worth, and the belief that perfection is required in all accomplishments in order to see oneself as anything but a failure. In regard to problems typically experienced by men, we may also add such notions as the importance of never admitting weakness or uncertainty, being in control of uncontrollable situations, having to win at all costs, the inseparability of emotional closeness with sexuality, and the myriad of other beliefs that come with the male role (Chapter 1, by O'Neil and Chapter 2, by Solomon in this volume). Instead of verbally trying to convince clients that these thoughts are unrealistic, the social psychological literature[73,74] suggests that the therapist can more effectively promote attitude change by having clients themselves offer arguments to support the unrealistic nature of these beliefs. Thus, the therapist plays devil's advocate not only in helping the client to agree that certain beliefs are unrealisic, but also to generate specific reasons for the unreasonableness of these views.

In the *third* step, clients are helped to understand that unrealistic self-statements mediate their own maladaptive emotions. In some cases, this awareness is gained spontaneously in the second phase. At other times, it may involve the systematic exploration of various emotionally arousing situations in the client's current life.

The *fourth* step of systematic rational restructuring involves actual practice in changing one's unrealistic expectancies by having clients use their feelings of emotional upset as a cue to reevaluate specific situations more realistically. Practice sessions can make use of imaginal presentations of anxiety-arousing scenes, where clients are instructed to "think aloud" so that the therapist can assist them in evaluating and modifying unrealistic assumptions. Following the use of this technique for imaginal rehearsal in the consultation session, clients are urged to apply this procedure in real-life situations.

Controlled therapy outcome research has indicated that this intervention procedure has been effective in dealing with various anxiety-related problems, such as test anxiety,[78] interpersonal anxiety,[76,77] and unassertiveness.[78] As mentioned above, it also appears to be particularly relevant in the treatment of the Type-A behavior pattern,[65] whereby men can learn to reevaluate the unrealistic standards that guide their self-destructive behavior. Moreover, it has clinically been found to be an effective component of marital therapy.[30,79]

COMMUNICATION AND NEGOTIATION TRAINING. Although the importance of communication training has been receiving increased attention within the behavioral literature, its origins exist in systems and family therapy, where the goal has been to deal with the problems of the identified client by working within the family system.[80–84] In addition to the overt content of a message, workers in this general area have been able to point to latent messages that serve to confuse the communication process. Such latent messages, which may be expressed by verbal or nonverbal means, often convey a sense of *domination* and *devaluation* that one or each partner imposes upon the other. Research on the topic of marital interaction has dramatically revealed how patterns of confused communication typically escalate, resulting in still further miscommunication.[85–87] Although one member of a dyad may have a given *intent* in sending a message, the *impact* that it makes on the receiver can often be quite discrepant. In the case of distressed marital relations, it often reaches a point where even neutral or positive messages are perceived as being negative.[88]

In working with couples clinically, it has often been observed that men struggle both mentally and emotionally in an attempt to get in touch with their feelings and express them openly. One sometimes observes that a statement beginning with "I feel" is often followed by the word "that," changing the statement more toward an expression of thoughts rather than emotions (e.g., "I feel that you shouldn't be treating the kids that way.") However difficult it may be to learn to send nonaccusatory messages to others, it nonetheless can pay off handsomely by (a) avoiding the power struggle that might otherwise ensue; (b) communicating the feelings of vulnerability and caring of the sender; and (c) providing the receiver with descriptive feedback and at times a request for some means of satisfying the sender's needs.

In an attempt to teach individuals to communicate more clearly, the distinction is often made between the skill in *sending* messages clearly and the ability to *receive* them accurately. Gordon,[89] in his work on parent effectiveness training, has made the distinction between "you" and "I" statements. It is the "you" statement that not only communicates an overt message, but that also provides an accusation or putdown of the receiver. Thus, the man who feels both threatened and deprived by his wife's growing independence might react with "You're inconsiderate and selfish by only doing things for yourself and never caring about my needs." In such instances, the "real" message is often lost, and what the receiver reacts to is the sense of being dominated and devalued. The issue at hand, then, becomes not one of the sender's feeling of deprivation, but rather the power struggle in which each individual is defending his or her own sense of freedom. In learning to be clearer in sending messages to others, individuals must learn to make "I" statements, indicating what they feel and think in a given situation. Thus, as opposed to the "you" message given above, a clearer communication might involve: "When you're into your own thing, I often feel uncared for and left out. I'm also a little bit afraid that you won't have any need for me anymore." Clearly, such a deceptively simple communication is difficult for most men, and requires an awareness of one's own thoughts and feelings, as well as the willingness and courage to express them.

A second important skill associated with effective communication is learning how to listen. In discussing conflictual issues, the receiver all too often concentrates more on his or her own counterarguments than on what the sender is saying. The ability to "actively listen"[89] is both a crucial and difficult skill to learn. Having its roots in nondirective therapy, active listening involves the receiver's empathic reflection of what he or she has just heard. In following through with the above example, the receiver of the "I" message might respond with: "You're finding that my independence and involvement in my work sets me apart from you, and you're worried that this may cause me to care for you less." Such reflective statements (a) can serve to ensure that the receiver has heard the sender correctly; (b) conveys a sense of interest in and caring for the sender; and (c) can help to further clarify the sender's own thoughts and feelings about the situation. In learning both to receive and send messages more clearly, the *real issues* that have been undermining a relationship become much more apparent, thereby allowing for attempts at their resolution.

A variety of different methods have been developed for training individuals in effective communication.[79,83,89–92] Most of these procedures involve some initial educational phase, perhaps employing self-help literature,[29,89,93,94] modeling, coaching, behavior rehearsal, and homework. As a way of helping inexpressive men identify and verbalize their feelings, it is particularly helpful for therapists to prompt such communications by serving as an alter-ego, using their clinical sensitivity to articulate for/with the client those emotions he is having difficulty in identifying and expressing.

Closely associated with improved communication is negotiation, a process by which constructive alternatives to past distressful behavior are generated in an attempt to compromise and reach a consensus. It is a form of conjoint problem solving where each partner learns both to express his or her requirements and to listen to the other, to decide which points are open for compromise and which are not, and to arrive at mutually acceptable agreements. Clearly this can only take place after good communication skills are available, for a prerequisite to negotiation is the ability to directly state and communicate one's desires. A first step in negotiation training is teaching people to reveal *what* they want and *why* they want it. The training emphasizes the phrasing of requests in terms of positive changes (e.g., "I'd like to spend more time with you."), as opposed to demanding that negative behavior be stopped (e.g., "I don't want you to be spending so much time out of the house.").

If men can learn to share their disagreements constructively and to understand another's point of view, then they may not feel the need to defend their own position at all costs or to exaggerate it in an attempt to have it better understood. Once basic differences are understood and accepted, and not labeled as indicators of the innate badness of the relationship, individuals can reevaluate which aspects of their positions are most important to them and which are less important and, therefore, negotiable.

SEX THERAPY. Behavior therapy was first applied in the short-term direct treatment of various sexual dysfunctions in the 1950s. Wolpe[59] conceptualized sexual dysfunction as conditioned anxiety responses to the sexual situation and suggested that it might be profitably treated by systematic desensitization. The ultimate impact that behavioral interventions had on prevailing therapeutic treatment of sexual dysfunctioning came some years later, with the publication of Masters and Johnson's[33] *Human Sexual Inadequacy*. Although not originally acknowledged as being behavioral in orientation, Masters and Johnson's approach advocated that time-limited, directive counseling could be effectively employed to deal with such immediate causes of dysfunction as performance anxiety, lack of information, difficulties with sexual communication, and the adoption of a spectator role during sexual activity. This direct treatment approach, in addition to its emphasis on sensory awareness, also involves education, communication training, and anxiety reduction.

In Masters and Johnson's therapeutic model, the couple, rather than the individual, is considered mutually responsible for the dysfunction and its cure. The program, usually consisting of 15 sessions, begins with an extensive history taking, and proceeds with a graded series of sexual tasks for the couple to do at home. The initial exercises, known as "sensate focus," involve mutual pleasuring and have the triple purpose of (a) removing performance anxiety by creating a no-demand experience; (b) eliminating the spectator role and encouraging the couple to tune into their own sexual experiences and feelings; and (c) increasing sexual communication of what feels good to each individual. At first, breast and genitals are excluded from the exercise, but are gradually added to the sensual body massage. Later, intercourse is reintroduced. One can clearly conceptualize this gradual advance from sensate focus to intercourse as a form of in vivo systematic desensitization.[95,96]

There have been many modifications of the basic Masters and Johnson program since its introduction in 1970. However, in varying degrees, the following principles are used by most clinicians who follow the brief direct treatment approach:

Mutual Responsibility. The couple, not the individual, is considered mutually responsible for the maintenance of the dysfunction (if not the cause) and, therefore, for its cure. Care is usually taken to provide a distinction between "responsibility" and "blame."

Eliminating Performance Anxiety. The couple is told to avoid "keeping score," and to stop being goal oriented for erection, orgasm, ejaculation, or any particular end result. Instead, they are asked to focus on enjoying the process. Banning intercourse and giving them permission to engage in other sexual activities aid in this therapy process. Formal desensitization may be used where anxiety is severe.

Education. Many people suffering from sexual dysfunction have little knowledge of both basic sexual physiology and effective sexual techniques. In direct therapy, there is an emphasis on accurate knowledge of the sexual response cycle as well as general principles of effective sexual techniques. This knowledge is provided through verbal discussion, providing the couple with appropriate reading materials, and/or the use of educational films.

Attitude Change. Individuals seeking sex therapy typically hold many negative attitudes toward sexuality. Attitude change may be accomplished by assigning reading material that comments positively on sexuality, arranging consultations with sympathetic clergy, recommendations of lectures and workshops on sexuality and sexual values, and the use of the therapeutic relationship itself through encouragement and self-disclosure.

Increasing Communication. Inhibitions about discussing sex openly frequently make it impossible for dysfunctional couples to clearly communicate their sexual likes and dislikes to each other. Direct therapy encourages open communication about technique and response. This may be facilitated by having couples read explicit erotic literature, sharing their fantasies, seeing and discussing sexually explicit movies, guiding their partner's hands during sexual activity, and giving each other direct verbal and nonverbal feedback during sex.

Prescribing Changes in Behavior. Direct treatment of sexual dysfunction is characterized by the prescription of specific sexual behaviors to be performed by the couple in privacy. This directiveness often can also be used to encourage couples to change destructive lifestyles that may be contributing to sexual dysfunction. The actual program of assignment varies among therapeutic settings, and is usually characterized by the use of graded sexual assignments, many of which are specific to the various dysfunctions.

For example, in *premature ejaculation,* the man is encouraged to focus on the penis and feelings of pleasure. The pause technique[97] or the squeeze technique[33] is typically used, during which the male learns to experience a massive amount of stimulation without occurrence of ejaculation, thereby providing an opportunity to gain ejaculatory control. The man learns to recognize the point of inevitability, beyond which he cannot stop the ejaculatory process. At some period before this point is reached, he either pauses, or he squeezes the coronal ridge until the urge to ejaculate passes. Stimulation is then resumed once again.

The treatment for *erectile dysfunction* tries to take the focus off the penis and on to other forms of sexual and sensual stimulation. The graded sexual assignments progress from nonsexual massage to include genitals and breasts. The instruction is given to stop stimulation of the penis should an erection occur. Only when the penis is flaccid can stimulation be resumed. This procedure called the "teasing technique"[33] convinces the couple that if erection is lost, it can be regained. Next, penile insertion into the vagina is allowed, but only with the flaccid penis. Once the male has been unable to avoid an erection during vaginal containment, slow pelvic thrusting, and finally vigorous intercourse, can be prescribed.

A third male dysfunction, *inhibited ejaculation*, is treated by having the couple provide massive amounts of stimulation to the man's penis, introducing vaginal containment only at the point of orgasm for the male. Once this has been achieved and the man has ejaculated intravaginally, the timing of the penetration can be slowly moved back to an earlier period in time.

These "exercises" are introduced within a therapeutic context that also explores personal and interactional variables that may be contributing to the dysfunction. Further, a complete medical evaluation is a necessary part of the assessment procedure.

As the field of sex therapy continues to develop, several modifications and improvements to this basic program have occurred. Progress has been made in the classification and assessment of sexual dysfunction,[32,34,98–101] and a focus on new populations to treat. In the early sex therapy programs, clients with individual psychopathology and severe marital stress were systematically screened out, as were individuals with a medically complicated history. Now there is a greater focus on treating all of these problems. As already noted, *inhibited sexual desire* has become a major presenting complaint at sex therapy centers. While brief sex therapy seems to be effective in the treatment of excitement and orgasm phase dysfunctions, it is less so with "desire phase" dysfunctions.[102] The treatment of desire phase disorders is obviously dependent on those factors found to be most significant in the etiology of a particular case. In instances where aversion becomes severe, treatment techniques for phobias may seem appropriate. Biologic factors may also have etiological significance and require biologic intervention. Where the causes of low desire seem more psychologically remote, a lengthier and more flexible insight-oriented sex therapy may be necessary.

ASSERTION/EXPRESSIVENESS TRAINING. Ironically enough, the recent work that has been carried out in the area of assertion training, while often used to assist women to become more instrumental in their functioning, may also have great relevance to problems associated with the male sex role. Although the stereotypic male presumably should have minimal difficulty in standing up for his own rights, the relevance of assertion training for men becomes more apparent when one recognizes that many men are often more aggressive than they are assertive. The basic distinction between the two is that while both are directed toward having one's needs and desires fulfilled, aggressive behavior often accomplishes this at the cost of someone else's integrity. Assertion/expressiveness training may therefore be helpful to temper men's somewhat aggressive ways of having their needs met. It may also be indicated in working on distressed marital relationships by altering a husband's overtly aggressive or passive–aggressive manner of interacting, and can be useful in training the alcoholic to deal with interpersonally frustrating situations more effectively and in resisting peer pressures to drink.

Assertion/expressiveness training has rapidly become one of the most frequently used interventions by behavior therapists, and indeed by many who do not align themselves with this particular orientation. The typical definition of "assertiveness" is that it involves an appropriate expression of one's feelings and needs, done so as not to interfere with the rights of others.[40,68,103–105] For the most part, assertiveness has been useful to describe the individual's ability to stand up for his or her own rights. However, assertiveness has also been used to refer to the individual's ability to express positive emotions as well. When used in its broadest sense, assertion/expressiveness training bears great similarity to sensitivity training, both of which are directed toward open and direct expression of one's thoughts and feelings.

The concept "assertiveness" has been criticized as being too broad and at times misleading, and several writers have suggested alternate terms for describing the behavior patterns associated with this general construct. For example, Lazarus[68] refers to "emotional freedom" as the more general construct involving a "recognition and appropriate expression of each and every affective state" (p. 116). He uses the term "assertive behavior" to refer to emotional freedom involving those situations where one has to stand up for one's own rights, and "positive expressiveness" for the communication of warmth, caring, tenderness, and other positive emotions. Goldstein[104] prefers to eliminate the concept of assertiveness training in general, replacing it instead with "appropriate expression training." As a way of avoiding confusion, one may follow McFall's[106] recommendation that it is more fruitful to talk in terms of "competence training," with the specific content of this competence being defined by the task requirements of the situation at hand. Thus, one may have competence training involved in learning how to refuse unreasonable requests, competence training in situations requiring the initiation of a new course of action and, particularly relevant for the inexpressive male, competence training for self-disclosing feelings and thoughts, expressing one's warm and tender feelings toward others, and requesting interpersonal support and nurturance in situations where it might be appropriate.

The general goal of assertion/expressiveness training is to teach the individual to respond with appropriate content (e.g., "I'm afraid that I'll be too busy to help you out tomorrow," "I really appreciate what you've done for me," etc.), to use a compatible paralinguistic style (e.g., adequate voice tone, absence of speech dysfluencies), and to accompany this with effective nonverbal behaviors (e.g., good eye contact, appropriate facial expression). Assertion/expressiveness training involves a number of specific intervention techniques.[40] *Modeling* procedures may be used by the therapist, or perhaps a therapeutic aide, whereby appropriate ways of responding to particular situations are demonstrated for clients. In addition, clients may require *coaching*, so as to provide them with information on both what they may say or do in given situations, as well as guidelines as to how they might do it. *Behavior rehearsal* is most typically used for assertion/expressiveness training, in that clients engage in repeated role-playing sequences that simulate real-life situations within the consultation room. In order to obtain a fuller appreciation of what the other person in the interaction is likely to feel and think, one may make use of role reversals. *Feedback* is typically provided by the therapist, or by a recorded playback of the interaction, to allow clients to focus in on those things they liked about their handling of the situation as well as aspects of their response that they would like to change. Finally, *homework* assignments play an important role in the training process, so that clients may try out in real life what they have learned in the consultation sessions. It has also been found that a particularly effective method for increasing assertive behavior involves the combination of *cognitive restructuring* procedures along with the methods described above.[78,105,107–110] By including cognitive restructuring, individuals are able to reevaluate more realistically the consequences associated with their being assertive/expression, as well as to learn the appropriate behavioral skills for implementing the assertive/expressive response.

PSYCHOLOGICAL ANDROGYNY

Having described some ways by which men can change, the question of how such changes will influence their lives remains. What are the new rules that men can adopt in guiding their interactions with others as well as their views of themselves? Is it possible for men to be in touch with their feelings, be sensitive, insightful, gentle, and emotional while still retaining many of the more instrumental attributes that characterize the male sex role? If so, are such men better adjusted, more flexible, and less prone to the negative results of the male sex role? The concept of "psychological androgyny" refers to just such a blending of both masculine and feminine qualities.

In this new model of sex-role orientation, "masculinity" and "femininity" are considered as two dimensions, rather than mutually exclusive opposites.[111,112] Bem has proposed that there are indeed individuals who possess both masculine and feminine characteristics, that it is possible to be both assertive and yielding, both instrumental and expressive. According to Bem's theory of psychological androgyny, androgynous men should behave more flexibly and effectively in a wider variety of situations than rigidly masculine individuals. Persons who integrate both masculine and feminine characteristics, regardless of gender, can behave in an instrumental manner when appropriate and in an expressive manner when the situation dictates that response. Thus, the concept of psychological androgyny denotes a person who is basically more complete and actualized in the sense of maximizing personal potential.[113,114] The corresponding implication is that sex-typed individuals are more limited in their range of available responses as they move from situation to situation, and tend to behave in a narrow, stereotypic manner.

A number of studies have marshaled evidence that androgynous individuals are indeed more flexible in their social functioning, varying their behavior according to situational demands rather than sex-role stereotypes.[113,114–116]

There has also been evidence that androgynous individuals score higher on measures of adjustment and mental health, and possess greater self-esteem.[112,117,118] In a study on sex roles and social skills, Kelly et al.[119] found that androgynous subjects were consistently rated as most effective in social interaction role-play situations. The authors conclude that what has been called androgynous roles probably represents a diverse, extensive behavioral repertoire of social competencies across situations.

Despite this evidence, however, there are also some findings indicating that the androgynous male may not be psychologically better off than the sex-typed male. Antill and Cunningham[120] examined androgyny and self-esteem in 237 college students and found that it was the level of masculinity that contributed most to self-esteem among androgynous individuals. Bennett[121] similarly found a greater adjustment advantage for masculine-oriented subjects, whereby androgynous men were less oriented to the present, more vulnerable to external influence, and more prone to symptoms of serious emotional disturbances than masculine men. Bennett concludes that any apparent adjustment advantage of an androgynous orientation can be more accurately attributed to androgynous individuals' level of masculinity than to their balance of high masculine and feminine characteristics. In a set of studies that compared androgynous with sex-type individuals on several attitudinal, personality, and behavioral dimensions, Jones et al.[113] also found that flexibility in adjustment was generally associated with masculinity rather than androgyny.

It is not clear what to make of these conflicting findings. Bennett[121] suggests that many of the measures of adjustment used in the studies may be biased towards instrumentally oriented dimensions of psychological health. Although such definitions of adjustment clearly reflect the prevailing views of effective functioning within our society at large, it nonetheless may have prevented positive contributions of such feminine characteristics as expressiveness and intimacy from emerging. However, this is no less true of the studies finding higher self-esteem among androgynous individuals. Perhaps what we need is less of a general, traitlike measure of androgyny and a more situation-specific behavioral approach.[122] This may help us to "fine-tune" the assessment and be better able to identify individual behavior patterns that are sex-typed and androgynous in nature, and their relative effectiveness in various specific life situations. Given the heterogeneous nature of our society, its associated life tasks, and its ever-changing evaluative standards, this more detailed approach may help to shed light on the question of the adaptiveness of psychological androgyny.

Even in the absence of a detailed investigation of the issue, one may expect that a departure from established cultural patterns would cause some personal anxiety or strain for the "deviant" individual. Although the androgynous male may not have to work quite as hard as his sex-typed brother to maintain a behavior pattern consistent with external societal and internal standards, he may be working even harder to maintain his androgynous behavior *in the face of* such standards. Sex-role deviance is more severely punished in men than in women, as reflected in the finding that a man who expresses attitudes inappropriate to the male sex type is viewed as less socially attractive than is a women with masculine attitudes.[123] Other studies have similarly demonstrated that men tend to be clearly devalued by others when they display emotions or behaviors that counter the traditional male role.[4,113,124,128]

Relevant to this issue, a study by Babl[129] investigated the hypothesis that males defend against sex-role threat by exaggerating their masculinity and engaging in a greater amount of antisocial behavior. Babl found that stereotypic males did indeed respond anxiously to an audio tape where a decreased level of masculinity in college males was discussed, and subsequently reported exaggerated levels of masculinity endorsement and antisocial behavior. Androgynous males also reported anxiety, but their response was different in that they lowered their level of masculine endorsement. However, the very fact that the androgynous men also became anxious is noteworthy, especially in light of their self-acknowledged comfort to both masculine and feminine characteristics. Despite their androgyny, they apparently do remain emotionally susceptible to sex-role threat. Still further evidence that it may not be so easy for a man to be androgynous in today's society comes from the Jones et al. study,[113] which found that when individuals were given a chance to express a preference, both males and females indicated a strong desire to increase their capacity to behave in an instrumental fashion. Both feminine and androgynous males prefer to become more masculine, whereas masculine males indicated relatively little desire for change.

Where does this leave us? On the one hand, the stereotypic male may defend himself against behaviors designated as appropriate for the opposite sex, maintaining a self-image as masculine. In doing so, he may be denying a part of himself at the cost of narrowness, inflexibility, and a constant effort at living according to certain role constraints. On the other hand, the androgynous male may have to deal with society's response to his more flexible behaviors, as well as his own feelings about sex-role appropriateness. It is clear that no overall conclusion can be reached at this point in time, and the most appropriate behavior pattern for any given male must carefully take into account his particular life situation. Any changes that occur in the direction of psychological androgyny, for the individual or for society in general, are going to be slow and painful. Although young people are starting to move in the direction of androgyny, role redefinitions may present a particular dilemma for older men who are caught in the gap between lifelong learning and current pressures. These conflicting sources of influence can indeed be confusing and frustrating, as the rules are no longer clear for what one has to do to "be a man."

BEHAVIOR THERAPY AND THE LARGER SOCIAL SYSTEM

In using behavior therapy to deal with problems associated with the male sex role, there are broader societal issues that need to be considered. One of the hallmarks of the behavioral approach to clinical work is its functional nature, whereby effective and ineffective behavior patterns are defined in terms of their consequences. As a result of this orientation, behavior therapists face the potential danger of encouraging what is likely to be reinforced by the client's environment, thereby maintaining a societal status quo, which, *in itself* may at times be harmful in its effects.

For example, concerns have been voiced by Winkler[130] and Nordyke et al.[131] about a case of a five-year-old boy for whom reinforcement procedures were used to foster masculine dress, play, and "masculine aggression," and to minimize feminine behavior and "maternal nurturance".[132] Although the overall goal was to prevent future sexual deviance, these critics—who themselves are behavior therapists—suggest that the objectives were determined on the basis of value judgments and not any evidence that the child's behavior pattern was in itself problematic.

Gurman and Klein[133] have similarly argued that behavioral marital therapy may inadvertently establish therapeutic goals that cause individuals—particularly women—to more effectively fit into current societal standards. Although behavior therapists have presumably taken an "objective" stance on the issue of sex-role behaviors within marital relationships, Gurman and Klein maintain that such seeming neutrality nonetheless reinforces traditionally sexist societal values. As they suggest, the basic issue is not solely whether values enter into the practice of behavior therapy, but also whether behavior therapists acknowledge that this is happening. The real danger, they argue, lies with the cloak of objectivity, behind which one may inadvertently foster well-accepted behavior patterns that nonetheless are problematic.

The question of just how much sex role stereotypes affect the judgments of mental health workers has received increasing attention in recent years. In a review of research in this area, Whitley[134] concludes that therapists make use of very much the same sex-role stereotypes in defining mental health as do lay people. In making actual clinical judgments, however, most of the available evidence suggests that these stereotypes do *not* serve as a source of bias. It is difficult to interpret such negative results, as they may either reflect methodological inadequacies in these studies or a nonbiased approach in actual clinical decision making. Until it becomes certain that sex-role stereotypes do not, in fact, have any influence on clinicians' judgments, it is advisable for therapists to become more clearly aware of how such stereotypes can affect their clients' lives.

Inasmuch as societal standards are rapidly changing, and will also vary at any given time from one subculture to another, a functional definition of "appropriate behavior" requires frequent reevaluation. It should be emphasized, however, that employing such a functional definition serves as a double-edged sword. On the more positive side, behavior therapists may be better able to respond to, and to incorporate societal changes into their definition of effective behavior, as they are not locked into a particular theoretical conceptualization of normality. Being sensitive to the fact that different skills are needed for functioning in different life situations, a behavioral approach lends itself particularly well to the facilitation of an androgynous behavior pattern.

Nonetheless, behavior therapists continue to be limited by their own cultural conditioning, and the danger of inadvertently encouraging an intrinsically maladaptive lifestyle continues to exist. Behavior therapy, like other approaches to therapy, has relatively little to say about the maladaptive nature of society.

Such an awareness has typically come from outside of the therapeutic system, such as the influence of the feminist movement as well as the personal experiences of therapists themselves. Those who write about sex-role issues have come to understand them in a first-hand and very personal way.

In working with clients whose problems appear to be closely tied to sex-role issues, it is important for therapists to openly acknowledge the changing nature of society, to recognize how their own values may affect their clinical behavior, and to discuss with clients the possible consequences associated with various behavior patterns. In the absence of any hard data on such long- and short-term consequences, it is up to therapists to offer their best guess as to the ramifications of a given behavior pattern, using whatever information they have at hand to make such judgments. We would agree with Baer et al.[135] and Birk[136] that there is a very strong need for therapists to become aware of problems associated with the male sex role, the difficulties involved in achieving psychological androgyny, and the various environmental factors that may constrain men from behaving in nonstereotypic ways.

Within the past few years, there has been a growing sophistication among many behavioral clinicians that has helped them look beyond individuals and their immediate environment and to focus on the larger social system that is likely to elicit and reinforce certain problems. Thus, while the accepted means for dealing with behavior problems in children had been to routinely train the parent (typically the mother) in social learning and reinforcement procedures, this approach has started to give way toward a recognition that marital, and at times family therapy, might be called for in many instances. Recognizing that behavior therapy may at times be limited in scope, Weiss[137] has provided an insightful analysis of how a behavioral approach to marital therapy is most consistent with a more general systems approach. Behavior therapists have become keenly aware that while it is important to ensure that a person is capable of functioning in certain ways, it is equally crucial that certain environmental conditions be present for that behavior pattern to be maintained. Indeed, when considering the issues involved in changing certain behavior patterns associated with the male sex role, the question of maintenance is an essential one. Although men may experience numerous positive consequences as they develop more intimate and expressive ways of relating to others, there are also potential dangers. Berger[138] has astutely observed that "It is hard to live outside the old social forms without support and not feel crazy" (p. 643). As we have indicated earlier in this chapter, our culture tends to punish, rather than reinforce various "feminine behavior" patterns among men. Societal influences on appropriate male behavior are indeed powerful, creating social pressure that is "like a cobweb—strong but hard to see."[139]

While the feminist movement has caused men to begin to question some of their accepted roles, many men continue to be unaware of the forces that direct their lives. In helping to foster such awareness, we cannot over-emphasize the very important function of consciousness-raising groups. Lange and Jakubowski[104] have argued that experience in such consciousness-raising groups can play a most useful supplemental role in any program of assertion/expressiveness training. Not only can such groups help men to become better aware of those problems associated with what it means to be male in our society, but they also can provide the needed social support to encourage changes in the direction of greater psychological androgyny for those who would benefit from a move in this direction.

For the most part, men's groups have made use of the consciousness-raising guidelines that have been developed for conducting women's groups. We would agree with Farrell[140] and Vanacek[141] however, that certain basic changes need to be made for men's consciousness-raising groups, especially the involvement of a trained leader. Compared with women, men are typically more reluctant to become aware of the limitations that sex-role stereotypes play in their behavior, and are not nearly as motivated to openly explore these issues. Consequently, a leader becomes crucial in helping men break out of the patterns of competitiveness and inexpressiveness that all too often can undermine the goals of consciousness raising. Without such leadership, observes Vanecek, it is all too easy for men's groups to develop into "bull sessions," perhaps providing a sense of comraderie and personal support but offering relatively little awareness of those ramifications associated with their roles as "provider, protector, producer, and performer."

Consciousness raising, while extremely important in providing men with a general knowledge of attitudes and habit patterns that are associated with being male, may not be sufficient in actually bringing about change. As suggested by Horney,[142] a general awareness of certain attitudes does little to change individuals. In an observation most consistent with a behavioral orientation, she notes: "What counts is the individual becoming aware of *specific* ways in which these factors operate within him and how in *concrete detail* they manifest themselves in his particular life. . . ." (p. 342). We would maintain that in addition to consciousness-raising groups, behavior therapy offers intervention procedures that can provide men with the necessary therapeutic experiences to lead them to alter their stereotypic roles.

SUMMARY

This chapter has dealt with some of the issues associated with the male sex role and the problems that bring men into therapy. Although men suffer from the full array of psychological problems that one is likely to encounter clinically, this chapter has focused specifically on marital conflict, sexual dysfunctioning, and alcohol dependency, as well as the more general issues of male inexpressiveness and the Type-A behavior pattern. A brief overview of behavior therapy was presented, noting that this approach to clinical work reflects such general characteristics as an emphasis on operational definitions, the need for ongoing behavioral assessment, a focus on the here and now, a systematic approach to intervention procedures, the importance of empirical verification, and the view of therapy as training in coping skills. Among the behavioral intervention procedures that are likely to be relevant to problems associated with the male sex role, relaxation training, cognitive restructuring, communication and negotiation training, assertion/expressiveness training, and sex therapy were described. The predominant theme of this chapter has been that knowledge of the behavioral, cognitive, and emotional patterns associated with the male sex role, and the implications of such patterns within the larger societal context, can provide the therapist with an important guideline in working with men clinically.

ACKNOWLEDGMENTS

Preparation of this chapter was supported in part by Grant Nos. MH 24327 and MH 26631 from the National Institute of Mental Health. The authors would like to express their appreciation to Anita Powers Goldfried and Leslie Schover for their most helpful comments on an earlier version of this chapter.

REFERENCES

1. Bem SL: Psychology looks at sex roles: Where have all the androgynous people gone? Presented at a Symposium on Women, University of California at Los Angeles, Los Angeles, California, May, 1972
2. Parson T, Bales RF: Family, Socialization and Interaction Process. New York, Free Press, 1955
3. Jourard S: The Transparent Self. New York, Van Nostrand Reinhold, 1971
4. Derlaga VJ, Chaikin AL: Norms affecting self-disclosure in men and women. J Consult Clin Psychol 44:376–380, 1976
5. Lewis R: Emotional intimacy among men. J Soc Issues 34:101–121, 1978
6. Fasteau MF: The Male Machine. New York, McGraw-Hill, 1974
7. Hartley R: Sex role pressures in the socialization of the male child. Psychol Rep 5:457–468, 1959
8. Vinacke WE, Gullickson GR: Age and sex differences in the formation of coalitions. Child Dev 35:1217–1231, 1964
9. Szal J: Sex differences in the cooperative and competitive behaviors of nursery school children. Unpublished Master's thesis, Stanford University, 1972
10. Harrison J: Warning: The male sex role may be dangerous to your health. J Soc Issues 34:184–195, 1978
11. Waldron I: Why do women live longer than men? Soc Science Med 10:349–362, 1976
12. American Heart Association: Heart Facts. New York, American Heart Association, 1974
13. Roseman RH, Friedman M: Neurogenic factors in pathogenesis of coronary heart disease. Med Clin North Am 58:269–279, 1974
14. Friedman M: Pathogenesis of Coronary Artery Disease. New York, McGraw-Hill, 1969
15. Jenkins CD: Recent evidence supporting ecologic and social risk factors for coronary disease. New Eng J Med 294:987–994, 1033–1038, 1976
16. Rosenman RH, Friedman M, Straus R, et al.: A predictive study of coronary heart disease. JAMA 189:103–110, 1964
17. Rosenman RH, Brand BJ, Scholtz RI: Multivariate prediction of coronary heart disease during 8.5 year follow up in the Western Collaborative Group Study. Am J Cardiol 37:903–910, 1976
18. Chesney N: Cultural and sex differences in the Type "A" pattern. Presented at the Annual Meeting of the American Psychological Association, New York, Sept 4, 1979
19. Rahe RH, Hervig L, Rosenman RH: Heritability of Type "A" behavior. Psychosom Med 40:478–487, 1978
20. Rosenman RH: The role of behavior patterns and neurogenic factors in the pathogenesis of coronary heart disease, in Stress and the Heart. Edited by Elliot RS. New York, Futura Publications, 1974, pp 123–141
21. Utensky A, Faralli V, Heebner D, et al.: Elements of the coronary prone behavior pattern in children and teenagers. J Psychosom Res 20:439–444, 1976

22. Waldron I: The coronary-prone behavior pattern, blood pressure, employment and socio-economic status in women. J Psychosom Res 22:79–87, 1978
23. Waldron I: Sex differences in the coronary-prone behavior pattern, in Coronary-prone Behavior. Edited by Dembroski TM. New York, Springer-Verlag, 1978, pp 199–206
24. Seligman MEP: Helplessness. San Francisco, Freeman, 1975
25. Glass DC: Behavior Patterns, Stress, and Coronary Disease. Hillsdale, Lawrence Erlbaum Associates, 1977
26. Glick PC, Norton AJ: Perspectives on the recent upturn in divorce and remarriage. Demography 10:301–314, 1973
27. Lederer WI, Jackson DD: The Mirages of Marriage. New York, Norton, 1968
28. Scanzoni J: Sexual Bargaining: Power Politics in the American Marriage. New York, Prentice Hall, 1972
29. Gottman J, Notarius C, Gonso J, et al.: A Couple's Guide to Communication. Champaign, Research, 1976
30. Broderick J, Friedman JM, Carr E: Negotiation and contracting, in In Response to Aggression. Edited by Goldstein A, Carr E, Davidson W, et al. New York, Pergamon Press, 1981
31. Zilbergeld B: Male Sexuality: A Guide to Sexual Fulfillment. Boston, Little, Brown, 1978
32. Kaplan HS: Disorders of Desire. New York, Brunner/Mazel, 1979
33. Masters WH, Johnson VE: Human Sexual Inadequacy. Boston, Little, Brown, 1970
34. Kaplan HS: The New Sex Therapy. New York, Brunner/Mazel, 1974
35. Friedman JM, Weiler SJ, LoPiccolo J, et al.: Sexual dysfunctions and their treatment, in International Handbook of Behavior Modification and Therapy. Edited by Bellack A, Hersen M, Kazdin A. New York, Plenum, 1982
36. Calahan D: Implications of American drinking practices and attitudes for prevention and treatment of alcoholism, in Behavioral Approaches to Alcoholism. Edited by Marlatt GA, Nathan PE. New Brunswick, Rutgers Center of Alcohol Studies, 1978, pp 6–26
37. Efron V, Keller M, Gurioli C: Statistics on Consumption of Alcohol and on Alcoholism. New Brunswick, Rutgers Center of Alcohol Studies, 1974
38. Marlatt GA, Nathan PE: Behavioral Approaches to Alcoholism. New Brunswick, Rutgers Center of Alcohol Studies, 1978
39. Marlatt GA: Alcohol use and problem drinking: A cognitive–behavioral analysis, in Cognitive–Behavioral Interventions: Theory, Research, and Procedures. Edited by Kendall PC, Hollon SD. New York, Academic Press, 1979, pp 319–355
40. Goldfried MR, Davison GC: Clinical Behavior Therapy. New York, Holt, Rinehart, and Winston, 1976
41. Alexander F, French TM: Psychoanalytic Therapy. New York, Ronald, 1946
42. Garfield SL, Bergin AE: Handbook of Psychotherapy and Behavior Change. New York, Wiley, 1978
43. Frank JD: The present status of outcome studies. J Consult Clin Psychol 47:310–316, 1979
44. Goldfried MR, Merbaum M: Behavior Change through Self-Control. New York, Holt, Rinehart, and Winston, 1973
45. Thoreson CE, Mahoney MJ: Behavioral Self-Control. New York, Holt, Rinehart, and Winston, 1974
46. Goldfried MR: The use of relaxation and cognitive relabeling as coping skills, in Behavioral Self-Management: Strategies, Techniques and Outcomes. Edited by Stuart RB. New York, Brunner/Mazel, 1977, pp 82–116
47. Shoemaker J, Tasto D: Effects of muscle relaxation on blood pressure of essential hypertensives. Behav Res Ther 13:29–43, 1975
48. Deabler H, Fidel E, Dillenkoffer R, et al.: The use of relaxation and hypnosis in lowering high blood pressure. Am J Clin Hypn 16:75–83, 1973
49. Cox DJ, Freundlich A, Meyer, RG: Differential effectiveness of an electromyograph feedback, verbal relaxation instructions, and medication placebo with tension headaches. J Consult Clin Psychol 43:892–898, 1975
50. Davison GC, Tsujimoto RN, Glaros AG: Attribution and the maintenance of behavior change in falling asleep. J Abnorm Psychol 82:124–133, 1973

51. Nicassio P, Bootzin R: A comparison of progressive relaxation and autogenic training as treatments for insomnia. J Abnorm Psychol 83:253–260, 1974
52. Gatchel RJ, Hatch JP, Watson PJ, et al.: Comparative effectiveness of voluntary heart rate control and muscular relaxation as active coping skills for reducing speech anxiety. J Consult Clin Psychol 45:1093–1100, 1977
53. Goldfried MR, Trier CS: Effectiveness of relaxation as an active coping skill. J Abnorm Psychol 83:348–355, 1974
54. Chang-Liang R, Denny DR: Applied relaxation as training in self-control. J Counseling Psychol 23:183–189, 1976
55. Denny DR, Rupert PA: Desensitization and self-control in the treatment of test anxiety. J Counseling Psychol 4:272–280, 1977
56. Snyder AL, Deffenbacher JL: Comparison of relaxation as self-control and systematic desensitization in the treatment of test anxiety. J Consult Clin Psychol 45:1202–1203, 1977
57. Zeisset RM: Desensitization and relaxation in the modification of psychiatric patients' interview behavior. J Abnorm Psychol 73:18–24, 1968
58. Jacobson E: Progressive Relaxation. Chicago, University of Chicago Press, 1929
59. Wolpe J: Psychotherapy by Reciprocal Inhibition. Stanford, Stanford University Press, 1958
60. Goldfried MR: Systematic desensitization as training in self-control. J Consult Clin Psychol 37:228–234, 1971
61. Meichenbaum DH, Cameron R: Stress inoculation: A skills training approach to anxiety management. Unpublished manuscript, University of Waterloo, Ontario, 1972
62. Suinn RM, Richardson F: Anxiety management training: A nonspecific behavior therapy program for anxiety control. Behav Ther 2:498–510, 1971
63. Suinn RM: The cardiac stress management program for Type A patients. Cardiac Rehab 5:13–16, 1975
64. Roskies E: Considerations in developing a treatment program for the coronary-prone (Type A) behavior pattern, in Behavioral Medicine: Changing Health Lifestyles. Edited by Davidson P. New York, Brunner/Mazel, 1980, pp 299–334
65. Jenni MA, Wollersheim JP: Cognitive therapy, stress management training and the Type A behavior pattern. Cognitive Ther Res 3:61–75, 1979
66. Beck AT: Nature and relation to behavior therapy. Behav Ther 1:184–200, 1970
67. Beck AT: Cognitive Therapy and the Emotional Disorders. New York, International Universities Press, 1976
68. Lazarus AA: Behavior Therapy and Beyond. New York, McGraw-Hill, 1971
69. Meichenbaum DH: Cognitive Behavior Modification: An Integrative Approach. New York, Plenum, 1977
70. Mahoney MJ: Reflections on the cognitive learning trend in psychotherapy. Am Psychol 32:5–13, 1977
71. Goldfried MR, Decenteceo ET, Weinberg L: Systematic rational restructuring as a self-control technique. Behav Ther 5:247–254, 1974
72. Ellis A: Reason and Emotion in Psychotherapy. New York, Lyle Stuart, 1962
73. Janis I, King BT: The influence of role playing on opinion change. J Abnorm Soc Psychol 49:211–218, 1954
74. King BT, Janis IL: Comparison of the effectiveness of improvised versus non-improvised role-playing in producing opinion change. Human Relations 9:171–186, 1956
75. Goldfried MR, Linehan MM, Smith JL: The reduction of text anxiety through cognitive restructuring. J Consult Clin Psychol 46:32–39, 1978
76. Kanter N, Goldfried MR: Relative effectiveness of rational restructuring and self-control desensitization in the reduction of interpersonal anxiety. Behav Ther 10:472–490, 1979
77. Malkiewich LE, Merluzzi TV: Rational restructuring versus desensitization with clients of diverse conceptual level: A test of a client-treatment matching model. J Counseling Psychol 27:453–461, 1980
78. Linehan M, Goldfried MR, Goldfried AP: Assertion training: Skill acquisition or cognitive restructuring. Behav Ther 10:372–388, 1979

79. O'Leary KD, Turkewitz H: Marital therapy from a behavioral perspective, in Marriage and Marital Therapy: Psychoanalytic, Behavioral, and Systems Theory Perspectives. Edited by Paolino TJ, McCrady BS. New York, Brunner/Mazel, 1978, pp 240–297
80. Haley J: Marriage therapy. Arch Gen Psychiatry 8:213–234, 1963
81. Jackson DD: Family rules: Marital quid pro quo. Arch Gen Psychiatry 12:589–594, 1965
82. Jackson DD, Riskin J, Satir V: A method for analysis of a family interview. Arch Gen Psychiatry 5:321–337, 1961
83. Satir V: A Guide to Theory and Technique, rev ed. Palo Alto, Science and Behavior, 1967
84. Watzlawick P, Beaven JH, Jackson DD: Pragmatics of Human Communication: A Study of Interactional Patterns, Pathologies, and Paradoxes. New York, Norton, 1967
85. Gottman JM: Marital Interaction: Experimental Investigations. New York, Academic Press, 1979
86. Gottman JM, Markman H, Notarius C: The topography of marital conflict: A sequential analysis of verbal and nonverbal behavior. J Marriage Fam 39:461–477, 1977
87. Margolin G: A sequential analysis of dyadic communication. Presented at the Annual Meeting of the Association for the Advancement of Behavior Therapy, Atlanta, Georgia, December, 1977
88. Kahn M: Nonverbal communication and marital satisfaction. Fam Process 9:449–456, 1970
89. Gordon T: PET: Parent Effectiveness Training. New York, Wyden, 1970
90. Jacobson NS, Margolin G: Marital Therapy: Treatment Strategies Based on Social Learning and Behavior Exchange Principles. New York, Brunner/Mazel, 1979
91. Margolin G, Weiss RL: Contracts, cognition, and change: A behavioral approach to marriage therapy. Counseling Psychol 5:15–25, 1975
92. Weiss RL, Hops H, Patterson GR: A framework for conceptualizing marital conflict, a technology for altering it, some data for evaluating it, in Critical Issues in Research and Practice: Proceedings of the Fourth Banff International Conference on Behavioral Modification. Edited by Clark FW, Hamerlynck LA. Champaign, Research, 1973, pp 309–342
93. Gordon T: TET: Teacher Effectiveness Training. New York, Wyden, 1975
94. Gordon T: LET: Leader Effectiveness Training. New York, Wyden, 1977
95. Laughren TP, Kass DJ: Desensitization of sexual dysfunction: the present status, in Couples in Conflict. Edited by Gurman AS, Rice DG. New York, Ahrenson, 1975, p 285
96. Wright S, Perreault R, Mathieu M: Treatment of sexual dysfunction: A review. Arch Gen Psychiatry 34:881–890, 1977
97. Semans JH: Premature ejaculation. A new approach. Southern Med J 49:353–357, 1956
98. Sharpe L, Kurlansky JB, O'Conner JF: A preliminary classification of human sexual disorders. J Sex Marital Ther 2:106–114, 1976
99. Schover LR, Friedman, JM, Weiler SJ, et al.: A multi-axial problem-oriented system for the sexual dysfunctions: An alternative to DSM-III. Arch Gen Psychiatry, in press
100. LoPiccolo J, Steger JC: The sexual interaction inventory: A new instrument for assessment of sexual dysfunction. Arch Sexual Behav 3:585–595, 1974
101. Derogatis LR: Psychological assessment of sexual disorders, in Clinical Management of Sexual Disorders. Edited by Meyer J. Baltimore, Williams and Wilkins, 1976
102. Kaplan HS: Hypoactive sexual desire. J Sex Marital Ther 3:3–9, 1977
103. Goldstein A: Appropriate expression training: Humanistic behavior therapy, in Humanism and Behaviorism: Dialogue and Growth. Edited by Wandersman A, Poppen PJ, Ricks DF. Elmsford, Pergamon Press, 1976, pp 223–233
104. Lange AJ, Jakubowski P: Responsible Assertive Behavior: Cognitive/Behavioral Procedures for Trainers. Champaign, Research, 1976
105. Wolpe J, Lazarus AA: Behavior Therapy Techniques. New York, Pergamon Press, 1966
106. McFall RM: Behavioral training: A skill-acquisition approach to clinical problems, in Behavioral Approaches to Therapy. Edited by Spense JT, Carson RC, Thibault JW. Morristown, General Learning Press, 1976,pp 227–259
107. Alden L, Safran J, Weideman R: A comparison of cognitive and skills training strategies in the treatment of unassertive clients. Behav Ther 9:843–846, 1978
108. Carmody TP: Rational-emotive, self-instructional, and behavioral assertion training: Facilitating maintenance. Cognitive Ther Res 2:241–253, 1978

109. Thorpe GL: Desensitization, behavior rehearsal, self-instructional training and placebo effects on assertive–refusal behavior. Eur J Behav Anal Mod 1:30–44, 1975
110. Wolfe JL, Fodor IG: Modifying assertive behavior in women: A comparison of three approaches. Behav Ther 8:567–574, 1977
111. Bem SL: The measurement of psychological androgyny. J Consult Clin Psychol 42:155–162, 1974
112. Spence JT, Helmreich R, Stapp J: Ratings of self and peers on sex-role attributions and their relation to self esteem and conceptions of masculinity and feminity. J Personality Soc Psychol 32:29–39, 1975
113. Jones WH, Chernovetz ME, Hansson RO: The enigma of androgyny: Differential implications for males and females? J Consult Clin Psychol 2:298–313, 1978
114. Bem SL: Sex role adaptability: One consequence of psychological androgyny. J Personality Soc Psychol 31:634–643, 1976
115. Bem SL, Lenny E: Sex typing and the avoidance of cross-sex behavior. J Personality Soc Psychol 33:48–54, 1976
116. Wiggins JS, Holzmuller A: Psychological androgyny and interpersonal behavior. J Consult Clin Psychol 46:40–52, 1978
117. Carlson R: Sex differences in ego functioning. J Consult Clin Psychol 37:367–377, 1971
118. O'Connor K, Mann DW, Bardwick JM: Androgyny and self-esteem in the upper-middle class: A replication of Spence. J Consult Clin Psychol 46:1168–1169, 1978
119. Kelly JA, O'Brien CG, Hosford RL, et al.: Sex roles and social skills: A behavioral analysis of "masculinity," "femininity" and "psychological androgyny." Presented at the Annual Meeting of the Association for the Advancement of Behavior Therapy, New York, December, 1976
120. Antill JK, Cunningham JD: Self-esteem as a function of masculinity in both sexes. J Consult Clin Psychol 47:783–785, 1979
121. Bennett S: Further implications of masculinity and femininity for psychological well-being in women and men. Presented at the 87th Annual Meeting of the American Psychological Association, New York, 1977
122. Canter RJ, Meyerwitz B: Sex-role stereotypes: Behavioral investigation. Presented at the 87th Annual Meeting of the American Psychological Association, New York, 1979
123. O'Leary VE: Androgynous men: The "best of both worlds?" Presented at the Annual Meeting of the American Psychological Association, San Francisco, California 1977
124. Costrich N, Feinstein J, Kidder L, et al.: When stereotypes hurt: Three studies of penalties for sex-role reversals. J Exper Soc Psychol 11:520–530, 1975
125. Deaux K, Traynor J: Evaluation of male and female ability: Bias works two ways. Psychol Rep 32:261–262, 1973
126. Feather NT, Simon JG: Reactions to male and female success and failure in sex-linked occupations: Impressions of personality, causal attributions, and perceived likelihood of different consequences. J Personality Soc Psychol 31:20–31, 1975
127. Jacobson MB, Efferty J: Sex roles and leadership: Perceptions of the leaders and the led. Organization Behav Human Performance 12:383–396, 1974
128. Larronce D, Pavelich S, Storer P, et al.: Competence and incompetence: Asymmetric responses to women and men on a sex-linked task. J Personality Soc Psychol Bull 5:363–367, 1979
129. Babl JD: Compensatory masculine responding as a function of sex role. J Consult Clin Psychol 47:252–257, 1979
130. Winkler RC: What types of sex-role behavior should behavior modifiers promote? J App Behav Anal 10:549–552, 1977
131. Nordyke NS, Baer DM, Etzel BC, et al.: Implications of the stereotyping and modification of sex role. J App Behav Anal 10:553–557, 1977
132. Rekers GA, Lovaas OI: Behavioral treatment of deviant sex-role behaviors in a male child. J App Behav Anal 7:173–190, 1974
133. Gurman AS, Klein MH: Women and behavioral marriage and family therapy: An unconscious male bias? in Contemporary issues in behavior modification with women. Edited by Blechman EA. New York, Guilford Press, in press
134. Whitley BE Jr: Sex roles and psychotherapy: A current appraisal. Psychol Bull 6:1309–1321, 1979

135. Baer S, Berger M, Wright L: Even cowboys sing the blues: Difficulties experienced by men trying to adopt nontraditional sex roles and how clinicians can be helpful to them. Sex Roles 5:191–197, 1979
136. Birk JM: Relevancy and alliance: Cornerstones in training counselors of men. Presented at the Annual Meeting of the American Psychological Association, Montreal, Quebec, September 5, 1980
137. Weiss RL: The conceptualization of marriage from a behavioral perspective, in Marriage and Marital Therapy. Edited by Paolino PJ, McCrady BF. New York, Brunner/Mazel, 1978, pp 165–239
138. Berger M: Men's new family roles—some implications for therapists. Fam Coordinator 28:638–646, 1979
139. Tavris C, Offir C: The Longest War: Sex Differences in Perspective. New York, Harcourt, Brace, Jovanovich, 1977
140. Farrell WT: The Liberated Man. New York, Random House, 1974
141. Vanacek FR: Men's Awareness Training. Unpublished manuscript, 1980
142. Horney K: Neurosis and Human Growth. New York, Norton, 1950

Chapter 16

Male Inexpressiveness

Behavioral Intervention

DAVID A. DOSSER, JR.

INTRODUCTION

The male sex role became an important topic of study during the 1970s and promises to be a major subject for the 1980s. This subject has been explored from the perspectives of a number of disciplines, theories, and methodological approaches.

One aspect of the male sex role that has been studied in detail is the concept of male inexpressiveness, that is, the idea that males are generally less expressive of positive emotions than are females. A number of researchers have found this to be the case and have indicated that this is primarily due to socialization experiences through which males are taught which behaviors are socially appropriate or masculine. Perhaps more important, males may be taught which are socially inappropriate or feminine behaviors. In addition, there is evidence that inexpressiveness encumbers males with intrapersonal and interpersonal problems, and that many men desire to be more expressive than they are. This chapter presents one approach to helping inexpressive males to be more expressive, an approach called expressiveness training, based on the premise that if men learned to be inexpressive, they can learn to be more expressive. Taking a cognitive–behavioral approach and drawing from relevant existing programs, expressiveness training includes elements of assertiveness training, communication skills training, male consciousness raising, and cognitive restructuring strategies. Techniques utilized to develop expressiveness skills include lecture and discussion, behavioral rehearsal, role playing, modeling, coaching, and videotaped feedback. This training program is designed to develop both verbal and nonverbal expression of emotion skills, and can be used for group or individual training.

DAVID A. DOSSER, JR. • Department of Child Development and Family Relations, North Dakota State University, Fargo, North Dakota 58105

This chapter is divided into three major sections: (1) a review of research on male inexpressiveness; (2) a review of, and suggestions for, assessing expressiveness; and (3) a description of expressiveness training. The goals of this chapter are to provide counselors/therapists with: (1) a better understanding of male inexpressiveness and implications of this problem for males; (2) a better understanding of procedures to assess expressiveness; and (3) knowledge of a training procedure designed specifically for use with inexpressive males to enable them to become more expressive.

MALE INEXPRESSIVENESS

There has accumulated over the last 25 years, from a number of different areas and from independent research efforts, substantial evidence that males are generally less expressive of emotions than females. For the past ten years Balswick and his associates[1–13] have been studying the inexpressive male.

Evidence has accumulated which makes it fairly clear that males have a more difficult time expressing their emotional feelings than do females. For example, in research based upon samples of over 500 college students and 1200 high school students, males were found to be less expressive than females of the emotions of love, sorrow, happiness, tenderness, grief, delight, affection, sadness, joy, warmth, "the blues," and elation.

Research in the areas of assertiveness training and self-disclosure has been in agreement with the findings of Balswick and his associates. In an empirical investigation studying sex differences in assertive behavior, Hollandsworth and Wall[14] attempted to determine if women are generally less assertive than men as has been assumed. This assumption has been explained in terms of societal role differentiation which rewards women for relying on nonassertive behaviors. They found, in compiling the results from a number of assertiveness studies, several sex differences in assertive behaviors. Specifically, the results indicated that men reported themselves as being more assertive than women with bosses and supervisors, more outspoken when stating opinions, and more ready to take the initiative in social contacts with members of the opposite sex. Men appeared to be less assertive than women, however, in the expression of love, affection, compliments, and anger to one's parents. These results support the findings of Balswick and his associates.

Jourard initiated the study of self-disclosure and has completed many studies of various aspects of self-disclosure. Self-disclosure has been defined as any information about himself which Person A communicates verbally to Person B.[15] Jourard and his associates[16–19] have consistently found that men reveal less personal information about themselves than do women. However, in a literature review of self-disclosure, Cozby[15] cited a number of studies that reported no sex differences in self-disclosure, and concluded that the fact that no study reported greater male disclosure may be indicative of actual sex differences.

Most of the self-disclosure research has been concerned with "general" disclosure rather than disclosure of feelings or affective self-disclosure. A few studies, however, can be specifically related to Balswick's findings. Studying the disclosure of feelings in marriage, Levinger and Senn[20] obtained findings that supported their hypothesis that wives would tend to be higher than husbands in the proportion of feelings they disclose to their spouses. They used a self-disclosure questionnaire quite different from any previous instrument employed by other investigators. The effects of situational factors, sex, and attitude on affective self-disclosure were investigated by Highlen and Gillis,[21] who noted that only a few studies have focused directly on affective self-disclosure. These studies reported that females expressed more feelings than males. Highlen and Gillis reported results that are consistent with previous research; females disclosed more feelings than males to best male and female friends across conditions. In a later study,[22] these findings were replicated within the acquaintance intimacy level. Research has indicated that affective self-disclosure is a complex variable which seems to be sex-linked and situation-specific.[21]

In summary, many studies involving various aspects of assertiveness and self-disclosure support Balswick's contention that men express feelings less than women. These various studies also used several different assessment procedures which provide validation for Balswick's concept of the inexpressive male.

MALE SOCIALIZATION. If men are generally less expressive of positive emotions than are females, how does the tendency develop? Balswick and Peek[12] discussed the development of the inexpressive male and they believe children from birth are taught implicitly and explicitly how to be a man or a woman. Boys, they believe, are taught to value expressions of masculinity and to devalue expressions of femininity. According to these researchers, masculinity is largely expressed through courage, toughness, competitiveness, and aggressiveness, whereas femininity is, in contrast, largely expressed through gentleness, expressiveness, and responsiveness. They concluded that boys readily and easily learn to view outward expressions of emotion as a sign of femininity, and, as such, undesirable for a male. Certain words such as "tender," "sentimental," and "gentle" are even considered feminine while "aggressive," "hostile," and "angry" are masculine.[8] Bem[23] used this classification of certain adjectives as feminine or masculine as the basis for her sex-role inventory or androgyny scale.

In offering his explanation for the inability of many men to express their emotions, Phillips[24] looked to traditional male socialization, suggesting that this is a process which demands that males live up to an ideal concept of masculinity which emphasizes strength, control, and rationality, and which denies the expression of feelings, vulnerability, gentleness, and sensitivity. Phillips believed that much of male socialization focuses on what young men are *not* supposed to be like; furthermore, he believed that this leads to a denial of, and an active effort to avoid, feminine behaviors and attitudes. This can continue, Phillips believed, to the extreme of "homophobia," fear of appearing gay,[25] which leads some males to make an even greater effort to embody the rigid role prescriptions of the masculine stereotype.

According to Jourard,[17] the tendency of males to be less self-disclosing is the result of socialization, and the male role—as personally and socially defined—requires a man to be tough, objective, striving, achieving, unsentimental, and emotionally unexpressive. A man needs to guard against exposing his secrets and true self in order to avoid revealing his areas of weakness and vulnerability. If a man is tender or weeps or shows emotions, he will probably be regarded as weak and unmanly by others, and will likely regard himself as inferior to other men. The male role and self-structure will not allow a man to acknowledge or to express the entire breadth and depth of his inner experience, to himself or to others.[17]

PROBLEMS OF MALE INEXPRESSIVENESS. If men are truly less expressive than females because of socialization experiences, what difference does it make? A number of personal and interpersonal problems have been attributed to inexpressiveness and limited self-disclosure. In fact, Balswick and Peek[12] and Balswick[3,6] discussed the impact that male inexpressiveness has on marriage. Balswick[3] wrote:

> This male inexpressiveness is no laughing matter; it's a real tragedy for the man's wife, his children, and most especially for himself. Think of the wife who year after year, never hears the words "I love you." Consider the child who is never told "fine work, I'm proud of you." And think of the tragedy of the man himself, crippled by an inability to let out the best part of a human being—his warm and tender feelings for other people (p. 66).

A male's inexpressiveness can become highly dysfunctional to his marital relationship, according to Balswick and Peek.[12] Part of this difficulty is due to some changes in marriages and familes, such as increased mobility, smaller families, and separation from extended family ties. These changes have caused us to become increasingly dependent on spouse or family members for affection, communication, and friendship.[3] Society teaches the male to be masculine and inexpressive, and, at the same time, expects the male in intimate relationships to be affectionate and express feelings.

In a review of the literature on male socialization and the implications for marriage and family therapy, Phillips[24] suggested that the traditional socialization of males in our culture inhibits the development of basic characteristics and skills which are important aspects of the ability to engage successfully in intimate and family relationships. He called the inability of many men, as a result of socialization, to become intimate with another human being a "dysfunction in intimacy." His review of research and clinical evidence indicated that this dysfunction affects the majority of men as they attempt to be friends, lovers, husbands, and fathers. Phillips encouraged counselors and therapists to become aware of this dysfunctionality and how it may inhibit or sabotage relationship systems.

There are many examples of the problems of inexpressiveness and the advantages of expressiveness in the self-disclosure literature. Jourard[17] has described appropriate self-disclosure as a necessary condition for a healthy personality and has discussed the "lethal aspects of the male role." Convinced that men, owing to low self-disclosure, are beset with many psychosomatic disorders that do not affect woman as frequently, Jourard believed that manliness seems to carry with it a chronic burden of stress which could be a factor related to man's shorter life span, and that the ability to suppress and express emotion selectively is the pattern of emotional control most compatible with psychological health.

Other research has found self-disclosure to be related to various aspects of psychological health: (1) Mayo[26] found that normals self-dislose more than neurotics or normals with neurotic symptoms; (2) Halverson and Shore[27] found a relation between high self-disclosure and interpersonal openness and effectiveness; (3) Thase and Page[28] stated that high self-disclosure is related to positive mental health, self-awareness, and improved interpersonal functioning; and (4) Halpern[29] stated that research has demonstrated self-disclosure to be positively related to personal adjustment and successful counseling outcome. There seems to be no doubt that self-disclosure is important and desirable.

A further problem with male inexpressiveness is contemporary society's changing sex-role stereotypes. It is particularly difficult in 20th century American society to determine what is masculine or feminine because the accepted and preferred sex roles for many are not as clear-cut or stereotyped as they once were. These changes are due largely to an increasing emphasis on androgyny (being instrumental and expressive) which is slowly influencing socialization. Findings that suggested that androgynous individuals display more sex-role adaptability across situations and are able to engage in situationally effective behavior without regard to stereotypes have been reported by Bem.[30] She added that nonandrogynous subjects displayed behavioral deficits of one sort or another. She concluded with the thought that the androgynous individual may someday come to define a new and more human standard of psychological health.

Bem did not discuss expression of emotions specifically; she discussed sex-typed behavior in general. It seems safe to assume, however, that she would consider the inexprssive male as falling short of the desired androgyny. Osofsky and Osofsky[31] have maintained that androgyny, i.e., no sex-role differentiation, is a viable lifestyle option for many individuals, that personal benefits for females are logical, and that males could benefit from an opportunity for greater individual freedom and for more meaningful relationships with women. Both Bem and Osofsky and Osofsky suggested a need for a lessening of traditional sex-role stereotypes.

Furthermore, there has been evidence of an increased interest in the changes in male roles in the family. Recently several entire journals issues have addressed this topic and questions related to it, both theoretically and empirically (e.g., *Journal of Social Issues,* Pleck and Brannon,[32] *The Counseling Psychologist,* Skovholt et al.,[33] and *The Family Coordinator,* Lewis and Pleck[34]). These journal issues have presented a number of papers discussing the changes in men's roles, the impact on men and women of these changes, and the impact of these changes on children. All evidence seems to suggest that men are being called on more and more to be expressive as well as instrumental and that the inability for a man to be expressive is stressful for the male and the family.

MEN'S DESIRE TO BE MORE EXPRESSIVE. There is evidence that many men, owing to the interpersonal and intrapersonal problems with inexpressiveness and low self-disclosure, want to be more expressive and self-disclosing. Balswick[7] has reported findings that suggest that many, perhaps most, males in our society wish to become more expressive and are not satisfied with their inexpressive selves. Clinical evidence that men are interested in improving their expressive skills and have found benefits in so doing has been reported.[24] There is reason to believe that men will continue to desire to be more expressive as intolerance grows with the male's inability to be expressive as well as instrumental, and as the strong, silent type of male becomes less glorified. With these changes many males are concerned with their inability to express emotions, and this concern will no doubt grow with impetus from the women's movement as well as from an increase in criticism of male inexpressiveness from marriage counselors, assertiveness and sensitivity group leaders, and youth in general.[6] Many others[35–40] have echoed this desire for changes in the male sex role and have discussed the many and varied advantages of a less rigid male sex-role stereotype.

SUGGESTIONS FOR IMPROVING MALE EXPRESSIVENESS. Most writers have not suggested specific ways to facilitate increased male expressiveness and self-disclosure. Most of their recommendations have been general in nature. For example, Farrell[35] suggested the efficacy of male consciousness-raising groups for lessening the rigidity of traditional male sex-role stereotypes. He described the benefits of groups that focused on objectives such as (1) increasing the awareness of how men's behavior is restricted by stereotypes of masculinity and femininity; (2) increasing men's openness and ability to admit weakness and demonstrate softness; (3) reducing competition with other men; and (4) challenging and reexamining their attitudes toward women, other men, and themselves. There has been little empirical research on these groups and most of the information comes from anecdotal reports.

Most of the assertiveness training books have discussed the expression of feelings and the fact that expressing feelings is assertive.[41–47] These books and the behavior change strategies they described, however, have focused primarily upon the expression of negative feelings and have only touched slightly on the expression of positive or tender feelings, which are the most difficult for inexpressive males to express in close relationships. The use of assertion training groups for men to create a relatively nonthreatening environment which facilitated a beginning process of resocialization through teaching skills necessary for relationships has been described by Phillips.[24]

In addition, several studies have used training programs to increase affective self-disclosure or expressiveness. For example, Damgaard[48] explored the relative effectiveness of structured versus unstructured procedures for training groups in the expression of feeling–cause relations for a population of adult male psychiatric inpatients. The structured program consisted of small group (directed and improvised) role playing in feeling–cause statements with modeling and feedback by the therapist. The unstructured program consisted of group-directed discussion of topics selected by the group members. Damgaard reported that unstructured procedures were more effective in the identification and expression of positive feelings, and that structured procedures were more effective in the identification and expression of negative feelings. Boone[49] found roughly similar results using Damgaard's training procedures with undergraduate male and female education majors. A third study was conducted by Highlen[50] (also reported by Highlen and Voight[51]), who investigated whether social modeling and cognitive structuring multicomponent strategies were effective methods for increasing affective self-disclosure in single undergraduate college males. Specifically, Highlen assessed the impact of the two training strategies on (1) amount of affect expressed, (2) quality of affect, (3) concomitant level of anxiety, (4) skill necessary for affective self-disclosure, and (5) attitudes toward disclosing feelings. Her results indicated that cognitive structuring was only slightly more effective than social modeling, while both 50-minute, videotaped, training sessions were statistically more effective than the control groups. The training effect was not, however, maintained at the three-week follow-up, which suggests the need for longer, more intensive training addressing the issues of generalization and maintenance of training effects.

In summary, research has been reviewed which indicates that men are more inexpressive than females. Research has been presented which suggests reasons for male inexpressiveness. Studies have been cited which present the advantages of male expressiveness and the disadvantages of male inexpressiveness. Evidence has been presented that indicates men are interested in becoming more expressive. Finally, studies have been reviewed which offered suggestions as to how to help males increase their expression of emotion. Other approaches to helping men realize the advantages of a less rigid male sex-role stereotype exist, but this review considered only those most relevant to expressiveness training, the approach proposed in this chapter. An expressiveness training program will be thoroughly described in the final section of this chapter; however, prior to this, a discussion of the assessment of expressiveness will be presented. It is important to consider assessment in order to be able to determine the success of any treatment approach or training program.

ASSESSMENT OF EXPRESSIVENESS

Research on the expression of feelings has been conducted in a number of areas and from a number of perspectives, including the following: male inexpressiveness,[1,3,6,12] assertiveness,[14,52–54] self-disclosure,[21,22,51] and nonverbal behavior.[55–61] Although much has been learned about expressive behavior, further research is needed to increase the understanding of this important area including: the causes of inexpressiveness, situational variance in expressive behavior, the relationship between expressiveness and personality variables (e.g., self monitoring), and sex differences in expressive behavior.

Further research is in progress to assess the effectiveness of a cognitive/behavioral approach to expressiveness training on increasing the verbal and nonverbal expressions of emotion for a group of adult males.[62] A critically important and needed element of this ongoing research is an effective, valid, and reliable means of assessing both verbal and nonverbal expression of emotion. This section will review research attempts in the areas of assertiveness and self-disclosure to measure expressiveness or closely related constructs. This review will consider both self-report and behavioral approaches to assessing expressiveness. Finally, implications of assessment of expressiveness for counselors/therapists are considered.

IMPORTANCE OF ASSESSMENT. Before considering specific approaches related to the assessment of expressiveness, it would seem appropriate to consider the importance of assessment in research and applied settings. This will be followed by a brief review of the two main methods of assessment in use, i.e., self-report and behavioral.

Assessment has long been considered an important aspect of many approaches to counseling/therapy; in recent years, however, it has become increasingly important. This has been particularly true of counselors and therapists who have been sensitive to the increased emphasis on behavioral assessment in the 1970s.[63] In identifying clients for treatment, in selecting appropriate and specific treatment for clients, in determining the effectiveness of intervention strategies, and in determining the generality and duration of treatment effects, behavioral assessment is especially important.

Among others, Cromwell et al.[64] believed that more systematic and rigorous evaluation is needed because of the importance of diagnosis and evaluation in marital and family therapy. Diagnosis and evaluation are particularly helpful when they can be linked to the intervention process to enable the therapist to develop a useful plan of treatment for a family or couple. The extremely close relationship between assessment and treatment in behavior modification, in general, and in the social skills area in particular, has, of course, been stressed by numerous clinicians (e.g., Hersen and Bellack[65]).

The importance of assessment in assertion training has been emphasized by Jackubowski and Lacks,[66] who have suggested that appropriate assessment procedures aid the therapist in completing two essential tasks: (1) ascertaining whether the client would benefit from assertiveness training, and (2) deciding whether the client did, in fact, gain benefits from the treatment. Several authors have described the importance of behavioral assessment in determining whether the client's social skills deficit is a result of (1) a deficient learning history where the requisite responses never became a part of the client's repertoire, or (2) the disruptive effects of anxiety which inhibit the demonstration of available responses.[65,67,68] This level of assessment leads directly to the intervention program where, for the problem of dealing with deficient social responses, specific skills training would be appropriate. For the problem of dealing with the disruptive effects of anxiety, oversensitivity, misconceptions, or irrational beliefs, intervention would address those specific factors that interfere with the display of appropriate skills.

Another benefit from assessment is the ability to determine during treatment or training whether the client is making progress. When such an evaluation demonstrates that progress is limited, changes in the intervention plan can be made. Without such assessment and evaluative procedures, the ineffective treatment conceivably could be continued, possibly with considerable costs to client and counselor/therapist in terms of time, energy, and money.

In addition to being important for (1) identifying the client's problem, (2) identifying an appropriate and preferred treatment technique, (3) determining whether the treatment is working, and (4) deciding whether the treatment has been effective, evaluation is important in order to determine treatment effect generalization and durability. Many authors have discussed the importance of considering generalization and durability (e.g., Bodner,[69] Heimberg et al.,[70] Jackubowski and Lacks,[66] Kerlinger,[71]). One direct approach to considering generalization and durability is to use a follow-up evaluation that is designed to assess both elements. The follow-up evaluation can be designed to determine whether treatment effects do, in fact, generalize to other target persons, other situations, and settings by evaluating the client's performance with various target persons, situations, and settings. The duration of treatment effects can be determined by arranging for a follow-up evaluation at different intervals of time following the conclusion of treatment, with longer durations of time preferable. Both of these concerns are often overlooked in treating clients; attention to these concerns can enhance treatment by identifying the need for additional (or booster) treatment sessions. These concerns would not be met without carefully planned and comprehensive evaluations.

TYPES OF ASSESSMENT. With this brief introduction to the importance of assessment, the discussion will now turn to the two broad types of assessment procedures: self-report methods and behavioral methods. It is not the intent of this paper to describe the long-term, expansive, and continuing debate over the relative merits of each of these approaches to assessment. Only a few points will be made relevant to this issue; the reader is referred to other sources for a more thorough review of this issue.[72–76] It is important to note that most authors in the assessment area make the distinction between self-report and behavioral methods of assessment and present examples of each approach (e.g., Bodner,[69] Gambrill,[67] Hall,[77] Heimberg et al.,[70] Hersen and Bellack,[65] Jackubowski and Lacks,[66] Lange and Jackubowski,[46] Rich and Schroeder[78]).

Behavioral self-report and observer subjective report are two other methods of assessment that have been suggested by Olson.[79] These two additional methods, he claimed, help to bridge the gap between self-report and behavioral methods. In distinguishing between these four methods of research and assessment, Olson divided them on two dimensions: (1) reporter's frame of reference (Insider vs. Outsider) and (2) type of data (subjective vs. objective). Olson defined each method as follows: (1) self-report is subjective data from an insider's perspective; (2) behavioral is objective data from an outsider's perspective; (3) observer subjective report is subjective data from an outsider's perspective; and (4) behavioral self-report is objective data from an insider's perspective. Cromwell et al.[64] made the same distinctions when discussing diagnosis and assessment in marital and family therapy, giving primary attention to the self-report and behavioral methods since these methods are more frequently used. Due to this fact, this discussion will consider only these two primary methods.

Self-Report Methods. In areas related to expressiveness (e.g., assertiveness, social skills, and self-disclosure) many self-report methods of assessment exist. Hall[77] believed that the issues surrounding the validity of self-report data have been widely discussed, but that many questions relating to reliability, social desirability, and the usefulness of self-report methods as measures of social skills remain unclear. Despite these unanswered questions, self-report is a major approach to the assessment of assertiveness owing to the economy and quantifiability of self-ratings and self-report inventories. The difficulties of self-reported assessment, including its susceptibility to subject-induced distortion, have also been noted by Hollandsworth and Wall,[14] who argued that more direct and objective measures of behavior are needed at some point. They agreed with Mischel[72] that self-reports have the advantage of being as good a predictor of future behavior as any other nonbehavioral measure while being easily and inexpensively administered. Although self-report methods of assessment are important, necessary, and useful, Jackubowski and Lacks[66] have cautioned therapists to be aware of the contradictory findings with respect to how self-reports correlate with overt measures of assertion when attempting to evaluate the effectiveness of assertion training.

Behavioral Methods. Several authors have been less charitable toward self-report measures. For example, Warren and Gilner[54] have cited research which compared behavioral and self-report measures and concluded that assessment of behavior is more predictive of future events and more sensitive to changes due to treatment in assertive training than are self-report measures. Their findings also support the common finding that self-report measures do not correlate highly with behavioral data. A number of researchers have attempted to avoid the difficulties usually associated with self-report methods through the use of behavioral tasks and role-playing tests of assertiveness which attempt to make assessment samples as close to "real life" situations as possible.[77] While admitting the desirability of assessing behavior directly, it has been pointed out that the major limitation presently of role-playing assessment is that no validation studies have been reported.[78] Hollandsworth and Wall[14] and Hall[77] have discussed the limits of behavioral assessments, in that the influence of varying response types and situational contexts must be considered. However, this could be an overwhelming and expensive task unless the wide range of situations can be narrowed to those that exhibit a potential for productive investigation.[14]

Advantage of Using Both Methods. While arguments have continued for and against both self-report and behavioral methods of assessment, several authors have argued for the importance of both in combination for research and assessment.[64,79] The importance of approaching assessment from a subjective–self-report–insider frame of reference as well as from an objective–behavioral–outsider frame of reference in order to gain a comprehensive picture of interpersonal relationships has been stressed by Olson,[79] who argued that each offers a different and valuable perspective, and that their combination has benefits that have been too often ignored by researchers. That different methods provide different kinds of information and that from both a research and a therapeutic perspective, data from each can provide a more comprehensive understanding has been argued by Cromwell et al.[64]; they believe that, since these methods tap different perspectives (insider's and outsider's) and generate different types of data (subjective and objective), one should not expect agreement across methods. Conflicting data may be considered as additional sources of clinical information which the therapist might effectively apply during the treatment process. Self-report, overt behavioral, and physiological response measures have had consistently low relationships with one another in the assessment of social skills[65] and there appears to be no indication that any one approach is sufficient to adequately represent the social skills complex. This view is supported by Olson,[79] who believes that the insider's and outsider's perspectives are two mutually exclusive frames of reference with neither being sufficient alone.

APPROACHES TO ASSESSING EXPRESSIVENESS. Now turning to specific approaches related to the assessment of expressiveness, this discussion will consider research in the areas of assertiveness and self-disclosure. These areas seem, intuitively, to be related to each other and to expressiveness; an effort will be made to demonstrate the relationship between them conceptually, theoretically, and empirically.

Expressiveness in the past has been considered simply as the expression of emotions; an operational definition has not existed. Absent an operational definition, and borrowing from Lange and Jackubowski[46] and Highlen,[50] expressiveness will be defined as the direct, honest, appropriate, and self-referenced expression of positive and negative emotions with feeling words; expressiveness also includes clearly stating the cause for the feelings. This definition is used as a guide in the search for appropriate assessment procedures.

Expression of Emotion Scale. The need to turn to indirect measures of expressiveness arises from the paucity of assessment techniques designed to measure expressiveness directly. Balswick's Expression of Emotion Scale[4] is one such scale that has demonstrated utility. This scale contains 16 items with four items for each of the four feelings of love, hate, happiness, and sadness. The scale was developed using factor-analytic techniques which give strong support for the theoretical soundness of the four dimensions of emotions which make up its subscales. Balswick considers the results of the factor structure of the scale as support for the notion that the four items which make up each of the four dimensions of emotionality are actually measuring a variety of the same type of emotion.

A factor analysis of a related scale, the Emotion Scale,[4] which was developed and is usually administered concurrently with the Expression of Emotion Scale produced similar results. It, too, is made up of the four subscales of happiness, sadness, hate and love but purports to measure feeling rather than expression of feeling. Like the *Expression of Emotion Scale,* it contains 16 items, four for each of the four feelings.

Respondents are asked to respond to each of the 16 statements in both of the Likert-type scales by selecting one of the four forced categories of "Never," "Seldom," "Often," or "Very Often." By giving weights to the response categories of from 1 (never) to 4 (very often), the potential scale scores for the Emotion Scale and the Expression of Emotion Scale are from a low of 16 to a high of 64. The potential scale scores for the subscales range from 4 to 16. According to Balswick, the 16 statements of the Emotion Scale seek to measure the degree to which each of four different types of emotions are present in the subject. The 16 statements on the Expression of Emotion Scale seek to measure the extent to which these same emotions are expressed by the subject.

Balswick considers his two scales as a beginning attempt at establishing some quantitative measurements of emotions, and has argued that the best way (within the situation of survey research) to measure something as abstract as emotionality and the expression of emotions is by directly asking people the extent to which they feel certain emotions and express these emotions to others. Balswick believes that the direct way in which the scales attempt to measure emotionality and the expression of emotions should give us confidence in their face validity, and has concluded that the scales could easily be adapted to consider situational and role differences in the feeling and expression of emotions, which he believes would further develop an understanding of the sociology of emotions (Balswick, research in progress). He has noted that other emotions could be included to provide a better understanding of feelings and expressions of emotions.

These scales have been the basis of a number of studies and have proved to be useful in studying sex differences in expression of emotions.[1,4–6,8,9,13] The scales, however, have not yet been subjected to a rigorous examination concerning reliability and validity. This fact would limit the use of the scales as measures of therapeutic changes with pre- and posttesting. The beginning steps have been taken to determine the reliability and validity of the Expression of Emotion Scale and the Emotion Scale, and research in this area is continuing. Results thus far have been promising for test-retest reliability and disappointing for concurrent validity. Specifically, these results indicated that the test–retest reliability coefficients for the Expression of Emotion Scale were .83 at one week for adults (n = 34) and .72 at six weeks for college students (n = 33)(Davidson and Dosser, unpublished data, 1979). In terms of concurrent validity, no significant correlations were found between expression of emotion scores and behavioral ratings of expressiveness for a sample of adult correctional officers (n = 35)(Dosser, Balswick, and Davidson, unpublished data, 1979). Research is in progress to further test the validity of Balswick's measure with other populations.

Assertiveness. In the absence of other available assessment procedures that would measure expressiveness directly, the construct of assertiveness seemed, on the basis of several definitions, to be related to expressiveness. Assertiveness is an area that has recently enjoyed immense popularity, both in the scientific community as the basis of much research and writing, and with the general public. It is also an area that, because of its behavioral theory and methodology, lends itself readily to research, evaluation, and assessment. Because of this fact, many self-report and behavioral approaches to assessing assertiveness have been developed. Those most clearly relevant to expressiveness will be reviewed following a review of published definitions of assertiveness and of established components of assertiveness.

Definitions of assertiveness. Salter,[80] one of the earliest to describe assertive techniques, proposed six techniques of general use to patients in increasing excitation (assertiveness). These were as follows:

1. *feeling talk,* which includes the utterances of spontaneously felt emotions;
2. *facial talk,* or the display of emotion on the face;
3. *contradict and attack,* which includes expressing disagreement with others;
4. *the use of I* to achieve ownership of feelings and statements;
5. *express agreement when praised,* which includes accepting praise and volunteering self-praise when reasonable;
6. *improvise* or make spontaneous responses to immediate stimuli.

Though these do not really define assertiveness, they certainly present what Salter believed excitation to be. A more direct, early definition of assertiveness was presented by Wolpe and Lazarus,[81] who defined assertiveness in a broad sense to include "all socially acceptable expressions of rights and feelings" (p. 39).

In a later work Wolpe[68] stated, "Assertive behavior is defined as the proper expression of any emotion other than anxiety towards another person" (p. 81). He distinguished between "hostile" (e.g., "Please don't stand in front of me"; "I can't stand your nagging"; "Your behavior disgusts me") and "commendatory" (e.g., "I like you"; "I love you"; "That was a clever remark") assertive statements. He further noted that the presenting problems of clients might include an inability to express affection, admiration, or praise because he/she finds such expression embarrassing.

In conceptualizing assertiveness in order to develop a self-report measure of assertiveness, Galassi et al.[82] identified three types of assertiveness: (1) *positive assertiveness,* consisting of expressing feelings of love, affection, admiration, approval, and agreement; (2) *negative assertiveness,* including expressions of justified feelings of anger, disagreement, dissatisfaction, and annoyance; and (3) *self-denial,* including overapologizing, excessive interpersonal anxiety, and exaggerated concern for the feelings of others. Lange and Jackubowski[46] provided a definition that was similar to Galassi et al., but they concentrated on the issue of each person's rights in the interaction, i.e., "Assertion involves standing up for personal rights and expressing thoughts, feelings, and beliefs in direct, honest, and appropriate ways, which do not violate another person's rights" (p. 7).

Other definitions of assertiveness have considered the issue of reinforcement. Warren and Gilner[54] conceptualized assertive behaviors as including the expression of all feelings and as seeking to optimize reinforcement in the social environment. They attempted to integrate positive assertions and rights (or negative assertions) by defining assertiveness as "direct communication congruent on verbal and nonverbal levels of where the individual stands both cognitively and affectively, expressed in a manner which respects the rights of the listener." Others[65] have defined social skills (including assertiveness) as "an individual's ability to express both positive and negative feelings in the interpersonal context without suffering consequent loss of social reinforcement" (p. 512). In keeping with an emphasis on reinforcement, Rich and Schroeder[78] offered a functional definition of assertive behavior. For them, it was "the skill to seek, maintain, or enhance reinforcement in an interpersonal situation through an expression of feelings or wants when such expression risks loss of reinforcement or even punishment." They believed that the degree of assertiveness was measured by the effectiveness of the individual's responses in producing, maintaining, or enhancing reinforcement.

These definitions have stressed different aspects of assertive behavior (e.g., rights, types of assertive behavior, reinforcement, expression of feelings, etc.). There are many other definitions and approaches to conceptualizing assertive behavior that could have been reviewed, but they are similar to those presented.

There are, however, a few definitions that focus only on demands, refusals, contradictions, expressing opinions, and other behaviors that seem to be almost aggressive. These definitions and conceptualizations seemed less appropriate to the issues at hand and so were excluded. It is believed that those definitions presented represent a good cross-section of extant definitions and conceptualizations of assertive behavior.

Difficulties with the concept of assertiveness. Hall[77] discussed two major difficulties with the concept of assertiveness. The first relates to determining the parameters of assertive behavior. He noted the problems related to the additivity of negative and positive components to achieve a total score of assertiveness. Hall believed that multidimensional assessment instruments of assertiveness are necessary and that adding scores from different dimensions to achieve a total score is confusing. The second conceptual difficulty affecting assessment of assertiveness is the problem of defining assertiveness as either a personality trait or as a situation-specific response. Both of these difficulties, and particularly the trait versus situation controversy, have led to confusion in defining, conceptualizing, and assessing assertive behavior. The latter problem has also been discussed by other authors with arguments for both the trait and situation-specific point of view.

Assertive behavior has been considered to be a broad personality trait, i.e., a generalized response tendency (e.g., Salter[80]). It has also been considered as an expression of a response which has situational specificity. The existing evidence supports the latter point of view, or assertiveness as a situation-specific response.[78]

One of the studies providing empirical evidence for the response specificity of assertive behavior attempted to explore the role of the social–interpersonal context in determining whether a response is assertive or not assertive. Behaviors which are socially appropriate in one circumstance may be inappropriate in another, Eisler et al.[53] concluded. They substantiated the hypothesis that assertive behavior is functionally related to the social context of the interpersonal interaction, and as they had expected, found that the content of the responses changed depending upon whether the situation required positive or negative assertion. In addition, Eisler et al. found that the nature of the situation produced significant differences on six of the seven nonverbal interactional variables that they considered. On this basis, Eisler et al. concluded that, in general, the results support a stimulus-specific theory of assertiveness, i.e., "an individual who is assertive in one interpersonal context may not be assertive in a different interpersonal environment."

Other empirical evidence that has been interpreted as support for the situation-specific nature of assertive behavior is provided by the factor analyses of assertive self-report measures. These studies have without exception found many factors instead of one major assertive factor. For example, a factor analysis of discomfort scores[83] found 11 factors accounting for 61% of the variance in one study with each factor accounting for from 7% to 3.9%. The researchers concluded that the emergence of a number of relatively equally weighted factors is supportive of the theory of situational specificity in relation to assertive behavior. In similar studies of another assertiveness measure, the Rathus Assertiveness Schedule (RAS),[84] similar results were found.[85,86] This evidence strongly suggests that attempting to measure or identify a global concept of assertiveness is useless.

In the closely related area of social skills, the importance of a situation-specific conception of social skills that involved the coordinated delivery of appropriate verbal and nonverbal responses was stressed.[65] Finally, Lazarus,[87] based upon his clinical experiences, divided the main components of assertive (or emotionally expressive) behavior into four separate and specific response patterns: (1) the ability to refuse; (2) the ability to make requests; (3) the ability to express positive and negative feelings; and (4) the ability to initiate and continue conversations.

In summary, the evidence and the opinions of most researchers seem to support a situationally specific conception of assertive behavior. This has important implications for both the assessment and the training of assertiveness. Those interested in assessing assertiveness or in training others to be assertive should consider only very specific components of assertive behavior, including specific types of assertions, specific situations, specific target persons, specific verbal content, and specific nonverbal components. These points will be expanded in the final section on implications for counselors/therapists.

Positive aspects of assertive expression. As can be seen from the definitions of assertive behavior which have been presented, the expression of positive feelings (e.g., love, affection, caring) is considered by many to be an assertive act. In spite of this, a great deal of the research, writing, and training has dealt with aspects of assertive behavior other than positive expressions of emotion. This same point has been made in noting that some definitions of assertiveness do not include the expression of positive emotions. Lazarus[88] found it unfortunate that the bulk of research on assertive behaviors has tended to place undue emphasis on the ability to attack or contradict people verbally. Apparently, the same concern led Hollandsworth[89] to attempt to provide some behavioral guidelines for differentiating assertion and aggression. In differentiating assertive and aggressive behavior, Lange and Jackubowski[46] noted that assertive behavior is "responsible" in that it does not violate the rights of the other person. Addressing this same issue, Lazarus[87] asked, "Is it not far more effective to educate people in applying the obvious and subtle nuances of *positive* reinforcement?" (p. 698). Lazarus stated,

> Time spent teaching people how to emit forthright expressions of love, adoration, affection, appreciation, and the specific verbal and nonverbal facets of compassion, tenderness, warmth, and other positive feelings often undermines the need for angry responses and righteous indignation.

Most studies to date have been concerned mostly with assertive behavior in a narrow sense, and have not considered the positive aspects of assertive expression, according to Eisler et al.[53] Based upon their research, they believed that "positive assertive expression, or what Wolpe[67] has termed 'commendatory' behavior, appears to be a real phenomenon that should broaden the scope of assertive training" (p. 355), and that few experimentally validated procedures exist for training individuals to increase their expression of positive feelings. Along these same lines, Warren and Gilner[54] pointed out how the research literature has begun to consider both positive and negative feeling expression in the study of assertiveness and how this effort has been hampered by a lack of adequate measures. Finally, other authors have suggested that considerably greater attention needs to be directed toward assessing the expression of positive feelings.[65,90]

In summary, many authors have called for and have noted the increased emphasis on positive feeling expression in assertive training. Some have even considered it more advantageous[87] to concentrate on positive feelings in assertion training. In spite of this upsurge of interest in the expression of positive feelings, there still exists a paucity of validated procedures to train people to express positive feelings more effectively, as well as measures of positive assertion that have been studied for reliability and validity. In the following review of self-report and behavioral assessment procedures for assertive behavior, the primary emphasis will be upon those procedures which can be used to assess the expression of both positive and negative feelings and which possess adequate reliability and validity. Following the warnings against combining positive and negative components of assertiveness to obtain a total assertiveness score,[77] only those measures of assertiveness that allow the computation of separate positive and negative feeling expression scores will be considered, and in keeping with the evidence for the specificity of assertive behavior, only those assertiveness measures that tap assertiveness in a broad range of situations will be considered. Based upon the definitions and conceptualizations of assertiveness presented above, it seems appropriate to approach the assessment of expressiveness by way of assertiveness.

Self-report measures of assertiveness. In considering self-report measures of assertiveness, journal articles and chapters related to the assessment of social skills and assertive behavior were reviewed.[46,65–67,69,70,77,78] Nineteen different measures were discussed that attempted to measure assertiveness directly or indirectly; only eight measures, however, were consistently discussed. The Rathus Assertiveness Schedule (RAS),[84] the Conflict Resolution Inventory (CRI),[91] and the College Self-Expression Scale (CSES),[82] were most frequently presented and reviewed in these sources. The following five measures were also frequently reviewed: (1) the Assertion Inventory,[83] (2) the Adult Self-Expression Scale (ASES),[92] (3) the Wolpe–Lazarus Assertiveness Scale (AS),[81] (4) the Lawrence Assertive Inventory (LAI),[93] and (5) the Constriction Scale (CS).[94] In terms of articles and chapters presenting and reviewing them, these eight assertiveness measures would seem to be the most popular and impressive.

Another important consideration of the usefulness of an assertive measure is the frequency with which it has been used in the past. According to Hall,[77] the most frequently used self-report assertiveness measures are the Wolpe–Lazarus AQ, the CSES, the ASES, and the RAS. He writes, "With the exception of the CSES, ASES, and RAS, there are insufficient data available to provide definitive evaluations of assertiveness inventories" (p. 339). Hall believed that the decision to use any of the inventories should be based on the nature of information desired and the use to which that information will be put as well as the psychometric properties of the instrument. Rich and Schroeder[78] differed with Hall by concluding that of the seven assertiveness inventories developed in recent years, only the CRI and, to some degree, the Assertion Inventory have shown demonstrable validity and usefulness in screening and assessment. They suggested that most instruments are less desirable because of the failure to correlate the instruments against external behavioral criteria, and that the poor correlations between the instruments and behavioral criteria resulted at least partially from failures to adequately define the response class to be measured. They suggested the use of a behavior-analytic approach to determine empirically the difficult situations for a specific response class (e.g., McFall and Lillesand[91] and Lawrence[93]).

Jackubowski and Lacks[66] reported that the LAI is overly long, too specific, and subject to responding in a socially desirable way. They further criticized the RAS for its relation to social desirability and aggression. Jackubowski and Lacks believed the CSES to be the most suitable measure of a variety of assertive responses, although they noted that its validity is questionable. They listed its strong points as being its brevity, its apparent independence of social desirability and aggressiveness, and the positive reaction of students to it. They also suggested that the CRI is a methodologically sound measure of the specific assertive behavior of refusing requests.

Based upon these opinions concerning the popularity, usefulness, reliability, and validity of various self-report measures of assertive behavior, and the specific interest of this paper in the assessment of expressiveness, the CSES, the ASES, and the Assertion Inventory will be considered in greater detail (Table I). The RAS was eliminated because, although it is frequently used and has demonstrated high reliability and validity, it has been criticized for measuring aggression as well as assertion,[66] because it attempts to measure a global tendency to behave assertively rather than a situation-specific response,[77,78,86] and because of questionable methodology in determining validity.[66,77,78] The CRI was eliminated from consideration because of its specific focus on "refusing requests," a factor which would seem to have little relation to the present interest of assessing expression of emotion. The Wolpe–Lazarus Assertiveness Questionnaire, although popular, is not considered owing to limited evidence of its reliability and validity. It is interesting to note, however, that many of the items in other instruments come from the Wolpe–Lazarus instrument. The Lawrence Assertiveness Inventory and the Constriction Scale are both excluded because of their limited use and limited research in addition to reasons listed previously.

The College Self-Expression Scale: The CSES[82] is a 50-item self-report inventory designed to measure assertiveness in college students. It uses a five-

Table I. Characteristics of Selected Self-Report Measures of Assertiveness

Name of scale	Authors	Number of items	Format	Types of assertiveness measured	Consideration of different situational contexts	Developed for which population
College Self-Expression Scale	Galassi et al.[82]	50	5-pt. Likert 0–4	1. Positive 2. Negative 3. Self-denial	yes	College
Adult Self-Expression Scale	Gay et al.[92]	48	5-pt. Likert 0–4	1. Expressing personal opinions 2. Refusing unreasonable requests 3. Taking initiative in conversation and in dealing with others 4. Expressing positive feelings 5. Asking for favors	yes	Adults
Assertion Inventory	Gambrill and Richey[83]	40	Subjects rate: 1. Degree of discomfort on 5-point scale 2. Probability of displaying behavior on 5-point scale 3. Problem situations by circling the item	1. Turning down requests 2. Expressing personal limitations 3. Initiating social contacts 4. Expressing positive feelings 5. Handling criticism 6. Differing with others 7. Service situations 8. Giving negative feedback	yes	College

point Likert format (0–4) with 21 positively worded and 29 negatively worded items. The scale attempts to measure three aspects of assertiveness: positive, negative, and self-denial. Positive assertiveness includes expressing feelings of love, affection, admiration, approval, and agreement. Negative assertiveness consists of expressions of justified feelings of anger, disagreement, dissatisfaction, and annoyance. Self-denial includes excessive interpersonal anxiety, exaggerated concern for the feelings of others, and overapologizing. The scale assesses assertive behavior in a variety of interpersonal contexts: family, relatives, strangers, authority figures, business relations, like and opposite sex peers. As with many other scales, items were, in part, derived or modified from work by Lazarus,[88] Wolpe,[68] and Wolpe and Lazarus.[81] Galassi et al.[82] contended that low scores on the scale are indicative of a generalized nonassertive response pattern (the total score is obtained by summing all items after reversing those negatively worded items). Test–retest reliability coefficients for two samples ($n = 182$) of college students were .89 and .90. As a test of validity Galassi et al. correlated their scale with items from the Adjective Check List (ACL)[95] and found positive correlations with items that typify assertiveness. They also found significant negative correlations with items consistent with nonassertiveness. Other scales were predicted to be unrelated to response on the CSES and this was the case. Galassi et al. were impressed with the nonsignificant correlation of the CSES with aggression, which suggested that it does not fall to the same difficulty as do some other scales in confusing assertiveness and aggressiveness. Finally, Galassi et al. reported a low, but significant, correlation between supervisor ratings on assertiveness and the ACES scores ($r = .19$, $p < .04$) with a sample of 121 student teachers.

Hall[77] pointed out that no subscales are available for the CSES and that the validation research has utilized a total score. He also cited the administration and scoring manual of the CSES[96] which suggested that attention to individual items rather than a total score might prove useful to clinicians, since assertiveness is considered to be learned and specific to the situation. This use of this scale might prove particularly useful to persons interested in assessing expressiveness.

Other evidence for the validity of the CSES has come from the studies of Galassi and Galassi[97] and Galassi et al.[98] In the first study, concurrent validity was studied by correlating CSES scores of student teachers with assertiveness ratings of their supervisors and by correlating scores of dormitory residents with ratings of resident hall assistants. Correlations of $r = .19$ ($p < .05$) and $r = .33$ ($p < .005$), respectively, were obtained. These correlations might have been depressed due to untrained raters and the limited possibility for interaction between subjects and raters, Galassi and Galassi suggested. A second part of this study using contrasted groups produced results as predicted (for the most part) and demonstrated the ability of the CSES to differentiate groups. Specifically, students who sought counseling for personal adjustment were significantly less assertive than noncounselees and vocational-educational counselees. In the second study, Galassi et al.[98] compared the CSES to behavioral performance criteria, concluding:

> that assertiveness as measured by the CSES reflects a combination of verbal and non-verbal behaviors including eye contact, assertive content of verbal responses, and subjectively experienced anxiety (p. 451).

In summary, the CSES seems to meet the criteria for a useful self-report measure of assertiveness. It might well be possible to use the subscales of negative and particularly positive assertion to get a better assessment of emotional expressiveness. This is apparently what Galassi and Galassi[96] had in mind when suggesting that clinicians focus on particular items of the CSES. The major limitations of the CSES would seem to be that it was written expressly for a college population and some of the items reflect this fact and would thus be inappropriate for noncollege samples.

The Adult Self-Expression Scale: The next self-report measure to be considered is the ASES,[92] which is in many ways similar to the CSES, except that it is intended for and validated on adult samples. It includes 48 items from a number of interactional situations which consider assertive behaviors including: expressing personal opinions, refusing unreasonable requests, taking initiative in conversations and in dealing with others, expressing positive feelings, and asking for favors. The ASES uses the same format and scoring procedure as the CSES. It uses many of the same or rewritten items from the CSES and for a sample (n = 194) of subjects with a mean age of 24.5 years the ASES correlated highly (r = .88) with the CSES. With subjects over 30 and married this correlation fell to .79. Gay et al.[92] reported two- and five-week test–retest reliability correlations of .88 and .91, respectively.

Validation procedures comparing the ASES to the ACL produced results which were similar to those with the CSES, according to Gay et al. They reported a factor structure which supported the two-dimensional model (including interpersonal situations and assertive behaviors) used to construct the scale. Evidence for concurrent validity for the scale is found in the fact that subjects seeking personal-adjustment counseling scored significantly lower on the ASES than did subjects in general.[92] The validation studies on the ASES are the most stringent and complete validation research that has been carried out on any measure of assertiveness; the ASES is a scale with moderate discriminant validity and relatively strong convergent and construct validity.[77] These qualities, Hall concluded, along with the self-scoring answer sheet and applicability to wide-ranging populations, make the ASES a very useful research tool. He noted, however, that the value of the ASES would be greatly enhanced with research on older populations and with the development of subscales based on situational and behavioral dimensions.

The ASES seems to be a valuable and useful scale for those interested in a reliable and valid measure of assertiveness. As with the CSES, its best use for assessing expressiveness might come from focusing on certain items, related groups of items, or factors until subscales are developed. An advantage of the ASES is its applicability to older and noncollege populations.

The Assertion Inventory: The final self-report measure of assertiveness to be reviewed is the Assertion Inventory,[83] a 40-item inventory which provides respondents with an opportunity to note for each item (1) their degree of discomfort; (2) their probability of engaging in the behavior; and (3) situations they would like to handle more assertively. The degree of discomfort and probability of engaging in the behavior are indicated using five-point scales, The situations the respondents would like to handle more assertively are indicated by checking the appropriate items. Also, selected demographic information is collected at the end of the inventory. According to Gambrill and Richey,[83] the 40 items for this instrument were developed from a number of sources including reports from students and clients, as well as a review of the literature to determine frequently occurring assertion difficulties. This constitutes a difference between this scale and others which were developed from old or rewritten items from other scales, particularly Wolpe and Lazarus.[81] Gambrill and Richey stated

> The 40 items fell into the following categories: (a) turning down requests; (b) expressing personal limitations such as admitting ignorance in some areas; (c) initiating social contacts; (d) expressing positive feelings; (e) handling criticism; (f) differing with others; (g) assertion in service situations; and (h) giving negative feedback (p. 551).

Many of the items were varied as to the relationship between the people involved (strangers, acquaintances, or intimates) in order to accommodate the belief that assertive behavior may vary according to people involved and the situation.

For this scale, discomfort and response probability scores are computed by adding responses on each dimension; difference scores for each person are determined by subtracting discomfort from response probability. Normative data were collected from four samples of college students and one sample of women attending assertion training. Gambrill and Richey report Pearson correlations for test–retest reliability at five weeks of .87 for discomfort and .81 for response probability, which they concluded indicated high stability of scores over time. They reported few sex differences except for certain specific items.

Gambrill and Richey reported validity in terms of the ability to differentiate between a clinical group and a normal population based upon scores on the inventory. The scores also reflected significant differences within the clinical group before and after training. They concluded, however, that additional data are needed regarding the relationship between scores on the Assertion Inventory and independently assessed performance on criterion tasks.

Other authors also mentioned the limited evidence of the validity of the Assertion Inventory. For example, Rich and Schroeder[78] pointed out that the validity of the scale may be limited because comparisons of scores on the Assertion Inventory with behavioral measures of assertiveness have not yet been reported. Although Hall[77] recognized that the inventory requires additional validation research in terms of behavioral measures, he believed that "the nature of the inventory and the information provided by it suggest its great potential as a research and clinical instrument for use with college students and relatively well educated adults" (p. 337). Finally, he suggested the use of factors, identified by a factor analysis of discomfort scores, as the basis for subscales that could provide behaviorally specific information on various types of deficits in assertive behavior.

In considering self-report measures of assertiveness, the ASES, the CSES, and the Assertion Inventory seem to possess the minimal requirements of reliability and validity. They also focus, at least with some items, on the expression of feelings. None of these scales, however, purport to measure only expressiveness. All of these scales consider assertiveness to be situation specific and allow measurement of specific situations with specific target persons that might cause subjects difficulty. These scales are also easy and quick to administer and score. They will probably be most useful, in terms of assessing expressiveness, if counselors/therapists will consider those particular items, groups of items, or factors which deal with the expression of feelings.

The selection of the most appropriate scale would, of course, depend upon the specific need and use for it. Hopefully, the descriptions of the three scales just presented will prove useful to those who might wish to use a self-report measure to identify a client's deficit in expressing feelings or to determine whether or not the client has improved his/her ability to express his/her emotions as the result of some therapeutic intervention. Other scales might also be useful for a particular purpose; the intent of this paper is certainly not to suggest that those scales reviewed here are the only ones of value. Scales and inventories are constantly appearing in the literature, and counselor/therapists are encouraged to be alert for those that may hold promise. Finally, as was stated previously, the assessment of expressiveness, to be most valuable, should include both a self-report and a behavioral component. Behavioral approaches to assessing assertiveness which hold promise for assessing expressiveness will be considered next.

Behavioral approaches to measuring assertiveness. All of the articles or chapters previously considered which reviewed the assessment of assertiveness included behavioral approaches as well as self-report. There are several behavioral measures which assess assertive behavior in analog social situations that are similar, with minor variations, in the general approach each takes, but each represents methodological advances in the behaviors that are observed and rated (e.g., Eisler et al.,[53] Eisler et al.,[52] McFall and Marston,[99] Warren and Gilner[54]). The measures usually consist of from 6 to 32 situations which are presented verbally or in writing to the subject in narrative fashion. The subject is provided with a prompt from a role-playing antagonist, actor, or confederate. As the subject responds, his/her response is audio- or videotaped and then rated retrospectively by independent judges in terms of overall assertiveness and in terms of more specific verbal and nonverbal component measures of assertiveness. These ratings are typically made on 7-point or 5-point Likert scales.

Behavioral approaches have been used successfully to identify behavioral deficits or treatment needs, to indicate therapeutic gains, and to address the issues of duration and generality of treatment effects. These last two concerns, unfortunately, are often overlooked in assessment, but behavioral approaches to assessment make it easier to consider them. Before considering specific behavioral measures and evidence of their reliability and validity, it might be helpful to consider behavioral assessment of assertiveness more generally.

Hall[77] stated:

> There is strong support in the behaviorally oriented literature for the use of role playing as both an assessment and therapeutic approach along with a long-standing orientation in assessment to make assessment samples as close to real-life situations as possible (p. 339).

After reviewing several behavioral measures, Hall concluded that the use of role-playing techniques in the assessment of assertiveness provides an opportunity to gain complete and precise information about an individual's behavior in situations that approximate "real life." The completeness and the preciseness of the information that is gathered are both enhanced by behavioral measures because they greatly expand what can be measured as compared to self-report. This would be particularly true with videotaped role-play situations where both verbal and nonverbal components of assertiveness can be assessed. Videotape rating also increases precision because it permits repeated viewing, which makes possible the consideration of more components of behavior and more time for accurate and reliable rater judgments.

Behavioral assessments differ in the extent to which they approximate "real life"; Rich and Schroeder[78] suggested three ways behavioral assessments have been accomplished which differ in this respect and are listed in decreasing order of verisimilitude: (1) direct observation in naturalistic settings; (2) observations in contrived behavioral settings; and (3) role playing. They also pointed out that the more an approach approximates "real life," the more difficult it is to carry out. Obtaining observations in most naturalistic settings, for example, is hampered by the difficulty of obtaining adequate samples of behavior and by ethical considerations. Some attempts have been made to use diary or self-reports with subjects recording their own behavior, but Rich and Schroeder concluded that these approaches are usually problematic with questions of reliability.

Contrived behavioral tasks permit adequate samples of behavior for large comparisons and also permit some degree of standardization and control over antecedent stimulus conditions, according to Rich and Schroeder. With this approach a confederate behaves in a preprogrammed and consistent way with all subjects: for example, measuring a subject's ability to refuse by using a surreptitious phone call from a confederate with the expressed purpose of soliciting volunteers, selling subscriptions, or getting help with coursework (e.g., McFall and Lillesand,[91] McFall and Marston,[99] McFall and Twentyman[100]). This approach also suffers from ethical concerns since the subject is usually deceived as to the real purpose of the interaction.[70,78,90] In fact, subjects often do not even realize that their actions, at that point, are part of a study. Some authors (e.g., Heimberg et al.[70]) have suggested that subjects could be advised that they will be observed unobtrusively during or after the study, without specifying a time or place, as a resolution to this ethical problem. Subjects would then consent to this arrangement without precise knowledge. Other authors have argued against the need or desirability of using deception in social-psychological research based on ethical and methodological concerns (e.g., Hersen and Bellack[90]). Another difficulty with contrived behavioral tasks is that, although they do offer some control and standardization, control over extraneous influences still presents a problem.[78]

The third method of behavioral observation described by Rich and Schroeder that is useful for assessing assertiveness is role playing. This is by far the most frequently used assessment method and it is also frequently used for training purposes (e.g., Lange and Jackubowski,[46] McFall and Lillesand[91]). This method typically involves identifying problematic situations for the subjects, simulating them in a standardized, semiautomated procedure, and then audio- or videotaping the subject's response. Subjects are usually instructed to imagine the situation as real and to respond as he/she would in real life. Although role playing is a useful and popular outcome measure, its major limitation is the lack of evidence of validity.[78] Related to this is the difficulty with the unnaturalness of role playing for many subjects; there is the question of whether the subject is really "in role."[77,78] Another problem with role playing is the possibility that subjects in assertiveness training do not become more assertive, but merely more skilled and comfortable with role playing after practice with role playing on the pretest and during the training.[78] In addition, questions of test–retest reliability have not been addressed with most behavioral measures.

The three methods of behavioral assessment of assertiveness just discussed have all been used successfully to some extent, but have all experienced the problems which were discussed. In addition, Bodner[69] believed that the validity of role-playing behavioral assessment techniques may be questioned because of their artificiality and "since preparation, practice, and demand characteristics are uncontrolled extraneous variables" (p. 94). To overcome these problems, the use of game simulation models that place subjects in a standardized goal-directed task which allows for assertive behaviors to be profitably emitted was suggested. Since the format is goal directed with a standardized format, there is a reduction in artificiality with more accurate and valid assessments.[69]

Three additional problems associated with using observational measures were described by Rich and Schroeder[78]:

1. Observational measures are often biased when subjects are aware they are being observed. This can be controlled to some extent by not letting the subjects know which specific behaviors are being assessed.

2. A second problem concerns the demand characteristics of the experimental situation. Here the concern is that the subject's behavior will change based on what he/she believes the experimenter wants. Hall[77] presented evidence that supports the need for varying the instructional demands (low and high demand) to control for demand characteristics. Varying the instructional demands allows the experimenter/clinician to assess not only what the client will do in assertion situations but also what the client can do under maximal demand for the same situation. A client who responds assertively only in high-demand situations would be inhibited although he/she obviously possesses the skills to be assertive. Although this addition would provide useful information, it also would require more situations, would greatly extend the time involved in assessment, and could introduce complicating factors such as fatigue.[77] The best approach to take to control demand characteristics is unclear, except to consider demand

characteristics when establishing instructions for subjects and to explain the study to the subject in a less specific sense without violating ethical considerations through deception.

3. The third problem comes from the fact that behavioral observations, by necessity, require the use of observers or raters. Raters may be biased in their ratings, e.g., by their attempts to conform to their understanding of the experimenter's expectations, and also by "halo effects" that occur when raters rate a subject they had rated previously. These problems can be controlled to some extent if raters are naive to experimental hypotheses and if they are unaware of the subject's situation (e.g., pretest, posttest, control group, experimental group).

For a more thorough discussion of the problems of reliability in observational research, the reader is referred to Hollenbeck,[101] who discussed observer bias, observee bias, circumstances of assessment, observer decay and drift, and influences on reliability stemming from the design of the scoring system.

A major problem in the behavioral assessment of assertiveness has been developing a clear delineation of the components of assertiveness in order for observers to focus on the essential aspects of behavior.[77] This problem is made even more difficult by the situational influences on assertiveness and the varying types of behavioral expressions that have been called assertive. Still another problem with most behavioral attempts to measure assertiveness is that the emphasis has been on measuring the ability to refuse requests and the expression of negative feelings. Greater attention needs to be directed toward assessing the expression of positive feelings.[90]

The problems listed above were considered in reviewing the behavioral approaches to assessing assertiveness; those that hold the most promise (none are problem free) for assessing expressiveness are presented below (Table II). In each case evidence of reliability and validity, if available, is presented as well as the procedures to be followed in using the measure. Also, a brief description of the research design for studies done on these measures is presented so that the reader can judge the results. There are many behavioral measures available, but since in many ways they are similar, only the best examples are presented although none match Hall's[77] ideal of a behavioral assessment battery that would

> utilize highly specific behavioral measures, allow for the assessment of assertiveness under varying situations, require the expression of different types of assertive behavior, include variations in instructional demands, and measure the role involvement of the subject (p. 350).

The Behavioral Role-Playing Test: One of the first behavioral tests developed to measure assertiveness was the Behavioral Role-Playing Test,[99] a test which employed 16 role-playing situations requiring assertive responses, to study the effects of behavior rehearsal on the assertiveness of college students. The 16 situations on the test were selected on the basis of an extensive examination of over 2000 situations which called for assertive behavior. This list was screened and condensed to 80 situations which were tested on a sample of 60

Table II. Characteristics of Selected Behavioral Measures of Assertiveness

Name of test	Authors	Number of situations	Type of situations	Type of presentation	Type of recording	Verbal ratings	Nonverbal ratings	Additional subject ratings
Behavioral Role-Playing Test	McFall and Marston[99]	16	Negative	Audiotape	Audiotape	Most assertive between pre- and posttest	None	Subject's anxiety 5-pt. scale; subject's satisfaction with response 5-pt. scale
Behavioral Assertiveness Test	Eisler et al.[52]	14	Negative	Female role model	Videotape	Overall assertiveness	9 behavioral components	None
Behavioral Assertiveness Test—Revised Male	Eisler et al.[53]	32	Positive and negative Familiar and unfamiliar Male and female	Male and female model	Videotape	Overall assertiveness, negative content, positive content	7 behavioral components	None
Behavioral Test of Tenderness Expression	Warren and Gilner[54]	15	Positive	Audiotape	Audiotape	1–4 scale for assertive tender response	None	Partner's rating form for use with couples

undergraduates. Following a factor analysis of the results, those situations with the highest factor loadings and which were rated as most difficult were administered to another sample of 45 undergraduates. Finally, McFall and Marston selected and developed the 16 situations for their behavioral test.

The stimulus situations were presented to subjects on audiotape; a bell served as the cue for the subject to make a response. Subjects were instructed to respond to each situation as if it were actually happening to him/her. Subjects' responses were tape recorded and rated later by five judges. For rating purposes, subjects' pre- and posttest responses were paired and the "blind" judges then independently used a paired-comparison procedure to determine which response in each pair was more assertive. The consensus of these judgments was taken as an index of each subject's improvement as a function of treatment with greater than chance preference of raters for posttest response indicating improvement. Subjects also rated each situation using 5-point scales (1 = not at all, to 5 = very much) to indicate: (1) how anxious they would feel if they were actually in the situation; and (2) how satisfied they would feel with the response they made.

The 16 role-play situations included interpersonal situations with friends, employers, and strangers. They included, for example: (1) friends interrupting your studying; (2) the laundry losing your cleaning; (3) a waiter bringing you a too-rare steak; (4) your boss asking you to work overtime when you already have plans. The format for the presentation of each stimulus situation included a description of the scene by the narrator followed by several statements to which subjects were instructed to respond. In one situation, subjects were supposed to imagine that they are in a long line outside a theatre two minutes before showtime, wondering whether there will be enough tickets left, when two people walk up to the person in front of them in line and begin talking. Then, subjects were presented with the following statements requiring their response:

> *Newcomer:* Hey, the line's a mile long. How about if we cut in here with you?
>
> *Person in line:* Sure, come on, a couple more won't make any difference.
>
> *Narrator:* And as the two people squeeze in line between you and their friend, one of them looks at you and says:
>
> *Newcomer:* Excuse me. You don't mind if we cut in, do you? (McFall and Marston,[99] pp. 297–298).

McFall and Marston presented no data to indicate interjudge reliabilities or the specific criteria used by judges to determine assertiveness. They did find, however, that the measurements were to some extent accurate indices of assertiveness levels since there was a significant difference between experimental and control groups in terms of judges' preferences of posttest responses.[77] The Behavioral Role-Playing Test has been important in the development of behavioral approaches to assessing assertiveness since it served as the model for other behavioral tasks.[77,90]

The methods of the Behavioral Role-Playing Test are relevant and important to the assessment of expressiveness; the situations, however, are less appropriate since they deal primarily with negative situations, e.g., refusal, expression of negative feelings, etc. In fact, McFall and Marston reported a correlation of $r = 0.76$ between improvement scores on two refusal-to-salesman situations and overall improvement scores. They used this as a basis for regarding refusal to salesman items as representative of assertive situations in general.

The Behavioral Assertiveness Test: Eisler et al.[52] extended the work of McFall and Marston[99] by developing the Behavioral Assertiveness Test (BAT) in a study of male psychiatric patients. The BAT contains 14 standard role-play situations of interpersonal encounteres requiring assertive responses and simulating real-life situations. A live role model was used by Eisler et al. to prompt subject's responses to each situation. The female role model enacted the roles of the patient's wife, sales clerk, waitress, etc., while reacting to the subject's responses, as she was trained, in a neutral, matter-of-face manner to prevent performance feedback. The BAT was administered to subjects in a videotape studio; all instructions and narrations were administered through an intercom system from an adjoining room.

In the instructions that each subject received he was told that the purpose of the procedure was to find out how he might react to some ordinary everyday situations that might occur outside the hospital and that the idea was for him to respond just as if he were in that situation at home, in a store, or in a restaurant. The instructions explained that the television camera was in the room so that he could be observed and that usually people find that they can relax in front of the camera in a short time. Each subject was requested to imagine that he was in each situation that was described and that when the role model spoke to him, he should say what he would normally say if he were actually in that situation. Each subject was then asked if he had any questions. Then, after two practice situations, the 14 situations of the BAT were administered and videotaped. The following represents an example of one of the 14 situations from the BAT including the short narration followed by the role model's statement, which serves as a cue for subject's response[52] (p. 296):

> *Narrator:* You're in the middle of an exciting football game. Your wife walks in and changes the TV channel as she does every time you're watching a good game.
>
> *Role Model Wife:* Let's watch this movie instead; it's supposed to be real good.

Eisler et al. used two trained judges with several months' practice to rate a series of verbal and nonverbal components of assertive behavior independently; judges were not specifically informed that ratings were related to assertiveness. Nine behavioral components were derived by asking several experienced clinicians to list specific behaviors they believed to be related to judgments of assertiveness and selecting those most frequently listed. The components used by Eisler et al. were the following: *nonverbal behavior* (duration of looking at role model, frequency of smiles); *speech characteristics* (response duration, latency of response, loudness of speech, fluency of speech); and *content and affect* (compliance content, content requesting new behavior, affect). Judges also rated the overall assertiveness of each subject using criteria adopted from Wolpe[68] and Wolpe and Lazarus.[81]

Eisler et al. report interrater reliabilities based on percentage of agreement for compliance and affect of 100% and 99.3%. Pearson produce–moment correlations were computed between the two sets of ratings on the other component measures and they ranged from .96 to .99. Five of the behavioral measures (response latency, loudness of speech, duration of response, compliance, and requests for new behavior) differentiated high- and low-assertive subjects as determined by overall assertiveness ratings. High- and low-assertive subjects were also differentiated by scores on a modified Wolpe–Lazarus assertiveness questionnaire.

Although the BAT is empirically derived, it is limited, since it focuses only on "hostile" assertiveness with responses directed only toward female role models. Reliability is reported and is impressive for judges, but test–retest reliability is not evaluated. The most important contribution of the BAT is the initial effort by Eisler et al. to isolate key verbal and nonverbal components of assertiveness. Again, as with the previous behavioral test, the BAT is more important and relevant for the assessment of expressiveness in terms of its methods (particularly the consideration of nonverbal components) than in terms of the specific situations used, since they are limited to negative assertiveness.

The Behavioral Assertiveness Test–Revised Male: The BAT was revised by Eisler et al.[53] to explore situational determinants of assertive behavior with 60 unselected psychiatric patients who were married, divorced, or separated. The Behavioral Assertiveness Test—Revised Male (BAT-RM) used 32 assertive situations that varied in social–interpersonal context by dividing the scenes along a familiarity–unfamiliarity dimension. In half of the scenes the target of the assertiveness is unfamiliar to the subject; in the other half the target is familiar to the subject. The situations were also divided along the sex dimensions with half of the scenes involving a male role model to prompt the subject's response and half using a female role model. Finally, and most importantly for our concerns, the situations were varied in terms of the type of assertive responses required, with half requiring positive (commendatory) assertive responses and half requiring negative (hostile) assertive responses. Thus, there were four scenes in each of the eight categories of stimulus scenes (three variables, two levels each: positive–negative; male–female; familiar–unfamiliar) to make up the 32 situations in the BAT-RM. The following two scenes are examples from Eisler et al.[53] (p. 342):

Male—Negative—Unfamiliar Scene:

Narrator: You go to a ball game with reserved seat tickets. When you arrive you find that someone has put his coat in the seat for which you have reserved tickets. You ask him to remove his coat and he tells you that he is saving the seat for a friend.

He says: I'm sorry, this seat is saved.

Female—Positive—Familiar Scene:

Narrator: Your wife has just bought a new outfit and is trying it on. You really like it and think she looks very nice in it.

Your wife says: Well, how do I look in this outfit?

A female research assistant played the role in all scenes involving a female interpersonal partner, and a male research assistant role-played all scenes having a male interpersonal partner. One-half of the subjects responded to the scenes involving female role models first and the other half responded to scenes involving a male role model first. Scenes within sex of role model were presented in a random order for each subject.

The 32 assertive situations were presented to subjects in a furnished room containing video equipment and a two-way intercom system. Each subject was escorted into the video studio and seated next to either the male or female role model. Both role models had been trained to deliver a predetermined prompt to the subject after the experimenter delivered the narration of the scene from the control room. The role model made no reply to the subject's response until the next scene started.

Each subject received instructions over the intercom which told him that the purpose of the procedure was to find out how he reacts to some everyday situations that might occur outside the hospital and that the idea was for him to respond just as if he were in that situation at home, at work, at a store, or in a restaurant. The narrator explained that each subject was to imagine that he was actually in the situation described to him and that in order for the situations to seem more like real life Miss Jones would play the part of a woman in the scenes and Mr. Smith would play the part of a man in the scenes. Each subject was instructed to respond to the actor or actress in the way that he would if he were in that situation. Finally each subject was told that some scenes were such that he would feel irritated or annoyed if he were actually in that situation. At this point the experimenter tested the subject's understanding of the instructions with a practice negative situation. If it appeared the subject understood, the experimenter gave additional instructions for the positive situations: "In other scenes you might feel appreciative or friendly toward the other person" (p. 344). Then a practice positive scene was narrated by the experimenter and attempted by the subject. Finally, the experimenter said, "Remember, try to express your true feelings whatever they might be. Also, be sure to express yourself as fully as possible" (p. 344). Subjects' responses to each of the 32 situations of the BAT-RM were videotaped and rated retrospectively.

The ratings were made independently by two trained judges who had over a year of experiences rating videotapes of components of assertive behavior. Eisler et al.[53] broadly categorized the components of social–interactive behavior in terms of (1) nonverbal behaviors; (2) positive content; (3) negative content; and (4) overall assertiveness. Ratings of nonverbal behaviors considered (1) duration of eye contact; (2) smiles; (3) duration of reply; (4) latency of response; (5) loudness of speech; (6) appropriate affect; and (7) ratio of speech disturbances to duration of speech. Ratings of negative content considered (1) compliance; and (2) request for new behavior. Ratings of positive content considered (1) praise; (2) appreciation; and (3) spontaneous positive behavior. Overall assertiveness was also rated by two other raters who were unfamiliar with the purpose of the study and who had familiarized themselves with Wolpe's[68] definitions of "hostile" and "commendatory" assertiveness. For content measures and smiles, raters tallied, for each subject, the presence of the behavior in each of the eight categories of scenes; for the other measures, the subject's score was obtained by taking the average over the four scenes in each of the eight categories. The scores were combined across all categories of scenes for each subject to analyze the data for differences between high- and low-assertive subjects. Interrater reliabilities were computed using percentage of agreement for the five measures of speech content, number of speech disturbances, and frequency of smiles. For these measures the percentage of agreement was over 95% across all situations. Pearson produce–moment correlations were computed between the two sets of ratings for the other continuous measures. Correlation coefficients were all greater than .94. Eisler et al.[53] attributed these exceptionally high reliabilities to the specificity of the criteria outlined for each measure, the fact that only one measure was rated for each videotape playback, and the fact that the raters had so much experience making similar ratings.

Results of the study indicated that, just as in the previous study, high- and low-assertive subjects were differentiated on the basis of 9 of the 12 measures of interpersonal behavior and on the basis of self-reported assertiveness measured by the Wolpe–Lazarus Assertiveness Questionnaire.[81] Results also indicated that interpersonal behavior in assertive situations varied as a function of the social context of the interpersonal interaction. Eisler et al.[53] found, as they had expected, that content of speech, or what one says, will differ in relation to whether the situation requires positive or negative assertive behavior. They also found, however, significant differences on six of the seven nonverbal components of assertive behavior when comparing responses to negative and positive assertive situations (i.e., the negative scenes elicited significantly different interpersonal behavior on nonverbal response measures). There were also differences in the types of assertive responses made to men and women role models across the situations when considering measures of speech content. The authors concluded that the results support a stimulus-specific theory of assertiveness; i.e., an individual who is assertive in one interpersonal context may not be assertive in a different one.

The importance of considering situational variance and determinants in the assessment of assertiveness was clearly demonstrated by this study. While this understanding is important, it is also problematic as long as the specific components which primarily influence assertive behavior are not clearly delineated. As Hall[77] points out, attempting to take all possible situational factors into account would produce an immense assessment battery. An assessment battery of this type would, no doubt, be unwieldy, difficult to use and score, and inappropriate for most uses. One solution to this problem is to design an assessment battery specifically for the population you wish to assess, which includes types of assertions, targets, and situational contexts that are problems for them.[46] This approach would be appropriate for assessing expressiveness using the methods developed by Eisler et al.[53]

Of the measures considered so far the BAT-RM is most appropriate for assessing expressiveness. One weakness, however, is that, although it does consider positive assertions, it does not consider some of the other types of positive assertions such as expressions of affection, liking, etc. Combining a greater emphasis on positive assertive behavior with the methods developed by

Eisler et al. for assessing the verbal and nonverbal components of assertive behavior would seem to be the best approach to the behavioral assessment of expressiveness. This point will be expanded later under implications for counselors/therapists.

The three behavioral approaches to the assessment of assertiveness presented thus far represent, in the opinion of the author, the behavioral approaches most relevant to assessing expressiveness. Each, beginning with McFall and Marston,[99] presents an advancement in the methodology of measuring behavioral components of assertiveness; each has served as a model for other behavioral tests. McFall and Marston's work was important not only because it was one of the earliest attempts at developing a behavioral measure of assertiveness, but also because it served as the prototype for other attempts. Eisler et al.[52] added to this seminal effort by introducing the identification and measurement of the behavioral components which are important to assertive behavior. A most important extension here was the development of the method for measuring nonverbal components using videotape. Finally, Eisler et al.[53] added to these two earlier two efforts by including the consideration of situational influences, including type of assertive behavior (positive and negative), on assertive behavior in their test, and by demonstrating the importance of considering these influences. Each of these methods, then, has been important in its own right, but together they represent a good historical overview of the research with behavioral approaches to assertiveness. Further, they have all been presented, hopefully, in sufficient detail to allow readers to use them (whole or in part). Certainly, as has been previously mentioned, the methods can be used with different situations which might be more applicable for a particular assessment need. This would be the suggestion for those wishing to assess expressiveness. Also, the research methods used to design and test the measures have been explained in detail to allow the reader to judge the results, particularly as they relate to reliability and validity.

While those behavioral tests which were presented are considered by the author to be the most relevant to assessing expressiveness and to represent a good sample of methodological approaches to the behavioral assessment of assertiveness, they are not, of course, free of methodological problems. In addition, there are other behavioral tests available, many of which were considered and eliminated for a number of reasons, but usually because they were not considered useful for assessing expressiveness. A very brief description of some of the more frequently cited behavioral tests which were not presented can be found in Hall[77] and Hersen and Bellack.[90] The reader is encouraged to review these references for alternative measures to make his/her own determination as to the appropriateness of other tests for his/her own assessment needs.

The Behavioral Test of Tenderness Expression: A final behavioral test of assertiveness will be presented which holds particular promise for the assessment of expressiveness. It is the Behavioral Test of Tenderness Expression (BTTE).[54] Based on the contention that assertiveness includes, and needs to stress to a greater extent, the expression of positive feelings, this test was designed to measure positive assertion in intimate heterosexual peer relationships.

The BTTE was tested on 41 couples who had dated at least 9 months or were married. The test was also checked for reliability and validity.

Warren and Gilner compiled a pool of 55 role-play items from several sources which covered areas of positive assertion including praise, appreciation, self-disclosure, sincere apologies, empathy, support, tolerance, interest in the intimate older person, and expression of positive feelings of loving, liking, and enjoyment. 15 of these items were selected for inclusion on this test of the BTTE. No further explanation or description of the items is given except for three sample items from the BTTE.[54] The following represent two of these sample items from the BTTE (p. 180):

> Your boy friend (girl friend) or spouse, one afternoon, comes in obviously very upset and says, "I am so tense and nervous these days I just don't know what it is. To top it off, I feel so insecure sometimes I just don't know what to do." What would you say?

> You are sitting at home, just beginning to read the afternoon newspaper, when in walks your boy friend (girl friend) or spouse with a record you've wanted. "Hi, I thought I'd bring you a little something." What do you say?

The 15 items which were selected are presented to the subjects individually on a tape following a series of taped instructions. Subjects were told to "Respond as if your partner, ________, were here in the room with you." Each subject's response was audiotaped. According to Warren and Gilner, the BTTE, including instructions, took 15 minutes. While one member of the couple took the BTTE the other member was seated in another room taking several self-report measures. Each partner then listened separately to the tapes of their partner's test responses and rated the response on the Partner's Rating Form.

Rating of subject's responses were made, using a three-page manual of rating guidelines, by two judges who replayed the audiotapes independently. The content of the responses was rated using a 1–4 scale with 1 being the least expressive and 4 being the most expressive. The criteria used by raters were as follows[54]:

1. punishing response to the partner or no response;
2. attention only to the partner, "umhumm," or other neutral verbalizations which attend only to the factual situation at hand;
3. minimal tender expressive response, some recognition of feelings, and expression to the other person; and
4. fully assertive tender response, full expression of feelings, and response to the partner's need.

Each response was rated from 1 to 4 and these scores were summed to yield an overall expression score. Each judge rated all 82 subjects on the 15 items (p. 131).

An interrater reliability of .86 was obtained using a Pearson product–moment correlation. The internal consistency of the BTTE was assessed with the α coefficient to measure split-half reliability, and an α coefficient of .79 was obtained. Concurrent validity was measured by the partner's ratings of taped behavior and was high, indicating that test behaviors were typical of usual behaviors at home in similar situations. The BTTE was found to be unrelated to social desirability and to be moderately correlated with self-report measures of expressiveness. Warren and Gilner concluded that the BTTE is a potentially useful instrument for the measurement of positive assertive behaviors, which possesses high interrater reliability and concurrent validity, and moderate internal consistency and correlations with self-report measures. An advantage of the test is that it takes only 15 minutes to administer, and, although each response must be rated, the rating criteria are direct and reliable.

The BTTE does then provide a useful behavioral approach to assessing assertiveness that is closely related to expressiveness. The shortcomings of the BTTE are similar to those of most behavioral measures in that, although some evidence of interrater reliability, concurrent validity, and internal consistency is presented, no evidence of test–retest reliability is available. Related to this is the fact that no evidence is presented to indicate the BTTE is sensitive to subtle pre- and posttest differences following training of treatment. Another shortcoming is that the BTTE does not consider nonverbal components of assertive or expressive behavior. The BTTE, however, could be easily expanded to do this by using video- rather than audiotape and using the procedures outlined by Eisler et al.[53] to rate nonverbal behaviors. Even with these shortcomings, the BTTE is an important and useful instrument, for those readers interested in assessing expressiveness, primarily because it is the first test to focus solely on positive expression of feelings.

Use of behavioral methods for assessing generalization. As was briefly mentioned previously, one of the advantages of including behavioral methods of assessment is that they are appropriate and useful for assessing generalization of treatment effects. Hersen and Bellack[90] presented five methods that have been employed to examine generalization:

(1) This first method simply involves assessing the subject's performance before treatment on a behavioral role-playing test. Training then proceeds using half the items for training practice and then the behavioral role-playing test is readministered. Performance on the items not included in the training provides a measure of generalization (e.g., McFall and Lillesand[91]).

(2) A second method, involving generalization across stimulus persons uses another role model with whom the subject has not previously interacted as a substitute for the original role model in some behavioral role playing task. This method allows the assessment of the subject's performance with different persons as a measure of generalization.

(3) The third method presented by Hersen and Bellack consists of making unobtrusive naturalistic observations. This method requires some means of observing and rating the subject's performance in a naturalistic setting without being unethical or obtrusive. This approach has been used in hospital settings with some success (e.g., Hersen et al.[102]) but it is difficult to carry out in noninstitutional settings. One approach that has been suggested is the use of unstructured periods of time during training or treatment for interaction between subjects which are unobtrusively videotaped (with subjects' permission) and retrospectively rated for expressiveness.

(4) The fourth and fifth strategies suggested by Hersen and Bellack involve deception. In one, a confederate, blind to research conditions, engages the subjects in several interpersonal situations. In the other, a situation is arranged where, for example, subjects are shortchanged or underpaid for their research participation and their reactions are videotaped and rated. McFall and Marston[90] developed one of the first and most widely employed methods of assessing generalization using deception. It was presented earlier under contrived behavioral situations and involves a telephone call to the subject's home to make an unreasonable request of some sort. The response of the subject is recorded and later rated. Several variations on this theme have been attempted with some success, although the use of deception has been criticized and questions have been raised as to whether these very specific follow-ups are adequate tests of generalization.[90]

After reviewing these five methods of assessing generalization, Hersen and Bellack concluded that observations in naturalistic settings are to be preferred for at least two reasons: (1) the ethical issues are minimized, particularly if at the beginning of the treatment the subject consents to being unobtrusively observed in a variety of settings; and (2) obviously the naturalistic setting has greater face validity as a measure of generalization since it more closely resembles actual situations. They suggested that one intriguing possibility for assessing generalization is to specifically evaluate those target behaviors modified during treatment (e.g., eye contact, duration of speech, making requests, etc.) in settings outside of treatment under naturalistic conditions. Hersen and Bellack[90] concluded that "much research is needed to identify the most relevant measures for assessing generalization in addition to determining the relationship between measures of generalization and within-treatment role-playing tasks" (p. 539).

In summary, behavioral approaches to assessment of assertiveness have been presented which, in the author's opinion, are useful for assessing expressiveness. These measures were presented in sufficient detail to allow readers to use them and to determine whether they would be appropriate for their assessment needs. An effort was made to explain how these behavioral measures of assertiveness could be adapted to assess expressiveness. Also, the importance of considering behavioral approaches to assessment as well as the problems inherent in behavioral assessment were presented. Most of the behavioral approaches presented involved role-playing tasks rather than naturalistic observations or contrived behavioral tasks, simply because role-playing tasks have been more frequently used, have been more systematically studied, and are easier and more direct to use. Again, as with self-report measures, the selection of tests to be presented was based on the author's judgment as to which were most applicable to assessing expressiveness. The reader is encouraged to consider other tests. There appears to be no "best way" to use behavioral approaches derived from assertiveness tests to measure expressiveness.

Physiologic measures exist that could possibly be useful but these were not presented because they are seldom used or researched and because in many cases they require equipment not readily available to most counselors/therapists. The reader is referred to other sources for more information on physiological measures (e.g., Cimenero,[63] Hersen and Bellack,[90] Kallman and Feurstein,[103] Rich and Schroeder[78]).

In attempting to identify and present methods of assessing expressiveness, methods from assertiveness were considered because by definition assertiveness includes expressiveness, i.e., assertiveness is the expression of both positive and negative feelings. In addition, assertiveness was considered because it is an area that is methodologically advanced and well researched with many assessment methods available. Both self-report and behavioral approaches have been presented with suggestions as to how they could be adapted to measure expressiveness. Assessment methods taken from the assertiveness literature would seem to be promising as methods of assessing expressiveness. There are also other psychological constructs which would seem to be related to expressiveness and which have developed and tested assessment methods. The other construct that seems to be the most related to expressiveness is self-disclosure, and it will be considered next.

Self-Disclosure. Research on self-disclosure has been extensive in recent years[51,104] with this construct serving as the focus of considerable theoretical and empirical inquiry as an interpersonal process related to counseling and psychotherapy.[105] Much of this research has included the development of assessment methods as well as tests of the reliability and validity of these methods.

Definitions of self-disclosure. The concept of self-disclosure comes primarily from existential and phenomenologic theory, according to Chelune,[104] who observed that to disclose means to show or make known. Self-disclosure, then, "is the process by which we make ourselves known to other persons by verbally disclosing personal information" (pp. 278–279). In discussing the "transparent self," Jourard[106] stated, "Self-disclosure is the act of making yourself manifest, showing yourself so others can perceive you" (p. 19). Pointing out that self-disclosure is limited to verbal disclosure, Chelune[107] noted the first step in conceptualizing self-disclosure is taken by limiting the scope of inquiry to verbal disclosures.

Another frequently used and cited definition of self-disclosure came from Cozby[15]: "Self-disclosure may be defined as any information about himself which Person A communicates verbally to a Person B" (p. 73). Even this broad definition places rigid boundaries on what is labeled self-disclosure, Chelune[107] noted, pointing out that "self-disclosure must meet the following three operational criteria: (a) it must contain personal information about Person A; (b) Person A must verbally communicate this information; and (c) Person A must communicate this information to a target Person B" (p. 2). Other definitions of self-disclosure which are more restrictive of the verbal disclosures that are considered self-disclosure exist, but those definitions presented are the most accepted and frequently cited.

Some investigators[51] chose to focus on a specific type of self-disclosure, e.g., affective self-disclosure, "a speaker's voluntary verbal statement made as an initiator or respondent in a dyadic interaction that expresses his emotions in feeling terms, is present oriented, and self-referenced" (p. 22). In other words, affective self-disclosure is the expression of feelings to others. This specific type of self-disclosure has become increasingly important in the counseling process as evidenced by the growing number of studies on this topic (e.g., Highlen and Baccus,[108] Highlen and Gillis,[21] Highlen and Johnston[22]). Out of this body of research have come methods to assess affective self-disclosure, some of which will be reviewed below.

Based upon the definitions just presented, self-disclosure, and certainly affective self-disclosure, would seem to be related to expressiveness. One of the ways a person can let someone know more about himself is to tell them how he feels. Some of the private, personal, or intimate information about a person that can be revealed to someone else is his feelings. So, conceptually, self-disclosure and expressiveness seem to be related. There is support for this belief since Balswick (unpublished data, 1977) has reported correlations in the .90's between his Expression of Emotion Scale and a modified 15-item Jourard self-disclosure questionnaire.

Difficulties with the concept of self-disclosure. In the midst of the research on self-disclosure, numerous inconsistencies have been reported.[15,107] Thus, Highlen and Voight[51] have noted that the construct of self-disclosure is extremely complex and is difficult to explain empirically. When so many definitions of disclosure include different subsets of self-disclosing behaviors, confusion results. Also, cross-study comparisons are difficult owing to the use of different methods of assessment; this probably contributes to some of the contradictory findings in the self-disclosure literature.[109]

Some of the complexity with the concept can be seen by examining the factors that affect self-disclosure. Chelune[104] saw self-disclosure as a function of both input variables (social-situational factors) and the personality characteristics of the discloser. Input variables which have affected self-disclosure include (1) the target person or recipient of the disclosure, including the relationship between the target and the discloser, the verbal and nonverbal behavior of the target, liking for the target person, and sex of the target person; (2) setting condition or situation; and (3) topic of the self-disclosure. Characteristics of the discloser that have affected self-disclosure include sex differences; birth order; age; and several personality measures, e.g., extroversion and sociability. With so many variables related to self-disclosure it is easy to see why there have been conflicting results and why some investigators (e.g., Chelune,[104,107] Cozby[15]) have advised caution in assessing self-disclosure.

To further complicate matters, self-disclosure is not considered to be a unitary construct.[15,104,107] Chelune[104] states

> As an interpersonal behavior, self-disclosure is thought to include five basic dimensions: (a) amount or breadth of personal information disclosed; (b) intimacy of the information disclosed; (c) rate or duration of disclosure, (d) affective manner of presentation, and (e) flexibility of the disclosure pattern (p. 283).

Chelune[107] cautioned that researchers must carefully consider which of these aspects of self-disclosure they desire to assess and then be certain not to generalize beyond the parameters considered. Unfortunately, researchers often make unqualified statements about differences in self-disclosure between subjects or between situations, he believed, based on unidimensional assessment measures. In order to address this issue researchers must decide whether to study self-disclosure as a unidimensional or multidimensional construct. Chelune[107] stated, "Whenever possible, future research should also attempt to use assessment devices that measure more than a single self-disclosure parameter" (p. 8).

Another question for consideration in selecting an appropriate definition of self-disclosure according to Chelune[107] is

> whether the focus of the study will be on individual differences in self-disclosure across social-situational contexts, or, conversely, on the conditions or situations that influence self-disclosure across individuals (p. 4).

This involves choosing a "trait" or "state" view, the same concern apparent with the construct of assertiveness.

Just as with assertiveness, this "state versus trait" controversy is unsettled. There has been, however, a movement toward a more temperate position on the issue[107] where "complex human behaviors such as self-disclosure are currently assumed to be multiply determined through the interaction of both person and situational variables" (p. 5). One important change here is that trait or person variables are no longer seen as rigid and enduring but rather as "stylistic consistencies." Situational factors affecting self-disclosure and individuals' "stylistic consistencies" in self-disclosure are both important, valid, and useful approaches for advancing knowledge in self-disclosure.[107]

A new finding has appeared in recent social-personality literature that may help overcome some of the limitations of taking either a state or trait position. This involves recent evidence that suggests that individuals differ in the extent to which their social and expressive behavior is consistent or variable across situations. This dimension is called *self-monitoring*.[110–112] High self-monitors are considered to be very sensitive to situational cues as to what type of behavior is appropriate in a situation and to observe and control their behavior carefully in accordance with those cues. Hence, they show considerable variability from situation to situation. On the other hand, low self-monitors are considered to be less attentive to situational cues so that their behavior is more consistent across situations. Chelune[107] concluded that such a construct could explain why the amount of variance explained in comparisons of self-report, self-rating, and actual behaviors rarely exceeds 50%.

A similar, though independently derived, construct for self-disclosure called self-disclosure flexibility has been proposed[107]:

> self-disclosure flexibility . . . refers to the ability of a person to modulate his or her characteristic disclosure levels according to the interpersonal and situational demands of various social situations, for example, the topic of disclosure, the target person, and the setting condition (p. 286).

This concept has implications for the state versus trait issue with individuals with low self-disclosure flexibility (i.e., consistency in disclosure levels across situations) most likely to show traitlike relationships between broad indices of self-disclosure and other measures of personality. Conversely, individuals with high self-disclosure flexibility (i.e., high situation-to-situation disclosure variability) are most likely to appear "trait-free." Chelune[107] concluded that readers and researchers should be aware of the limitations of either a state or a trait view of self-disclosure on the generalizations and predictions that can be made; people differ in the extent to which their self-disclosing behavior is either situation-specific or trait-determined; and self-disclosure flexibility has potential for controlling these differences and could be a bridge between the "state versus trait" distinctions in self-disclosure.

The issues and difficulties arising from the use of different subsets of self-disclosing behavior, different methodological strategies, and different parameters of self-disclosure are integrally related to the choice of an assessment technique.[107] According to Chelune,[107] when empirically defined, self-disclosure is "simply whatever the assessment device measures" (p. 8). He saw several considerations that are involved in selecting an assessment instrument including: the question to be addressed; whether to use self-disclosure as a dependent or as an independent variable; and which situational and personality variables to consider.

All of these difficulties with the concept of self-disclosure must be considered, to some extent, by someone wishing to assess self-disclosure. This is because, as has been presented, the particular definition of self-disclosure used suggests the appropriate assessment technique. The researcher must decide which aspects of self-disclosure to consider, whether a trait or state approach to self-disclosure should be taken, whether it should be used as an independent or dependent variable, whether self-report or behavioral methods should be used, and whether a uni- or multidimensional approach should be taken. These questions can only be answered by the individual researcher based upon his/her own interests, needs, abilities, and resources.

Self-report measures of self-disclosure. Chelune[107] believed that the data derived from self-report measures provide the answers to a number of explicit or implicit questions: When? To whom? On what topic? To what degree? Under what circumstances? By whom? The question of *when* divides self-report measures into two classifications: history measures—self-evaluations of past disclosures—and expectation measures—self-evaluations of willingness to disclose. Chelune concluded that history measures may be confusing since no time unit is specified and that expectation measures can be interpreted to represent current dispositions to disclose and as such are better predictors of actual disclosing behavior than most history measures. The question of "to whom?" has been answered by researchers with a number of target persons including the following: mother, father, male friend, female friend, a stranger, an acquaintance, a best friend, closest family member, therapist, best-liked-girl in class, least-liked-girl in class, and better-liked parent. One understudied aspect of this area, according to Chelune, has been the effect of the experimenter on self-disclosure or the experimenter as a target. "On what topic?" has generally included variations in intimacy of topic content with findings to indicate that intimacy level affects self-disclosure, although explanations for this finding vary. "To what degree?'' has been answered usually in terms of past extent of disclosures using a three-point scale, frequency with which the items were discussed, and willingness to disclose on specific items. ''Under what circumstances?'' has been, according to Chelune, perhaps the most overlooked question in self-report assessment procedures since the typical self-report inventory does not specify the situation or setting for the subject. Subjects are left on their own to describe the settings and this is a source of variation between subjects. Finally, the question ''by whom?'' is another area needing more research since the typical subject has been an undergraduate introductory psychology student. The above-listed questions represent some of the major situational and personality variables that are often embedded in self-report measures; they should be considered, according to Chelune, by anyone wishing to assess self-disclosure.

The Jourard Self-Disclosure Questionnaire: The earliest and most widely used self-report instrument to assess individual differences in self-disclosure has been Jourard's Self-Disclosure Questionnaire (JSDQ).[19] The JSDQ consists of 60 items with 10 items in each of six content areas: attitudes and opinions, tastes and interests, work, money, personality, and body. It measures the amounts of past self-reported disclosure to each of four target persons: the mother, the father, a male friend, and a female friend. Subjects responded to each item by indicating the extent to which the information has been revealed to each target by using the following three-point scale[106]:

0: Have told the other person nothing about this aspect of me.
1: Have talked in general terms about this. The other person has only a general idea about this aspect of me.
2: Have talked in full and complete detail about this item to the other person. He knows me fully in this respect and could describe me accurately.
X: Have lied or misrepresented myself to the other person so that he has a false picture of me (p. 4).

Subjects' ratings of each item are summed (X's are counted as zeros) yielding a total self-disclosure score. In addition, scores for each target person and for each topic category can be obtained by summing the scores for that target person or topic category. Subjects were given the following instructions in completing the questionnaire[106]:

> The answer sheet which you have been given has columns with the headings Mother, Father, Male Friend, Female Friend, and Spouse. You are to read each item on the questionnaire, and then indicate on the answer sheet the extent that you have talked about that item to each person; that is, the extent to which you have made yourself known to that person. Use the rating scale that you see on the answer sheet to describe the extent that you have talked about each item (p. 4).

Examples of items from each of the six topic categories are presented below[106]:

1. *Attitudes and opinions*—My personal views on drinking.
2. *Tastes and interests*—My likes and dislikes in music.

3. *Work (or studies)*—What I find to be the most boring or unenjoyable aspects of my work.
4. *Money*—How much money I make at my work, or get as an allowance.
5. *Personality*—What it takes to get me feeling real depressed and blue.
6. *Body*—How I wish I looked: my ideals for overall appearance (p. 189).

In reviewing research on the reliability and validity of the JSDQ, Chelune[104] stated that the general psychometric quality of this instrument is considered to be quite good. Jourard and Lasakow[19] reported an overall split-half reliability coefficient of .94 with 70 unmarried white college students. Cozby[15] stated that the JSDQ appears to be independent of intelligence which is evidence of discriminant validity. The fact that nurses who scored high on the questionnaire were rated a year later as higher in the ability to establish and maintain relationships with patients and as more open with nursing faculty has been seen as evidence for construct validity of the JSDQ.[16] Further evidence of construct validity exists in the finding that self-disclosure is related to three operationally and conceptually independent aspects of interpersonal functioning (conceptual complexity, authoritarianism, peer nominations) and to behavior ratings of interpersonal flexibility and adaptability.[27]

While the reliability and construct validity of the *JSDQ* have been generally considered to be sound, there is little evidence of the predictive validity of the instrument as a measure of general disclosingness.[15,104] According to the reviews by Cozby[15] and Chelune,[104] researchers have been unable to find significant relationships between the JSDQ and actual disclosure in a situation, ratings of actual disclosure made by peers, ratings of intimacy of self-descriptive essays, ratings of disclosure in group settings, and time spent talking and ratings of intimacy in structured interviews.

Numerous explanations have been offered for the poor predictive validity of the JSDQ. Usually these explanations have included the fact that the JSDQ measures subjects' past history of disclosure to parents and same- and opposite-sex friends, while when actual disclosure is measured, the subject is disclosing to an experimenter or to peers whom the subject has never met.[15] Jourard,[106] in answering the question "Are self-disclosure questionnaires valid?" (p. 168), concluded that there was evidence to support the construct, concurrent, and predictive validity of the instrument. On discussing the predictive validity, he argued that previous tests of the questionnaire's predictive validity demonstrated that the JSDQ did not predict the classes of behavior these tests studied, but this was not to say that the JSDQ was not valid. Jourard then presented evidence of the predictive validity of the JSDQ.

The primary value of the JSDQ for the assessment of expressiveness lies in the method and format developed by Jourard and in the use of the questionnaire as a more global measure of disclosure, believing that general self-disclosure is highly correlated with affective self-disclosure. The value of the method and format of the original JSDQ can be seen by the fact that almost all other self-report measures of self-disclosure are modifications of the JSDQ. In fact,

Jourard[106] developed two self-report inventories similar to the JSDQ, a 25-item and a 40-item self-disclosure questionnaire, both of which have been used successfully. The modifications made in the general format of the JSDQ by other researchers have usually been in one or more of the following respects: instruction set, number of items, rating scale, or target person.[104] It would seem that one modification that could be made would be to consider only disclosure of feelings using the general format and methods developed by Jourard. This, in fact, is very similar to the Expression of Emotion Scale,[4] which was mentioned previously. In addition, other variations might prove useful for specific assessment needs. Some extensions of Balswick's scale designed to consider situational differences in expressiveness that were based on the format developed by Jourard will be presented later.

Other self-report measures of self-disclosure that consider intimacy of disclosure, situational influences, and child and adolescent disclosure are presented in reviews on self-disclosure by Cozby[15] and Chelune.[104] These other self-report measures might be of some use to the reader, and the reviews provide some general information on their format and purported use. Since these measures deal with more specific aspects of self-disclosure, it was believed that some readers might wish to consider these aspects in terms of expressiveness and thus, could benefit from a cursory knowledge of their methods. The reader is referred directly to the references for more information on these questionnaires.

In summary, the JSDQ was presented because it has been the model for most other self-report measures of self-disclosure and because it is still frequently used in one form or another. Also, the methods developed by Jourard are applicable for assessing expressiveness through self-report. Other self-report methods were not presented since they were less relevant to expressiveness; for the most part, the other questionnaires are only modifications of the JSDQ anyway. A number of problems that exist with self-report measures of self-disclosure were discussed, but the primary value of self-report methods continues to be their economy of administration and scoring. They also, as mentioned previously, provided another source of data from a perspective different from behavioral measures, which leads to a more comprehensive picture of self-disclosing behavior.

Behavioral measures of self-disclosure. One of the advantages of using behavioral measures is that they make it possible to assess self-disclosure from another perspective, that of the recipient or independent observer rather than the discloser. Chelune[104] believed that this was important because the use of behavioral measures increases the amount and types of information that can be gathered. He urged caution, however, in comparing and generalizing results from behavioral measures since they often use different judgment criteria. Chelune divided behavioral measures of self-disclosure into observational measures and objective measures. A brief summary of Chelune's description of these approaches will be presented and will be followed by a behavioral approach to measuring affective self-disclosure, which holds particular promise for assessing expressiveness.

Observational Measures: Chelune described four approaches to observational measures that are frequently used: (1) projective techniques, (2) peer nominations, (3) self-descriptive essays, and (4) rating systems. The use of projective techniques includes the use of subjects' responses to TAT cards and standardized approaches to rating subjects' sentence completions for self-disclosure. The peer nomination technique is a popular sociometric method employed as a means of ranking individuals within a group for self-disclosure (e.g., Halverson and Shore[27]), although its validity is questionable for large groups. Self-descriptive essays are used for scoring the depth of self-disclosure from essay questions (on the same content as the JSDQ) which subjects answer. The final observational measures described by Chelune are the rating scales, which usually include the use of scales to rate verbal behavior from interviews or groups.

These observational measures of self-disclosure might prove useful to readers wishing to assess expressiveness. Certainly, their methods could be applicable to the assessment of expressiveness when the researchers were interested in observing and rating interviews or segments of verbal behavior. In fact, some of the scales included expression of feelings categories. The reader is referred to Chelune for more information on this approach to assessing self-disclosure.

Objective Measures: In describing objective measures, Chelune[104] stated, "Two parameters of self disclosing behavior, amount and duration, readily lend themselves to objective measurement" (p. 301). Amount of disclosure is defined as the number or breadth of the items of information disclosed; duration refers to the time spent disclosing aspects of the self. Chelune examined some of the objective procedures used to assess these two dimensions. Measures of amount have included: number of words subjects used to describe themselves; breadth of disclosure based on topical content; and content analyses techniques. Measures of duration of self-disclosure have included: time spent talking (which is based on the assumption that the more a person talks the more he/she will disclose); reaction time (i.e., amount of latency in seconds a subject takes before responding to an interview topic); and silence quotient (i.e., summing all silent pauses over three seconds in length [excluding reaction time] and then dividing this sum by the total duration of the responses to an item).

These objective measures, much like the observational measures, hold value for those interested in assessing expressiveness, primarily because their methods might be applicable to the assessment of expressiveness as secondary measures. No research is available to support their use for this purpose although similar methods have been used to assess assertiveness (e.g., Eisler et al.[53]). They were presented from Chelune's[104] review to allow readers the opportunity to consider the possibility of using them to meet their assessment needs. The reader is referred to that review for more complete information on these methods including procedures and research on reliability and validity.

Chelune[107] stated that observational assessment techniques might require more time to train judges and run subjects through an experimental setting than self-report devices, but they greatly reduce the embedded social-situational factors that can add unexplained variance to the system. He identified problems, however, with this approach in that the data which are obtained are unique to the experimental condition used to obtain the data, and that several person-perceptual variables remain embedded in observational techniques. One of the difficulties inherent in using objective techniques, he believed, is that, since objective metrics define self-disclosure in terms of specific elements, they may not respond to self-disclosure as a total phenomenon. Chelune[107] concluded,

> Researchers must carefully weigh the advantages of increased control against the possibilities that the operational definition and derived data will not adequately reflect the phenomenological behavior we describe as self-disclosure (p. 26).

Affective Self-Disclosure: One final behavioral approach to assessing self-disclosure will be presented. This method was designed for assessing affective self-disclosure.[21,22,51] With this performance test each subject listened to and verbally responded to from 8 to 16 audiotaped situations which were presented in random order. These situations simulated dyadic interactions between subjects and their best male and female friends (intimacy level of target can vary, e.g., to acquaintance as in Highlen and Johnston[22]). Subjects made responses both as initators and as respondents to situations calling for positive and negative feelings, so that subject role (initiator, respondent), type of feeling (positive, negative), and sex of best friend (opposite, same) were crossed factors in the audiotaped performance test.

The following written and verbal instructions were presented to subjects at the start of the performance test[21]:

> In this experiment, you will be recording your responses to typical situations which arise in people's lives. It is important that you try to IMAGINE THAT YOU ARE ACTUALLY IN THE SITUATIONS and talking to your best male or best female friend. It is also important that you try to EXPRESS YOUR TRUE FEELINGS that you would experience if you were in that particular situation with your best friend (p. 279).

In addition, subjects were instructed to take a few seconds and write down the names of their best male and female friend to help them keep in mind the people they are to be imagining in the situation during the experiment. Subjects were presented with two practice situations in order to acquaint them with the task; the responses to practice situations were not evaluated. An example of one experimental situation used by Highlen and Gillis[21] illustrating the combination of initator, positive feeling, and same-sex best friend is as follows:

> Your boyfriend has broken off with you, and you want to be alone for the evening. After much persuasion, your best female friend convinces you to go to a movie with her that you didn't particularly want to see. Much to your surprise as the movie ends, you find that you've really enjoyed the evening. You turn to your friend and say . . . (p. 271).

Highlen limited subjects' responses to 15 seconds, after which time the next situation began. A self-report concomitant anxiety scale was also used following each response. Subjects were asked to rate the anxiety they would actually feel if they were saying their response to their best friend on a 1–7 Likert scale, ranging from very calm and relaxed to extremely nervous.

Two trained raters rated the performance tapes for affective self-disclosure with each response receiving a score from 0 to 3. A response had to contain an affect word used as a verb, adverb, or adjective appropriate to the positive or negative affect present in the stimulus situation. Criteria used by Highlen and Gillis[21] to assign points were as follows:

1. affect present and appropriate, 1 point;
2. statement self-referenced (I, me, my, mine), 1 point;
3. reason for affect given, 1 point, (p. 272).

Using this rating system interrater reliability coefficients in the 90's and an interrater agreement of 94% were obtained. In studies to date Highlen and her associates have demonstrated the efficacy of this performance test for assessing training effects and exploring situational variables in affective self-disclosure.

A new addition designed to assess the use of voice tone to express feelings was added in the Highlen and Johnston[22] study. This procedure was derived from the anecdotal observation that subjects relied heavily on voice tone as well as hand and facial gestures to convey their feelings, suggesting that subjects rely on more than verbal content. In order to assess the proportion of subjects using appropriate vocal inflection without affective content to those making affective verbalizations, two raters evaluated each tape for presence or absence of affective content and tone. Highlen and Johnston[22] assigned each response to one of the following categories:

1. content and tone present (the person makes an affective statement, and the tone of voice is sincere);
2. content present, tone absent (the person makes an affective statement but speaks in a monotone and/or sounds insincere);
3. content absent, tone present (vocal expression is appropriate for the situation, but affect words are not used to convey feelings);
4. content and tone absent (the person does not make an affective statement, and the tone of voice does not convey feelings or is inappropriate for the situation) (p. 256).

A Pearson product–moment correlation coefficient for jointly rated tapes of .92 was reported. Highlen and Johnston using this procedure found that "Subjects consistently relied on tone of voice to convey their feelings instead of using appropriate content" (p. 257).

Of all the behavioral methods reviewed, those developed by Highlen and her associates would seem to have the most promise for assessing expressive behavior. They consider expressive behaviors in a wide range of situations with apparent reliability and some evidence of concurrent validity based upon correlations with self-report measures of attitudes toward disclosing feelings. The performance test is also easy and quick to administer, reliable and straightforward to rate, and does not require unusual equipment. The performance test has demonstrated usefulness as a pre- and posttest measure to assess subtle training effects; however, no test–retest reliability was presented. A shortcoming of the procedure is that, although it does consider voice tone, it does not consider the wide range of nonverbal behaviors that would be possible with videotape. This would seem to be the logical extension of Highlen's work and this idea will be expanded in the final section.

Affective Communication Test. The Affective Communication Test (ACT)[113] is a recently published and somewhat different approach to assessing expressiveness with demonstrated reliability and validity. The ACT is a 13-item self-report scale designed to measure individual differences in nonverbal expressiveness or what is sometimes called "charisma." The authors of the scale, Friedman et al.,[113] developed it in an attempt to explicate the concept of expressiveness and its psychological implications including the personality and social characteristics of expressive people. They hoped that the development of the ACT would help to expand the knowledge of expressiveness by overcoming two factors which have limited the study of expressiveness: (1) the conceptual ambiguity of expressiveness; and (2) the absence of standard, convenient measuring instruments.

The development of the test began with an attempt by Friedman et al. to refine the concept of expressiveness by asking students and associates to generate behavior-related self-report items that they thought would measure expressiveness. These items were tested, refined, and condensed on several groups of students and ambiguous items, and those showing little variance were thrown out. Item intercorrelations were computed on the remaining items, and those which led to high internal consistency and test–retest reliability were used to construct a shorter 46-item test with several versions. Friedman et al. then recruited college students to fill out this questionnaire. Items that were ambiguous were removed, and markedly skewed or low-variance items were deleted from the scale. Finally, interitem and item total correlations were computed on the remaining items and a reliable scale was constructed.

For each of the 13 items on the ACT the subject indicates on a 9-point scale from −4 to +4 the extent to which the statement is true or false about him or her. Friedman et al.[113] presented an example of their scale by stating, "For example, the first item (which is answered on a scale of 'not at all true of me' to 'very true of me') is 'When I hear good dance music, I can hardly keep still'" (p. 336). Other items include: "My laugh is soft and subdued"; "I can easily express emotion over the telephone"; and "I often touch friends during conversations" (p. 335). The ACT is scored by adding the scores on the individual items after eliminating negative numbers by adding five points to each item and reversing the scores for the six items worded in the opposite direction. Friedman et al. noticed that, although the scale was developed on and was expected to be used with college students, there is no evidence that the ACT is not valid with other populations, and researchers should not refrain from the cautious use of the ACT with other groups.

Friedman et al.[113] presented evidence of the reliability and validity of the ACT that resulted from several studies. They stated, "The reliability of the ACT is excellent, especially for a research tool (as opposed to a standardized, applied test) and one of such short length" (p. 336). This conclusion was based upon evidence of internal consistency for the scale indicated by a coefficient alpha equal to .77 (for a sample of 289 undergraduates) and test–retest reliabilities for 2 months of .90 (for a sample of 44 students) and for one week of .91 (for a sample of 38 students). Evidence of the validity of the ACT was found in the "significant and nontrivial relationship" (r = .39) between the ACT scores and ratings of expressiveness by friends of subjects. This led Friedman et al. to state, "Although a short, self-report measure, the ACT seems valid in the sense that it reflects the perceptions of others concerning one's expressiveness" (p. 337).

The authors of the scale then explored the relationships between the ACT and measures of interpersonal relations, measures of personality, and nonverbal communication skills. They found as they had predicted that the ACT was significantly related in the expected manner to lecturing, political charisma, stage acting, acting class, acting experience, occupation, future occupation, and sales, as measured by a nine-item questionnaire addressing these issues. In addition, in a study with 25 family practice residents, they found a correlation (r = .52, $p < .01$) between the ACT and physician popularity, indicating that expressive physicians were more likely to have more patients. The authors explored the relationship between the ACT and established personality measures by correlating it with: (1) the Personality Research Form; (2) the Eysenck Personality Inventory; (3) the Marlowe–Crowne Social Desirability Scale; (4) the Machiavellan Scale; (5) the Taylor Manifest Anxiety Scale; (6) the Rotter Internal–External Locus of Control Scale; (7) the Coopersmith Self-Esteem Inventory; and (8) the Snyder Self Monitoring Scale. The results indicated that the ACT was highly related to the personality trait *exhibition* and related in the predicted fashion to other Personality Research Form traits. The ACT was also related to extraversion and slightly negatively correlated with neuroticism, both of which were measured by the Eysenck Personality Inventory. The correlations of the ACT with the other scales showed it to be (1) related to social desirability (r = .22, $p < .06$), self-esteem (r = .27, $p < .05$), and internal control (r = .28, $p < .05$, individuals with an internal locus of control tended to be more expressive); (2) slightly related to self-monitoring (r = .21 and r = .14, both ns); and (3) not related to Machiavellianism (r = .08, ns); and manifest anxiety (r = −.17, ns). Based upon these results, Friedman et al. stated, "As a psychometric instrument (a personality test) the ACT does well, particularly given the limitations of an economical self-report measure" (p. 343). Finally, in an attempt to explore the relationship between the ACT and nonverbal communication skills, the authors of the scale correlated it with the ability to send various emotions accurately, which was measured following Ekman et al.[58] They found that expressiveness was related to posed emotional sending ability for females but not for males. Friedman et al.[113] concluded on the basis of all these studies that the ACT is a valid and useful instrument for refining the construct of expressiveness.

In summary, the ACT seems to meet the criteria for a useful and important measure of expressiveness which attempts to measure nonverbal expressiveness by way of self-report and has demonstrated reliability and validity. One advantage of this measure is its brevity (13 items) and ease of administration and scoring. There seems to be no doubt that this instrument holds great promise for research on expressive behavior and for the assessment of expressiveness. Although the authors of the scale do not discuss it, the ACT would also seem to be potentially useful for assessing expressiveness in a clinical setting when used in conjunction with some of the other methods discussed thus far. In addition, the ACT provided further evidence for male inexpressiveness because, according to Friedman et al., in two large samples (n = 287 and n = 311) mean scores for females were slightly higher than for males.

IMPLICATIONS FOR COUNSELORS/THERAPISTS. The expression of emotions has been the subject of many types of research efforts from Balswick's[2,3,6] explorations of male inexpressiveness to Highlen's[21,22] examination of the specific parameters influencing affective self-disclosure. Inexpressiveness has been considered a problem for persons in intimate relationships and marriages[3,12,17,24] and in the counseling process.[108] Treatment programs have been suggested to help people, particularly males, become more expressive.[24,51,62] In order to identify clients needing these sorts of treatment approaches and to evaluate the client's progress during and after treatment, reliable and valid methods of assessing expressiveness are needed. The purpose of this paper has been to explicate the need for assessment, the types of assessment methods, the problems with various types of assessment, and some specific, reliable, and valid methods that could be used to assess expressiveness.

The implications from this review for counselors/therapists who are interested in addressing client's problems with inexpressiveness are many and will be summarized below. The first is that assessment is important and useful for: (1) identifying the client's problem; (2) identifying an appropriate and preferred treatment technique; (3) determining whether the treatment is working; (4) deciding whether the treatment has been effective; and (5) determining treatment effect generalization and durability. There are two major approaches to assessment, self-report and behavioral, each with advantages and disadvantages. There is an advantage in using both approaches in combination since they provide different kinds of information. Furthermore, from a research and therapeutic perspective, data from both can provide a more comprehensive understanding of the behavior studied.[64,79,90]

The most direct measures of expressiveness are the Expression of Emotion Scale[4] and the Affective Communication Test,[113] both of which have been used in a number of studies. Other than these measures, it is necessary to go to closely related psychological constructs to find useful assessment methods. Assertiveness and self-disclosure are two constructs that, based on definitions, are conceptually similar to expressiveness. Also, they both possess tested self-report and behavioral assessment methods that hold promise for assessing expressiveness. The best examples of these were presented with a discussion of problems inherent in their use and suggestions regarding their adaptation for assessing expressiveness. The implication here for counselors/therapists is that methods are available for assessing expressiveness although some adaptations might be necessary (e.g., focusing on specific items or factors which deal with positive assertiveness on self-report measures of assertiveness).

Based on this review, more general implications regarding assessment include the suggestion that assessment methods should consider situational variability. Evidence was presented that indicated that assertiveness, self-disclosure, and expressiveness are not "traits," i.e., each is affected by situational variables. Another suggestion is that the assessment method used should be multidimensional in order to measure expressive behavior adequately. Based upon research on the assessment of both assertiveness and self-disclosure, it is important to consider both verbal and nonverbal behavioral components of behavior when assessing expressiveness. Evidence of the reliability and validity of a number of self-report and behavioral measures that could be used to assess expressiveness was presented; these concerns with reliability and validity need to be considered in choosing an assessment method. Finally, the nature and design of the assessment method used and the operational definition of expressiveness are closely related, and both limit the generalizations that can be made from the data.

It is now possible using the suggestions and implications contained in this review to describe what an appropriate and useful method of assessing expressiveness would be and to give an example. The assessment method would be (1) multimethod—self-report and behavioral; (2) multidimensional—measure more than one parameter of expressiveness; (3) consider both verbal and nonverbal components of expressiveness; (4) adequate in terms of reliability and validity; (5) appropriate for addressing generality and duration; and (6) relatively quick and easy to administer and rate or score. The example of the suggested approach to assessing expressiveness includes the following self-report components: (1) Balswick's[4] Expression of Emotion Scale; (2) The Expression of Emotion Scale varied by target person; (3) The Expression of Emotion Scale varied by situation; (4) 16 situations (which were borrowed from Highlen[50]) requesting subjects' response to situations which vary in terms of sex of target (same, opposite), type of feeling required (positive, negative), and role of subject (initiator, respondent); and (5) the Self-Monitoring Scale.[110] It also includes a behavioral section which consists of the subjects' videotaped responses to the same 16 situations from the self-report section, which are interacted with a male or female role model. The Affective Communication Test[113] could easily be included here and would provide additional information. It had not been published, however, when research with this combination of assessment methods was started.

The instructions to the subject and the format for the self-report portions of this assessment can be found in Appendix A. The self-monitoring section is included to address the issue of whether the inexpressiveness is due to a skills deficit or to an inhibited response. This issue could be resolved if the results show the subject is high on self-monitoring and he/she demonstrates much situational variability. In this case the treatment approach should address the reasons for the inhibited response in particular situations rather than general skills training. The entire self-report section has taken subjects between 20 and 45 minutes to complete. The written responses to the 16 situations are rated in a manner similar to that used by Highlen and Gillis.[21] Their procedure has demonstrated adequate interrater reliability and research is underway to determine the reliability of this adaptation; reliabilities calculated during rater training have been promising. With the new Expression of Feeling Rating Scale, expressiveness is rated on a five-point scale as follows: 5—clear, self-referenced feeling with clear reason for the feeling given; 4—clear self-referenced feeling with no or unclear reason for the feeling given; 3—unclear feeling or a response to feeling in an indirect, unclear, or confusing way; 2—response to content, cognitive statement, or affect that is other referenced; 1—irrelevant response or response with inappropriate feeling; 0—no response. An additional measure of expressiveness, number of words, is also computed.

The behavioral section of this assessment method is best administered several days after the self-report to minimize contaminating effects. This procedure requires the use of videotape and is best conducted in an experimental room with two-way mirror. For ethical reasons, the subject is advised of the videotaping, but the equipment should be as inconspicuous as possible. Also an effort should be made to help subjects feel comfortable and relaxed with the videotaping prior to beginning the procedure. One additional advantage with this assessment procedure is that, since the same 16 situations are used in both the self-report and the behavioral sections of the assessment, it is possible to compare self-report and behavioral data directly.

The following instructions are presented verbally and in writing to each subject at the start of the session:

> In this study, you will be asked to respond to typical situations which arise in people's lives. It is important that you try to imagine that you are actually in the situations, and are interacting with your best male or best female friend. It is also important that you try to express your true feelings that you would experience if you were in that particular situation with your best friend. Take a few seconds now to think of the name of your best female friend and your best male friend to help you keep in mind the people you are imagining you are with in these situations. Try throughout this experience to imagine the actor as your best male friend and the actress as your best female friend. In order to better imagine the situations that will be described, you could think about what it would feel like to be in the situation, where it would occur, and what you would see, hear, and smell. Then, when you are certain that you understand the situation and can imagine it, you may proceed to respond to the actor or actress. Try to respond just as you would to your best friend. Remember, express your feelings as well as you can. After each situation, I will explain the next situation and you will have time to get ready. In some of the situations, you will respond first, and, in others, you will respond after the actor or actress speaks to you.

When the subject demonstrates an understanding of the instructions, the situation is presented on a card which is given to the subject. After the subject has a chance to understand and imagine the situation, an actor or actress enters the room and the subject responds. The situations are presented to the subjects in a random order to control for any order response bias and proceed from one situation to another until all 16 situations have been presented and responses to each have been obtained. Although subjects' responses are not limited by time, each response ends with their first response, and does not include any further interaction with the actor or actress.

Two practice situations are presented to ensure that subjects understand the instructions, to acquaint each subject with the task, and to further relax them. These situations are very similar to the experimental situation, and can be videotaped for later use in rater training. Further explanation is offered at this point to those subjects who experience difficulty in following the instructions.

Videotaping commences at the conclusion of the introduction of the situation and when the first words are spoken by either the actor/actress or the subject. At the end of the subject's response to each situation, the actor/actress states the number of the situation for the videotape and audiotape. This allows the specific situation to be identified for rating purposes.

Following each response to the situation and once the video equipment is turned off, each subject is asked to rate the anxiety he/she would actually feel if he/she had made that response to his/her best male or female friend. A 1–7 Likert scale, ranging from "very calm and relaxed" to "extremely nervous" is used to report anxiety for each situation (e.g., Highlen[50]). The entire behavioral portion of this assessment procedure takes approximately 20 to 30 minutes per subject to administer. The rating, although requiring raters and video equipment, is reliable and straightforward.

Two trained raters rate the performance audiotape as described above for affective self-disclosure and also for length of response (number of words). Two additional raters are trained to rate nonverbal expression of emotion by observing the videotapes. Reliability measures should be calculated for these raters.

Each of the 16 videotaped responses for each of the participants is rated using methods similar to those used to assess nonverbal components of assertive behavior. Eisler et al.[52] and Eisler et al.[53] suggested eight nonverbal units of behavior that are useful for this study: duration of looking, smiles, duration of reply, latency of response, loudness of speech, fluency of speech, affect, and overall assertiveness. The scale suggested for use in this assessment procedure has been adapted from Eisler et al.[52] This scale consists of the following eight behaviors: loudness of speech, affective voice tone, fluency of speech, animation of body, latency of response, facial expression, distracting behavior, and overall expressiveness. Each of these categories is on a scale from 1 to 11 (see Appendix B for all scales and definitions).

For all behavioral measures the participant's score is obtained by taking the mean value averaged over the 16 situations. It should be noted that the adapted measurement and scoring procedure has been used for a sample of 35 correctional officers with acceptable reliability (reliabilities for the three raters corrected by the Spearman–Brown Prophecy Formula ranged from .69 to .88) and demonstrated ability for scores to differentiate between high- and low-assertive subjects (Dosser et al., unpublished data, 1979). With only brief training of raters in the above-mentioned pilot study, the scale proved useful and reliable. Other nonverbal rating methods exist (e.g., Ekman et al.,[58] Izard,[59,114] Mehrabian[61]), but they are more complex and less straightforward.

Research results support the contention that rating videotape, rather than live behavior, will not affect the reliability of the ratings. For example, Eisler et al.[115] concluded that videotaped observation of nonverbal interaction for the behaviors they studied (looking and smiling) is highly reliable and equal to reliabilities obtained by observing the interactions live. They also suggested a distinct advantage to the use of videotapes, in that it can be viewed more than once to facilitate precision in defining and measuring behaviors.

The assessment procedure just described for measuring expressiveness can be used in whole or in part, although using only part limits the data and the generalizations possible from the data. It is expected, however, that most counselors/therapists would use only a part of this suggested assessment package, primarily because of time constraints. This procedure is believed to be appropriate for counselors/therapists to assess treatment effects, identify inexpressive clients, etc., as well as for researchers attempting to further explore expressive behavior. It is composed of parts that have previously demonstrated reliability and validity, although the entire procedure has not yet been tested; however, research is underway to test the effectiveness of this procedure. Further research is needed to increase the understanding of expressive behavior including: the causes of inexpressiveness, situational variance in expressive behavior, the relationship between expressiveness and personality variables (e.g., self-monitoring), sex differences in expressiveness, and the relative effectiveness of various techniques of increasing expressiveness. For this type of research to be conducted a reliable and valid method of assessing expressiveness is necessary. Hopefully, this review and the assessment procedures suggested will stimulate research toward this end.

In addition, this review has implications for training/treatment approaches dealing with inexpressiveness. Research has been presented which not only addresses the assessment of expressiveness, but in addition, explicates the parameters of expressive behavior. In designing the training/treatment program, the counselor/therapist should be sensitive to situational variability in the expressive behavior of his/her client. Training/treatment at any one time should be directed toward only very specific components of expressive behavior including specific types of expressive content, specific situations, specific target persons, specific verbal behaviors, and specific nonverbal behaviors. In other words, training/treatment should be just as specific as assessment. Based on this review, it should be evident that taking a global or "trait" approach to training/treatment should be as confusing as taking a similar approach with assessment.

These points can easily be incorporated into a training/treatment program which uses assessment before, during, and after the intervention to indicate the client's particular deficits at that point. For example, modeling, behavior rehearsal, and coaching can be developed to address a client's problems with particular target people and situations. The client can then attempt to be expressive in a similar but slightly different situation, which is videotaped. The tape can then be reviewed by the clinician and the client to identify further deficits needing more attention and to teach the client to be more expressive verbally and nonverbally.

The nonverbal components of expressive behavior can be taught from two perspectives. First, the client can be taught with videotaping to express his/her feelings more appropriately by using the various nonverbal components of expressive behavior (e.g., facial expression, gestures, voice tones, body posture).

Procedures of this sort have been suggested in assertive training (e.g., Serber[116]) and could be similarly conducted for expressiveness training. The other perspective involves teaching clients to discriminate the nonverbal communication of emotion from others. These two perspectives are closely related since, in order to improve his/her nonverbal communication, he/she must learn to discriminate nonverbal communication. This perspective is also closely related to more general social skills in that responding to someone's feelings, which is dependent upon the ability to discriminate feelings, is an important communication and relationship skill.

The final issue related to training/treatment that was presented involves the necessity of addressing both skills deficit and skills inhibition reasons for inexpressiveness. As was mentioned previously, assessment methods which consider situational variability and self-monitoring differences in expressive behavior can assist the counselor/therapist in identifying a particular client's reason for inexpressiveness. A comprehensive training/treatment program must address both issues by teaching skills and by identifying and challenging whatever is inhibiting the expressive behavior. One approach that has been suggested for doing this is using a cognitive/behavioral approach to teach people to be more expressive.[62] This expressiveness training procedure is similar to procedures used in assertive training except that it focuses on the expression of positive feelings. It uses skills training techniques from assertive training such as modeling, behavior rehearsal, coaching, and role playing. In addition, it uses cognitive restructuring procedures to address irrational beliefs or overlearned socialization messages that inhibit expressive behavior. This training procedure will be thoroughly described in the final section of this chapter.

In summary, this section on assessment has implications for counselors/therapists who are interested in assessing expressiveness, and for counselors/therapists who are interested in treating clients with inexpressive difficulties. Suggestions have also been made that pertain to research on expressiveness and ways to use assessment procedures to advance the understanding of expressive behavior.

EXPRESSIVENESS TRAINING

Previous attempts to address changes in the male sex role have included unstructured consciousness-raising groups,[35] assertive training groups for "resocializing" men,[45] and numerous approaches to both individual and group counseling/therapy. In addition, several training programs[48,50] have been developed to increase affective self-disclosure or expressiveness. All of these programs have experienced some success in helping men to adapt more flexible attitudes and to develop more effective behaviors. The research on these programs, however, has indicated the need for improvements in these efforts to lessen the rigidity of traditional sex-role stereotypes. The expressiveness training program described in this chapter was designed to make use of those components from other programs that had been shown to be effective and to improve upon those that did not work as well.

The design of this training program is based upon the suggestions made in previous research. For example, the training is longer in duration as suggested by Highlen[50] to increase treatment effects and their maintenance. It includes a more structured and systematic approach to treatment as suggested by the behaviorists, as well as unstructured activities as suggested by Damgaard[48] to improve generalizability and to aid the development of positive feeling expression. The unstructured portion of this program (approximately 30 minutes each week) is very similar to a consciousness-raising experience and, as such, allows the participants to learn that their problems and concerns are not unique and to share their thoughts and feelings with others. Many structured training programs do not include time for this; it is seen as valuable in this approach to expressiveness training. In addition this training uses videotape as an instructional tool as suggested by Serber[116] and Eisler et al.[117] to improve both verbal and nonverbal expressiveness skills. In addition to teaching skills, it attempts to address the erroneous or irrational beliefs that inhibit men's expressive behavior through cognitive restructuring procedures.

A training approach was selected for treating male inexpressiveness for several reasons. First, the author believes there is value in taking a training approach rather than a strict counseling/therapy approach; this value arises from the fact that many inexpressive males are not good candidates for most types of counseling/therapy and would be extremely reluctant to enter personal, marital, or family counseling/therapy because to do so could be seen by themselves and others as an expression of weakness and vulnerability, feelings the male has been taught not to express. This concern would be lessened, however, with a training program since many men are learning new skills. Highlen[50] experienced success in obtaining volunteers for her training sessions for increasing affective self-disclosure by advertising her program as communication skills training for improving the ability to express feelings. Such a strategy would seem to be useful for attracting more clients to training.

The belief that the problem described above is real and worthy of consideration has been reinforced by the author's training and research experiences. The author's findings have been that the least expressive men (as assessed by the assessment procedures described in the previous section of this chapter) are the least likely to be interested in programs dealing with "feelings." There are several explanations for this, some of which were discussed previously in describing male socialization. Part of the problem, no doubt, arises from a fear of the unknown and of changing that is typical of many clients. Other aspects of the problem involve exaggerated and irrational ideas that men might have about the nature of such programs,including the idea that they are run by "radicals" who want to "put them down" and who will try to get them to change their personalities and behavior drastically. Another exaggerated and irrational idea that men have expressed is that participating in such "men's groups" is tantamount to homosexual behavior and so they resist participating. This is an important reason for utilizing a skills approach combined with cognitive restructuring to encourage changes in men's behavior and beliefs and for addressing primarily one specific element, expressive behavior, and doing so in a very systematic fashion. Expressiveness training is less threatening to inexpressive males than other approaches since it affords the opportunity to improve expressiveness skills in an unthreatening, accepting environment, while addressing behavioral deficits systematically through successive approximation with much reinforcement directed toward more satisfying behavior. Even though the primary effort is focused on changes in behavior and skills, attitudes and beliefs are not ignored since attention is placed on cognitive strategies and unstructured consciousness raising. Issues related to rigid sex-role stereotypes and the ways in which they limit men's behavior are addressed in order to provide encouragement to try new ways of behaving.

For those men with particularly intense or severe personal, marital, or family problems, the training serves to motivate them to take advantage of group or individual counseling/therapy through the cognitive restructuring activities which challenges the beliefs that men must always be strong, tough, expert, and competent. It also serves to refute the belief that participating in counseling/therapy is indicative of weakness. The assessment before, during, and after the training is used to identify clients with more serious problems and is helpful for suggesting the most appropriate counseling/treatment techniques.

Additional advantages of the training approach to treatment of inexpressiveness include the ability to affect a group of men at once thus making it possible to use the group's dynamics, support, and the increased opportunities for modeling. In addition, expressiveness training can be used as a preventive as well as a treatment program, thus increasing its potential efficacy with widely diverse groups. Although this training is usually conducted with groups of men, it is also appropriate for inexpressive women, and the techniques and procedures can be used with individuals as well as with groups. Finally, this program teaches specific skills which can be added to the client's behavioral repertoire to be used or not used as the client so desires in different situations. No assumption is made that males should always be expressive in every situation. Instead, the primary assumptions of expressiveness training are (1) men can learn to be more expressive; (2) many men want to be more expressive in various situations with various individuals; and (3) many men can benefit intra- and interpersonally from becoming more expressive.

In summary, expressiveness training utilizing techniques and procedures borrowed from assertive training, communication skills training, and male consciousness-raising groups is suggested as a means of increasing male expressiveness. Suggestions made by researchers to improve training techniques that were tried previously were considered in designing this particular approach. The particular techniques and procedures that it includes have been shown to be useful and were believed to be the most likely to attract and to have a significant impact upon inexpressive males. Although inexpressiveness is only one aspect of stereotypic male sex-role behavior, it has important implications for males in terms of their relationships with women, children, as well as other males.

OVERVIEW OF ASSERTIVE TRAINING. A general introduction to assertive training is presented since many of the techniques and procedures used in expressiveness training are taken from assertive training. Salter and Wolpe are usually given the credit for initiating the use and study of assertive training.[46,118] Although Salter's Conditioned Reflex Therapy[80] was the first attempt to describe assertiveness (excitation) and to suggest the advantages of behaving in an assertive fashion, Wolpe[68,119] is generally given credit for having the greatest impact on the current development of assertive training,[46,118] because, according to Rimm and Masters,[118] in 1958, when Wolpe published his first work, psychiatric and psychological establishments were probably more amenable to considering a learning-based or behavioral approach than in 1949, when Salter published his work. Also, the early acceptance of Wolpe's systematic desensitization and the theoretically close tie of assertive training to it facilitated the acceptance of assertive training. Finally, this was a period when many people dismissed Salter's ideas, failing to appreciate the merit in his approach because of his attacks on psychoanalysis and because his procedures and ideas were in sharp contrast to those of many conservative clinicians. Wolpe was using assertive training when Salter's book appeared and was encouraged by Salter's writings[118]; although both Wolpe and Salter stressed the importance of assertive behavior, there are important differences between their approaches, according to Rimm and Masters. Wolpe did not assume that every client is in need of assertive training although he employed it frequently, and he stressed the situational variability of assertive behavior whereas Salter viewed assertiveness (excitation) as a generalized trait.

The popularity of assertive training has greatly increased since the initial efforts of Salter and Wolpe, and may be viewed as a natural outgrowth of several cultural changes that occurred in the sixties, e.g., the increased value placed on personal relationships, the wider range of socially acceptable behavior requiring skills to make choices about how to behave, and skills to act on and defend the choices made.[46] Lange and Jackubowski[46] believed that the seventies, with an increased emphasis on personal effectiveness and growth, created the cultural context in which the interest in assertive training has grown—"not as a passing fad, but rather as a set of effective procedures whose time has come" (p. 2). Assertive training, they believed, meets a strong and pervasive cultural need.

The original work of Salter and Wolpe has been greatly refined and expanded over the years. Today assertive training is frequently used and frequently researched as a treatment approach for a number of problems. Clinical applications of assertive training have included anxiety, obsessive–compulsive disorders, maladaptive interpersonal behaviors, aggressive and explosive behavior, and with chronic psychiatric patients.[70] In addition, assertive training techniques and procedures have been used with a number of populations including the following: (1) college students (e.g., McFall and Lillesand[91]); (2) women (e.g., Jackubowski-Spector[120]); (3) men (e.g., Phillips[24]); (4) job seekers (e.g., McGovern et al.[121]); (5) anxious clients (e.g., Cautela[122]); (6) psychiatric patients (e.g., Serber[116]); (7) aged clients (e.g., Corby[123]); (8) severely disabled clients (e.g., Grimes[124]); and (9) correctional officers (e.g., Duncan[125]). Hersen and Bellack[65] noted that "assertive training appears to work for such disparate problems as hysterical crying spells, marital discord, neurotic depression, alcoholism, urinary retention, pedophilia, withdrawal in chronic schizophrenia, and self-mutilating behavior" and concluded that "its application universally helped dysfunctional individuals to acquire particular social skills (depending on their specific skills deficits) that enable them to cope more effectively with their environments" (p. 563). Assertive training, then, has become very popular and has been used with a number of populations for the treatment of a number of problems. It has also been the subject of numerous research efforts which have demonstrated the efficacy of assertive training as a therapeutic technique when compared to no-treatment control groups (e.g., Rathus[126]), attention placebo groups (e.g., McFall and Marston[99]), and other types of therapy (e.g., Lazarus[127]). Even with all the research on assertive training, generalizations are limited due to the absence of a standard treatment package.[78]

General Approach to Assertive Training. Assertive training is different from most other approaches to treatment in that it does not represent a universally agreed upon set of procedures.[118] In fact, some researchers believe that assertive training is not a unique or even well-defined behavioral training procedure since assertiveness defines the target rather than the nature of the training procedures.[78] To demonstrate the variety of techniques and procedures included in assertive training, Rich and Schroeder[78] stated:

> Assertiveness training has included hierarchical presentation of stimulus situations, operant shaping, constructive criticism, role playing, role reversal, playback of responses, response practice, homework assignments, postural and vocal analysis training, therapist exhortation and lecturing, modeling, relaxation, fixed-role therapy, exaggerated role taking, instructions, coaching, external reinforcement, and self-reinforcement (p. 1085).

They pointed out how further confusion arises when therapists use different "brand names" to refer to roughly the same procedures.

Although there is no agreement as to the set of procedures that constitute assertive training, this is not surprising, according to Lange and Jackubowski,[46] because the way in which assertive training is conducted must vary as the needs of clients vary. In other words, different groups of people require different assertive training techniques. Despite the lack of general agreement on the procedures which constitute assertive training, there is a need to define what assertive training is, and, in the view of Lange and Jackubowski, it generally incorporates the following four basic procedures:

1. teaching people the differences between assertion and aggression, and between nonassertion and politeness;
2. helping people identify and accept both their own personal rights and the rights of others;
3. reducing existing cognitive and affective obstacles to acting assertively, e.g., irrational thinking, excessive anxiety, guilt, and anger; and
4. developing assertive skills through active practice methods (p. 2).

Lange and Jackubowski concluded that assertive training is a semistructured training approach which emphasizes the acquisition of assertive skills through practice, whether the practice is direct by way of role-playing alternative assertive responses or indirect by vicariously acquiring assertive skills through observing models demonstrating assertive behavior.

Other general approaches to assertive training exist, although they are similar in some ways to the procedures just described. Another useful way of conceptualizing assertive training procedures was suggested by Galassi and Galassi,[44] who believed that the procedures of assertive training may be tailored to meet the unique requirements of the client, but that the repeated and systematic use of the training procedures is important. In their plan, following self-assessment, there are four major steps the client should follow to learn assertive behavior:

(1) The first of these steps is appraising the situation, which includes (i) determining the rights and responsibilities of the parties in the situation; (ii) determining the probable short- and long-term consequences of possible courses of action; and (iii) deciding how to behave in the situation.

(2) Experimenting with new behaviors and attitudes in practice situations is their second step. This step includes the following three components: (i) trying out the new behavior in situations provided by the trainer; (ii) practicing situations developed by the client; and (iii) disputing erroneous beliefs and counterproductive attitudes, and replacing them with more accurate and productive beliefs.

(3) The third step in the plan developed by Galassi and Galassi is for the client to evaluate his/her behavior, which includes: (i) determining the anxiety felt in the situation; (ii) evaluating the verbal content; and (iii) evaluating how the message was delivered.

(4) Implementing new behavior in everyday interactions is the final step in this plan. It includes the following: (i) completing homework assignments and prerehearsed interactions; (ii) behaving assertively in naturally occurring interactions; and (iii) recording and evaluating homework assignments, prerehearsed, and naturally occurring interactions. This four-step plan contains the four basic procedures suggested by Lange and Jackubowski[46] and provides a more detailed description of the procedures to be used.

Another general approach was suggested by Rich and Schroeder[78] who attempted to define the components of assertive training in order to decrease the confusion caused by the variety of approaches to assertive training. They stated that training procedures can be categorized by function into the following categories: response-acquisition operations, response-reproduction operations, response-shaping and strengthening operations, cognitive-restructuring operations, and response-transfer operations. They described each of these five categories and presented the assertive training procedures that are contained in them.

Response-acquisition operations. Three conditions which might result in deficits of assertive behavior and which might require different response-acquisition procedures were presented by Rich and Schroeder: (1) when an individual fails to discriminate adequately when to behave assertively, even though he/she possesses assertive skills; (2) when an individual's assertive responses are inhibited by emotional or cognitive variables; (3) when the individual simply does not possess adequate assertive skills.

Discrimination training to help the client learn when to respond assertively helps in the first condition. Disinhibition procedures are recommended for the second condition; while the third would require skills training of novel responses. Modeling and instructions are two response-acquisition operations that have been reported in the literature. Modeling procedures have included the use of live models, taped models, videotaped models, filmed models, and imagined models to present effective assertive behavior. As Rich and Schroeder have stated,

> The modeling literature suggests that modeling effects may be enhanced by modeling displays that are vivid, novel, and that contain several models of the same age and sex as the observer; by displays showing models of high status, competence, and power; by models rewarded for engaging in assertive behavior; and by displays that contain narration and instructions to attend to relevant cues and that minimize competing stimuli (p. 1086).

In addition, rewarding the observer for matching the model's behavior enhances response acquisition, while too limited exposure to the model is a primary cause of failure in modeling attempts. The use of instructions has varied from using general performance rules to using specific task instructions describing the specific verbal content and nonverbal aspects of the suggested response.

Response-reproduction operations. Response practice, behavioral rehearsal, and role playing are procedures from the assertiveness literature that Rich and Schroeder categorize under response-reproduction operations. They preferred the term "response practice" and suggested that is has varied along two dimensions: overt–covert and directed–improvised. Overt response practice provides the advantage of motivating disinterested clients, may be more effective for response generalization, and may be more effective in training nonverbal components of assertive behavior. Rich and Schroeder believed the advantages of covert response practice include: it may be less threatening to the client, more flexible and economical, and more effective in treating the more complex cognitive problems. Directed and improvised response practice differ in the extent to which specific instructions are given to clients regarding the type of response desired. In directed practice, the client is provided with a model to match or with a script of appropriate responses to practice. Very general performance rules are provided with improvised practice and the client is instructed to improvse an appropriate response with his/her current behavioral repertoire. While the effectiveness of these two procedures has not been compared, according to Rich and Schroeder, they suggested that directed response practice may be better for socially inhibited and less competent individuals and improvised response practice may be better for persons with unpracticed response repertoires.

Response-shaping and strengthening operations. The response-shaping and strengthening operations used in assertiveness studies include audio-feedback, video-feedback, self-feedback, therapist coaching, and group reinforcement. In self-feedback the client is responsible for evaluating his or her own behavior and total responsibility for detecting discrepancies and needed changes rest with the client. With therapist coaching, the client is given specific instructions based upon the therapist's observation and evaluation of the client's behavior regarding flaws in his/her behavior and needed changes to correct the flaws. In addition, Rich and Schroeder suggested the need for including both external and self-reinforcement systems in strengthening operations, even though the strongest reinforcement likely occurs as a consequence of successful attempts at assertiveness in real-life settings.

Cognitive-restructuring operations. Within the category cognitive-restructuring operations Rich and Schroeder included (1) giving a rationale about the importance of assertive behavior; (2) using strong therapist exhortation that assertive behavior is good, healthy, and appropriate; (3) using rational–emotive procedures; and (4) using projected consequences. The first two procedures are designed to convince clients that assertive behavior is highly desirable, if not essential. Rational–emotive procedures are used to teach clients how irrational beliefs and negative self-statements inhibit assertive behavior, and to teach them how to challenge these beliefs. The procedure of projected consequences involves helping the client to realize the likely consequences of assertive behavior in order to change the client's unrealistic fear of negative consequences and failures to an anticipation that his or her assertive behavior will be successful.

Response-transfer operations. Rich and Schroeder noted that provisions for the transfer of training to real life are notably lacking in many behavioral training programs. They believed that without provisions and opportunities for clients to test their newly acquired assertive skills under real-life conditions that are likely to produce reinforcing consequences, transfer will probably be minimal. Homework assignments are often used to enhance transfer of training to real life. These assignments usually consist of instructing clients to use assertive skills outside of training and to monitor and record their progress for discussion during the next training session. Graded structure is usually employed in these assignments such that clients attempt to be assertive in less challenging situations which are likely to produce rewarding consequences before attempting more difficult and anxiety-producing assignments. In addition, Rich and Schroeder suggested that persons in the client's real-life environment can be trained to reinforce the client's newly acquired assertive skills, which will facilitate generalization and transfer.

In summary, three general approaches to assertive training have been presented. Each approach represented what the authors of that approach believed to be the essential elements of assertive training. The approaches suggested by Lange and Jackubowski,[46] Galassi and Galassi,[44] and Rich and Schroeder[78] were similar in some respects with some overlap, but each represented a different way of conceptualizing assertive training. Rich and Schroeder provided the most complete organization of components of assertive training; their categories included those components considered as necessary by the authors of the other two approaches. They concluded that their system of classification can be considered a minimal and standard treatment package for assertiveness training. In other words, any assertive training program should contain procedures to address response-acquisition, response-reproduction, response-shaping and strengthening, cognitive-restructuring, and transfer to real life. In addition, Rich and Schroeder presented frequently used assertive training procedures that are contained in their categories. Next, it will be important to briefly review research on these procedures that has demonstrated the usefulness of these procedures. The reader is referred to reviews of assertive training for more complete information (e.g., Lange and Jackubowski,[46] Heimberg et al.,[70] and Hersen and Bellack[90]).

Assertive Training Research on College Samples. Research on assertive training procedures has been extensive with many attempts made to establish the efficacy of a number of procedures alone or in combination with other procedures for a number of problems and with a number of populations. The most frequently cited research studies involving college students as subjects are the three by McFall and his associates.[91,99,100] In the first of these studies McFall and Marston[99] found that subjects exposed to behavior rehearsal, either with or without performance feedback, improved significantly more on behavioral, self-report, and physiological measures of assertiveness than did subjects given placebo therapy or no treatment. There were some indications, though not statistically significant, that behavioral rehearsal in combination with performance feedback resulted in the strongest effect.

In a later study, McFall and Lillesand[91] compared the effects of overt rehearsal plus modeling and coaching with covert rehearsal and coaching, and with assessment-placebo control. The results indicated the superiority of the two treatment programs with covert rehearsal, modeling, and coaching yielding the most improvement on self-report and behavioral measures of assertiveness.

In a third study, McFall and Twentyman[100] assessed the additive effects of behavior rehearsal, coaching, and modeling on behavioral and self-report measures of assertiveness. The results indicated that behavior rehearsal and coaching individually, but more so in combination, contributed significantly to increased assertive behavior. Observing a model, however, did not add to the combined effects obtained with behavior rehearsal and coaching. In addition, no differences were found between the three types of behavior rehearsal used: covert rehearsal, overt rehearsal, and a combination of the two.

Other research done with college students has been frequently cited. In two studies with female college students, Rathus[126,128] demonstrated the effectiveness of assertive training groups. In the first study Rathus[126] compared a group receiving assertive training with a placebo-discussion group and a no-treatment control group. In this study, assertive training consisted of instructions, behavior rehearsal, coaching, feedback, and homework assignments. The results indicated that the assertive training group was superior to the two control groups on self-report and behavioral measures of assertiveness. In the second study, Rathus[128] demonstrated the superiority of an assertive training group when compared with placebo-treatment and no-treatment control groups. In this study, assertive training consisted of observing videotapes of assertive models and behavior rehearsal of new responses.

In an additional study, Friedman[129] explored the comparative effectiveness of the following six procedures with unassertive college students: modeling, modeling plus role playing, directed role playing, improvised role playing, assertive script, and a nonassertive script. Subjects in the modeling plus role playing and the improvised role playing groups improved the most from pre- to posttest on a behavioral task requiring assertive behavior. No differences were found, however, between the six groups on a self-report measure; this was probably due to the fact that training was for only one session.

Assertive Training Research on Psychiatric Patients. Other studies have been completed on the effectiveness of assertive training procedures with psychiatric populations. Lazarus[127] explored the effectiveness of behavior rehearsal when compared with nondirective therapy and with direct advice for nonassertive psychiatric outpatients, and found that behavior rehearsal produced the greatest improvement. Three other studies with psychiatric patients have been conducted by Eisler, Hersen and their colleagues.[130–132] Eisler et al.[130] demonstrated the superior effectiveness of modeling, which included observing a videotaped assertive model, for increasing assertiveness when compared with practice in role-played situations and no treatment. In addition, no differences were found between the practice-control and no-treatment groups, suggesting that practice alone without specific instructions, coaching, or modeling is not sufficient for psychiatric populations.

In another study, Hersen et al.[131] compared the following five groups on self-report and behavioral measures of assertiveness: test–retest control, practice control, instructions, modeling, and modeling plus instructions, and found that modeling, instructions, and modeling plus instructions were the most powerful procedures for increasing assertive behavior. For more complicated components of assertiveness, modeling plus instructions was the most effective treatment whereas for more simple behavioral changes, instructions alone was just as effective as modeling plus instructions. In addition, neither test–retest control nor practice-control groups showed any improvements or dependent measures.

In a third study, Hersen et al.,[132] studying the generalization of effects of assertiveness training, confirmed the superiority of modeling plus instructions for increasing assertive behavior, and again found no difference between test–retest and practice-control groups. Including special instructions for generalization did not increase, however, the effectiveness of the modeling plus instructions treatment combination.

Evaluations of Assertive Training Procedures. After reviewing the research on the effectiveness of assertive training procedures Heimberg et al.[70] reached the following general conclusions: (1) almost any training procedure with college students has produced marked increases in assertive behavior when compared to placebo and no-treatment controls; (2) self-report measures have been less sensitive to increases in assertiveness, probably due to the limited treatment used in most analog studies; and (3) behavior rehearsal, coaching, and modeling have been the most effective components. They also noted that with college students, modeling adds little to the effectiveness of the combination of behavior rehearsal and coaching, but modeling has been found to be an effective independent treatment. In addition, they concluded that research with psychiatric patients has supported the above conclusions except for the different finding that modeling is instrumental in producing change in psychiatric patients with the combination of modeling, focused instructions, and response practice appearing to be most powerful with this population. Gambrill[67] and Hersen and Bellack[90] came to similar conclusions subsequent to their reviews. For example, Hersen and Bellack concluded that with college students, the most active assertive training procedures appear to be behavioral rehearsal, coaching, modeling (overt and covert), and performance feedback; modeling and instructions appear to be the most potent component techniques for psychiatric patients.

In summary, a general introduction to assertive training was presented since much of expressiveness training is based upon assertive training techniques and theory. A brief history of the development of assertive training was presented as well as a description of some of the ways it has been used in the past. General approaches to assertive training including a conceptual framework with which to categorize assertive training procedures by function was presented in order to identify the components necessary for successful assertive training programs. Finally, the research evidence supporting the efficacy of specific assertive training procedures was presented in order to identify which specific procedures have been most potent for particular populations and which should be included in a training program. Before describing the specific component procedures of expressiveness training, it is important to explore the many parallels between assertive training for women and expressiveness training for men.

ASSERTIVE TRAINING FOR WOMEN. Much of the popularity of assertive training was generated through the interest in and successful use of programs designed for women. As the impetus from the Women's Movement increased, women became more interested in learning how to recognize and stand up for their personal rights and how to communicate their feelings effectively. In fact, some authors believe that assertiveness as a personal quality has become a major focus of the Women's Movement. In response to this interest, assertive training programs were developed to meet the unique needs of women which have resulted largely from their socialization experiences. Usually these assertive training programs for women focused on overcoming socialization experiences that in many cases taught them to be, or at least to appear to be, passive, dependent, nuturant, docile, emotional, submissive, weak, intellectually inferior to men, content with inferior positions in society when compared to men, etc.

The assertive training programs for women dealt specifically with such skills as expressing anger, making requests, refusing requests, expressing negative feelings, recognizing and standing up for basic personal rights, and doing all of these things without feeling guilty. Some women's assertive training groups have focused on specific concerns such as assertiveness in regard to sexuality and assertiveness in professional positions. One of the first people to focus on assertive training procedures for women was Jackubowski. Since her initial efforts, she has continued to be active in presenting assertive training to women by writing articles, monographs, and films, and by conducting training programs for women across the country. Assertive training, then, has served an important and useful function for women, and its application for women has been the basis of much writing and research. Understanding the background of assertive training for women is important because expressiveness training is based upon the idea that just as assertive training has helped many women to overcome somewhat the limits placed upon them by sex-role socialization, it can similarly help men, thereby making such programs important and necessary.

Parallels between Programs for Women and Men. The parallels between assertive training for women and expressiveness training for men are many, although the specific goals and objectives are different. Where training programs for women have focused on expressing negative feelings such as anger, and refusing and making requests, programs for men focus on expressing positive feelings and demonstrating affection. Ideas were presented previously which suggested that expressing positive feelings is an assertive act, and one that is underemphasized in research and training. The similarities between programs for men and women arise from the assumption that sex-role socialization is related to many of the assertiveness problems experienced by both sexes and from the fact that the same basic assertive training procedures are applicable to both groups. Other similarities in the need for assertive training and in the procedures applicable for men's and women's groups can be found by reviewing a cognitive/behavioral approach to assertive training for women.[133]

Socialization. Wolfe and Foder[133] presented their ideas for an assertive training program designed specifically to modify assertive behavior in women. Many of the points they made supporting the need for a cognitive/behavioral approach for women are equally valid for men. For example, they concluded that when women follow the nurturant docile "programming" of the female role and deny their own needs in order to devote themselves to winning the approval and love of others, they develop severe deficits in assertive behavior. The same can be said for men who follow the strong and silent "programming" of the male role, except that the assertive deficits are in expressing positive feelings. Likewise, women are often afraid to be assertive for fear of being "selfish," "too masculine," "aggressive," or of being rejected by others. Men, on the other hand, are afraid to be assertive through expressing positive feelings and affection for fear of being "feminine," "weak," "passive," or of being rejected by others.

Irrational beliefs. Another of the foundations of the training program suggested by Wolfe and Fodor is their belief that

> the most important factor blocking women's effective assertion of their rights and feelings is a welter of irrational beliefs, inculcated early in life, that leaves them anxious and fearful—of losing others, of hurting others' feelings, of being too aggressive or of unleashing a flurry of catastrophic retaliations (p. 46).

This again, could also be said of men except that their irrational beliefs would leave them anxious and fearful of appearing weak, gay, feminine, or vulnerable if they were to be more expressive of their positive emotions. Wolfe and Fodor suggested that any successful assertive training program for women must focus on identifying and challenging the irrational belief systems which inhibit assertive behavior. This would also be true for expressiveness training for men.

Skills training. Women need direct training in specific skills that are lacking in their response repertoires. This training is analogous, Wolfe and Fodor believed, "to other kinds of 'remedial' learning, with women belatedly receiving experience in and reinforcements for the sorts of self-actualizing behaviors their male peers were directly training in since infancy'' (p. 46). On the other hand, inexpressive males need ''remedial'' learning with a chance to receive experience in and reinforcement for expressive behaviors that their female peers were trained for since infancy. These expressive behaviors can be seen as ''self-actualizing'' for men just as negative assertive behaviors have been seen as ''self-actualizing'' for females.

Training procedures. Similarities between the assertive training program for women and expressiveness training for men can also be found in the training procedures used by both programs. Expressiveness training uses many of the same procedures suggested by Wolfe and Fodor who suggested a two-pronged training program emphasizing (1) direct training of skills with behavior rehearsal plus modeling and group feedback; and (2) cognitive restructuring with consciousness-raising and the identification and challenging of ''irrational ideas.'' Expressiveness training uses the procedures suggested by Wolfe and Fodor as well as other procedures.

In summary, much can be learned from the experiences of women with assertive training that is relevant for men in terms of general approaches and specific procedures. Many men can benefit from expressiveness training just as many women have from assertive training. In addition, there are many parallels between the two approaches including their rationales and suggested procedures. Although the major portion of expressiveness training procedures is adapted from Lange and Jackubowski,[46] encouragement for using them and additional suggestions for training procedures are found in Wolfe and Fodor.

DESCRIPTION OF EXPRESSIVENESS TRAINING. Expressiveness training does not represent the creation of new treatment procedures. Rather, it is the use of established and tested procedures which have been borrowed from other areas, particularly assertive training, to address a particular problem, male inexpressiveness, in a new, structured, and systematic way. No effort is made to claim originality for the development or use of these treatment procedures, independently or in combination. If there is any originality it would have to come from the compilation of a number of training and treatment procedures taken from a number of areas and the adaptation of them for treating male inexpressiveness with a comprehensive training package. In other words, there is value in suggesting the need to focus on expressiveness training procedures for inexpressive males and in suggesting an appropriate training package.

The term ''expressiveness training'' is used to discriminate between this approach to training which utilizes assertive training procedures to increase the expression of positive feelings by inexpressive males, and other standard assertive training programs for men which stress expressing negative feelings and identifying and standing up for basic personal rights. In addition, although expressiveness training is largely taken from assertive training and is largely composed of assertive training procedures, it also uses procedures taken from communication skills training and from consciousness-raising groups. These additions to expressiveness training from other treatment approaches are important and add to the potency and adaptability of the treatment program.

While specific procedures in a particular sequence will be suggested, expressiveness training is not limited to the procedures described in this chapter. In fact, expressiveness training should vary according to the particular skills, training, and resources of the counselor/therapist as well as the needs and progress of the client. Hopefully, the presentation of this approach will encourage other counselors/therapists/researchers not only to use this treatment approach but also to improve it through research and suggestions for changes.

For more information on assertive training, the reader is referred to Lange and Jackubowski[46] for an extremely comprehensive and useful presentation of cognitive/behavioral procedures for trainers. Their discussion includes often forgotten topics of evaluation of training programs and ethical issues involved in training others in assertive skills.

Expressiveness training follows the suggestions made by Rich and Schroeder[78] regarding the components necessary to constitute a minimal and standard treatment package. It contains procedures that address each of the five categories of functions suggested by Rich and Schroeder. To address response-acquisition, expressiveness training uses modeling (live and video) and instructions. Expressiveness training also includes discrimination training, direct skills training, and disinhibition or cognitive restructuring procedures to address each of the conditions which might lead to deficits in expressive behavior. The discrimination training uses lecture, discussion, videotaped presentations, and exercises to help the clients learn when it is appropriate to be expressive, as well as how to be expressive. This procedure will be described in more detail under cognitive restructuring procedures. For response-reproduction operations the training uses overt, covert, directed, and improvised response practice. Therapist coaching, group feedback, self-feedback, and video-feedback are all used in expressiveness training to address response-shaping and strengthening. The cognitive restructuring operations include lectures that present the values of expressiveness, group discussion and support for attempting new behaviors and challenging inhibiting beliefs, and rational-emotive procedures to challenge irrational beliefs. Homework assignments and unstructured consciousness-raising exercises are used to address response transfer and generalization.

Although the procedures used during training can vary from group to group and client to client, all expressiveness training programs should include procedures from each of the five functional categories developed by Rich and Schroeder. In addition, it is usually most important to include exercises at the first of the group's sessions that are designed to help the group members relax and feel comfortable. The specific uses of these procedures for expressiveness training will be described next. These procedures are described in detail elsewhere[46,67] and only the specific uses for expressiveness training will be discussed.

Beginning Exercises. As with any group experience, it is important to allot some time, early in the training, for the group members to get to know one another. Many exercises exist that can be used for this purpose; the important considerations in selecting an exercise are: (1) that it allows group members to learn each other's names and something about each other; (2) that it provides an opportunity for each group member to self-disclose something about themselves; (3) that it provides an opportunity for each member to take a risk by trying to do something he would not routinely do; (4) that each member is reinforced for his efforts during this exercise; and (5) each member is aware of the accepting attitude of the trainer, who establishes him/herself as a model during the first exercise.

One of the most basic, frequently used, and effective opening exercises includes self-introductions, self-descriptions, and positive self-affirming statements. In this exercise, each group member is asked to introduce himself to the group and to tell the group any things about himself he considers important, interesting, and most descriptive. The trainer models these behaviors and then asks the group members to begin. It is usually best not to identify a particular group member to begin or to point out subsequent members. Instead, the trainer can say, for example, "Who would like to go next?" and leave members to decide when they want to speak. This approach has two advantages. First, it establishes an atmosphere of freedom for group members and places responsibility on them for working during the training. The second advantage is that it provides the trainer with additional information on group members in terms of their anxiety, their ability, and their willingness to participate in group activities. The trainer should reinforce the clients' efforts by listening and responding to their statements. At this point, group members can be encouraged to ask each other questions or to make comments on the introduction and descriptions of other members in order to allow further exchange and interaction between group members. Finally, the group is asked to make a positive self-affirming statement. Again, the trainer models an appropriate statement and then reinforces members as they respond. This exercise is particularly useful for helping the clients to risk trying assertive behavior early in the training. It is also useful because with many clients the reluctance or inability to make a positive self-affirming statement is related to the negative thoughts and beliefs that inhibit their expressive behavior.

Many other frequently used exercises exist, for example, asking each group member to share three positive and three negative characteristics of himself. Other exercises can be found in Lange and Jackubowski.[46] The level of self-disclosure and risk-taking can be varied to match the group based upon pretest information so as to avoid asking too much of the group too soon. The objectives of the initial exercise are to create an atmosphere of acceptance and support that is conducive to risk taking and to encourage the client to take responsibility for changing his behavior. If these objectives are met, it will facilitate the remaining activities since when the group members are relaxed and comfortable they will be better able and more willing to learn and to try new behaviors. At the conclusion of this exercise, the group members should feel invested in the group and committed to it because they will have already risked and self-disclosed and observed the risk-taking and self-disclosure of the other group members.

Response-Acquisition Procedures. Instructions. The first response-acquisition procedure involves instructions used in expressiveness training to make the exercise or task explicit for the client. Instructions can be very general or very specific in nature, but, when necessary, the instructions should be as specific as required to provide the client with a clear understanding of the task. This is particularly true when the tasks involve complex behaviors or a complex sequence of behaviors. When nonverbal behaviors are stressed, it is important to provide the client with instructions that point out the specific nonverbal components of expressiveness to be attempted (e.g., "This time try to express your feelings again and be careful to maintain eye contact, speak distinctly and loud enough, and replace the continuous, nervous smile with a full smile at the end of your statement").

Instructions are also important in conjunction with the cognitive restructuring procedures, and they should clearly tell the client when and how to use cognitive procedures in behavior practice. In addition, instructions can be more general in nature, later in the training, when the trainer is interested in fading out specific instructions so that the client will be able to perform the behaviors on his own. This is an important consideration in terms of generalization of training effects.

Modeling. The other response-acquisition procedure is modeling, which is extremely important in expressiveness training for three reasons.[46] First, the use of models provides the clients with specific and clear information on how to be expressive. Modeling plus instructions should give clients adequate cues to the specific components of behavior required to be expressive and should lead to the acquisition of expressive behaviors. The use of models becomes more important as the complexity of the behavior being taught increases and is of particular value for teaching the nonverbal components of expressive behavior. The second, and perhaps most important, benefit of modeling for expressiveness training is the opportunity to present examples of males being successfully expressive and being rewarded for it. This is especially important because it not only presents the model of effective expressive behavior, but also it communicates to the client that expressive behavior is appropriate for males. This is advantageous in overcoming some of the beliefs and attitudes that inhibit expressive behavior. In other words, modeling provides "permission" for clients to engage in similar behaviors and reduces their apprehensions about becoming expressive.[46] Finally, modeling reinforces the existing expressive behavior of clients.

Modeling can be formal or informal. In most assertive training groups, modeling is done informally and unsystematically with the trainer or group members serving as live models and demonstrating alternative assertive behaviors for another group members.[46] This type of modeling is usually used in a behavioral rehearsal, role-reversal sequence where the trainer or a group member takes the role of another person in the group and demonstrates appropriate assertive behavior for a particular situation.[46] This type of informal modeling is appropriate for expressiveness training and can be very useful for demonstrating expressive behaviors especially when used in conjunction with formal modeling procedures.

Formal modeling procedures are more systematic and involve highly structured video or audio modeling tapes.[46] The use of video modeling tapes is suggested for expressiveness training since they allow the presentation of verbal and nonverbal expressive behaviors. These videotapes can be constructed to present any type of expressive behavior and can, in addition, contain narration which can provide instructions and an example of the model's positive self-statements in conjunction with cognitive restructuring procedures. In addition, the narration can contain specific instructions to attend to relevant cues which can minimize competing stimuli.[78] Additional advantages of modeling videotapes include the following: (1) they can be watched more than once to focus repeatedly on the same component of expressive behavior until the client assimilates the material; (2) they can be watched more than once to focus on more than one component of expressive behavior; (3) they allow the presentation of identical stimuli to the entire group, and (4) they usually hold the attention of clients more than audiotapes would.[46]

An effective combination of formal and informal modeling procedures might include the initial presentation of formal modeling videotapes with practice to follow. During the behavior practice, informal models from the group (or the trainer) could provide additional demonstrations of a particular aspect of expressive behavior. The use of both formal and informal modeling with videotape and live models allows the most flexibility in the presentation of effective expressive behaviors.

There are, however, some potential dangers in using modeling. Lange and Jackubowski[46] pointed out that modeling, if used crudely and in an authoritarian manner, may hinder clients' progress since they may learn only to mimic and memorize rather than integrate the modeling. This can lead to clients becoming overly dependent on modeling and not developing the skills to respond in an expressive manner on their own when confronted with novel situations. Another potential danger with modeling is that, if the trainer is not careful, inappropriate behaviors may be modeled and reinforced. The trainer should be very attentive to this possibility especially when preparing modeling videotapes. Lange and Jackubowski discussed constructing modeling tapes and the reader is referred there for more information. Briefly, the tapes should present models, the same sex and close to the same age as the clients, who appear confident and competent while behaving in an expressive fashion in novel, vivid, and interesting situations. In addition, they should keep the clients' attention, contain narration and instructions, and present reinforcement for the model's behavior. A final danger with the use of modeling is that the modeling sequence may present overly complex behaviors which can be confusing, if not overwhelming, to the client observing the model. Related to this problem is the possibility that video modeling may present too many distracting stimuli leading the client to focus on features of the model's behavior that are not relevant. These problems can lead to feelings of failure for the client when he is unable to successfully reproduce the model's complex behavior. These problems can be avoided by carefully considering constructing modeling videotapes, by focusing on only very specific behaviors and short sequences of behavior, and by considering the group's skill level and then presenting a modeling sequence commensurate with their skill level.

Additional problems that can occur with informal modeling include the inadvertent reinforcement of inappropriate behaviors when a client is chosen as a model and is unable to adequately demonstrate the desired expressive behavior. This can be controlled by carefully selecting clients to serve as models for the rest of the group and by the use of trainer coaching and feedback to shape the models' performance and to focus on the desirable aspects of the performance. The trainer can also serve as an informal model when there might be a question as to whether any of the clients in the group can successfully demonstrate the desired behavior. When excessive problems occur with the use of informal modeling, the trainer can replay the videotaped model to eliminate any confusion.

In summary, modeling and instructions can be used in expressiveness training to help the client acquire expressive responses. Instructions can be general or specific in nature according to the complexity of the task and the stage of the training. Modeling and instructions can be used together to specify what constitutes an effective expressive response and to guide the client's response practice. Modeling can be formal or informal and the utilization of both in an expressiveness training program provides the most flexibility. Research was presented which supports the efficacy of modeling procedures for assertive training, although additional research is needed to determine the exact contribution that modeling makes to expressiveness training and the most potent type of modeling for expressiveness training. It seems certain, however, that modeling is a useful and necessary component of any expressiveness training program.

Response-Reproduction Procedures. Response practice is the procedure used in expressiveness training to aid the client in learning to reproduce expressive responses. Response practice is the term suggested by Rich and Schroeder[78] to include behavioral rehearsal and role playing. They suggested that response practice can vary along two dimensions: overt–covert and directed–improvised. Expressiveness training makes use of overt, covert, directed, and improvised response practice.

Directed and improvised response practice. During the early stages of training while the clients' skills may be limited and whenever a client is particularly inhibited or incompetent, the use of directed practice, with explicit instructions and modeling, is stressed. As the training continues and the clients' skills increase, it is often appropriate to change to improvised response practice, where the clients are given only very general instructions and told to improvise an appropriate expressive response. This strategy slowly removes the client from the control of or the need for explicit instructions or models in order to respond appropriately. This fading process allows the client to behave independently, thereby increasing the generalization of training effects since he will not always be able to receive instructions or view a model prior to attempting expressive behavior. The combination of directed and improvised response practice can, of course, be varied to meet the client's needs. For example, if a client experiences some difficulty in an improvised response practice situation, the trainer can supply instructions or a live or videotaped model to assist the client in practicing the response. When the client successfully completes the directed practice situation, the trainer can assign a similar improvised situation. This process can continue until the client is able to improvise effective expressive responses.

Overt and covert response practice. The use of both overt and covert response practice procedures is suggested in expressiveness training in order to maximize training effects. Overt response practice involves the client actually practicing the response, out loud, and in view of the trainer and the rest of the group. This is usually accompanied by some form of feedback, and has the advantage of being observable by others. Covert response practice, on the other hand, is when the client imagines himself behaving in an expressive fashion in a particular situation. Since this type of practice cannot be observed by others, the feedback is limited to self-feedback. Both overt and covert response practice have been shown to be effective in assertive training with overt better for nonverbal behaviors and response generalization, and covert more effective for complex cognitive behaviors.[78] McFall and Lillesand[91] suggested the use of a

> combination of covert and overt training in which *Ss* initially engage in nonthreatening covert rehearsal in order to develop competence, and subsequently shift to more life-like overt responses in order to foster transfer to extralaboratory situations (p. 322).

The combination of overt and covert response practice would seem to offer the advantages of both approaches without creating any negative effects.

Suggested response practice format. In expressiveness training, the combination of overt and covert response practice with each practice situation is suggested. The general response practice format includes giving the client explicit instructions and presenting him with a model of a small segment of expressive behavior. The total situation should be broken into small workable segments for practice to avoid confusing the client, increasing the client's anxiety, or setting him up to fail. The client then is instructed to covertly practice the response and to evaluate his behavior himself (self-feedback) and to decide what needs to be changed in order to match more closely the instructions and the model's presentation. If a client is overly anxious or is unable to perform to his own satisfaction at this point, the process can be repeated with increasingly more specific instructions, more observations of the model, and smaller segments of behavior to be practiced, until the client is satisfied with his ability to reproduce the desired segment of expressive behavior.

When the client is satisfied, he is instructed to overtly practice the response. This procedure too can continue, with additional instructions, observations of the model, and additional covert rehearsal, until the client's reproduction of the expressive response is adequate without excessive anxiety. Once one segment of the response has been mastered by the client, additional segments are practiced, first covertly, then overtly, until the client can successfully reproduce the entire scene while considering all components of expressive behavior. As the training continues, the practice segments can become longer and can require more complex behaviors to match the client's increasing skill level. Several types of feedback are, of course, provided for the client, in addition to his own opinions of his behavior, in order to shape his response successively closer to the desired expressive response. In addition, the client's behavior is reinforced to strengthen the expressive response.

Whenever possible, it is advantageous to have a female assistant for male trainers so that the clients can practice their responses to women, since many of their expressive difficulties are with women. In addition, it is useful and helpful to use a graded structure of situations for the clients' response practice. These situations can be developed by the trainer or generated from personal difficulties by the clients. In both cases, it is helpful to have situations ranked in terms of difficulty, so that easier situations can be practiced first. This should be the case for situations practiced during the training and for any homework assignments. When easier situations are attempted first, the clients can experience success, reinforcement, and competence, which will increase their confidence and minimize their anxiety about attempting subsequent tasks.

Advantages of this response practice format. The combination of overt and covert response practice procedures has several advantages. First, it allows the client to become accustomed to covertly practicing his response before delivering it. This allows the client to combine response practice with cognitive techniques to relax him and to challenge any thoughts or beliefs that might inhibit his behavior. It also provides the client with an opportunity to decide whether an expressive response is appropriate for that particular situation based upon his ability to discriminate when expressive behavior is appropriate. In addition, this combination teaches the client to evaluate his own behavior, thereby not making him totally dependent upon the feedback of others. Finally, the use of overt practice allows the client to practice in conditions that more closely approximate real-life situations and in conditions where others can respond to the client's verbal and nonverbal behavior.

When other group members are involved in the client's response practice, it increases the complexity of situations that can be practiced and allows the client to learn how others would likely respond to his expressive behavior. This is of particular importance since many clients have unrealistic and overly negative expectations about how others will respond to their expressive behavior. It is also possible to have group members role-play various negative reactions the client might receive so that the client can learn to handle the negative responses he fears.[46] Role reversal can also be used so that the client can experience what receiving an expressive response is like, which is especially valuable when the client is unsure or worried about the impact of his expressive behavior.

In summary, response practice is the procedure used in expressive training to ensure that clients can reproduce the expressive responses which are taught. Expressiveness training makes use of directed, improvised, overt, and covert response practice in order to maximize treatment effects. Situations are broken down into small segments, which are practiced and mastered consecutively by the clients until the entire situation can be successfully reproduced. Less difficult situations are attempted first by each client in order to maximize the client's chance for success.

Response-Shaping and Strengthening Procedures. Since first attempts at using a newly acquired skill are likely to be gross, awkward, and inefficient, it is important to include procedures in the training program that are designed to refine and stabilize the response.[78] For expressiveness training the response-shaping procedures include self-feedback, video-feedback, feedback from other group members, and trainer coaching. Feedback from all of these sources is used in order to give the client an accurate picture of his performance and information on how his response could be improved.

Self-feedback. With self-feedback, the client evaluates his own performance based upon the criteria that he learned with the response-acquisition procedures. In other words, the client reviews his behavior and decides how well it matched the desired behavior that was described in the instructions or presented by the model. Self-feedback is important particularly for covert response practice, but also because self-evaluation and self-feedback take on additional importance when the client begins to use newly acquired skills outside the training setting. Then he encounters novel situations requiring further response-shaping based upon the reactions of others to his expressive behavior and upon his own evaluation of its effectiveness, and he is without the benefit of video, group, or trainer feedback. With self-feedback the client is able to continue to shape his own expressive behavior to more closely approximate the desired and effective expressive behavior in particular situations. The problem with self-feedback is that until the client has developed some skill in expressiveness and has had some experience using expressive skills, he may not be a very good judge of his behavior.

Videotaped feedback. Videotaped feedback is suggested whenever possible for expressiveness training since much of expressive behavior is nonverbal. The use of videotaped feedback allows the client to see himself as others see him, and it allows him as well as others to evaluate how well he expresses himself nonverbally. Videotaped practice situations can be viewed more than once to focus more thoroughly on any one component or to focus on several components. The major problems with the use of videotaped feedback are that it requires the use of special equipment and that it requires extra time to record, rewind, and view the videotape. An additional problem can occur if the task is too difficult for the client and the tape of his failure is viewed. This can very easily heighten the client's anxiety, embarrass him, and destroy his confidence to try new behaviors, suggesting the need to wait until the clients have demonstrated their ability and skills with other forms of feedback before using videotaped feedback.

Group feedback. The use of group feedback is also stressed in expressiveness training. With group feedback, other members of the group evaluate the client's performance and then provide him with feedback on their impressions. Using group feedback is important because it keeps the other group members involved and because it helps them learn what an affective expressive response is because they are called on to judge the responses of others. They can make better responses themselves when they can identify what constitutes an affective response. Group feedback also enhances the modeling effects during response practice because it ensures that group members will be more closely observing what goes on. In addition, group feedback allows clients to learn that there is more than one effective expressive response to any particular situation. The major problem with group feedback is that, if it is not carefully structured, it can include many personal biases and prejudices of the group. It can also disintegrate into arguments and "getting back" unless the trainer provides structure for the feedback, models appropriate feedback, and shapes the feedback of the group members.

Trainer coaching. Trainer coaching is the final type of feedback suggested for expressiveness training. Coaching should be viewed as providing suggestions or alternative ways of responding rather than demanding a specific response. Coaching is extremely valuable because the trainer is usually the most knowledgeable and objective observer in the group. Coaching is very similar to instructions except that it occurs after the response practice and is based on the trainer's evaluation of how well the client's response matched the desired response and how the client's response could be improved. The problem with coaching is that the client can very easily learn to listen to trainer only and to depend on the trainer's feedback. This problem can be avoided if the trainer stresses the value of the other types of feedback and incorporates the other types of feedback into his/her coaching suggestions. Again, it is important that the trainer not accept the role of unquestioned expert, but instead continually stress that there are many types of acceptable expressive responses to any situation.

Positive feedback. No matter what type of feedback is used it is important that the first attempts at feedback stress the positive. This is important no matter how bad the client's response might be. Something positive can be said about it, and it should be said before moving to ways of improving the response. Things that the client did wrong should not be stressed, but rather suggestions as to how the response could be improved should be made. The feedback should be given as a suggestion rather than as an order or an absolute. The suggested format for feedback is (1) self-feedback; (2) video-feedback; (3) more self-feedback; (4) group feedback; and finally (5) trainer coaching (throughout and after the other types). The client should be given ample opportunity to evaluate his own behavior before others evaluate it, and the trainer coaching should occur during the other types of feedback in order to shape that feedback. It also should occur after the other types of feedback in order to pull them all together so the client can try again.

Reinforcement. Reinforcement is a major consideration with expressiveness training in terms of response strengthening and durability. Once the response has been acquired and the client can reproduce it, it still needs to be shaped by feedback and strengthened by reinforcement of that response. Expressiveness training uses self-reinforcement, reinforcement by the group, trainer-reinforcement, and reinforcement from the real-life setting. Self-, group-, and trainer-reinforcement are used in conjunction with self-, group-, and trainer-feedback. Other types of more tangible reinforcement in addition to social reinforcement can be used as the trainer desires, including reinforcement schedules or contracts. It is probably true, however, that the greatest reinforcement for the client will come from his ability to successfully express himself in real-life situations where he could not before. The most important point concerning reinforcement is that successive approximations of the desired behavior are reinforced, rather than waiting until total mastery of the response is obtained by the client.

In summary, feedback and reinforcement constitute the response-shaping and strengthening procedures suggested for expressiveness training. Feedback includes feedback from self, the group, videotape, and the trainer. Feedback should always emphasize the positive aspects of the client's behavior before turning to areas requiring improvement, and feedback should always come first from the client about his own behavior. Reinforcement comes from self, the group, the trainer, and others outside the group. Finally, reinforcement should always be given no matter how small the improvement.

Cognitive Restructuring Procedures. Cognitive restructuring is such a large area with so many techniques and procedures suggested in the literature that this section can only briefly present a few cognitive restructuring procedures that are appropriate for expressiveness training. This presentation is not intended to imply that other cognitive strategies would not be useful, but only to give the reader some ideas for including cognitive restructuring procedures in his/her counseling/therapy with inexpressive males. The primary cognitive-restructuring procedures used in expressiveness training include (a) a justification or rationale for expressive behavior; (b) trainer exhortation that expressive behavior is good and important; and (c) rational–emotive procedures developed by Ellis.[134–138]

Lectures and discussions. The presentation of the rationale is primarily by lectures and discussions designed to present what inexpressiveness is, how it is learned through male socialization experiences, what the values of expressiveness are, what the problems of inexpressiveness are, and how males can learn to become more expressive. The major point in these lectures and discussions is that males learn to be inexpressive through male sex-role socialization experiences, that males experience inter- and intrapersonal problems because of inexpressiveness, that males can learn to become more expressive through expressiveness training, and that males can benefit from becoming more expressive. Throughout these lectures the trainer is in essence exhorting the client to become more expressive and stressing the value of expressive skills for use when the client desires. Hopefully, these procedures will slowly change the clients' opinions and beliefs about male expressive behavior, at least to the point where they will be responsive to attempts by the trainer to get them to try new expressive behaviors.

Associated with these lectures and discussions in expressiveness training are several others on assertive training. These are included because of the strong ties between the two types of training. These lectures include trainer exhortations about the value of assertive behavior and the fact that expressiveness is assertive. They also include lectures and discussions on general socialization messages that inhibit assertive behavior and the differences between aggressive, passive, and assertive behavior. Exercises for clients are included whenever possible to augment the lectures and discussions.

Discrimination exercises. Three exercises are of particular importance and address discrimination skills. The first involves the ability to discriminate between aggressive, passive, and assertive behaviors. This exercise uses a videotaped presentation and lecture to describe the three types of behavior and the differences between them. This videotape can be constructed by the trainer or videotape and films of this sort can be purchased. Lange and Jackubowski[46] and Galassi and Galassi[44] both presented excellent discussions of this topic. After the lecture, the videotape, and the discussion are completed, the clients take part in the discrimination exercises that demonstrate their ability to discriminate between the three types of behavior. These discrimination exercises use written and videotaped examples of behavior which the client attempts to label as assertive, aggressive, or passive based upon his understanding of these different types of behavior. The goal of this type of discrimination exercises is to help clients distinguish between aggressive, passive, and assertive behaviors so that they can learn to act more assertively by replacing passive and aggressive behaviors with assertive behavior. The fact that male expressiveness is assertive rather than passive or aggressive is stressed in these exercises.

Another type of discrimination exercise is included to address one of the causes of deficits in expressive behavior. This exercise is designed to ensure that clients can discriminate between when it is appropriate to be expressive and when it is not. These issues can be addressed through lecture, discussion, exercises, and videotaped presentation. The lecture should present the general boundaries of appropriate expressive behavior based upon societal expectations. Generally speaking, much more expressive behavior in a wide range of settings is acceptable than most inexpressive males realize. Next, specific circumstances can be discussed by the group in terms of whether expressive behavior is appropriate. Finally, the exercises include a chance for each client to identify several situations where he would like to be more expressive and it would be appropriate, and several situations where it would be inappropriate for him to be expressive. Videotapes could be constructed to further address this issue. Hopefully, this exercise will help each client discriminate when expressive behavior is appropriate for him and in which situations he would like to learn to be more expressive. In addition each client should learn the difference between the boundaries society sets on what is appropriate expressive behavior for males and the boundaries he sets for himself.

The third type of discrimination exercise comes from communication skills and involves the ability to discriminate between feelings, both personal feelings and those of other people. This skill is taught using lecture, discussion, and written and video exercises. The lecture and discussion present the importance of this skill for effective communication skills. The written and video exercises give clients an opportunity to assess their ability to read or observe the statements of persons and then decide how they feel. The reasons for suggesting these exercises include the belief that learning to discriminate between the feelings of others will make males more sensitive to their own feelings and that they will learn that other people have feelings very similar to their own. These exercises are particularly important for males who do not think on an affective level. This is true about many inexpressive males, even to the point where they have difficulty just naming more than a few basic feelings. If they cannot identify their feelings, it will certainly be difficult to express them.

Additional lectures and discussions. Additional lectures and discussions are included in expressiveness training to address two issues: (1) the verbal and nonverbal components of expressiveness, and (2) some basic communication skills that are relevant for expressiveness training. The verbal components of expressiveness are presented in a lecture and discussed, and then videotape is used to present and discuss the nonverbal components. Exercises can also be included here so that clients can experiment with the various components. Videotape can be used to see if clients can identify various emotions which are communicated nonverbally and to see if clients can effectively communicate various emotions nonverbally. The particular verbal and nonverbal components that are stressed in these exercises can vary, but both verbal and nonverbal components need to be addressed to some extent. The communication skills that are relevant to expressiveness training, in addition to discriminating feelings, are listening, empathy, and responding skills. These are included to help the client communicate his feelings in a more systematic and effective fashion. Listening and empathy are discussed so that the client can express himself more effectively based upon his perception of the other person's feelings. These skills blend nicely with with feeling discrimination skills. Responding skills help the client to better phrase his responses to others about their feelings. Numerous response structures could be used and the trainer can construct them to meet the client's needs. The most basic and probably the most useful response format is, "I feel ________ because ________." With this format, the feeling and the reason for the feeling are filled in the blanks. Early in training this structure is usually useful and helpful for the client, although later the client may come to view the structure as restrictive and limiting. At the point where the client's skills no longer require the aid of the structure, it can be eliminated and the client can use his creativity to improvise expressive responses.

Rational–emotive procedures. In addition to lecture, trainer exhortation, videotaped presentations, and exercises designed to encourage the client to become more expressive and to convince the client that expressive skills are valuable, more specific cognitive restructuring procedures are used in expressiveness training to challenge beliefs that inhibit expressive behavior. While there are many cognitive strategies that might be helpful in expressiveness training, rational–emotive procedures are suggested. These were developed by Ellis[134–138] and they provide the means for the client to challenge the irrational ideas and negative self-statements that inhibit expressive behavior and to replace these with more effective ideas and self-statements. Lange and Jackubowski[46] presented an entire chapter on cognitive restructuring procedures for assertive training, and many of them are relevant for expressiveness training. They also presented outlines for several exercises designed to develop an assertive belief system based upon rational–emotive procedures including introductions to those procedures and principles, to rational self-analysis, and to rational–emotive imagery. The reader is referred to Lange and Jackubowski, Galassi and Galassi,[44] or to Ellis for specific rational–emotive procedures. It is very important, however, to include these cognitive procedures in an expressiveness training program since there is reason to suspect that many inexpressive males possess expressive skills but inhibit them because of their perception of what is appropriate behavior for males. In addition, it is important to consider the inhibiting effect of anxiety, and relaxation techniques can be taught to clients to help overcome excessive anxiety.

Different clients may have different beliefs and self-statements that inhibit their expressive behavior, but some of the most common are based on male socialization messages. These include the following: (1) "Males should not express their feelings for to do so is feminine." (2) "Males should always appear confident, strong, and competent and should never express vulnerability." (3) "It is always important for males to compete." (4) "Males should never touch or express affection for other males because to do so is homosexual." (5) "Males must very carefully avoid any behavior that would appear to be homosexual." (6) "There is strength in keeping feelings of pain and hurt inside and not letting anyone know you feel them." and (7) "My wife and children expect me to be strong and silent and could not accept me if I were more expressive." This list certainly does not represent all the irrational and erroneous beliefs that might inhibit males' expressive behavior. Clients can generate their own personal lists during the course of training and then challenge these beliefs. The important point is that these beliefs must be successfully challenged before the client's behaviors will change.

In summary, cognitive restructuring procedures are a necessary part of expressiveness training. The specific procedures used in expressiveness training include presenting the rationale for expressiveness training through lecture and discussion, using trainer exhortations that expressive behavior is good, important, helpful, and useful, and using rational–emotive procedures for challenging the irrational beliefs and negative self-statements that inhibit expressive behavior. These cognitive procedures are very compatible with other procedures described so far and should be used in conjunction with these other procedures.

Response Transfer Procedures. Rich and Schroeder[78] noted that many training programs do not include provisions for the transfer of training to real life. Further, they believed that without such provisions and opportunities for clients to test newly acquired skills in real-life conditions that are likely to produce rewarding consequences, the transfer is likely to be minimal. For these reasons, response transfer procedures are suggested for expressiveness training, including (1) homework assignments; (2) unstructured consciousness-raising exercises; and (3) procedures for ending the group.

Homework assignments. Many types of homework assignments are used in expressiveness training, but they all have as their objective to increase expressive skills and to encourage the use of expressive skills outside the training setting. The homework assignments should be on a graded structure to ensure that clients are not given assignments beyond their skill levels. The first several homework assignments usually are related to the clients' belief systems and involve reading on inexpressiveness, assertiveness, and rational–emotive principles and procedures. Then as the clients' skills increase, they are given specific assignments to practice expressive skills outside the training situation, to carefully monitor their expressive behavior, and to report back to the class on their progress or problems. It is extremely important to begin each training session by discussing the homework assignment from the previous session. If this is not done, the trainer may not know if the client is experiencing difficulties in practicing the behaviors or in understanding the material that has been presented. Other types of homework assignments can be used to meet particular client's needs, but some use of homework assignments is recommended.

Unstructured discussions. Unstructured consciousness-raising exercises are suggested for expressiveness training in addition to the structured training procedures in order to allow time for group dynamics and group support to augment the training effects and because research has indicated that unstructured procedures are better for the expression of positive feelings and for the generalization of training effects.[48,49] These unstructured sessions have topics for each session, but do not have a group leader. They usually occur during the final 30 to 45 minutes of each training session and involve an unstructured discussion of the topic. Suggested topics include (1) feelings about being in the training group; (2) reducing competitive feelings; (3) masculinity; (4) self-disclosing vulnerability; and (5) expressing affection. It is most important that these groups be more than just an extension of the structured training sessions. Hopefully, the unstructured nature of these discussions will allow the men to experience the commonality between their feelings and those of other men and to feel the support of the other men for them as they struggle to improve their expressive skills.

Ending the group. Finally, in terms of response transfer, it is important to end the group with a discussion of how the clients' newly acquired behavior will affect the other people in their lives. This is important in order to avoid or minimize problems that clients might have following the conclusion of training. Other steps can be taken by the trainer to address response transfer including follow-up evaluations of training effects and the use of "booster sessions" when they are suggested by the follow-up evaluation or when the client requests them. The final lecture and discussion should also stress the importance of continued covert response practice, self-evaluation, self-feedback, and monitoring of expressive behavior with the use of a log or some other record-keeping procedure. If these considerations are addressed, the client's successful use of expressive skills should continue beyond the end of the training program.

In summary, response transfer procedures need to be considered. The response transfer operations suggested for expressiveness training include homework assignments, unstructured consciousness-raising exercises, and a lecture and discussion on generalization to end the group. If these procedures are used, response transfer should be maximized, but the use of follow-up evaluations and "booster sessions" is suggested when needed.

Summary. The final section of this chapter has presented specific procedures that would be included in an expressiveness training program for emotionally inexpressive males. These procedures followed the suggestions of Rich and Schroeder[78] concerning which training functions must be addressed in a minimal and standard training package. The procedures presented are merely suggestions and other procedures could be included. Any expressiveness training program must, however, address both skills deficits through direct skills training and inhibiting belief systems through cognitive restructuring procedures. While these procedures would routinely be used within the context of a training group, most of them could just as well be used with clients in individual counseling/therapy. The primary purpose in suggesting this approach to working with inexpressive males is to encourage other counselors/therapists to use these procedures. While preliminary attempts at using these procedures with men's assertive training groups have been encouraging, further research is needed to establish the efficacy of this approach and to identify the most potent procedures and combinations of procedures. Hopefully, this section will stimulate research of this sort and will provide counselors/therapists with some direction in working with inexpressive males.

SUMMARY

This chapter has presented research evidence from a number of areas that suggested that males are generally less expressive of positive emotions than are females. It has suggested that male inexpressiveness is due to male sex-role socialization. It has suggested that male inexpressiveness leads to inter- and intrapersonal problems for males and that many males desire to become more expressive. This chapter has stressed the need for a greater focus on the assessment of expressiveness both in research and in counseling/therapy, and it has suggested appropriate assessment procedures. Finally, this chapter has presented one approach to working with inexpressive males, an approach called expressiveness training, which is based on the premise that if men learned to be inexpressive they can learn to become more expressive. Expressiveness training takes a cognitive-behavioral approach and draws from relevant existing programs including assertive training, communication skills training, cognitive restructuring procedures, and male consciousness-raising exercises. The training program uses a number of procedures designed to address both verbal and nonverbal expressiveness skills, and it can be used for group or individual training.

The chapter was divided into three major sections: (1) a review of research on male inexpressiveness; (2) a review of, and suggestions for, assessing expressiveness; and (3) a description of expressiveness training. The goals of the chapter were to provide counselors/therapists with (1) a better understanding of male inexpressiveness and implications of this problem for males; (2) a better understanding of procedures available to assess expressiveness; (3) knowledge of a specific training program designed for use with inexpressive males to help them become more expressive; and (4) encouragement for further research on the etiology of and implications of male inexpressiveness and on the efficacy of this suggested training approach to treating male inexpressiveness.

ACKNOWLEDGMENTS

Portions of this chapter were presented at the annual meetings of the National Council on Family Relations in Boston, 1979, and in Philadelphia, 1978, and at the annual meeting of the American Psychiatric Association in Atlanta, 1978. Portions of this chapter served as part of the author's doctoral candidacy exam and appreciation is expressed to the author's doctoral committee, Jack O. Balswick, Charles F. Halverson, Sharon Price-Bonham, Raymond K. Yang, and Timothy F. Field, for their helpful suggestions. Appreciation is also expressed to James C. Walters for editorial comments on earlier drafts of this chapter.

APPENDIX A: SELF-REPORT ASSESSMENT OF EXPRESSIVENESS

1. SITUATIONAL EXPRESSIVENESS.* On this section of this questionnaire, you will be writing your responses to typical situations which arise in people's lives. It is important that you try to *imagine that you are actually in the situations* and talking to your best male or best female friend. It is also important that you try to *express your true feelings* that you would experience if you were in that particular situation with your best friend. Take a few seconds now and write down the name of your best female friend and your best male friend to help you keep in mind the people you are to be imagining in the situations. In order to better imagine the situations you could think about what it would feel like to be in that situation, where it would be, and what you would see, hear, and smell. Then, after carefully reading each situation, write down exactly what you would say in the space provided. Try to write it just as you would say it. Remember, express your *feelings* as well as you can.

Situation 1: It's the worst day of your life. You overslept and missed an important class and then got back a test on which you had done poorly. Then on the way to an important afternoon meeting your car breaks down. Finally, your plans for the evening, which you had been very excited about, fall through, and you are left with nothing to do except think of the terrible day. Your best *male* friend comes by and says: "How's it going?" and you say ________________

____

____

Situation 2: Your grandfather has been very sick for a long time, and you have just returned from visiting him at the hospital. He looked very bad, didn't even recognize you, and had clearly deteriorated. This has upset you so much that you need someone to talk to. You go to your best *male* friend and say ___

____

____

Situation 3: You have worked very hard preparing an exotic and delicious dinner for your best *female* friend and had looked forward to enjoying it with *her*. You had arranged for her to arrive at 7:30 p.m. At 9:30 p.m., after the dinner has been ruined, *she* arrives and says: "Gee, I'm really sorry I'm late, I got busy with my studies and forgot about our plans." You respond to *her* by saying ______

*These situations are borrowed from Highlen.[50]

Situation 4: You're giving a party, and the behavior of one of your best *female* friends has become increasingly objectionable and obnoxious over the course of the evening. You're upset with *her* behavior, so you go over to *her* and say ______

Situation 5: A *female* friend is taking a carpentry course and has really struggled with it. Secretly, you think it's kind of a crazy thing for *her* to do, but for your birthday *she* brings you a really nice coffee table that *she* made. After *she* gives you the gift, you say ______

Situation 6: Your best *male* friend has finally convinced you to go to a play with *him*. Much to your surprise as the play ends, you find that you've enjoyed it and *his* company immensely. This evening has reminded you how much *his* friendship means to you. You turn to *him* and say ______

Situation 7: Your best *female* friend's parents have just filed for divorce. Your friend is really upset and feels torn between them. You and *she* talk several hours, and you assure *her* that *she* can still love both of them. *She's* visibly relieved and says, "Thank you so much. I really needed to talk to someone, and you've helped a lot." You reply ______

Situation 8: You're camping with your best *male* friend. It's night, and you're sitting together by the fire watching the stars. *He* turns to you and says . . . "Hey! Isn't this fantastic?! Thanks for asking me to come. Listen, I think you're a really special person—I care for you a lot." You respond by saying

---

____

____

____

Situation 9: It's the worst day of your life. You overslept and missed an important class and then got back a test on which you had done poorly. Then on the way to an important afternoon meeting your car breaks down. Finally, your plans for the evening, which you had been very excited about, fall through, and you are left with nothing to do except think of the terrible day. Your best *female* friend comes by and says: "How's it going?" and you say ______________

____

____

____

Situation 10: Your grandfather has been very sick for a long time, and you have just returned from visiting him at the hospital. He looked very bad, didn't even recognize you, and had clearly deteriorated. This has upset you so much that you need someone to talk to. You go to your best *female* friend and say __

____

____

Situation 11: You have worked very hard preparing an exotic and delicious dinner for your best *male* friend and had looked forward to enjoying it with *him.* You had arranged for *him* to arrive at 7:30 p.m. At 9:30 p.m., after the dinner has been ruined, *he* arrives and says: "Gee, I'm really sorry I'm late, I got busy with my studies and forgot about our plans." You respond to *him* by saying _____

____

____

Situation 12: You're giving a party, and the behavior of one of your best *male* friends has become increasingly objectionable and obnoxious over the course of the evening. You're upset with *his* behavior, so you go over to *him* and say __

____

____

Situation 13: A *male* friend is taking a carpentry course and has really struggled with it. Secretly, you think it's kind of a crazy thing for *him* to do, but for your birthday *he* brings you a really nice coffee table that *he* made. After *he* gives you the gift, you say ______________________________

____

____

____

Situation 14: Your best *female* friend has finally convinced you to go to a play with *her*. Much to your surprise as the play ends, you find that you've enjoyed it and *her* company immensely. This evening has reminded you how much *her* friendship means to you. You turn to *her* and say ______________________

____

____

____

Situation 15: Your best *male* friend's parents have just filed for divorce. Your friend is really upset and feels torn between them. You and *he* talk several hours, and you assure *him* that he can still love both of them. *He's* visibly relieved and says, "Thank you so much. I really needed to talk to someone, and you've helped a lot." You reply ______________________

____

____

____

Situation 16: You're camping with your best *female* friend. It's night and you're sitting together by the fire watching the stars. *She* turns to you and says . . . "Hey! Isn't this fantastic?! Thanks for asking me to come. Listen, I think you're a really special person—I care for you a lot." You respond by saying

____

____

____

2. BALSWICK'S FEELING SCALE AND EXPRESSION OF FEELING SCALE. Please respond to the next items by circling the number which best describes how often the following occur:

1 = Never 2 = Seldom 3 = Often 4 = Very often

1. I feel *anger*.	1 2 3 4
2. I feel *love*.	1 2 3 4
3. I feel *sorrow*.	1 2 3 4
4. I feel *happy*.	1 2 3 4
5. I feel *tenderness*.	1 2 3 4
6. I feel *grief*.	1 2 3 4
7. I feel *delight*.	1 2 3 4
8. I feel *hate*.	1 2 3 4
9. I feel *affection*.	1 2 3 4
10. I feel *resentment*.	1 2 3 4
11. I feel *sad*.	1 2 3 4
12. I feel *joy*.	1 2 3 4
13. I feel *rage*.	1 2 3 4

14. I feel *warmth.* 1 2 3 4
15. I feel *blue.* 1 2 3 4
16. I feel *elation.* 1 2 3 4
17. When I *do* feel *angry* toward people I tell them. 1 2 3 4
18. When I *do* feel *love* toward people I tell them. 1 2 3 4
19. When I *do* feel *sorrow* I tell people. 1 2 3 4
20. When I *do* feel *happy* I tell people 1 2 3 4
21. When I *do* feel *tenderness* toward people I tell them. 1 2 3 4
22. When I *do* feel *grief* I tell people. 1 2 3 4
23. When I *do* feel *delight* I tell people. 1 2 3 4
24. When I *do* feel *hate* toward people I tell them. 1 2 3 4
25. When I *do* feel *affection* toward people I tell them. 1 2 3 4
26. When I *do* feel *resentment* toward people I tell them. 1 2 3 4
27. When I *do* feel *sad* I tell people. 1 2 3 4
28. When I *do* feel *joy* I tell people. 1 2 3 4
29. When I *do* feel *rage* I tell people. 1 2 3 4
30. When I *do* feel *warmth* I tell people. 1 2 3 4
31. When I *do* feel *blue* I tell people. 1 2 3 4
32. When I *do* feel *elation* I tell people. 1 2 3 4
33. I pretend to feel *anger, hate, rage* or *resentment.* 1 2 3 4
34. I pretend to feel *love, tenderness, affection* or *warmth.* 1 2 3 4
35. I pretend to feel *sadness, sorrow, grief,* or *blue.* 1 2 3 4
36. I pretend to feel *happiness, delight, elation,* or *joy.* 1 2 3 4
37. I find it easier to express my feelings to strangers than to someone I know real well. 1 2 3 4
38. I find it easier to express my feelings to a group than to an individual, one-on-one. 1 2 3 4
39. I find it easier to express my feelings to children than to adults. 1 2 3 4

3. BALSWICK'S EXPRESSION OF FEELING SCALE VARIED BY TARGET PERSON. Following are a list of 16 feelings which you might feel toward another person. Simply indicate how often you tend to *tell* each type of person each of the following types of feelings.

1 = Never 2 = Seldom 3 = Often 4 = Very often

	Father	Mother	Female friend	Male friend	Female stranger	Male stranger
1. When I *do* feel *angry* toward this person I tell him/her.	1 2 3 4	1 2 3 4	1 2 3 4	1 2 3 4	1 2 3 4	1 2 3 4
2. When I *do* feel *love* toward this person I tell him/her.	1 2 3 4	1 2 3 4	1 2 3 4	1 2 3 4	1 2 3 4	1 2 3 4

3. When I *do* feel *sorrow* toward this person I tell him/her.	1 2 3 4	1 2 3 4	1 2 3 4	1 2 3 4	1 2 3 4	1 2 3 4
4. When I *do* feel *happy* toward this person I tell him/her.	1 2 3 4	1 2 3 4	1 2 3 4	1 2 3 4	1 2 3 4	1 2 3 4
5. When I *do* feel tenderness toward this person I tell him/her.	1 2 3 4	1 2 3 4	1 2 3 4	1 2 3 4	1 2 3 4	1 2 3 4
6. When I *do* feel *grief* toward this person I tell him/her.	1 2 3 4	1 2 3 4	1 2 3 4	1 2 3 4	1 2 3 4	1 2 3 4
7. When I *do* feel *delight* toward this person I tell him/her.	1 2 3 4	1 2 3 4	1 2 3 4	1 2 3 4	1 2 3 4	1 2 3 4
8. When I *do* feel *hate* toward this person I tell him/her.	1 2 3 4	1 2 3 4	1 2 3 4	1 2 3 4	1 2 3 4	1 2 3 4
9. When I *do* feel *affection* toward this person I tell him/her.	1 2 3 4	1 2 3 4	1 2 3 4	1 2 3 4	1 2 3 4	1 2 3 4
10. When I *do* feel *resentment* toward this person I tell him/her.	1 2 3 4	1 2 3 4	1 2 3 4	1 2 3 4	1 2 3 4	1 2 3 4
11. When I *do* feel *sad* toward this person I tell him/her.	1 2 3 4	1 2 3 4	1 2 3 4	1 2 3 4	1 2 3 4	1 2 3 4
12. When I *do* feel *joy* toward this person I tell him/her.	1 2 3 4	1 2 3 4	1 2 3 4	1 2 3 4	1 2 3 4	1 2 3 4
13. When I *do* feel *rage* toward this person I tell him/her.	1 2 3 4	1 2 3 4	1 2 3 4	1 2 3 4	1 2 3 4	1 2 3 4
14. When I *do* feel *warmth* toward						

this person I tell him/her.	1 2 3 4	1 2 3 4	1 2 3 4	1 2 3 4	1 2 3 4	1 2 3 4
15. When I *do* feel *blue* toward this person I tell him/her.	1 2 3 4	1 2 3 4	1 2 3 4	1 2 3 4	1 2 3 4	1 2 3 4
16. When I *do* feel *elation* toward this person I tell him/her.	1 2 3 4	1 2 3 4	1 2 3 4	1 2 3 4	1 2 3 4	1 2 3 4

4. BALSWICK'S EXPRESSION OF FEELING SCALE VARIED BY SIZE OF GROUP. Following are a number of situations in which you might feel more or less free to express your feelings about another person. Simply indicate how often you are likely to express your feelings to others in the various types of situations.

1 = Never 2 = Seldom 3 = Often 4 = Very often

	When alone with the person	When in a small group	When in a large group
1. When I *do* feel *angry* toward people I tell them.	1 2 3 4	1 2 3 4	1 2 3 4
2. When I *do* feel *love* toward people I tell them.	1 2 3 4	1 2 3 4	1 2 3 4
3. When I *do* feel *sorrow* toward people I tell them.	1 2 3 4	1 2 3 4	1 2 3 4
4. When I *do* feel *happy* toward people I tell them.	1 2 3 4	1 2 3 4	1 2 3 4
5. When I *do* feel *tenderness* toward people I tell them.	1 2 3 4	1 2 3 4	1 2 3 4
6. When I *do* feel *grief* toward people I tell them.	1 2 3 4	1 2 3 4	1 2 3 4
7. When I *do* feel *delight* toward people I tell them.	1 2 3 4	1 2 3 4	1 2 3 4
8. When I *do* feel *hate* toward people I tell them.	1 2 3 4	1 2 3 4	1 2 3 4
9. When I *do* feel *affection* toward people I tell them.	1 2 3 4	1 2 3 4	1 2 3 4
10. When I *do* feel *resentment* toward people I tell them.	1 2 3 4	1 2 3 4	1 2 3 4
11. When I *do* feel *sad* toward people I tell them.	1 2 3 4	1 2 3 4	1 2 3 4
12. When I *do* feel *joy* toward people I tell them.	1 2 3 4	1 2 3 4	1 2 3 4
13. When I *do* feel *rage* toward people I tell them.	1 2 3 4	1 2 3 4	1 2 3 4

14. When I *do* feel *warmth* toward people I tell them.	1 2 3 4	1 2 3 4	1 2 3 4
15. When I *do* feel *blue* toward people I tell them.	1 2 3 4	1 2 3 4	1 2 3 4
16. When I *do* feel *elation* toward people I tell them.	1 2 3 4	1 2 3 4	1 2 3 4

APPENDIX B: NONVERBAL EXPRESSIVENESS RATING SCALES

A. LOUDNESS OF SPEECH. Loudness of speech is an important characteristic of assertive behavior. For purposes of this experiment, loudness of speech will be determined in comparison to the confederate.

11 very loud
10
9
8
7
6 equal to confederate
5
4
3
2
1 very low, not able to hear

B. AFFECTIVE VOICE TONE. This scale considers the communication of emotion through the voice tone, or the paralinguistic qualities of the voice.

11 full, lively, sincere, appropriate voice tone
10
9
8
7
6 not monotone, but not lively voice tone
5
4
3
2
1 very flat, unemotional, monotone; insincere voice tone

C. FLUENCY OF SPEECH. This scale considers how easily the speech flows. Fluent speech avoids fillers or interruptions such as "you know," "ah," "er," and inappropriate pauses.

11 very fluent, easily flowing speech with no fillers
10
9
8
7

6 somewhat fluent with some fillers but without frequent interruptions
5
4
3
2
1 not fluent at all, with speech frequently interrupted with fillers

D. ANIMATION OF BODY. This scale considers the communication of body language. It includes the consideration of gestures, body posture, and body movement.

11 very animated with use of gestures and posture appropriate to the situation
10
9
8
7
6 some use of gestures with some animation
5
4
3
2
1 no animation of body, remains still and stiff which is inappropriate to the situation

E. LATENCY OF RESPONSE. This scale considers how quickly the response follows the stimulus or the initiation of the situation.

11 no hesitation, immediate response
10
9
8
7
6 some hesitation, but response follows within a reasonable amount of time
5
4
3
2
1 too much hesitation; extremely slow to respond; inappropriate delay

F. FACIAL EXPRESSION. This scale considers communication through facial expression and changes in facial expressions. It considers specifically three important facial regions: the brow, the eyes and eye lids, and the mouth and lower face.

11 very expressive face with eyes, brow, mouth all appropriate for the situation; active and congruent
10
9
8
7

6 some expression facially, but not clear or congruent
5
4
3
2
1 totally inexpressive, blank face inappropriate to situation

G. DISTRACTING BEHAVIOR. This scale considers behaviors that limit the communication by distracting the speaker or the listener, or both. These behaviors include: nervous gestures, tics, inappropriate smiles; inappropriate body posture; playing with pencil; scratching; rattling change, etc.

11 no distracting behavior; nonverbal behavior appropriate
10
9
8
7
6 some appropriate; some distracting nonverbal behavior
5
4
3
2
1 very much distracting behavior; nonverbal behavior totally inappropriate

H. OVERALL EXPRESSIVENESS. This scale considers the global rating of expressiveness, integrating voice tone, facial features, and body movements to generate an overall impression of expressiveness.

11 very expressive
10
9
8
7
6 moderately expressive
5
4
3
2
1 not expressive

REFERENCES

1. Balkwell C, Balswick JO, Balkwell J: On black and white family patterns in America: Their impact on the expressive aspect of sex-role socialization. J Marriage Fam 40:743–747, 1978
2. Balswick JO: The effect of spouse companionship support on employment success. J Marriage Fam 32:212–215, 1970
3. Balswick J: Why husbands can't say I love you. Woman's Day 38:68, 150, 160, Apr 1974
4. Balswick JO: The development of an emotion scale and an expression of emotion scale. Presented at the Annual Meeting of the American Sociological Association, San Francisco, California, August 16 1975

5. Balswick JO: The effect of a broken home upon children's feelings and the expression of feelings. Presented at the Annual Meeting of the National Council on Family Relations, San Diego, California, October 19, 1977
6. Balswick J: Why I Can't Say "I Love You." Waco, Word Books, 1978
7. Balswick JO: Male inexpressiveness. J Soc Issues, in press
8. Balswick JO, Avertt C: Differences in expressiveness; Gender, interpersonal orientation, and perceived parental expressiveness as contributing factors. J Marriage Fam 38:121–127, 1977
9. Balswick JO, Balkwell J: Religiosity, orthodoxy, emotionality. Rev Religious Res 19:282–286, 1978
10. Balswick JO, Balkwell J: Emotional expressiveness: Learned from parents. Presented at the Annual Meeting of the Southern Sociological Society, New Orleans, Louisiana, March 21, 1978
11. Balswick JO, Peek C: The inexpressive male and family relationships during early adulthood. Sociol Symp 4:1–2, 1970
12. Balswick JO, Peek C: The inexpressive male: A tragedy of American society. Fam Coordinator 20:363–368, 1971
13. Sleven K, Balswick JO: Sex difference in perceived parental expressiveness. Sex Roles, in press
14. Hollandsworth JG, Wall KE: Sex differences in assertive behavior: An empirical investigation. J Counseling Psychol 24:217–222, 1977
15. Cozby PC: Self disclosure: A literature review. Psychol Bull 79:73–92, 1973
16. Jourard SM: Age trends in self-disclosure. Merrill-Palmer Quart 7:191–197, 1961
17. Jourard SM: The Transparent Self. Princeton, Van Nostrand, 1964
18. Jourard SM, Landsman MJ: Cognition, catharsis, and the dyadic effect in men's self-disclosing literature. Merrill-Palmer Quart 6:178–186, 1960
19. Jourard SM, Lasakow P: Some factors in self-disclosure. J Abnorm Soc Psychol 56:92–98, 1958
20. Levinger L, Senn P: Disclosure of feelings in marriage. Merrill-Palmer Quart 13:237–249, 1967
21. Highlen PS, Gillis SF: Effects of situational factors, sex, and attitude on affective self-disclosure and anxiety. J Counseling Psychol 25:270–276, 1978
22. Highlen PS, Johnston B: Effects of situational variables on affective self-disclosure with acquaintances. J Counseling Psychol 26:255–258, 1979
23. Bem SL: The measurement of psychological androgyny. J Consult Clin Psychol 42:155–167, 1974
24. Phillips RA: Men as lovers, husbands, and fathers: Explorations of male socialization and the implications for marriage and family therapy, in Synopsis of Family Therapy Practice. Edited by Simpkinsen CH, Platt LJ. Olney, Family Therapy Practice Network, 1978, pp 142–147
25. Weinberg GH: Society and the Healthy Homosexual. New York, St. Martin's Press, 1972
26. Mayo PR: Self disclosure and neuroses. Br J Soc Clin Psychol 1:140–148, 1968
27. Halverson CF, Shore RE: Self-disclosure and interpersonal functioning. J Consult Clin Psychol 33:213–219, 1969
28. Thase M, Page RA: Modeling of self-disclosure in laboratory and non-laboratory interview settings. J Consult Psychol 24:35–40, 1977
29. Halpern TP: Degree of client disclosure as a function of past disclosure, counselor disclosure, and counselor facilitativeness. J Counseling Psychol 24:42–47, 1977
30. Bem SL: Sex-role adaptability: One consequence of psychological androgyny. J Personality Soc Psychol 31:634–643, 1975
31. Osofsky JD, Osofsky HJ: Androgyny as a lifestyle. Fam Coordinator 32:411–418, 1972
32. Pleck JH, Brannon R (eds): Male roles and the male experience. J Soc Issues 34:1–199, 1978
33. Skovholt TM, Gormally J, Schauble P, et al. (Eds): Counseling men. Counseling Psychol 7:1–79, 1978
34. Lewis RA, Pleck JH (Eds): Special issue: Men's roles in the family. Fam Coordinator 28:425–652, 1979
35. Farrell W: The Liberated Man. New York, Random House, 1974
36. Komarovsky M: Dilemmas of Masculinity. New York, Norton, 1976
37. Lyon HC. Tenderness Is Strength. New York, Harper and Row, 1977
38. Petras JW: Sex: Male/Gender: Masculine: Readings in Male Sexuality. Port Washington, New York Alfred, 1975

39. Pleck JH, Sawyer J: Men and Masculinity. Englewood Cliffs, New Jersey, Prentice-Hall, 1974
40. Sargent AG: Beyond Sex Roles. New York, West, 1977
41. Alberti RE, Emmons ML: Your Perfect Right: A Guide to Assertive Behavior. San Luis Obispo, Impact, 1970
42. Alberti RE, Emmons ML: Stand Up, Speak Out, Talk Back: The Key to Self-Assertive Behavior. New York, Pocket Books, 1975
43. Fensterheim H, Baer J: Don't Say Yes When You Want to Say No. New York, Dell, 1975
44. Galassi MD, Galassi JP: Assert Yourself: How to be Your Own Person. New York, Human Sciences Press, 1977
45. Jackubowski P, Lange AJ: The Assertive Option: Your Rights and Responsibilities. New York, Research, 1976
46. Lange AJ, Jackubowski P: Responsible Assertive Behavior: Cognitive/Behavioral Procedures for Trainers. New York, Research, 1976
47. Smith MJ: When I Say No, I Feel Guilty. New York, Dial Press, 1975
48. Damgaard JA: Structured versus unstructured procedures for training groups in the expression of feeling–cause relations. Unpublished doctoral dissertation, Duke University, 1974
49. Boone RA: An evaluation of structured procedures for training education majors in the expression of feeling–cause relations. Unpublished doctoral dissertation, Georgia State University, 1975
50. Highlen PS: Effects of social modeling and cognitive structuring strategies on affective self-disclosure of single, undergraduate males. Unpublished doctoral dissertation, Michigan State University, 1975
51. Highlen PS, Voight NL: Effects of social modeling, cognitive structuring, and self-management strategies on affective self-disclosure. J Counseling Psychol 25:21–34, 1978
52. Eisler RM, Miller PM, Hersen M: Components of assertive behavior. J Clin Psychol 29:295–299, 1973
53. Eisler RM, Hersen M, Miller PM, et al.: Situational determinants of assertive behaviors. J Consult Clin Psychol 43:330–340, 1975
54. Warren NJ, Gilner FH: Measurement of positive assertive behaviors: The behavioral test of tenderness expression. Behav Ther 9:178–184, 1978
55. Ekman P: Universals and cultural differences in facial expressions of emotion, in Nebraska Symposium on Motivation 1971. Ed by Cole JK. Lincoln, University of Nebraska Press, 1972, pp 207–283
56. Ekman P: Darwin and Facial Expression: A Century of Research in Review. New York, Academic Press, 1973
57. Ekman, P, Friesen WV: Unmasking the Face. Englewood Cliffs, New Jersey, Prentice-Hall, 1975
58. Ekman P, Friesen WV, Ellsworth P: Emotion in the Human Face. Elmsford, Illinois, Pergamon, 1972
59. Izard CE: The Face of Emotion. New York, Appleton-Century-Crofts, 1971
60. Mehrabian AE: Communication without words. Psychol Today 2:52–56, 1968
61. Mehrabian A: Nonverbal Communication. Chicago, Aldine-Atherton, 1972
62. Dosser DA, Balswick JO: Expressiveness training for emotionally inexpressive males. Presented at the Annual Meeting of the National Council on Family Relations, Philadelphia, Pennsylvania, October 19 1978
63. Ciminero AR: Behavioral assessment: An overview, in Handbook of Behavioral Assessment. Edited by Ciminero AR, Calhoun KS, Adams HE. New York, Wiley, 1977, pp 3–13
64. Cromwell RE, Olson DHL, Fournier DG: Diagnosis and evaluation in marital and family counseling, in Treating Relationships. Edited by Olson DHL. Lake Mills, Graphic Publishing, 1976, pp 517–562
65. Hersen M, Bellack AS: Assessment of social skills, in Handbook of Behavioral Assessment. Edited by Ciminero AR, Calhoun KS, Adams HE. New York, Wiley, 1977, pp 509–554
66. Jackubowski PA, Lacks PB: Assessment procedures in assertion training. Counseling Psychol 5:84–89, 1975
67. Gambrill ED: Development of effective social skills, Behavior Modification: Handbook of Assessment, Intervention, and Evalution. San Francisco, Jossey-Bass, 1977, 530–601

68. Wolpe J: The Practice of Behavior Therapy, 2nd ed. New York, Pergamon Press, 1973
69. Bodner GE: The role of assessment in assertion training. Counseling Psychol 5:90–96, 1975
70. Heimberg RG, Montgomery D, Madsen CH Jr, et al.: Assertion training: A review of the literature. Behav Ther 8:953–971, 1977
71. Kerlinger FN: Foundations of Behavioral Research, 2nd ed. Atlanta, Holt Rinehart, and Winston, 1974
72. Mischel W: Personality and Assessment. New York, Wiley, 1968
73. Sackett GP: Observing Behavior, II: Data Collection and Analysis Methods. Baltimore, University Park Press, 1978
74. Ciminero AR, Calhoun KS, Adams HE: Handbook of Behavioral Assessment. New York, Wiley, 1977
75. Walsh WB: Validity of self-report. J Counseling Psychol 14:18–23, 1967
76. Walsh WB: Validity of self report: Another look. J Counseling Psychol 15:180–186, 1968
77. Hall JR: Assessment of assertiveness, in Advances in Psychological Assessment IV. Edited by McReynolds P. San Francisco, Jossey-Bass, 1978, pp 321–357
78. Rich AR, Schroeder HE: Research issues in assertiveness training. Psychol Bull 83:1081–1096, 1976
79. Olsen DH: Insiders' and outsiders' views of relationships: Research studies, in Close Relationships. Edited by Levinger G, Rausch H. Amherst, University of Massachusetts Press, 1977, pp 115–135
80. Salter A: Conditioned Reflex Therapy. New York, Creative Age Press, 1949
81. Wolpe J, Lazarus AA: Behavior Therapy Techniques. New York, Pergamon Press, 1966
82. Galassi JP, Deleo JS, Galassi MD, et al.: The college self-exression scale: A measure of assertiveness. Behav Ther 5:165–171, 1974
83. Gambrill ED, Richey CA: An assertion inventory for use in assessment and research. Behav Ther 6:550–561, 1975
84. Rathus SA: A 30-item schedule for assessing assertive behavior. Behav Ther 4:398–406, 1973
85. Hull DB, Hull JH: Rathus assertiveness schedule: Normative and factor-analytic data, abstracted. Behav Ther 9:673, 1978
86. Law HG, Wilson E, Crassini B: A principal components analysis of the Rathus Assertiveness Schedule. J Consult Clin Psychol 47:631–633, 1979
87. Lazarus AA: On assertive behavior: A brief note. Behav Ther 4:697, 1973
88. Lazarus AA: Behavior Therapy and Beyond. New York, McGraw-Hill, 1971
89. Hollandsworth JG Jr: Differentiating assertion and aggression: Some behavioral guidelines. Behav Ther 8:347–352, 1977
90. Hersen M, Bellack AS: Social skills training for chronic psychiatric patients: Rationale, research findings and future directions. Compr Psychiat 17:559–580, 1976
91. McFall RM, Lillesand DB: Behavior rehearsal with modeling and coaching in assertion training. J Abnorm Psychol 77:313–323, 1971
92. Gay ML, Hollandsworth JG, Galassi JP: An assertiveness inventory for adults. J Counseling Psychol 22:340–344, 1975
93. Lawrence PS: The assessment and modification of assertive behavior, Unpublished doctoral dissertation, Arizona State University, 1970
94. Bates HD, Zimmerman SF: Toward the development of a screening scale for assertive training. Psychol Rep 28:99–107, 1971
95. Gough HG, Heilbrun AB Jr: The Adjective Checklist Manual. Palo Alto, Consulting Psychologists Press, 1965
96. Galassi JP, Galassi MD: Instructions for Administering and Scoring the College Self-Expression Scale. Chapel Hill, University of North Carolina, 1974
97. Galassi JP, Galassi MD: Validity of a measurement of assertiveness. J Counseling Psychol 21:248–250, 1974
98. Galassi JP, Hollandsworth JG Jr, Radecki JC, et al.: Behavioral performance in the validation of an assertiveness scale. Behav Ther 7:447–452, 1976
99. McFall RM, Marston AR: An experimental investigation of behavior rehearsal in assertive training. J Abnorm Psychol 76:295–303, 1970

100. McFall RM, Twentyman CT: Four experiments on the relative contributions of rehearsal, modeling and coaching to assertion training. J Abnorm Psychol 81:199–218, 1973
101. Hollenbeck AR: Problems of reliability in observational research, in Observing Behavior II: Data Collection and Analysis Methods. Edited by Sackett GP. Baltimore, University Park Press, 1978, pp 79–98
102. Hersen M, Turner SM, Edelstein BA, et al.: Effects of phenothiazines and social skills training in a withdrawn schizophrenic. J Clin Psychol 31:588–594, 1975
103. Kallman WM, Feuerstein M: Psychophysiological procedures, in Handbook of Behavioral Assessment. Edited by Ciminero AR, Calhoun KS, Adams HE. New York, Wiley, 1977
104. Chelune GJ: Nature and assessment of self-disclosing behavior, in Advances in Psychological Assessment IV. Ed by McReynolds P. San Francisco, Jossey-Bass, 1978, pp 278–320
105. Stokes J, Fuehrer A, Childs L: Gender differences in self-disclosure to various target persons. J Counseling Psychol 27:192–198, 1980
106. Jourard SM: Self-Disclosure: An Experimental Analysis of the Transparent Self. New York, Wiley, 1971
107. Chelune GJ: Measuring openness in interpersonal communication, in Self-Disclosure. Edited by Chelune GJ. San Francisco, Jossey-Bass, 1979, pp 1–27
108. Highlen PS, Bacchus GK: Effect of reflection of feeling and probe on client self-referenced affect. J Counseling Psychol 24:440–443, 1977
109. Chelune GJ: Self-disclosure: An elaboration of its basic dimensions. Psychol Rep 36:79–85, 1975
110. Snyder M: Self-monitoring and expressive behavior. J Personality Soc Psychol 30:526–537, 1974
111. Snyder M: Self-monitoring processes, in Advances in Experimental Social Psychology, Vol 12. Edited by Berkowitz L. New York, Academic Press, 1979, pp. 85–128
112. Snyder M: The many me's of the self monitor. Psychol Today 13:32–40, 92, 1980
113. Friedman HS, Prince LM, Riggio RE, et al.: Understanding and assessing nonverbal expressiveness: The affective communication test. J Personality Soc Psychol 39:333–351, 1980
114. Izard CE: Human Emotions. New York, Plenum Press, 1972
115. Eisler RM, Hersen M, Agras WS: Videotape: A method for the controlled observation of nonverbal interpersonal behavior. Behav Ther 4:420–425, 1973
116. Serber M: Teaching the nonverbal components of assertive training. J Behav Ther Exp Psychiatry 3:179–183, 1972
117. Eisler RM, Hersen M, Agras WS: Effects of videotape and instructional feedback on nonverbal marital interaction: An analog study. Behav Ther 4:551–558, 1973
118. Rimm DC, Masters JC: Behavior Therapy: Techniques and Empirical Findings. New York, Academic Press, 1974
119. Wolpe J: Psychotherapy by Reciprocal Inhibition. Stanford, Stanford University Press, 1958
120. Jackubowski-Spector P: Facilitating the growth of women through assertive training. Counseling Psychol 4:75–86, 1973
121. McGovern TV, Tinsley DJ, Liss-Levinson N, et al.: Assertion training for job interviews. Counseling Psychol 5:65–68, 1975
122. Cautela JR: A behavior therapy approach to pervasive anxiety. Behav Res Ther 4:99–109, 1966
123. Corby N: Assertion training with aged population. Counseling Psychol 5:69–74, 1975
124. Grimes JW: The effects of assertion training on severely disabled students/clients. J Appl Rehab Counseling 11:36–39, 1980
125. Duncan AS: The effects of assertive training on selected correctional officer behaviors. Unpublished doctoral dissertation, University of Georgia, 1976
126. Rathus SA: An experimental investigation of assertive training in a group setting. J Behav Ther Exp Psychiatry 3:81–86, 1972
127. Lazarus AA: Behavior rehearsal vs. nondirective therapy vs. advice in effecting behavior change. Behav Res Ther 4:95–97, 1966
128. Rathus SA: Instigation of assertive behavior through videotape-mediated assertive models and directed practice. Behav Res Ther 11:57–65, 1973
129. Friedman PH: The effects of modeling and role playing on assertive behavior, in Advances in Behavior Therapy. Edited by Rubin RD, Fensterheim H, Lazarus AA, et al. New York, Academic Press, 1971, p. 149–169

130. Eisler RM, Hersen M, Miller PM: Effects of modeling on components of assertive behavior. J Behav Ther Exp Psychiatry 4:1–6, 1973
131. Hersen M, Eisler RM, Miller PM, et al.: Effects of practice, instructions, and modeling on components of assertive behavior. Behav Res Ther 11:443–451, 1973
132. Hersen M, Eisler RM, Miller RM: An experimental analysis of generalization in assertive training. Behav Res Ther 12:295–310, 1974
133. Wolfe JL, Foder IG: A cognitive/behavioral approach to modifying assertive behavior in women. Counseling Psychol 5:45–52, 1975
134. Ellis A: Reason and Emotion in Psychotherapy. New York, Lyle Stuart, 1962
135. Ellis A: Growth through Reason. Palo Alto, Science and Behavior Books, 1971
136. Ellis A: Humanistic Psychotherapy: The Rational-Emotive Approach. New York, Julian Press, 1973
137. Ellis A: Disputing Irrational Beliefs (DIBS). New York, Institute for Rational Living, 1974
138. Ellis A, Harper RA: A New Guide to Rational Living. Englewood Cliffs, New Jersey, Prentice-Hall, 1975

Chapter 17

The Female Therapist in Relation to Male Roles

TERESA BERNARDEZ

INTRODUCTION

In looking at the extensive literature on psychotherapy over the years, it is striking to note that the treatment of male patients by female therapists has not received special attention. In fact, with the possible exception of some adolescent and homosexual patients, the therapist's gender has been considered irrelevant to the process and outcome of psychotherapy.

The scarcity of female psychotherapists with extensive training and credentials may explain, in part, the absence of the examination of cross-sex therapy of male patients. But particularly within the psychoanalytic field, a number of well-known and creative female therapists existed throughout the years who could have paid special attention to their experience with male patients. The author believes that the relatively egalitarian nature of the original psychoanalytic circles tended to create blind spots for the issue of gender and the difference it makes. Women, who were in the minority as psychoanalytic workers, would have a special investment in minimizing their differences with the dominant group. Psychoanalytic norms at the time tended to maintain that the therapist's gender made little difference since the transference would assume maternal or paternal characteristics regardless of the reality of the sex of the therapist.

In the last ten years, the explosion of women studies, sex-role research, and the examination of sex biases made the emergence of sex visible as an important variable to be considered.[1] Specifically with psychotherapy, the effect of the sex of the therapist on the patient and vice versa was studied and explored in relation to the treatment of women. An array of literature for females and psychotherapy emphasizes the advantages of female therapists for female patients and underline the historical fact that men in authority had been, in a major way,

TERESA BERNARDEZ • Department of Psychiatry, Michigan State University, East Lansing, Michigan 48824

responsible for setting a dominant–submissive interaction with women, an interaction compelled to be reproduced in the therapeutic situation.[2]

The literature on male roles began to appear in the mid 1970s, in connection with feminist questioning of sex-role prescriptions for women. The feminist criticism of male role socialization, with its emphasis on power, control, and domination, fostered a self-related inquiry on the part of men. Several authors[3–5] began to examine the restrictions imposed upon men by complying with stereotypic role expectations and the necessity to alter the socialization of the male. Their analysis carried—implicitly or explicitly—a connection between the socialization of the male for power and control (of the female, of other males) and the toll exacted from the individual in psychological and emotional spheres.

The sociocultural view of sex-role socialization has not been systematically approached by therapists within the male sex-role literature, however. Their views may be taken as agreeing with feminist views of the politics of sex-role distribution, but such is not always the case.[3] There seems to be a discrepancy and a lack of connection between the emphasis on the individual male and his suffering under restrictive and oppressive sex role prescriptions on the one hand and the analysis of social advantages males have acquired and preserved over the centuries on the other. The contradiction between the advantages in the social realm and the impairments in the emotional and psychological realms inherent in the male role have not been examined by psychotherapists. There has been no frontal confrontation with the ethical issues involved in the change of male role and the social implications of a profound alteration of the distribution of power and assignment of functions for both sexes, as authors in other fields have done.[6] Thus, psychotherapists want to change individuals towards maximizing their development, maturity, potentialities, creativity, and self-actualization; but they often ignore the implications these changes have for the collective matrix or rarely face the question of what is the responsibility of the collective matrix that gives rise to pathologic characteristics in men that may need to be changed before the individuals can function more freely and more productively in our society.[4,7] Male authors face the dilemma of sharing the feminist analysis made by women in which they are part of the dominant group[8] or else assume a stance in defense of the individual male suffering the restrictions of his role and disregard the sociocultural position of the male. The first position places men in an unusual situation for them: (1) as followers rather than leaders of women; (2) acknowledging the reality of domination and the impossibility of an egalitarian society with such division of power; and therefore (3) giving up their social power over women while they are still in control; that is, they voluntarily give up their social advantages. The second position involves a scotomization of the social processes that determine male role socialization. To help men with the restrictions imposed upon them without connecting them with the reasons that these restrictions originate in the social world, specifically their advantages and control over others, seems short-sighted.

But psychotherapists have not, until recently, been sufficiently aware and cognizant of the interactions between systemic forces and the individual. Male psychotherapists who are particularly invested in the changing definitions of masculinity and in enhancing the integration of "feminine" characteristics need to pay special attention to the dilemma of helping males who seek enlightenment and change in themselves but who want to maintain the social status quo. A systematic analysis of the advantages of the male should lead to an understanding of the intimate connection between rearing for domination and the suppression or underdevelopment of qualities of nurturance, empathy, affiliation, cooperation, affective awareness, and expressiveness.

In this regard, the two contradictions that psychotherapists of male patients face (between the liberation from restrictive definitions of masculinity and the giving up of masculine privileges) would be more apparent than real. A systems approach to the understanding of the common "pathology"* in contemporary men is the best guarantee that the integration of different aspects of the male patient will also reflect a different position vis-à-vis women and also a change in relation to status and power. One of the problems that therapists face in the marital treatment of men[9] is that the patient has to "give up" many of his advantages and thus is not motivated to change and is fundamentally resistant to the goals of psychotherapy. This is the result of an incomplete understanding of the interactions between spouses. The "advantages" of domination and power are deceptive and need to be uncovered step by step in the complex connection with the underlying anxieties and dependencies that they attempt to control. When the price connected with these advantages is recognized, there is less resistance encountered in changing.

FEMINIST VIEWS OF PSYCHOTHERAPY

The author's work with men in psychotherapy is formed by feminist assumptions regarding the enormous impact on behavior and experience of the socialization in the specific sex role. Just as much as the author does with women patients, she views the behavior and experience of men as reflecting in great measure unexamined assumptions about the nature of their identity and self-definition that conspire against their fullest development, freedom, and capacity to create. As a therapist, the author supports the notion that our culture specifically requires and rewards manners of relating to self and others that are at cross-purposes with growth and attainment of self-actualization.

With men as well as with women patients, the author examines in specific ways the "out there" as well as the inner self. Because of her conviction that the social milieu and the prescriptions engendered by socialization are responsible for a great deal of conflict with the male's inner struggles towards integration and affiliation with others, she presents the examination of the responsibility of the culture in engendering and preserving certain pathological states and behaviors to differentiate it from the responsibility of the individual in struggling towards solving the problem that sometimes adapting to such a world demands.

*I use this term advisedly. I am very much aware that it reveals the biases of the diagnostician in making the assessment. Pathology in this case is short for "the result of adaptation to restrictions imposed from without."

The individual is still responsible for his choices, but only when he is fully informed of the participation of his milieu in engendering the role prescriptions that he did not question. Once he is aware that his efforts at adaptation have led to his restricted freedom and stunted growth, he has real choice to make changes.

Keeping in mind that these restrictions are intricately connected with politics of domination and superiority that pervade the masculine world, *the important vehicle for change is to uncover the emotional origins of these developments in the actual life of the patient* and to provide the kind of relationship that would permit both a reexperiencing of those early situations in the life of the patient and a redefinition of the patient as person through the new experience of relating with the person of the therapist. Here the therapist lends her skills and neutrality as a professional, her awareness and insight as a feminist, and her personal experience and emotional support as a person.

It is in relation to the parents—the primary agents of sex-role socialization designated by society—that the patient receives his first crucial information about his sex-role behavior and about the world's attitudes and expectations about the sexes.[10] To the extent that the parents adhere to and adapt to the culture's expectations, our patients struggle with the parents' transmission of roles in a personal and specific way. It is in this realm, in the emotionally charged atmosphere of early and important relationships, that the understanding and change of socialization has the affective impact that touches the individual.

The author does not wish to minimize the importance of learning about sex roles in other situations. A great deal of change happens as a result of education, analysis, and rational understanding. But the roots of prejudice are profound and to reach the depth from where understanding and change spring, the author believes that it is important to rely on the complex connections with the early emotional life of the individual man. It is in this connection that it is vital for men, in the author's opinion, to understand their relations with their mothers. Their attitudes towards women stem from this primary relationship. It is here that we will see in which particular way the restrictions acquired by men were important for their survival, who encouraged what, and how and when our patients learned issues of dominance and control.

The Woman Therapist's Position

Because of the intimate connection between socialization and the primary relationship with the parents as agents of socialization, the examination of this relationship is rich and rewarding. It is in the midst of it where the ironies and paradoxes of domination and control arise. Consider for instance, the paradigmatic situation of the mother of the male child. She is the object of power and control in relation to the child himself but her position in the surrounding social world is in great contrast to that. In it, she is secondary, often without voice, discriminated against. Her balance or conflict between these two spheres, her role as a mother (a potentially powerful source of self-esteem and skills), and her devaluated role as a person vis-à-vis men inevitably mark her relationship with her child. The mother is aware of the high value of the male in the world and may look upon the male infant in many ways as a precious, valued "property." Depending upon whether she identifies with him and seeks satisfaction through him or identifies him with the resented male dominant and whether she is aware or not of her conflicts in regard to men, her relationship with the child will be more or less problematic.

Since the relationship with a woman is the primary relationship in most of our patients' early lives, the most affectively strong components, the more lasting and irrational feelings are experienced with and in relation to her. The mother's crucial role in the differentiation phases of early development[11] make her a key person in the acquisition of gender identity. The woman therapist is in an ideal position to observe, through the transference reactions, the reliving of this primary relationship and to work through, with the patient, in the midst of the most charged relationship, the conflictual origins of the patient's socialization as a male and to understand the connections of this role with his past and present interactions with women. The paradoxical nature of the relationship of the male child with his mother in this culture has an important bearing on the vicissitudes of male gender identity. Although the child is in a powerless and dependent position vis-à-vis the mother, as a male he may be regarded by the mother as belonging to a superior or powerful sex. By virtue of his maleness, the child is assigned, in the mother's mind, to the valued male sex but also to the dominant sex. The reality of male dominance in our culture is a fact and the author's assumption is that the mother would respond to it in one way or another. She may be resentful, compliant with it, resigned, or openly defiant, but whatever her stance, it would color the ways in which she would regard the male child, her expectations of him, and her conception of his role. Although the intricacies of the mother–child relationship are not the only ones responsible for the eventual outcome of gender-role identity, they are the conflictual foundations of the male role. Because of their early origins, these interactions cannot be recalled in the way later relationships can. As a result, it is in relation to the female therapist that these conflicts can be reexperienced and reconstructed.

In what follows, the author will attempt to delineate the areas in which the prevailing conceptions of masculinity in our culture have led to detrimental outcomes. She will then try to clarify how these restrictions can be transformed through the analysis of the material that comes up in relation to the woman therapist. For this purpose, the phases which most male patients move through in the therapy with a female therapist will be described. The description will reveal major dynamics involved in the socialization of the male in our society and the transformation of the social self of the patient that is possible within the therapeutic relationship. It is also here where the integration of the original conflicts of the patient and the social prescriptions surrounding him have to be elucidated in their complicated and interlocking nature.

MALE ROLE RESTRICTIONS—SOCIAL DETERMINANTS

The restrictions that the male role places on men in this culture have been described by several authors.[4,12–14] Again, these are characteristics predominant in men in this culture at this time. Not all men find themselves in these dilemmas but they are frequent enough that they can be designated as culture-specific for the male role. A review is offered here with some additions.

FATHERING ROLE. Men do not rear children and their relationships with infants are distant at best. With older children, their relationships tend to be limited in time and emotional involvement.[15] As a consequence, men do not experience what is gained by raising human beings: exercise of tender care and nurturance, flexibility, capacity for empathy, adaptability in teaching immature human beings, developing of nonverbal skills, immediate sense of the value of human life, and connection with less rational human beings (and therefore connections with the more irrational–emotive aspects of the self).

AWARENESS AND EXPRESSION OF AFFECT. Because they are reared for positions of domination and control, men are trained to block emotional expression of a variety of affective states.[16] Their socialization tends to diminish the awareness and expression of sadness, fear, longing, and tenderness.[17] These limitations of awareness have the consequence of dislocating intuitive channels of behavioral guidance for which an integration of affective experience is crucial.

DENIAL OF DEPENDENCY NEEDS. Of particular importance among the affective states "forbidden" to men is that of dependent longings, be those of normal or pathologic intensity. The strong association between this prohibition and the difficulties men show in loss and separation will be discussed separately. The capacity for grieving is handicapped when dependency is not permitted.

FRIENDSHIPS WITH OTHER MEN. Close, affective bonds of intimacy with other men are warded off because of homophobic concerns ubiquitous in the culture. A system that encourages dominance of other males and aggressive competition contributes to the emotional isolation of males from one another.

FRIENDSHIPS WITH WOMEN. The necessity to sexually objectify females in our culture makes it difficult to have a variety of relationships with women as persons, particularly egalitarian and nonexploitative kinds of relationships. This lack of experience with women contributes to the devaluation or idealization of women common among men.

DESTRUCTIVE AGGRESSIVENESS. The socialization of males to fight and compete for positions of superiority and power are further helped by their underdeveloped capacities to nurture and their depreciation of tender and compassionate feelings. The result is a predominantly destructive discharge of aggressive energy with a frequent absence of genuinely self-assertive behavior.

SEXUAL PERFORMANCE. Performance anxiety is common in males, whose socialization increases the chances that they will focus on the mechanics of sexual activity and that they will isolate their affective life from their sexual experience. Their socialization in the sexual area is in direct opposition to that of females in our culture and seems aimed at rendering heterosexual couples incompatible or limited to the pleasures of physical discharge. The erosion of eroticism in men appears to go hand in hand with the increasing aggressivization of sexual activity.

WORK AND ACHIEVEMENT COMPULSION. In many men, the frantic pursuit of achievements at the expense of other aspects of their lives, the excessive identification of work with self-worth, and the centering of identity in the occupational sphere are characteristics that have been frequently described.[18] The author is making a distinction between this compulsion and the healthy investment in serious work. The latter is often less conflictual in males than in females.

The following conflictual themes have not been previously described but the author sees them as distinctive of males in this culture.

INFLATED SELF-ESTEEM. In part due to their dominant position in the culture, many men have a false sense of their worth. Their power is often the result of a higher social status or advantaged economic position. Because of their subordinate position, women have often lied to men about the man's assets and liabilities, contributing to the men's inflated self-esteem. The majority of men are at least subliminally aware of the fact that women are not free, in most cases, to give an objective or honest appraisal of the man they see. The desire to preserve this false sense of power and the distrust of subordinates' intentions in eliciting it with praise leads to a conflict specific of men. Superficially self-confident, many men have underlying problems with their self-appraisal.

GUILT OVER DOMINANCE. Many men feel collective guilt over the fate of women in this society. This sense of guilt is often unconscious and appears to be related to unconscious desires to maintain women in a submissive position. Some of these wishes in men are consciously rejected but in many cases appear with relative ease in consciousness, being justified by the anger men feel over the prominence that women play in their personal lives. In men who have a highly developed sense of justice and social concerns about civil rights, the position is one of guilt over the passive stance most men have taken in regards to the most obvious features of women's issues (discrimination in employment and education, physical violence against women). Considering the active participation that many white men took in the struggle for the civil rights of Black people, the absence of a similar move to transform the situation of women requires an explanation.

SYMBIOTIC DEPENDENCY ON WOMEN. As a result of their socialization, men are in a difficult position to nurture themselves and to achieve autonomy. Bernard's analysis[19] of current statistics indicating that married men are in better psychological health than single men leads to the conclusion that the capacity to function emotionally appears diminished in men when they are not attached to a woman partner.[20] Many of the restrictions already described as part of the masculine role conspire against the capacity for self-caring. The dependency on women, not frequently acknowledged by men, is evident in observations of couples and in male reactions to separations, particularly when the female takes the initiative in terminating the relationship. The counterpart of the symbiotic dependence of many women on men is found in men's reliance on women for nurturance, the maintenance of their emotional life, the neutralization of aggression through the erotization of women, and the continuous enhancement of their self-esteem. The envy of women—born in the author's opinion from their prohibitions in identifying with them—contribute to their excessive dependence. Lerner[21] has masterfully described the central role of envy in the devaluation of women.

THE DYNAMICS OF MALE ROLE SOCIALIZATION

The problems that men experience as a consequence of their socialization seem to stem from two major dynamic sources: (1) the prohibition of identification with mother; and (2) the identification with a distant, hostile, or brutal father.

These features appear pervasively in the backgrounds of men in therapy. Our social mores reinforce the negative identification with women and further encourage compliance to the masculine group with its social advantages and payoffs. Of these, *the prohibitions in identification with the female are of special importance in the successful treatment of men and the dramatic alteration of stereotypic male characteristics.*

The early experience of affective closeness with a woman (the mother) and the tender reliance on and identification with the primary love object that normally occurs in the first year of life are the origins of the capacity for empathy, the development of emotional expressiveness, and of awareness of internal feeling states. The premature loss of the connection with the mother that takes place in a male child's life and the prohibition of dependency on the mother before these longings can be naturally resolved and outgrown is, in the author's opinion, responsible in great part for the disavowal and loss of those affective capacities. The socialization of the male child (encouraged both by mother and father) towards a premature withdrawal from the relationship with mother leads to the loss of the early identification with her, now considered a threat to identity as a male. Dependency needs that are unresolved are defended against by denial and counterdependent moves.

These unresolved dependencies in the male and the repression of the love for the mother play a role in later affiliations with women. The replacement of the "original mother" is often thinly disguised in the male's relentless search for a wife who is dedicated to him and whose faithfulness and safety are beyond doubt. Mr. L.S. kept his wife constantly under his thumb. He was seen as an authoritarian man by his children. He expected complete submissiveness from his wife but was often enraged at her excessive dependence on him. This behavior turned out to be directed towards the mother of his childhood. The patient had behaved towards her in an endearing and submissive way. He had felt his mother had betrayed his love by subjecting him to his brutal father's discipline. The mother had encouraged a loving relationship with her son which she often asked her husband to disrupt. The patient in his marriage behaved like his own father, condemning the dependency of his wife (as father had done with the patient's dependency on mother) while encouraging absolute compliance. But the wife was also the representative of the mother, now powerless and in his control.

When this patient could recall his warm attachment to his mother and live through his disappointment with her and the loss of such an important relationship, his relationship with his wife made a dramatic turn. This occurred in connection with the abandonment of the identification with the feared aspects of his father, closely connected with the circumstances of the disruption of his early relationship with mother. In working through the disappointment and anger of this patient towards his mother, it was possible for him to recover the times when he was close and affectionate towards her in a nonconflictual way. This made possible the following steps:

1. Reevaluation of the relationship with acceptance of dependent and loving feelings;
2. Awareness of loss and grieving of the lost attachment;
3. Review of identification with father out of fear;
4. Recovery of the early identification with mother and with it the armamentarium of emotional responsiveness and expressiveness tied to the primary relationship with a woman; and
5. Separation of the marital relationship from the original source of the displacement.

These early situations, often responsible for later conflicts, are first manifested in the transference. The woman therapist has easy access to this aspect of the transference and is in a potentially ideal position to act as intermediary between past object relations and the present ones.

ADVANTAGES OF THE FEMALE THERAPIST

In addition to the capacity to evoke the early transference reactions to mother and with them the conflictual core of later relationships with women, the female therapist offers the possibility of identification with her. The resolution of the prohibitions of identification with the female are also a major part of the work of the male therapist but here the sexes have different although equally important advantages. The male therapist helps to resolve this prohibition through the patients' identification of the therapist's masculine and feminine aspects. The female therapist offers a direct route to the identification with the repressed and forbidden aspects of the patient's own identification with his mother through the reproduction and resolution, in the transference, of the conflictual themes that promoted such repression. The female therapist encourages this through the experience and expression of feelings until then forbidden, reassuring him with her very presence and acceptance of the patient's fears. The tolerance of dependency when it reappears in the therapeutic relationship permits the understanding of the original situation with the mother and leads to the gradual resolution and working through of feelings of shame and inferiority accompanying the awareness of dependent longings. The female therapist is in an advantageous position to help her patient work through feelings of anger, envy, and disappointment at mother. Although much in these conflicts involves clearly personal dynamics, it is important to stress that the author has repeatedly seen what she regards as culture-specific conflicts in so many of her male patients that she tends to consider them the product of a fairly common conflict (in this culture) in the developmental experience of the male child. The disappointment in the mother concerns her abandonment of the male child to the "masculine society" and her inability to rescue, in him, the very characteristics of sensitivity, affection, and gentleness that she helped arouse.

The male child has a particular painful conflict vis-à-vis his mother. Not infrequently, the mother resents the limitations of her position at home and in the family and makes the child aware of and sympathetic to her dissatisfaction. On the other hand, the male child is conscious at some level that he belongs to the very group who hold mother's position down; that is, that father in particular and men in general are perceived as responsible for mother's unhappiness and restrictions. If mother is not aware of these feelings and does not struggle with them consciously, she is likely to displace her ambivalence towards men onto her male child, on the one hand expecting him to "compensate" her for her restricted life, on the other hand disliking him for belonging to a group that holds superior positions over women. Mr. N.N. berated his mother for not being satisfied with his achievements. Although he was a doctor, he was not a physician like his mother would have preferred. In connecting the apparent differences between his comfortable and somewhat liberating relationship with the author and that with his mother, the author commented that she was a doctor so that he did not have to do that for her and maybe this time it would be possible for him to choose what he liked rather than follow his mother's prescription. After seeing his mother's possible dissatisfaction with her own life more clearly, his resentment gave way to an awareness of his mother's plight.

The male child might feel the conflict of the mother more or less intensely. The author had seen many a patient of hers exceedingly aware of mother's unhappiness and intensely wishing to do something about it. But the very thing that might temporarily alleviate her unhappiness (to achieve the achievements she might have wished for herself) conspires against his own choices and independent development and may also bring with it the envy that mother may experience towards the advantages of men. This particular dilemma is repeated again and again in the adult life of the patient with the woman he marries: he feels that he "owes" it to her to succeed and achieve even if those are not his goals, because she is not free to carry out her personal ambitions.

This conflict unfolds within the transference to the female therapist. The patient is often unaware of the ambivalent feelings he has towards his mother regarding his sex-role assignment and he has also repressed his early awareness of the mother's dilemma as presented above. In order to uncover the origin of the particular conflict with the mother two elements seem necessary: the development of the conflicts with mother within the transference reaction and the awareness of the conflictual themes connected with the male sex role and the mother's conflicts with her sex role in the therapist. The attitudes of the mother should be understood in connection with her specific gender dilemmas in this culture and not just as the expression of her own personal dynamics.

THE SEXUALIZATION OF LOVING FEELINGS. The female therapist has the advantage that her sex offers her to permit the live resolution of this common defense in men. The patient's prohibition of loving feelings toward the mother, his anger at her, and his fear of submissiveness to her converge in the desire to "possess" and make the therapist "his own." The desire for domination and revenge is mixed with the longing for closeness and intimacy which has had to be warded off and devalued.

THE ACCEPTANCE AND INTEGRATION OF HOMOEROTIC FEELINGS. The male patient's experience of love for other men is also frequently sexualized. The homophobic characteristics of the culture make the awareness of these feelings unacceptable to many men. The female therapist has a particular advantage in the working through of homoerotic feelings; the patient is reassured by his positive relationship to her of the predominance of his heterosexuality and of his pleasure in it. Often, homosexual feelings are most threatening to men when they simultaneously experience rejection from or towards females. The loving connection with the female therapist permits awareness and evaluation of the feelings towards men and the discovery of bonds of affection and longings for closeness and intimacy not tolerated before. The encouragement of feelings of solidarity and affection by the female therapist is aided by interpreting the obstacles to intimacy with other men just as a male therapist would do. But in the case of the female, the specific ways in which her sex can be used to advantage are (1) in increasing the tolerance and new understanding of homoerotic feelings aided by the presence of the heterosexual bonding within the therapeutic relationship; and (2) the specific support and encouragement given by a woman of close egalitarian relations with men. The freedom from concerns with dominance and submission connected with the masculine mystique is achieved through the clarification of their origins in the patient's life and in the culture.

THE TREATMENT PROCESS: PHASES AND DILEMMAS

The author's clinical experience throughout 22 years of psychotherapy practice in various settings reveals a change in the requests for treatment expressed by many men. Their awareness of the changing situation of women and of their own sex-role behavior has been heightened. The wish for "liberation" from male role restrictions is present virtually in all requests she receives for psychotherapy.

Gradually, psychotherapists have begun to consider the pervasive influence of sex-role behavior in their patients. The radical departure from traditional therapies has been in emphasizing that the gender role of the patient fundamentally affects his behavior and experience[22] and that the outcome in therapy is in part dictated by the biases about sex roles that the therapist consciously or unconsciously holds. On the other hand, the behavior of the patient is also affected by the sex of the therapist.

Women have brought this fact to public awareness and female therapists have written extensively about the implications of the male therapists treating females and the advisability of female therapists for treating a multiplicity of female problems.[23,24] Recently, male therapists have similarly described their work with male patients with an emphasis on the commonalities of male role conflicts and of specific ways of understanding and helping male patients.[12,13]

The analysis of specific differences, advantages, and disadvantages of the therapist's sex in relation to the male patient have not been discussed in much detail. Toomer[25] reviews the sparse research literature on the effects of sex of therapist on client's behavior as well as the studies of therapists' biases on judgments concerning the mental health of males and females. The fairly consistent finding regarding the effects of sex of the counselor is the effect of the female sex on the male's self-disclosure and expression of feelings. Particularly after the initial sessions,[26] increasing satisfaction and discussion of feelings is found. Though both women and men seem to prefer male counselors,[27,28] preferences for females are greater when understanding personal problems is required. The male counselor is preferred for authoritative advice. Sex of therapist was found a more important variable than race[29] in encouraging self-experience. Black clients explored themselves to a greater extent with a female regardless of racial similarity. Male patients expect therapists to be more directive, analytic, and critical while females anticipate nonjudgmental and accepting styles.[30] On the other hand, male mental health professionals, while rating males more positively than females, tend to expect more traditional male behavior from their male patients than females would. If we add to this that highly authoritarian males tend to hold more stereotypical views and devalue women as authorities,[31] we can hypothesize that males with more stereotypic sex-role behavior are likely to choose male therapists whose expectations of masculine roles are more traditional.

The author's experience with patients with strongly stereotypic male traits is that despite initial discomfort and devaluation of the female therapist, they are more likely to change sex-role behavior with a female, particularly if the female has authoritative characteristics the patient identifies as desirable (greater experience, age, status, credentials). However, a study of male participants in a group conducted by female leaders[32] found self-actualization increased in those males with lower scores of authoritarianism and profeminist attitudes.

In describing her experience with the psychotherapy of male patients, the author wants to pay special attention to her observations of the effect that her gender appears to have in the process of treatment. She sees female therapists as having different but just as specific advantages as male therapists have to help patients resolve the variety of conflicts associated with their roles as males and females.

In a good number of cases the male patients the author sees in psychotherapy had indicated that her sex was an important determinant of their choice (credentials and other requirements being equal). The other half who consciously did not consider her sex relevant in their selection did seem to have, upon closer examination, important reasons in their past to wish to encounter a woman therapist. It is therefore impossible for the author to know whether the conflictual themes that she sees so often in the lives of her patients and those of other women therapists are relevant only for the patients who consciously or inadvertently seek a woman because of certain conflict clusters in their background.

The histories of the author's male patients reveal that they have often had an intense and important relationship with their mothers, that the love for their mothers is often "buried," and that they share similar unresolved conflicts and unfinished attempts at separation from them that become central in their therapy with the author. Men have not been allowed to "love" their mothers and/or to identify with them. Premature separations with enforcement of stereotypic role behavior[33] leave the male unable to resolve dependency longings, to work through individuation and separation phases effectively, and to be able to integrate the tender affection and the sexual components of the relationship. The relationship to a female therapist allows, through the medium of the transference, an affectively alive reiteration of those conflicts with the opportunity for working through and resolution.

Self-disclosure and expression of feelings appear to be greater for male clients in the presence of a female counselor.[26,29,34,35] To regain the early affective vocabulary, often learned next to mother in the first years of life, is more of a natural process with a woman therapist. This new "language," different from that commonly used by men, allows continuous reexperiencing and communication of the forbidden affects of the mother–son relationship.

Initial Phase. The author has noticed with curiosity that in addition to the attentive kindness and benevolence with which she tends to listen to patients, an attitude of delicacy towards the male patient is often aroused in her. The patient experiences himself as a delicate creature with sensitivities that are considered precious rather than being treated contemptuously as had often happened to him in the past. An element of a "corrective emotional experience" seems to be initially appropriate to permit the evocation of the very emotions that had been buried by shame, sternness, or hostility.

Men tend to emphasize their experiences of anger, resentment, frustration, distaste, contempt, and other negative emotions. Their communication style tends to be logical, hyperrational, and directive. The author's emphasis is to allow by example, focusing, and interpretation the prominence of affective experience. The interpretation of anger as a defense against other affects, when appropriate, greatly facilitates their emergence (primarily feelings of hurt, aloneness, loss, and abandonment). The tolerance and permission of the therapist and the understanding that anger is a "comfortable" emotion and that serves as a defense against "soft," tender, and vulnerable feelings the patient experiences with fear and shame relax the barrier blocking core experiences.

In the initial interviews, the differences between male and female patients are striking. Female patients seldom express their anger while they find it relatively easy to express their feelings of loss and sadness. Female patients have specific prohibitions about angry feelings and the therapist's awareness of this sex-role restriction often helps her in the interpretation of the "hidden" affect.

The important elements in the initial phase of treatment are the following:

1. The establishment of a bond of tender and respectful feelings established between therapist and patient;
2. The focusing on increasing affective awareness;
3. The interpretation, when appropriate, of negative emotions as defenses against forbidden feelings;

4. The interest of the therapist and encouragement in reaching painful affective experiences, previously blocked, and allowing understanding of these in connection to the prohibitions of masculine role; and
5. Dealing with fears of passive-dependent impulses by interpreting the intolerance towards this inner experience and the responsibility of the culture in this regard.

LOSS AND GRIEF. After phobic fears of passive-dependent impulses and the angry stance of defense have been partially dealt with, it is common to encounter the reexperience of losses and feelings of regret that had not been allowed acknowledgment and resolution. Frequent recollections of abandonments, in the recent past and in childhood, the loss of friends and loving relations, seem to emerge, forming a tapestry of the painful losses in the patient's life. The importance of permitting the patient ample room for the experience and examination of these feelings is fundamental to the specific understanding in that person's life, of the brutal effect in the life of the male of stereotypical assumptions about his role built up all along the way. This understanding permits the patient a reevaluation of his life, his attitudes, and his future that also integrates the role his social milieu plays in it. Until the patient is aware of how pervasive (and common to other men) his training as a man is in dictating choices and behavior and in sculpting his experience, his awareness is limited and his capacity to change is determined in part by his continuous compliance with the social order. It is the author's belief that an examination of the personal cannot be isolated from the examination of the cultural role in his indoctrination, for the patient will have to make a choice between defying the assumptions of his role assignment or maintaining his compliance with this order. This choice is to be made consciously, now that the patient realizes that his behavior as a man had been determined by his social engineering and is not part of what a person is.

This phase is also fundamental because in reexperiencing losses and in mourning them appropriately, the patient's prohibitions about crying can be overcome, yielding to sadness and the realization of his vulnerability and helplessness. The emotional life of the patient begins its integration with his understanding of his past and present in this important phase. The expression of the deep emotional crises that the patient never followed to their completion leads to the awareness of the constrictions of emotional expression contained in his role and mobilizes the freedom to express himself. But if in this phase the recognition of the losses and the importance of one's socialization in preventing its awareness and integration is important, it is just as fundamental to clarify the details and meanings of these experiences. The patient's feelings of loss are profoundly marked by his loss of connection with his mother first and his awareness of the loss of a relationship with his father. In the themes of abandonment, the patient's real tragedy is often disguised: *the loss of a part of himself, that assigned a "feminine" character, with all its affective richness is buried with the premature separation from the mother.* Although the family dynamics of the author's patients are singular and varied, this is a persistent theme. The disguised nature of this loss is also characteristic: men are forbidden to express the loss of the "feminine" self and are not conscious of the content nor of the prohibition. The therapist's role is to connect the signs that lead to its existence to have it available for examination. For this and other reasons, this phase offers unusual difficulties to therapists. The therapist's own biases about the role of men and their reactions to deep sorrow and mourning of the "female self" engender conflictual feelings in the therapist whose own socialization has not been deeply examined. Despite their greater tolerance, female therapists also tend to retreat from the full expression of sadness and loss in male patients because they are extremely sensitive to a man's weeping. For the females, the experience goes against their expectations of masculine strength and invulnerability and arouses primitive guilt about destructive wishes towards men. The female identifies with the "guilty mother" of the patient's fantasy which happens to coincide with the "guilty mother" of the female fantasy and cannot allow full expression of the patient's sorrow.

Although these feelings of loss recur throughout treatment, the major breakthroughs occur after the mourning of the lost self. In ways not different from the female patient, the male patient has to come to grips with the awareness of his compliance with an order in which he was an accomplice to his own victimization. The compensation for his loss of his genuine and feeling self appears now more obvious: power and domination. When experienced in this context, these masculine gains are seen as empty and undesirable. We can come here to an important understanding of the characteristic male defenses: The author interprets the desire to control and dominate as an attempt to trade in on the advantages of the male but primarily as *the desire to control and dominate the femaleness in himself, the core of feelings towards which the male patient has been encouraged to feel distrust, contempt, and shame.*

If we contend that an important function of the male role is to maintain in check the domination of the male self over the femaleness of the man and to keep buried at all costs the awareness of the losses, regrets, and feelings associated with this demise, we are beginning to see male socialization in its personal, dynamic implications. In this context, the male's desire for the domination of the female has at its depth a connection with the lost feminine identification and the impulse to control its emergence. In addition, revenge against "female abandonment," as well as the attempt to prevent its reoccurrence, fuels the desire for female domination. This dynamic aspect of the male's domination is displayed in the cultural context as well and reinforces the individual's participation in it.

In this connection, it is important to emphasize that the anger at the abandonment of the mother involves similar feelings toward the abandonment by the father as well. The propensity in our culture to indict mothers[36] for the failure of both parents is pervasive and an important issue to clarify with our patients.

Love in the Transference. This phase of treatment, crucial to resolve the impediments of the identification with the female and to understand the anger towards women, poses specific problems for the female therapist. Many patients show a tendency to sexualize the relationship with the therapist to ward off feelings of love and dependency and to express anger in a disguised form. The therapist may feel pressed to discourage these feelings rather than work with them because of the discomfort aroused if her own sexual feelings are evoked. Females appear to have less tolerance than men in this area and exhibit greater prohibitions about experiencing sexual attraction or loving feelings to their patients.[37,38] They have less propensity to act out their own countertransference as well.

Yet it is when the early feelings towards the mother are evoked in the transference that a major part of the task of understanding and working through the male patient's feelings towards his mother (which color his relations to women) and recovery of the early identification with her is possible. The author is primarily talking about the appearance of the unambivalent, egocentric love more characteristic of early developmental phases. The transference reaction seems the only vehicle capable of evoking and thus helping the patient recover this forbidden stage of the relationship to the mother. While the sexualization of the therapeutic relationship is often associated with the covering up of aggressive feelings, the patient attempting control and domination of the therapist and devaluing her as a mere sexual object, it is just as often a defense against tender feelings and accompanying fears of submission.

Mr. M.O. used his erotic feelings towards the author as a resistance in treatment. Because of his history of maternal abandonment and promiscuous behavior that seemed a revenge against women and a defense against involvement and potential abandonment, the author interpreted his fear of his tender feelings towards her as causing this characteristic response in him. The result was the recovery of very loving feelings that made him feel he was "soft in the head" and utterly vulnerable. He had felt that his mother had exploited his feelings to make him compliant and that she then abandoned him. At all costs, this scene was not to be repeated again. In his life with women he would leave them or betray them as soon as he began to feel involved. In the therapeutic relationship he was attempting to control the author in case she did what his mother had done. By staying within this reaction it was possible to recover the extraordinary sensitivity and the richness of his affection toward his mother.

The loving feelings evoked in this phase are a powerful motive for change. The patient feels loved and special, daring and powerful and yet intensely vulnerable but not afraid. These feelings help the patient take bold steps in involvements with others, try new experiences, and experience in turn the reactions of other people towards him. This offers an opportunity for the patient to express love openly and unashamedly and to understand his defensive behavior in the past. It is important to underline that the erotization of the positive transference is much more likely to happen in connection with a female therapist[39] and as such it presents the problems and the opportunities discussed in a cross-sex situation only.

ANGER AND INDIVIDUATION. The disappointment within the special relationship with the therapist/mother and the frustration of the expected everlasting love leads to the awareness of anger and hate in the transference. The early situations of disappointment and abandonment are evoked at this time. Patients often complain of the ungenuine nature of the therapist's love. Others feel that the therapist is not dedicated enough or is not responsive to the patient's loving feelings. The fantasy of the ideal mother is brought to an abrupt end. Vacations of the therapist and/or the therapy bills often trigger these reactions. Rebellious behaviors, acts of covert retaliation, and sexual acting out are sometimes expressions of the anger that the patient cannot express openly and vigorously towards the therapist. With some of the author's patients, this angry phase starts when she introduces the option of working with her and a male cotherapist in a series of conjoint therapy sessions. This evokes the infantile situation in which the presence of the male was brought in to separate the child from the mother. The importance of the reoccurrence of the anger in relation to the therapist is to facilitate the understanding of the experience in the past, to clarify the responsibilities of both parents and of the social system in some of the tragic events that took place, and to heal wounds not previously acknowledged. This anger is very different from the "comfortable" state that many patients show in their early contacts with the therapist. For one thing, it is directed toward the therapist, the very person who is also seen as helpful and nurturant. It threatens the disruption or in some cases, the actual destruction of the positive relationship with the therapist. Although it has defensive aspects too, this experience of anger is in much closer connection with the dependent wishes of the patient and with his loving feelings as well. The task is to encourage the assertion of individual rights and the voicing of the anger directly without negating the other aspects of the experience. This situation, often anxiety-provoking for both patient and therapist, is another milestone in the continuous process of individuation which the patient has not had enough opportunity to go through in the past. Anger serves the purpose of separation and differentiation when placed at the service of relevant personal needs and when positive feelings are expressed as well. The patient in fact utilizes for his differentiation and autonomy the very characteristics of the therapist that he had found helpful. Parting with the woman therapist is hopefully different from the traumatic parting from the mother; the feminine aspects that are valuable are preserved within the patient, his autonomy is increased, and his anger has been voiced, heard, and understood.

As Miller[40] and Bernardez[41] have pointed out, men require change and improvement in their helpful expression of anger. The fact that their socialization has permitted them greater freedom with negative affects and more tolerance of competition, rivalry, and aggression, does not mean that it has taught them how to combine it with loving aspects of the self to prevent destructiveness. The anger of men at women has several determinants, but the most frequently encountered is the betrayal of the son by the mother; the boy child feels that he has been delivered to the male world for survival and that the mother did not protect the vulnerable aspects of the child nor fight for him no matter how impossible this may have been for the mother because of her own situation of subordination.

At this time in the treatment, the illusions and omnipotent fantasies regarding the mother can be realized. The fantasy of the perfect mother[42] is elucidated and a sympathetic view of the mother, her position in the family and at large also becoming clearer, can emerge. It is important to allow the development and expression of the feelings of anger and disappointment first before attempting to explain mother's behavior or her position. The feelings of the patient about her betrayal are very real and they do not change with an intellectual understanding of her role and that of father in it. But it is just as important for the patient to learn of her actual plight since it is not different from that of other women and his responsibilities and those of men in them are to be examined.

If his mother defended the "feminine" characteristics of her boy child she would be considered a destructive mother who made a "sissy" out of her son. If she allowed him to be dependent until more appropriate times for his autonomy she may be accused of tying her son to "her apron strings." In either case, she would be blamed for his destiny. This double bind and unfair assignment of responsibility tends to increase the resentment that women may harbor towards men and that may be expressed toward the male child.

Male patients express similar feelings of anger toward their mothers. Among the most common complaints:

1. The premature separation and neglect of dependency;
2. The manipulation of the child for purposes of power;
3. The devaluation of "feminine" characteristics in him;
4. The encouragement of submission to the "masculine" world with the destruction of the "feminine" self; and
5. The pressure to perform for her and achieve for her.

If the resentment is not uncovered and worked through in the original situation, chances are that the relationship with other women will be dictated by defending against their possible domination, rejection, or exploitation.

RELATIONSHIPS WITH WOMEN. The relationship with the female therapist allows a direct look at some of the male patients' assumptions about females, blind spots, biases, and difficulties. That relationship can be used as a major tool to examine and change attitudes towards the female, particularly after the strongly affective phases of the work in the maternal transference have been dealt with. The author pays specific attention to limitations in the sexual life of the patient that seem connected with his socialization: the prohibition of sensuous, passive pleasure, the compulsion to perform, the inability to connect emotional and sexual life, the tendency to discharge anger through sexual behavior, and attempts to devalue, exploit, or dominate women.

In many of the author's patients, the dependent relationship with the woman is thinly disguised. Although the patient may take a controlling or dominant position in some aspects of the relationship with the woman, the patient feels often controlled by her because of his excessive dependence on her. Often the wife is the representation of the mother of childhood who is now placed at one's service. The dread of grown women that many men express in their choice of very young females seems based on their association with the pre-Oedipal mother, the dreaded, powerful, and unreliable object. When the male patient no longer fears this association because his anger and his fear of submission have been squared away, a notable improvement in his relationships with women ensues. The fear of being dominated by women *again* is often connected with the need to dominate them. In so doing, the patient also attempts to keep control of the forbidden female self. The culture reinforces these tendencies because these fears are collective.

Mr. M.J. noticed with surprise a change in his relationship with his wife. She had become gentle and receptive. She had not been hypercritical of him as she used to be. He had discovered that it was possible for him to listen to her and to be attentive to her needs. He also had noticed that he had dealt with her criticism of him in a more realistic manner. It was with surprise that he concluded that she was changing in reaction to him and his changes. He was no longer embattled to prevent her possible domination by controlling her and was satisfying more of her needs. Their sexual life became more active and pleasurable with the patient noting that they were more spontaneous and playful. Through the changes in his wife and their relationship he discovered the changes he himself had undergone, particularly in his domineering and critical stance.

RELATIONSHIPS WITH MEN. The female therapist does not have the valuable advantages of role modeling relationships with the same sex that the male therapist has. But her role in encouraging and enhancing the male patient's new bonds of solidarity, intimacy, and tenderness with other men, is very important. Many conflicts with men originate in the difficult period in which the child is forced to deny aspects of himself to be acceptable to the masculine world. The male patient's relationship with his father becomes clearer once his feelings towards his mother have been separated from those towards his father. But in the same way in which the patient also saw his father through his mother's eyes, the therapist's interventions reveal the father in again a new light, that of the man perceived by the woman therapist. Here, the equanimity of the therapist is quite important. A compassionate and objective neutrality on the part of the therapist is necessary for the male patient to understand the often tragic fate of the "distant" father and to be able to empathize with him. But it is just as important to note the father's responsibility for the mother's abandonment of the child rather than assign total responsibility to the mother. This issue is crucial to understand the dynamics of domination in a live way. If the patient understands how domination of the female worked in his own family and what were the dreadful effects on him as well as on his own parents, he may have a very different attitude toward his own tendency to exercise similar power over others.

As Solomon[12] has pointed out, changes in the patient's sex-role behavior will bring about conflicts since this society rewards a defensive stance in males and devalues his feminine-like qualities. The author finds that her patients' new behaviors are first confined to their relationship with her. But soon the interactions with women seem to change the most and with less anxiety than anticipated. It is with men who are not friends or intimates that the new changes take the longest to be expressed with comfort. The female's role of encouragement and admiration of change is an important source of support. The female has played the role of acknowledging, affirming, and supporting his sexual differentiation in his life. It is possible that the female therapist plays this role again in this new differentiation.

CONJOINT WORK WITH MALE THERAPISTS

The use of therapists of both sexes in the treatment of families and mixed groups has been a regular characteristic of family and group therapy. Some authors have advocated the advantages of having both sexes in the treatment of individual patients.[43,44] Yet, the specific effects and indications of the therapist's gender for the male or female patient have been focused on[45] but have not been separately evaluated. The majority of authors working with conjoint therapy point to the valuable presence of the couple with all the implications for the patients' potential resolution of his position in triadic relations. Because the effects of the gender of the therapists have not been evaluated separately, many therapists working in cross-sex teams tend to obscure those effects or be totally unaware of them.

The author has found it valuable in the individual treatment of patients to introduce a male colleague and work as a therapeutic couple for a limited number of sessions. The male therapist provides a ready-made role model for identification. If he is loving and warm, expressive and receptive and at the same time he is assertive, clear in his identity, nonstereotypic in his reactions, and neither threatened by women nor controlling of them, he provides the integration of "feminine" and "masculine" characteristics required for growth. Male patients seem to identify more readily with male therapists who have attractive personal characteristics, a solid sense of their own authority, and the flexibility, humanness and freedom from the defensive characteristics of the stereotypic male role.

Introducing a male therapist for discrete periods of time has the following advantages:

1. To study, observe, and work with the separate transferences to male and female;
2. To give the patient an opportunity to reexperience and work through conflictual feelings in relation to his parents as a couple;
3. To facilitate the working through of problems with the father in the presence and with the support of his female therapist;
4. To permit identification with a male comfortable with masculine and feminine characteristics; and
5. To help in the individuation phase with the female therapist and in the expression of anger and disappointment at having to give her up.
6. To witness and experience a cooperative, egalitarian, and respectful relationship in the therapeutic couple.

SUMMARY

The dilemmas common to contemporary men that have a bearing in the restrictions of male roles are as follows:

(1) The prohibitions against feminine identification: The rejection of female models for identification in men deprive them of valuable "feminine" charac-

teristics and encourage their dependency on women for the opportunity to express and develop those aspects of the self.

(2) The flight from dependency: The premature separation from maternal objects of dependency is encouraged in little boys in our culture. Men are socialized to deny dependent needs which are displaced onto adult women partners. Relations with women are often permeated with unacknowledged and displaced dependent needs that have not been resolved. The fear of abandonment by women is part of this complex picture.

(3) The irrational belief in and fear of mother's (and women's) omnipotent destructive power: This unconscious belief operates in men to detract from relations of equality with women and to encourage efforts to dominate them.

(4) The defense of sexualization: The tendency in men to sexualize relations of intimacy is seen as a way to preserve autonomy and dominance and of defending against the fear of passive longings and of tender, affectionate feelings.

In relation to the female therapist, the male patient can reexperience the early and conflictual relationship with his mother. The recovery of the early love for the mother and the rescuing of the female identity of the patient is regarded as the central task of the treatment. Other phases of the treatment that are essential in acquiring and integrating lost capacities in males deal with the awareness of losses and the grieving of such losses and the anger and individuation phase dealing with the separation from the female therapist. The psychotherapy of men aims at the acquisition of awareness of affective strivings and expressiveness of emotional needs, the reclaiming of nurturance and tenderness that neutralize destructive aggression, the ability to mourn and grieve, the resolution of dependency towards women, the integration of affectionate and sensuous components in the sexual life of the patient, and the resolution of the need to dominate and control women. The integration of the early dynamics of socialization with the cultural prescriptions is elucidated.

The transference reaction is the vehicle used to understand the patient's dynamics of his early socialization as a male. This live understanding, coupled with an awareness of the social and cultural prescriptions infringing upon the patient, is utilized in the therapy to allow him to exercise choice in what was previously automatic or ego-syntonic behavior. Conjoint work with a male therapist for a discrete number of sessions has specific advantages to work through phases of separation and integration of male and female characteristics in sex-role identity.

REFERENCES

1. Brodsky A, Hare-Mustin R: Women and Psychotherapy: An assessment of research and practice. New York, Gilford, 1980
2. Chesler P: Patient and patriarch: Women in the psychotherapeutic relationship, in Women in Sexist Society: Studies in Power and Powerlessness. Edited by Gornick V, Moran B. New York, Basic Books, 1971, pp 362–392
3. Farrell W: The Liberated Man. New York, Bantam Books, 1974

4. Goldberg H: The Hazards of Being Male. New York, New American Library, 1977
5. Filene PG: Him/Her/Self: Sex Roles in Modern America. New York, Harcourt Brace Jovanovich, 1974
6. Dinnerstein D: The Mermaid and the Minotaur. Sexual Arrangements and Human Malaise. New York, Harper and Row, 1977
7. Wong MR, Davey J, Conroe RM: Expanding masculinity: Counseling the male in transition. Counseling Psychol 6:58–61, 1976
8. Fasteau MF: The Male Machine. New York, McGraw-Hill, 1974
9. Rice DG: The male spouse in marital and family therapy. Counseling Psychol 7:64–67, 1978
10. Stroller RJ: Sex and Gender: Vol I. The Development of Masculinity and Femininity. New York, Jason Aronson, 1975
11. Mahler M: The Psychological Birth of the Human Infant. New York, Basic Books, 1975
12. Solomon K: Therapeutic aspects of changing masculine role behavior. World J Psychosynthesis 11:13–16, 1979
13. Stein TS: The effects of women's liberation on men. Presented at the 132nd meeting of the American Psychiatric Association, Chicago, Illinois, May 16, 1979
14. Stevens B: The sexually oppressed male. Psychother: Theory Res Pract 11:16–21, 1974
15. Tavris C, Offir C: The Longest War: Sex Differences in Perspective. New York, Harcourt Brace Jovanovich, 1977
16. Balswick JO, Peek CW: The inexpressive male: A tragedy of American society, in The Forty-Nine Percent Majority: The Male Sex Role. Edited by David, DS, Brannon R. Reading, Massachusetts, Addison-Wesley, 1976, pp 55–58
17. Skovholt T: Feminism and men's lives. Counseling Psychol 7:3–10, 1978
18. Gould R: Measuring masculinity by the size of the paycheck, in The Forty-Nine Percent Majority: The Male Sex Role. Edited by David DS, Brannon R. Reading, Massachusetts, Addison-Wesley, 1976, pp 113–118
19. Bernard J: The Future of Marriage. New York, World Publishing, 1972
20. Pleck JH: Men's power with women, other men and society: A men's movement analysis, in Women and Men: The Consequences of Power. Edited by Hiller D, Sheets R. University of Cincinnati Office of Women's Studies, 1977, pp 12–23
21. Lerner H: Early origins of envy and the devaluation of women: Implications for sex role stereotypes. Bull Menninger Clin 38:6:538–533, 1974
22. Maffeo P: Conceptions of sex role development and androgyny: Implications for mental health and for psychotherapy. J Am Med Women's Assoc 33:255–230, 1978
23. Chesler P: Women and Madness. New York, Doubleday, 1972
24. Sturdivant S: Therapy with Women. A Feminist Philosophy of Treatment. New York, Springer, 1980
25. Toomer JE: Males in psychotherapy. Counseling Psychol 7:22–25, 1978
26. Hill CE: Sex of client and sex and experience level of counselor. J Counseling Psychol 22:6–11, 1975
27. Boulware D, Holmes D: Preferences for therapists and related experiences. J Consult Clin Psychol 35:269–277, 1970
28. Clayton V, Jellison JM: Preferences for the age and sex of advisors: A life span approach. Dev Psychol 11:861–862, 1975
29. Granthon R: Effects of counselors' sex, race and language style on black students in initial interviews. J Counseling Psychol 20:553–559, 1973
30. Tinsley EH, Harris DJ: Client expectations for counseling. J Counseling Psychol 23:173–177, 1976
31. Adorno TW, Frenkel-Brunswik E, Levinson D, et al.: The Authoritarian Personality. New York, Harper and Row, 1950
32. Follingstad D, Kilmann PR, Robinson E, et al.: Prediction of self-actualization in male participants in a group conducted by female leaders. J Clin Psychol 32:706–712, 1976
33. Maccoby E, Jacklin C: The Psychology of Sex Differences. Stanford, Stanford University Press, 1974
34. Fuller F: Influence of sex of counselor and of client on client experssion of feeling. J Counseling Psychol 10:34–40, 1963

35. Brooks L: Interactive effects of sex and status on self-disclosure. J Counseling Psychol 21:469–474, 1970
36. Abramowitz CV, Abramowitz SI, Weitz LJ, et al.: Sex related effects on clinicians' attributions of parental responsibility for child psychopathology. J Abnorm Child Psychol 4:129–138, 1976
37. Hoffman M: Sex differences in empathy and related behavior. Psychol Bull 84:712–722, 1977
38. Abramowitz SI, Abramowitz CV, Roback HB, et al.: Sex related countertransference in psychotherapy. Arch Gen Psychiatry 33:71–73, 1976
39. Wittkower ED, Robertson BM: Sex differences in psychoanalytic treatment. Am J Psychother 31:66–75, 1977
40. Miller JB: Aggression in women and men. Presented at the Annual Meeting of the American Academy of Psychoanalysis, New York, New York, December 1, 1979
41. Bernardez Bonesatti T: Women and anger: Conflicts with aggression in contemporary women. J Am Med Women's Assoc 33:215–219, 1978
42. Chodorow N: The fantasy of the perfect mother. Presented at Michigan State University, East Lansing, Michigan, April 18, 1980
43. Carter CA: Advantages of being a woman therapist. Psychother: Theory Res Pract 8:297–300, 1971
44. Kell W, Burow J: Developmental Counseling and Therapy. Boston, Harcourt Brace Jovanovich, 1974
45. Bernardez Bonesatti T, Stein TS: Separating the sexes in group psychotherapy: An experiment with men's and women's groups. Int J Group Psychother 29:493–502, 1979

Chapter 18

Epilogue

RICHARD L. GRANT

AN INVITATION TO THE READER

You have now arrived at virtually the same place I was when, having read the penultimate drafts from the contributors, I paced the floor searching for what I might say to you. During this book's development, months went by where thoughts about what I had agreed to do were banished from consciousness. Finally, with all the drafts before me and a "While You Were Out" phone message from Ken Solomon on my desk, I either had to say something to you or quit. Finding myself uncharacteristically decidophobic, I needed help. Support for either side of my ambivalence was clearly in order. So I called Ken and explained. The direction of his encouragement is obvious. With expected humanistic understanding, Ken, having read previously written portions of this epilogue, urged me to persist.

Following, then, are my two major reactions to the book distilled from the melange of feelings, thoughts, and opinions engendered in me by the chapters I read. Next, I describe the change that has been taking place in my perspective about men over the last several years, especially as they impact my views about psychotherapy. Finally, I present my understanding of the term "androgyny" and how I believe it relates to psychotherapeutic endeavors.

I would truly be pleased if this very personal view could elicit sufficient reaction to lead you to change this monologue into a dialogue by writing to me about your perspectives. Whether supportive or critical, such contact can only have a salubrious effect on my growth as a person, therapist, and man. And such an effect is, I'm sure, the *raison d'être* of this book.

DISPARATE REACTIONS TO THE BOOK

The contributions to this volume were both stimulating and disquieting to me. The expansion of our knowledge about men appeals to my belief in the

RICHARD L. GRANT • Department of Psychiatry, University of Colorado Health Science Center, and Southeastern Colorado Family Guidance and Mental Health Center, La Junta, Colorado 81050

value of information in expanding our repertoire of choices in an ambiguous world. The excitement I feel in learning things I did not know was once again rekindled as I read. There was also a more private satisfaction that a group of which I was part was getting some specific and deliberate attention in its own right.

What troubled me then? As a militant eclectic, confessed devil's advocate, and self-appointed men's apologist, I had misgivings about the almost crusading sense of advocacy for change in men implicit and explicit in the writings. Intimations of scapegoating males, a strong theme in the feminists' orchestration for societal change, are reflected inappropriately in the writings. Psychoanalytic theory is greatly overrepresented in contrast with other schools of psychological thought. To me, sweeping overgeneralizations from the data abound. All these from the same authors who say we are just beginning to scratch the surface of the knowledge we may yet come to know about ourselves.

These two elements of the book, scientific knowledge and perhaps biased exhortations for change, begged integration. To attempt this, I tried to discern the goals and nature of this collection. Earlier, I surmised that change, growth, progress (however it should be phrased) is the basic goal of this book. But what kind of change, in whom, for what purpose, with what consequences? Without answers to these questions, I was unable to achieve even a modicum of closure between my two reactions to the book.

If change is the goal, then the kinds of changes that might result from reading this book could be scientific, sociopolitical, intrapersonal, interpersonal, professional, or perhaps, others. Each of these roles is potentially, if not actually, part of each reader's persona and should somehow be impacted by aspects of these chapters. After all, this is one of those unusual books that integrates the three kinds of literature described in Chapter 1, by O'Neil: popular, nonempirical social scientific, and research. In company with most psychological literature, and in contrast with compilations on nonpsychological topics such as physics, engineering, or biology, which appeal most to the scientific and professional roles played by people, the readers are invited regularly to consider the implications of these writings for their intrapersonal, interpersonal, and political roles as well. I doubt if even the most objective of scientists could read these chapters without some reflections on their personal existence, on the discrepancies between their real and ideal selves, on which of these selves may need revamping, or on their nascent or activist concerns for society and its direction.

Experiencing at this point the exhilaration of an "ah ha" phenomenon, I saw emerging the central issue around which I could integrate both information and misgivings. This book, for me, is primarily a resource for psychotherapists. Oh yes, seekers of intrapersonal and interpersonal growth will find nourishing fare, sociopolitical activists will discover support for their favorite concerns, and scientists, social and psychological, will clearly applaud the expansion of knowledge and its sequela: even more questions to be studied. But, it was now clear to me that I wished to speak as a psychotherapist to that part of any reader's professional role that is also psychotherapist. To do this I have described the personal odyssey I undertook on the way on the two conclusions reached after reading the chapters.

The first conclusion is that ideologies supporting political activism for pro-humanistic social change, however desirable, may not be best suited to the conduct of individual or family psychotherapy, at least with certain people.

The second conclusion is that men, their behavior, their motivations, and their turmoil need as much empathic, nonpejorative acceptance and understanding by our scientists and political activists as by our psychotherapists.

I have not before seen so clearly how my desire for a more humanistic society with reduced sexism and racism might prejudice the effectiveness or appropriateness of my psychotherapy. Nor have I felt more strongly that it is not men but an undecipherable combination of genetics and environmental learning that has brought us all to our current condition. To hold or intimate that men disproportionately contributed to our condition appears to be both unfounded and bad tactics.

A Change in Perspective

Were I to have written this Epilogue several years ago, my perspective, sad to say, would have been narrower than that I am now able to offer. I say this is sad because at that time, I recall experiencing a smug satisfaction with my views about men and with my thoughts on how to bring about the changes I perceived to be needed. I admit to having fallen victim to the popular mode of thinking seen in a preponderance of recent discussions that might be characterized as myopic certitude. With self-conscious, ineluctable pride, I characterized my views and behavior as progressive, emancipated, unsexist, benevolent, and liberated. At least I thought so. I even thought that the changes needed in society should be reflected in the psychotherapy I did.

The direction for the future was obvious to me and the hypothesis on which it was based simple. Men are equal victims with women of an unthinkingly evolved system that cast them into complementary roles. Instead of a virtual symmetry befitting the apparently logical equality of the sexes, human potentials were split into pairs where one role was distinctly different from the other. Each was necessary but associated or identified predominantly with only one gender. The earliest paradigm for the complementarity of gender roles concerned reproduction with its impregnation and child-bearing distinctions. With the waning of pure animal-like subsistence living, other roles became differentiated, again on physical grounds. Larger size and strength on the one hand, contrasted with their opposites. Women also needed some protection during the gestational cycle. There followed such logical role differentiations as hunting versus cooking and fighting versus sustenance. From these roles there evolved a set of role distinctions based not primarily on physical attributes, but rather on the roles that had come about because of those attributes: Toughness versus succor, independence versus dependence, and ultimately dominance versus submission are the residuals of our heritage.

There is some evidence to suggest that male and female brain anatomy and biochemistry are different in ways that might affect behavior.[1] Mankind, however, is thought to be much better able than other animals to use intelligence to override perhaps instinctive gender-dimorphic behavior. For this discussion, I am going to assume that most gender-specific stereotypic behaviors do not have an underlying biological imperative. They just evolved.

What began as a logical partition of roles became unthinkingly extended by succeeding participants. Distinctly different self-concepts evolved for males and females and came to have a life of their own and an ability to shape and influence behavior. The role-distinct behavior generated by the different self-concepts then reinforced the inappropriate nonphysically based self-concepts in a type of reverberating circuit removed from its source.

Yes, I said, that is how it came about. That is how we got to the mid-Twentieth Century. Many of the gender-role distinctions were inappropriate, that is, not based on any current reality other than the also inappropriate self-concepts that fueled the behaviors and were reinforced by them. Sexism was in full flower and everyone was its victim. Given this atavistic pattern, it seemed logical that the historical trends in the Western world toward redress for the underdog would eventually discover and alter sexism's inappropriatenesses. The so-called Women's Movement continues to be that effort.

It is an interesting historical conjunction that sexism and racism are both under attack at the same time. Both movements have long histories replete with important events, but the last two decades really mark the burgeoning of awareness, and most importantly, legislation (society's mechanism for legitimization), aimed at eliminating inequities without basis in fact. In the last two decades the Black Movement was quickly followed by the Women's Movement and the Hispanic Movement. In these efforts for equality the "oppressor" was associated almost always with the male gender and usually the Caucasian race. But, I reasoned, males were as conditioned and driven by their history as the rest.

I accept as a given that movements must push against something in the way adolescents must push away from their parents. Today, we can see an inexorable dialectic process in action concerning the place of men in our culture. The thesis of that process, concerning men and social relationships, is how things have been; the antithesis is how things might or even "should" be; the synthesis is how they evolvingly are. Perhaps to risk being teleologic, the purpose of the antithesis is to alter the status quo. By casting the role men have fulfilled as the thesis, then the pressures and forces for change in the relationships between men and women are the antithesis. Men have not been the instigators in this process, but the dialectic imperative nevertheless will see to change in men and their roles. No real alteration in a social system will leave any essential subset unchanged. The task then is for men to chart a course during this evolution to a different definition of the interacting roles of men and women.

It seemed males had two choices. They could resist and fight the accusations, thus confirming the perjoratives about them and providing usefully more impetus to the growing independence of the "minorities," or agree and identify with the theses of those groups. Between this Scylla and Charybdis there seemed little opportunity to establish a separate identity that was desirable. However difficult, "reasonable" men decided that we needed to quit doing certain things and begin doing certain other things. In almost every case, the impetus for change stemmed from problems defined by the "minorities." Men were reactive rather than proactive, but not necessarily in disagreement with the goals.

In this atmosphere of cultural self-reconditioning and with the reinforcement of "minority" representatives and the small "liberal" subculture closest to me, I gradually attempted to take on those ideals given earlier along with their behavioral expressions. It seemed perfectly clear that I, as a white male, was no better than a Mexican–American, Indian, Black, or woman. With the zeal of a convert approaching enlightenment, I embraced the philosophies and took on those attributes that were aimed at the assumed desirable and attainable goal of equality or symmetry. I shared household duties. I welcomed women calling me for a date. I made active efforts to hire and work with minorities. I decided to sit down to urinate because it made less of a mess to clean. I split lunch checks. I gave "boys" toys to girls and vice versa. And more importantly, it seemed to me essential to promulgate these ideals. As a psychiatrist, my treatment approaches at the very least suggested the importance of expunging unentitled dominance in males and of encouraging assertiveness in women. I believe subassertiveness leads to depression through the mediation of a sense of helplessness. I believe domination, as contrasted with leadership, leads to depression through helplessness' partner, alienation.

But the Holy Grail of equality seemed not within my personal grasp or sphere of influence. How, I asked, was it possible for a disagreement or argument between two men or two women to be reasonable and legitimate (nonsexist) when an argument with an opposite-gender partner earns the label "sexist?" Could one have a confrontation with a partner over control that solely came out of a bilateral philosophical stance of equality? Further, the question of whether males as a group had any abiding and unique core philosophy or role, other than the procreative one, nagged me more and more. Could maleness be defined without reference to femaleness? Is there a reasonable set of roles for males that will not be the Punch for some Judy?

These were interesting questions to me; both personally and professionally. As a member of the American Psychiatric Association (APA), I had access to colleagues for whom these questions should be especially germane. Yet, my peers did not seem to be addressing them. Yes, recognition and leverage for Blacks, Hispanics, and women has increased in the APA, hopefully to a meaningful level. Yet, I did not hear the males, especially the overwhelmingly white male majority of the APA, addressing these questions at their annual meetings. The Gay Caucus of recent years was on the right track but seemed limited to a movement for legitimization of personal freedom in sex-object choice. As a forum for a broad exploration of maleness, it would not appeal to most male members of the APA.

It was at this point of my thinking in 1977 that Norm Levy and I instigated the idea of an Open Forum at the APA annual meetings. This is a mechanism whereby a topic is announced, meeting space is provided, and any interested members or guests may come and take part in a discussion of the announced topic. The idea for using the Open Forum came from Ann Chappell, an active participant in the Women's Caucus of the APA. Our Open Forum, "On Being a Male," in 1977 attracted a small but enthusiastic group. As an outgrowth of that beginning, Norm, and later Ken Solomon, have organized Special Scientific Sessions at succeeding APA meetings on issues related to males. This book incorporates some of the invited papers those Special Sessions brought together.

These sessions, attended by people interested in the topic, provided some continued support for my own evolving goals and my chart of a course as a person and psychiatrist. The social and behavioral scientists who presented papers elucidated interesting facets of the role of being a male in contemporary society. My faith in the importance of gathering data was affirmed. Striving for egalitarianism continued worthwhile. Expansion of my understanding of aspects of being male could only augment my approaches to psychotherapy. My own personal direction seemed confirmed.

This takes me up to the summer of 1979 when I was asked to contribute to this volume. That request became an occasion to review my thoughts. Out of my rethinking and reformulating came the discovery that my position, despite my desires, was really a very narrow one. This was so for two reasons.

First, and easiest to define, any views I held about what might be a desirable direction for males were coming from a person totally unrepresentative of males and very much insulated on a day-to-day basis from the normal or predominant concerns of men. Twenty-five years of formal education and training, being in a vocation providing psychological mindedness, challenge, complexity, and high satisfaction, being white and aspiring to upper-middle-classness, and having only an untroubling number of doubts about ability, or capacity for emotional expression, appropriate dependency/independency, and sexuality separate me almost completely from the mainstream. Like perhaps all the male authors in this book and many of their subjects or the responders of studies they report, I am unable to assume that I have access to anything but a very limited and skewed view of males.

Further, the sample of patients I have seen over 17 years of providing psychotherapy as part of an academic medical career did not help. Being almost exclusively white and seeking fee-for-service psychotherapy made the men I saw as limited as I myself was. It was not until mid-1978, when I became medical and clinical director of a rural comprehensive community mental health center, that I came more intimately in contact with what might be more widely held concerns and problems facing men. This did not come just from clients in the mental health center, but also from the remarkably increased contact I had with men (and women) in the community at large. Playing softball and poker, meeting with the Ministerial Alliance, contacting men in the Elks, Kiwanis, or Lions, buying and caring for a horse, going hunting, going to Mexican-American fiestas, dancing in honky-tonks, and engaging in the social life of a small community exposed me to attitudes, beliefs, and behaviors that heretofore rarely, if ever, impinged on my limited personal interactions.

Besides being unrepresentative of males, and not regularly or meaningfully exposed to the full range of male concerns, my view was further narrowed by a second factor. I had confused the concepts of egalitarianism, equality, and symmetry. I had thought that there was a close parallelism in the application of these concepts to individual interpersonal relationships and to such fields of human interaction as politics, employment and business, sports, religion, and the law. Sexism, the mistaken belief that skills and attributes can be determined solely from the fact of gender, affects choices and judgments in all these fields as well as in social and interpersonal relationships. Decisions based on a sexist frame of reference can equally misjudge men and women. In the fields of specialized human endeavor mentioned, it seems reasonable that, as nearly as possible, judgments should be made on the real assets and deficits of the individual in question. The question is not can men be effective seamstresses but, can this person be effective at sewing? Equal opportunity, as uninfluenced by sexism as possible, is the goal. In that sense, men and women should have parity, be viewed as equals. For completeness, the term racism could be substituted for sexism and dealt with in the same manner. Whether sexism or racism is the question, the term and goal of equality is appropriate, I thought.

Not only did I find racism and sexism flourishing, I began to wonder if I had found their Source. My "modern, liberated, and progressive" views suddenly belonged in quotation marks because they were so stereotyped and limited. Where, I asked myself, was the appropriate sustaining goal-directed role or roles for the men I was meeting? That could give purpose and meaning to their choices of behavior? That could provide a rationale for behavior that was not just reactive or defensive? That could create a sense of purpose, meaning, and loving acceptance of oneself?

My fellow men found my views foreign, impractical, disruptive—in a word, wrong. When I thought of the consequences to them if they implemented the behaviors attendant on my views, I came to agree with them because the prevailing social network is highly punishing of deviance. Initially, I had looked on my fellows' reluctance to rid themselves of the inappropriate self-concepts and behaviors as reprehensible. A certain lack of empathy pervaded my responses. Fortunately, this is giving way to my searching anew for a sense of what a man is, what it is to be male and how I can contribute to my fellow man.

One of the first principles to go was that of the attainability of equality or symmetry in male/female relationships. Equality in the abstract, as in equal opportunity, is obviously desirable. Yet, equality is not a specific thing that can be applied to actual interpersonal relationships. Any two people interacting are in the abstract equal. Neither person has equality to give to another. Each has it until one or the other, or both, behaves unequally. It seemed to me that trying to translate the abstract concept of equality into interpersonal relationships obscured an identification of the process whereby satisfying and productive interpersonal interactions are maintained. Between the sexes, mutually satisfactory complementarity seems to be the essential ingredient for the continuance of supportive, growth-encouraging, loving, interpersonal relationships. By complementarianism, I mean the structuring of responsibilities and interactions according to present skills, goals for future skills, satisfaction, and reason. People engage in complementarianism by reciprocally behaving in a complementary manner with others in some of their interactions. An insistance on totally symmetric (equal) behavior precludes such collaboration.

By viewing interactions between any two people on Haley's continuum[2] from symmetrical to complementary, I could now see how equality or symmetry was an interfering concept. First of all, no two people are equal. They bring unique histories, personality styles, skills, attitudes, and goals to their exchange. Secondly, if there are differences needing resolution, the only way that will come about is for one or both parties to relinquish their need for equality or symmetry in favor of satisfactory complementariness. With troubled couples, the problem is not a lack of equality. Rather, the dilemma is that one or both is dissatisifed with the degree of complementariness. Useful treatment improves the degree of satisfaction either by a reappraisal and change in the attitude that led to the dissatisfaction or by changing one's own behavior sufficiently to get the other person to change. With some couples where the roles are strongly gender stereotyped, changes in those roles are virtually impossible. Restoring satisfaction to the complementariness is reasonable and accomplishable. Androgynous attitudes and behavior may seem appropriate for the future, but for most of the patients seen in our rural mental health center, they are inappropriate, maladaptive, and perhaps even distress-producing. I want to advise caution in applying the concept of androgyny to psychotherapy. The caution is against the disquieting militancy in the change-agency advocacy language of some of the authors in this book.

ANDROGYNY

As a way of managing my disquiet, I wish to digress into the well-accepted technique of cognitive restructuring. I hope the following explication of the concept of androgyny performs the same useful function for any reader who shares my concern as it did for me.

It will take more research, more writings, and more reflections before our knowledge concerning the differences between men and women will be at a level where recommendations for what might be ideal may be made with any certainty. Meanwhile, androgyny, or more clearly stated, psychological and behavioral androgyny, is put forward as the most current best guess as to a potentially ideal identity and set of behaviors for both men and women. Refining the concept of androgyny with the terms psychological and behavioral as it is apparently meant in today's context is important. The original definition of androgyny and its adjectival variant androgynous have in the past meant a union or melding of the physical aspects of the sexes. Usage of these terms over the years has gradually come to take on a behavioral and psychological interpretation. But, in order, to account for the various levels of dimorphic sex roles defined by Money,[3] especially the sex-irreducible and sex-derivative roles, it seems more clear to speak of psychological and behavioral androgyny. This, then, is a possible, if not desirable, set of beliefs and behaviors that allows for the presence of sex-irreducible, and perhaps even sex-derivative roles still to be clearly legitimate for both men and women. Changes in gender identity/role, the related psychological and behavioral aspects of a person, will obviously be most possible in Money's sex-arbitrary roles, less possible in the sex-adjunctive roles, still less possible for sex-derivative roles, and not at all possible for the sex-irreducible roles.

At the risk of stating the obvious: androgyny can never reduce the differences between the sexes to zero. At best, there will be a redefinition of what is pridefully and legitimately male or female with a reduction in the number of examples of sex-arbitrary, sex-adjunctive, and sex-derivative roles or behaviors that have previously been considered core elements in male and female gender identity/roles. As used here, my use of the concept androgyny embodies this redefinition and recognizes its differential penetrance into the various levels of sexually dimorphic roles. It carries no implicit or explicit threat of loss of core gender identity/role.

As a way of conceptualizing and simplifying the concept of androgyny, a metastructural model has been deduced from the many examples given by authors in this volume. The model represents the various dimensions of known or believed differences between men and women. Most of the differences are characterized by a continuum wherein a particular attitudinal or behavioral component is represented as occurring at a greater frequency or intensity in men as opposed to its frequency or intensity in women, or vice versa. Many authors in this volume comment that, except for sex-irreducible identity/roles, the differences between men and women are differences in frequency.

Figure 1 depicts this metamodel. The horizontal axis represents either frequencies or intensities of occurrence of the (any) behavior or attitude in question from low to high. The vertical axis gives the number of people, when measured by a hypothetical meta-instrument, who characteristically score at a given level

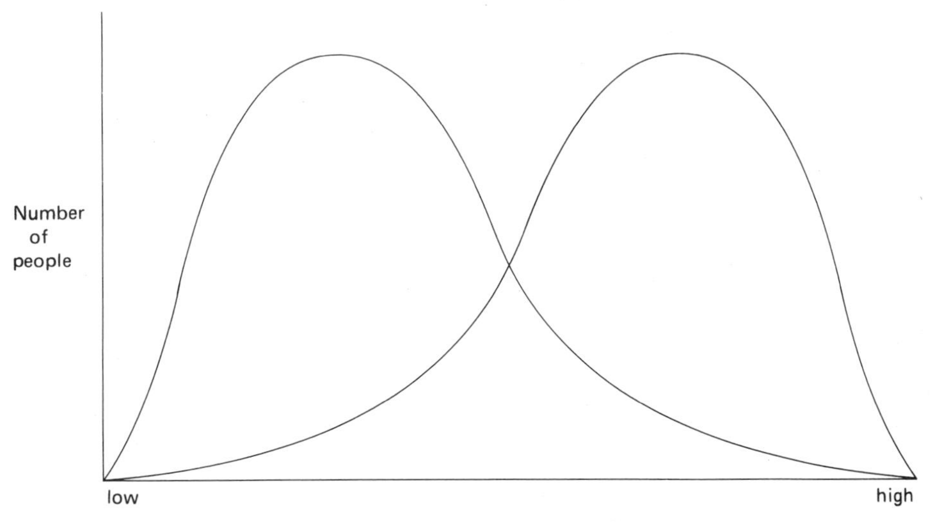

Figure 1. *Metamodel for male/female differences.*

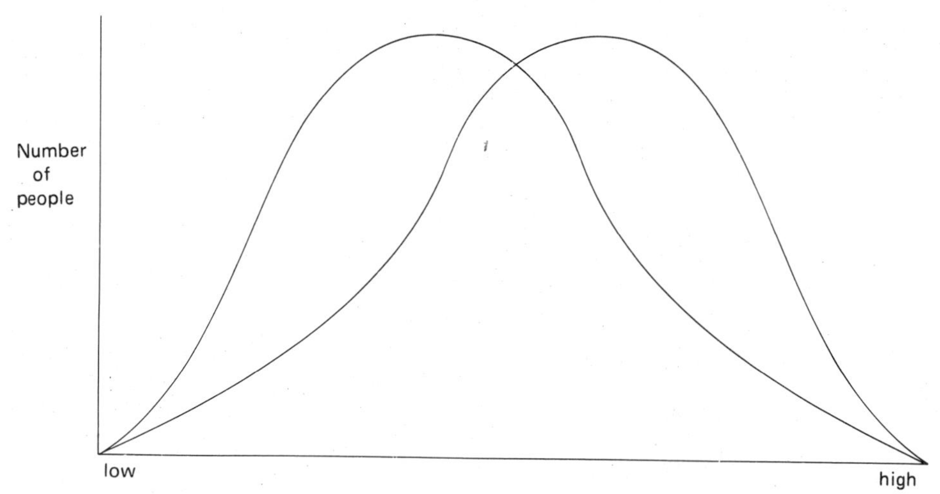

Figure 2. *Representation of male/female differences on self-disclosure. U.S. residents with grade 12 education.*

on the dimension being measured. The number of men and women at each level of intensity are represented separately to demonstrate both that as groups they are different and that there are some individuals from one group who are identical with individuals from the other group.

Culture, ethnicity, education, wealth, health, geographic location (urban–rural, north–south, Africa–United States), religion, and probably other demographic variables would affect the shape, overlap, and skewness of the figure. For instance, if Figure 1 represented the U.S. population as a whole on the dimension of self-disclosure, then Figure 2 shows a guess for the curves for all the residents of the U.S. with a completed 12th grade education or over when the same dimension, self-disclosure, is being measured. Men and women still differ but there is more overlap than on Figure 1. Such demographic influences on the concept of the differences between men and women are important elsewhere in this discussion and especially bear on psychosocial treatment philosophy and approaches. For this discussion of androgyny, such differences will be set aside.

Androgyny, like sexism, racism, feminism, or masculinism (if there is such a word or concept) is never distinguishable solely from the occurrence of a single discrete behavior. Each of these terms is a construct or judgment that is selected from several possibilities as a principle that best explains or accounts for the behavior involved. For instance, a man hired to do sewing work might be fired after two weeks work by a woman supervisor. His performance was substandard. One cannot label the firing sexist; it might just be smart. If one knew the supervisor to have stated that a man cannot handle the work or that women with equally substandard performance at two weeks were always kept on longer, then the inference of sexist behavior is warranted. In the absence of these two or other knowledgeable backgrounds associated with sexist beliefs, then the firing would have to be called something else, perhaps performancist, indicating a bias based on a performance priority belief.

This elaboration hopefully makes the point that a given behavior cannot be ascribed to an abstract category of behaviors without knowledge of the context, pattern, and motivation or intent of the behavior. A person cannot be said to be behaving androgynously from a given behavior. Only a knowledge of the patterns of that person's behaviors, the specific contexts of those behaviors, and the intent and motivation for the behavior would help us say that the person is behaving androgynously.

Returning to Figure 1, further elaboration on the model represented there is now possible. To continue the fantasy about instruments or measures that would yield such data, suppose the universe of continua which now differentiate men and women could be defined, or suppose a portion of that universe which would validly represent it could be selected. Suppose further that scores across those continua could be accumulated and that this process would yield a continuum score on which men and women in general would be differentiated. Each person represented then has a single composite score derived from the several representative continua chosen. The distribution of such composite scores could then be said to be represented in Figure 1. This now is a derived scale of androgyny. But where is androgyny? Obviously, somewhere in the center. Central scores represent a balance. With too high a score, a person is more stereotypically female. Likewise, with too low a score, a person is more stereotypically male.

Here we get to the crux of my concern and reservations about the androgyny movement and how its principles should impact psychiatrists and other psychotherapists. For this discussion, self-help groups, consciousness-raising activities, and personal growth endeavors are all assumed to be generically similar to the activites of psychotherapy. With some exceptions, no one specifically undertakes any of these activities without some desire for change in the self or others. This desire can be seen as motivated by some internal perception of distress. Any activity devoted to amelioration of this distress can then be said to have goals. As I discuss the goals of psychotherapy, I assume an identity between them and the goals of the other activities written of elsewhere in this volume and represented by the terms above.

Goals of Psychotherapy

What, then, are the goals of psychotherapy? Certainly, to become relatively capable of adjusting with minimal unnecessary distress to any given status quo is insufficient. This could apply to slaves, prisoners, sexist or racist discriminatees, other downtrodden, or any other group not now considered permissible in a humanistic, egalitarian society. Yet, most people presenting with distressing symptomatology are, in fact, in conflict with all or part of their own specific status quo or real world. Expanding their repertoire of behaviors to deal more effectively with their real world and to reduce their distress is a clearly desirable goal. It is a necessary but not sufficient definition of the goals of psychotherapy.

To enhance an individual's capacity to act effectively toward change of an undesirable up-til-then status quo appears to be also a necessary goal of psychotherapy. This imperative is stronger the more the particular conditions are non-humanistic, demoralizing, and symptom-producing for the individual.

These two goals, reduction of maladaptiveness and unnecessary distress and change agency, are in some ways inimical. A reduction of distress often mitigates the desire for change in the outside world. In fact, most people in psychotherapy stop when the first goal is met. Their personal distress is sufficiently reduced and they can handle their real world and do not perceive change in their environment as necessary. Others, especially as they incorporate social distress as a personally perceived distress, are more likely to pursue the goals of acting on their environment. As soon as that environment becomes expanded to include people and procedures out of their immediate personal experience, then their actions are more in the political than the psychological arena. Political activism is not one of the appropriate goals of psychotherapy.

It is at this point that two potential aspects of the psychotherapist may become confused. On the one hand, the therapist is dedicated to the alleviation of distress in individual patients. On the other, recognizing the impact of societal forces impacting patients and contributing to the personal distress of patients, the therapist may wish to be a change agent and political activist against such social inequities as discrimination, nonhumanistic interpersonal interactions, or other undesirable-isms. My role as therapist is more or less clearly distinguishable from my desire to change unwanted societal conditions. The arena for the latter is never in the consulting room.

CONCLUSION

My misgivings about that part of this book that seemed to suggest excessive enthusiasm in embracing androgyny are now set to rest. Psychotherapy is not the place for me to engage in social activist activities inappropriate to the ideosyncratic needs of each patient. As the clinical director of the mental health center, I find myself with a remarkable frequency pointing out to the clinicians the high level of antimale bias that pervades their case presentations and treatment planning. These clinicians are young, well educated men and women caught up, as I was, in an enthusiasm for redress of sexism's consequences. Unfortunately, it takes some effort in therapy to avoid using the victim/victimizer theme that has been part of the necessary social/political tactics to reduce sexism.

By reading these chapters, I am left with a greater desire to accept and care about men. I am sure there is an irreducible core gender identity/role for men. Many of those attitudes and behaviors once thought essential to being a male can now be viewed as unnecessary. I believe we can help our fellow men best with a gentle acceptance of where they are now and a nonpejorative invitation to growth.

REFERENCES

1. Weintraub P: The Brain: His And Hers. Discover 2(4):14–20, 1981
2. Haley J: Strategies of Psychotherapy. New York, Grune and Stratton, 1963
3. Money J: Love and Love Sickness. Baltimore, The Johns Hopkins University Press, 1980

Chapter 19

Counterepilogue

Wolfgang Lederer

It is an ungrateful task, after so many able and diligent scholars have carefully presented the sum and essence of their experiences and opinions, have properly documented them with quotations from the latest sources, and have in the end proclaimed their near-consensus—it is an ungrateful task now to come along and counter them, question their premises and conclusions, and assert that the very data they base themselves on can as easily be given the opposite interpretation. And yet, since this is the task this author has been assigned, he must put his mind to it and in the spirit of fairness, attempt to put forth the sense of the matter as he sees it, grateful to the editors for permitting this lone voice of dissent.

To begin then, let him review the image of man as it is presented or implied in the preceding pages. But let him immediately suggest that while the picture to be reviewed is astonishing in and of itself, the near-unanimity of the authors as to man's misdeeds and vile nature is such as to cause misgivings, unanimity of opinion being most often a matter of fashion, of like talking only to like, rather than of enduring wisdom or science.

And so: What a piece of work is man? How noble in reason! How infinite in faculty! In form, in moving, how express and admirable! In action, how like an angel! In apprehension, how like a god! But no: The author is quoting Hamlet here, when he should be quoting his fellow authors! They put it otherwise.

Man as He Appears to Our Authors

They say that man is *in and of himself,* limited by his sex role (O'Neil): Brutal in his muscular strength (Nadelson and Nadelson), he has a need to prove his masculinity (Balswick), to be a sturdy oak (Solomon). Hence, he is aggressive, assertive, and success-oriented (Stein) to the point of causing all international violence (Nadelson and Nadelson). He is and must be tough, cool, unemotional,

---

Wolfgang Lederer • Department of Psychiatry, University of California Medical School, San Francisco

invulnerable (Gould), a fearless fighter (O'Neil, Gould) who is yet afraid to cry (Solomon) and takes counterphobic risks (Solomon). He is a dolt without artistic appreciation (Boles and Tatro) and altogether destructive (Bernardez).

In his *dealings with other men* he has a driving need to add up to something (Solomon), yet he is impatient and noncooperative (Boles and Tatro), insensitive (Nadelson, Solomon, Boles and Tatro), nonaffiliative (Nadelson, Boles and Tatro), competitive (Balswick, Solomon, Stein, Norton), emotionally isolated (Bernardez), status conscious, interrupting and disrespectful, and avoiding of noncompetitive physical contact (Stein).

Toward women he is conventional in manner, but basically hostile (Solomon). He manages neither affection nor gentleness (Nadelson, Stein, Boles and Tatro); his genitals are separated from his emotions (Balswick, Gould), hence he is incapable of intimacy (Nadelson, Balswick, Solomon) and sexually inhibited (Gould). No wonder he tends to be a "detached avoider" or an "angry griever," unless he becomes a "devoted clinger" (Halle). In any case, he is immature (Halle), denies dependency (Solomon), tends to dominate (Nadelson, Stein), control (Solomon), and oppress (Stein, Bernardez) (often through the irritating qualities of logic and intellect [Stein]), and lacking altogether in introspection, he is incapable of self-disclosure or of sharing affective experiences (Stein). In fact, he seems to be totally inexpressive of emotion (Balswick, Solomon, Stein, Bernardez, Dosser, Wong) unless he explodes with repressed anger (Solomon).

As to his *children,* he does not love them (Boles and Tatro), is a nonnurturing (Lewis and Roberts), distant (Nadelson), and inadequate father (Stein).

No wonder then that he feels deeply *guilty* of being a man (Stein, Bernardez), feels heartily *sick* of his masculinity (O'Neil, Bernardez), and is overcome by a longing to *change* (Solomon, Stein). He wants to break through the emotional limitations of his sex role and stop being such a brute, and his salvation, we are told, is *androgyny:* for a man to be redeemed from the curse placed on him by his gender he clearly must strive to be as little like a man and as much like a woman, as he can manage. Men, in short, must learn how to "unbecome men" (Stein).

Let the author hasten to admit that the distillate from the preceding pages which he has just set forth presents a picture more strident, if not to say more absurd, than that given by any single one of the authors. Yet there is no denying that when this book speaks of "changing male roles," it is never neutrally descriptive. On the contrary, it openly admits a bias in favor of femininity, of which it mentions only the warmest, most endearing, most positive aspects (Nadelson, Stein), while the positive qualities of manliness are altogether omitted. The relationship between the sexes is uniformly seen as antagonistic, with man in the role of the oppressor and woman the victim: a currently popular, but not necessarily an accurate or a constructive point of view. It places man on trial much as the sons of Kulaks in Russia or the sons of intellectuals in China were put on trial: "You are by birth a member of that wicked class. Now admit to being an oppressor, an exploiter, a traitor. . . ."—and nothing but the most meekly humble confession will do.

Well: let us examine to what extent this inquisitorial approach may, or may not, be justified.

WHAT A MAN IS IN AND OF HIMSELF

Money, in his admirably concise and factual Foreword to this volume, makes clear the simple fact that the only sex-irreducible male function is that of impregnation; whatever else we consider male is sex-derivative or perhaps merely sex-arbitrary. All male roles, except the male sex role, can be performed by women as well, or by some women, at any rate; and to that extent a man is nothing special, or even largely superfluous, since his sex role, while essential, takes up such a minute part of his life. This potential superfluity of the man is a fact of immeasurable importance: a woman's sex role lasts much longer and is much more obvious than a man's, and to that extent she has an irreduceable function of greatest importance for the species cut out for her, whereas a man at all times, though much more today than in the past, must prove to himself and others the worthwhileness, usefulness, and indispensability of his existence. A man therefore, more than a woman, has always been and is today *in quest of a meaning*.

Money speaks of those qualities which are sex-shared but threshold-dimorphic: they appear in both sexes, but more in one than in the other. Men have always attempted to justify their existence and to find their meaning by accentuating and exploiting to a maximum those threshold dimorphic qualities which make them in certain respects more capable than women. What are they?

Men are on the average, from infancy[1] and childhood[2] on, more muscular, and stronger, and have more physical energy. They have an urge to make use of their leaner limbs to roam, explore, penetrate new territory, and pit themselves against the unknown and its terrors. Listen by way of a splendid example, to Sir Richard F. Burton's[3] rhapsody on the delights of the "solitary wayfarer" in the Arabian desert:

> Above, through a sky terrible in its stainless beauty, and the splendors of a pitiless blinding glare, the Samun caresses you like a lion with flaming breath. Around lie drifted sand-heaps, upon which each puff of wind leaves its trace in solid waves, flayed rocks, the very skeleton of the mountains, and hard unbroken plains, over which he who rides is spurred by the idea that the bursting of a water-skin, or the pricking of a camel's hoof, would be a certain death of torture,—a haggard land infested with wild beasts, and wilder men,—a region whose very fountains murmur the warning words "Drink and away!" What can be more exciting? what more sublime? Man's heart bounds in his breast at the thought of measuring his puny force with Nature's might, and of emerging triumphant from the trial.

Nineteenth century romanticism? Not at all. For the appeal of stresses and dangers that try the most manly of a man's mettle has never slackened, and from the very midst of our pampered suburbs, young men still set forth alone in search of adventure and hardship or brave it in the company of like-minded fellows. Some of them risk their necks surfing or hang-gliding and others of the author's young patients have, without fuss or fanfare, trekked alone through ever-dangerous Afghanistan or traversed the Sahara on foot. Men climb mountains for the hell of it, to test their mind and muscle and to conquer the universal enemy, fear, and to come in touch, at the outer boundaries of experience, with the mystery of being, with the spirit, with God.[4,5] And for all that they must be, they *want* to be, *hard,* not soft, male, all male, and alone or in all-male company.

Nor is this male quest limited by the boundaries of visible earth. That very same urge translates into any kind of exploration, penetration, or intrusion into the make-up of matter, the laws of the physical universe, the structure and growth of abstract thought, or of the mind itself. The territories man's restless energies are exploring extend into all dimensions.

The "territory," from the most literal to the most abstract sense of the concept, must not only be explored, it must be defended. Men have, as a phylogenetic heritage, built into them a readiness to compete for and defend their territory, for it is in, on, and through their territory that their women and children, their families, clans, and nations have their being. Nesting and parentalism, states Money, are more prevalent in girls than in boys. But he neglects to state the fact that men, by virtue of their physical strength and their instrumental orientation, are generally the ones who *build* the "nest" and that their roaming, insofar as it has the purpose of hunting and gathering, contributes essentially to parenting. From the earliest days of which we have any evidence to the present day, men have always defended and supplied the "nest" and have seen in this their most *meaningful* activity. All other manly activities are extensions, elaborations—or perversions—of this basic function which is, essentially, *to serve.* Johnson quotes Goethe as having come to the insight that "man is to serve woman; then she will serve him."[5] To serve: to serve the family, a cause, or God: that is beyond a doubt the object of life and the true source of happiness.[5] Anyone who does not grasp that man's basic mission and purpose on earth is to serve the biologic function[6] of woman, to serve her needs, well-being, and happiness[7] has missed the point entirely.

But if indeed man finds his most basic meaning (hence satisfaction) consciously or unconsciously in the role of protector and provider, then most of the qualities the author listed before as having been severely criticized suddenly turn out to be quite positive. For a man to be a tough, even a brutal, aggressive fighter is negative only if he uses these qualities merely for himself, and not in the service of his "nest," his family, tribe, or community. For him to go out and face danger is indeed quintessentially manly and he would be of no use to his family if he refused to do so. While in combat, and it does not matter whether against a mammoth, an armed intruder, an adversary in a court of law, or a business competitor, he must indeed not cry; he must be in fullest control of himself and of his emotions and faculties. Self-control, far from being the burdensome straightjacket which some of our authors claim it to be, is in fact one of the hardest won, one of the most effective and proudest[8] manly achievements.

It is quite true that in some instances self-control, like a weak and uncertain government, becomes excessively and cripplingly restrictive. But control in and of itself consists not just of "turning off"; it consists of turning on or off at will and as the situation may require. Just so, a man who has himself securely under control can also securely let go; he can, for instance, quite safely cry with joy or with grief, as many great men of all times, including ours, have done. And just so, it is often the strongest men who are, in intimate situations, most gentle.

Men, says one of our authors (Bernardez), are destructive; and that, she implies, is wicked indeed. No doubt she has in mind the inquisitive manipulations of little boys let loose in a living room full of bric-a-brac. Yes, men are destructive, and every boy on his way to manhood must learn how to master the violent side of himself, so that he cannot be overcome by his rage but can use the power in it for conscious purposes.[5] Yes, men are at times legitimately destructive: of enemies, enemy cities, governments, existing values, and even of nature. They are (it is absurd that one should have to point this out) also the ones who, in the first place, built those cities, established those governments, agreed on those values. They did not establish nature, but the survival of our species, like the survival of any form of life, required at times not only living in and with her, but also opposing her. And insofar as men have caused her excessive and unnecessary damage, it has already become and henceforth will have to be their concern to minimize or perhaps reverse the destruction. Strength (and, of course, not just muscle, but brain strength, intelligence) is morally neutral. It can be used to build and to destroy. It is the very scheme of nature that anabolic and catabolic processes must always go hand in hand, that there is no construction without destruction, that the new always, at least in part, destroys the old, *must* destroy the old if it is to find room to live.[9] What needs to be destroyed is, in human society, a matter of judgment; but a man who could not destroy, be he architect, lawyer, or farmer, could not protect and provide. He could also not create; he would hardly be worth his keep.

And speaking of creation: Men, we are told by two of our authors (Boles and Tatro), lack artistic appreciation. This author does not mean to do them an injustice; they are no doubt referring to a very limited stratum of a very limited society and not to men in general. It is indeed true that in these United States, where schooling has so largely been placed in the hands of women, both learning in general and learning about art in particular did, among schoolboys and among those who never grew beyond that station, acquire the odor of femininity, and that such a taint, by males still shaky in their manliness, would have to be eschewed. But there is a creative, feminine element in every man, that aspect of him to which the Jungians refer as the *anima:*

> Some men seem to have an enormous anima potential. . . . This is neither good nor bad in its own right. If they can bring this feminine side to good development, then they can be highly creative men and *no less masculine* [italics this author's] just because of their powerful inner component. These are the artists, the seers, the intuitive, sensitive men who are so culturally valuable in any society.[5]

In fact, most art in all ages and places, including the United States today, has been and is being produced by men; surely to attribute a blanket lack of artistic appreciation to men is therefore nothing less than absurd.

MEN DEALING WITH OTHER MEN

It is undeniably true that men, in their dealings with other men, are often competitive. But it is remarkable that, as often as our authors have stated this fact, they have not once asked why. Yet, boys compete with boys, bulls with bulls, male terns with male terns, male cichlids with male cichlids; one has to go pretty far down the evolutionary ladder to find males of a given species who do not compete. They all complete *against* each other—and *for* the female. In many species, right up to our closest cousins, the apes, winner takes all: all the females are impregnated by the dominant male and no other male can get near them. Nor are we far removed from that: winners of our day, whether they be boxers, rock stars, Chairmen of the Board, or just plain President, they are all surrounded by worshipful women who see something in them that they want, without, by and large, being able to tell what it is. But it is in men just what it is in other species: the winner, the strongest, the fastest, the most cunning, the most resourceful, the most powerful all have one thing in common, namely, superior germ plasm. The females of all species know, without any special instruction, that the best male is likely to make them the best offspring, and they know instinctively that this is important. The man who wins in competition is not only likely to be the best protector and provider, he will have the best children, or at least, the probabilities point that way. In actual fact, things are of course more complicated.

It still remains that fighting among men helps to select the fittest, hence has a very fundamental positive value. But it is not true that, because men compete, they are therefore "noncooperative," "nonaffiliative," or "emotionally isolated." Competition among men, as among boys playing baseball, soccer, or any other competitive sport, has always also had the function of mutual training, of mutual exploration and appreciation of positive qualities, in fact: of mutual bonding. He who fights me best will be my best comrade-in-arms, my best friend. This has been true at all times, from Enkidu who fought Gilgamesh[10] and became his inseparable companion, to the leading brawlers in a contemporary schoolyard or the prosecutor and defense counsel whose acrimonious court battles induce in them, if not affection and friendship, then that professional respect which is among the most precious gifts men can bestow upon each other. The friend, the buddy, the comrade, the associate, the sidekick, figures of immeasurable importance to men[8] (and totally ignored in the preceding chapters), are all likely to have had to prove their mettle in some contest, their loyalty in some battle, and they are often more intimately and more durably related to a man than anyone besides his wife.

It is absurd to call men nonaffiliative considering that, in the natural order of things, they, and not the women, had the opportunity and the need to join in hunting, work, and war parties and, later, in armies, administrations, trading ventures, and all the complicated apparatus of civilization which indeed they joined to establish. Meanwhile the women, for whose security and welfare these matters were wrought, could hardly move for having one baby in the belly, one infant at the breast, one toddler at the hand, and who knows how many bigger ones pulling at their apron strings. These things have changed now in the Western world, for good reason, and women are proving what really should never have been in doubt: that they can function in organizations as well or as badly as men. But it remains that if by affiliation we mean something beyond the kinships that nature provides, then it was men who developed it and to this day, in the service of society, find in it their major function and employ.

That within the social apparatus and hierarchy men, like chickens or baboons, seek status, is absolutely true and needs no defense. Only two categories of men or, for that matter, women, can ignore status: those who are already on top and are beyond challenge and those who, for whatever reason, despair of attaining it. The first have nothing to prove; the second lack the ability to prove themselves. All in between are more or less acutely, more or less clearly, in formal terms of rank and insignia or in the most subtly understated gesture and symbols, aware of and striving for status. And status, particularly if self-won, is generally, and by and large rightly, regarded as indicative of a man's worth.

Status, of course, can be unearned and undeserved. It may be unduly flaunted or infinitely abused. But status properly speaking, namely, the position in society which a man has won for himself or has been assigned, and based on which he fulfills his functions and obligations in relation to all those to whom organizational lines connect him, on whom he depends and who depend on his functioning in just that manner, requires of a man the exertion of his best faculties, most of which, again, have never once been mentioned in the preceding chapters. In his position a man must, above all, be able to work hard and conscientiously in the face of fatigue and distraction and despite ill health or physical pain. He must function despite and regardless of his frailties, sufferings, passions, excitements, or despondencies. Such functioning, which we call "professionalism," requires a maximal amount of self-discipline and loyalty and is duly rewarded by a sense of self-confidence and a feeling of pride. And since pride in his accomplishments, whatever they may be, is to a man what only can be equalled by a mother's pride in her children, therefore the scorn cast in the preceding chapters on those qualities that may justify manly pride is mischievous indeed.

As to the supposed insensitivity of man, what can one say about it? That it is a myth? Surely not. There have been and are insensitive men as well as women. But the very prevalence of men artists, writers, musicians, and psychologists should make it self-evident that not all men are insensitive, that in fact many men have been teachers and educators in the use of the senses, and not only of those which function through nerve endings, but also of those far more complex sensory functions which we call intuition, empathy, sympathy, tact, taste, spirituality, and inspiration.

But men do wage war! And, say our authors, it is male competition which leads to war (Lewis and Roberts). Surely, they say, if women were in leadership positions, they would bring to them more gentle qualities and, by implication, would avoid war? Well, history does not seem to bear that out. There is something about positions of power which seems to bring out the male side of women, their *animus*. The famous queens and women rulers of the past or the present (e.g., Elizabeth I of England, Catherine the Great of Russia, Golda Meir, or Indira Ghandi) showed and show no less animosity and fight, no less willingness to go to war than would men in their place. The explanation would seem to be that while personalities may trigger or shape wars, they do not cause them. Rather are wars caused by competition for "territory" in the literal or figurative sense, by competition for space, food, and security which arise from the circumstances and exist regardless of whether the rulers be men or women. That wars are hell, frequently achieve nothing, and should be abolished, on this men and women are in full agreement, particularly now that a man can no longer console himself for the dangers and hardships of the "front" by the thought that he is at least helping to keep his family safe "back home" or keeping the war "far away from our shores." But how wars are to be ended once and for all: that is a problem which will require the best brains and efforts of men *and* women and it is naive indeed to think that substituting one for the other would do the trick.

Men in Relation to Women

It is in this area that the catalogue of men's sins, crimes, and defects as listed by our authors is most voluminous. Foremost amongst the accusations is this: that men dominate, control, oppress and exploit women and that they do this solely for the men's own benefit. Where there is that much smoke there must be at least some fire; let us look for it.

The job market would seem to be the logical place to start. There is no doubt that in many occupations women, doing the same work as men and doing it equally well or better, are still paid less and promoted more slowly than their male co-workers. That this is, with rare exceptions, unjustifiable and therefore a scandal to be remedied as fast as possible, no fair-minded person can deny. On the other hand, it is necessary to point out that women are not the only "minority" to be so treated, but that each ethnic, national, racial, religious, or sexual group as it newly "immigrated" into the job market has met with similar exploitive discrimination by those already established and defending their vested interests. Such discrimination has always taken time, effort, and sometimes bloody fighting to erase, but it is a dog-in-the-manger, not a sexual, issue. The same "male chauvinist pig" who bullies women, condescends to them, and discharges his fear of them through dirty jokes is quite likely to have quite similar attitudes toward ethnic groups other than his own or against whosoever his special target for contempt happens to be. That such bigotry is based on fear of the stranger, strange ways, or competition, is easy enough to see.

Which leads to a wider and even more basic matter: men's fear of women not just at work, but in any social setting, in the home, and in bed. To this fear, which the authors of the preceding chapters have almost entirely ignored, this author devoted a whole book,[11] but here it will suffice to sketch briefly some of its roots.

The author has already pointed out that a man, in and of himself, is not much and that he cannot derive self-justification, self-respect, or the meaning and purpose of his existence entirely from within himself. He must, in some capacity, serve something or someone, which reduced to the barest rudiments simply means to serve the continuation of his family, tribe, nation, culture, and species. Most men have a longing to participate in this process by means of their most "sex-irreducible faculty," to quote Money. But to that end, they need a woman. How to get her? And how to get her to cooperate?

It is quite true that some men, despairing of their ability ever to attract a women and to make her like or even love them, resort to force. Rapists exist, always have existed, and what with the acrimonious contemporary sexual climate there are perhaps more of them today than during most other periods in history. But the overwhelming majority of men are not rapists (not in the street and not in the marriage bed) and never will be. To obtain a woman they have to woo her and that can be both too difficult and too easy.

Some of the very best and most valuable men do not know how to go about it at all. They are the Beast in his lonely castle or the frog at the bottom of the well, who need the love of a woman in order to become the princes they are capable of being; they are the wild man–animal Enkidu or Hesse's "Steppenwolf" needing to be civilized by a prostitute; they are the boy, Kay, of Andersen's "The Snow Queen," sitting on the "icy mirror of reason" and awaiting redemption through the love and devotion of the girl, Gerda; they are the Flying Dutchman, roaming the storm-tossed seas, they are the feverish student Raskolnikov; all needing and longing to be saved from their terrible isolation by the love of a woman and all feeling basically unworthy of such love and despairing that the woman they cannot, dare not, reach for will ever come and reach for them. They fear that she will not see the prince within them of whom they themselves are but dimly aware; they fear that she will only see the lonely beast and turn away with contempt and disgust. As Johnson[12] puts it most beautifully:

> At his best, a man knows who he is; and he knows he has a god, a magnificent being, somewhere within him. But when a woman lights the lamp and sees the god in him, he feels called upon to live up to that, to be strong in his consciousness . . . he seems to require this feminine acknowledgement of his worth. . .

Because he needs her so much and because she may deny him the validation he requires, he fears her and may defensively act more beastly the more desperate he is.

At the other end of the continuum from the lonely seekers are the seducers who value women the less the more easily they are won. But Don Juan is not validated by his conquests; he momentarily makes women feel intensely desired and important, but beyond that he does not take charge of their needs and it is the fulfilling of a women's needs that fulfills a man. This is most sadly apparent in today's "body shops" or "meat markets," where not even seductive skill is required, but a casual conversation and a drink lead within the hour to sexual intercourse—without true intimacy, without any but the most technical sexual expectations, that is: without love or loyalty, without expectation of understanding or of commitment, and without any hope for the future. Such encounters, at best, release sexual tension, but they have no redemptive magic. They do not render the partners unique and uniquely important as true lovers are to each other, and in this context men and women fear each other for the disillusionment, the emptiness, the return to loneliness of the next morning.

But most men do manage to win a woman and to settle down to the lifelong task of meeting her needs and demands, and the lifelong risk of failing her. Sexual performance, social, professional, and financial status, and all the fame and fortune that men supposedly preen themselves with, are in truth quite relative and valuable only insofar as they elicit her proud admiration; there is nothing but gall and ashes if she greets them with scorn. No man, it is said, is a hero to his valet; but no man can truly feel a hero unless he is a hero to his woman. He fears that she may deny him her admiration—from lack of understanding, from indifference, from hate, that her sharp tongue may slash his pride, her moods deprive him of his reward, her contempt defeat him utterly. These, and many others which the author can skip in this context, are his fears. How does he react?

He reacts in one of the infinite variety of ways that constitute the vast spectrum of human behavior. It is quite true that some men, scared, hurt, or both, withdraw emotionally, sexually, or both, and exhibit overt or covert hostility to women or to their woman. It is true that some men become bullies and brutes, like frightened dogs that bite at the least provocation. It is quite true that some men, like some women, are just plain no damn good. But to maintain that all men are unfeeling and inconsiderate clods, as most of our authors imply or explicitly state, is one of the weirdest aberrations to be found in psychological literature. It appallingly ignores that in the whole history of humankind nothing has been as inspiring or has brought as much happiness as the love between man and woman. Yet in all the preceding chapters, there is no mention of love!

The author knows it is not necessary to document his point, but listen, just by way of contrast, to Sherwood Anderson: "I thought I had got into something like a strange new world. It was paradise. I had become a man. I was one who had been singled out by a . . . girl."[13] "The night," he says elsewhere,

> can never be quite gorgeous, to its full possibilities, without the woman. . . . There are the nights that come when you are excessively alive. . . . There is the woman beside you asleep. How quietly and softly she breathes. . . . Now the mind and the fancy both race. You seem to feel and hear, with her breathing, the breathing of the earth under your house, breathing of trees. There is a river just down a short hill from the house. It also breathes softly. Now the moon is breathing, the stars breathing. Woman, woman. . . . Woman, you are earth beautiful. . . .

Or Henry de Montherlant,[14] extolling sexuality

> because of the respect you feel for your partner, and the friendship, tenderness, confidence, and protectiveness, in short all the kind feelings one creature can experience with regard to another. . . . And is it not a wonderful thing . . . that your whole thought should be concentrated on the pleasure you are going to give . . . rather than on the satisfaction you yourself are going to enjoy?

Or William Carlos Williams,[16] in a letter to his wife:

> But if . . . I was a disappointed and unhappy . . . boy, though this is true I am a most happy man. And the greatest thing which has caused that has been yourself. . . . For some uncanny reason you saw through me and you saw me good. I in my turn

> recognized in a flash of intuition that you were the queen of the world for me . . . that feeling went through my whole body like sweetest nectar. . . . There was the eternal in that and I knew it at once.

Or Raymond Chandler,[17] the tough writer of tough detective fiction, in answer to a letter of condolence about his dead wife:

> She was everything you say, and more. She was the music heard faintly at the edge of sound. It was my great and now useless regret that I never wrote anything really worth her attention. . . . Perhaps by now she realizes that I tried.

But men, say our authors, are "inexpressive of emotion!"

It may be objected that the author is quoting writers who, of course, are not representative of the generally inexpressive males. But then it must also be admitted that there is no correlation between depth of feeling and expression of feeling. Borderline individuals can pass from crying to laughing and back again with great ease, and the lack of residue from each emotion suggests that there is not much depth to it. Similarly, members of the "love generation" could express, in word and gesture, love and affection for others whom they hardly knew and towards whom they did not act in the consistently considerate and caring manner which would substantiate their profession of love or friendship. On the other hand, many men and women are capable of deep feelings they do not usually display, but of which they give proof at appropriate occasions by means of important actions involving effort, and courage, and self-sacrifice. It is thus by no means certain that an easy display of emotions is truly desirable or truly significant. Rather, emotionality must be counted among the styles of conduct as they may be characteristic of individuals, families, or entire ethnic groups. Emotionality considered normal and desirable in one family or nationality may be indicative of disturbance in another. Americans, derivative of ethnic groups from all over the world, can hardly be expected to conform to any one behavioral stereotype nor to adopt any such stereotype as ideal. One man cries easily and another one does not. It is not a question of whether it is better to cry or not to cry, but whether, for each of these two men, his particular behavior is ego-syntonic and satisfying. Nor does one or the other necessarily serve our society better.

The same can be said for talking. "Falling in love," says Johnson,[12] "is the Western way of being touched by the splendor or the power of a god." But how easily cannot the splendor, the magic, the whole marvelous mutual idealization of lovers be *talked* to death, be *communicated* and *analyzed* out of existence! What would life be like without secrets, without mystery, without a playground for fantasy and imagination? Every therapist has seen couples who far from suffering a lack of verbal expression, have talked and communicated their feelings for each other into boredom and irritation, until no corner of their souls remained unexamined and unsullied. No, verbal expression and self-revelation, while precious faculties, are not fail-safe paths to closeness and understanding, and in their excesses can be as harmful as excessive reticence and inexpressiveness.

What really matters is not how well a man expresses his love, but how deeply he feels it. And if it is true that love transforms a man and makes him the best he can be, then how much more its crowning achievement, its *ultimum mysterium,* the truly awesome miracle of "unto us a child is given . . ." Listen to the old curmudgeon, Malcolm Muggeridge[18]:

> It was at this time that Kitty first became pregnant. I found the whole process utterly wonderful; her stomach gradually swelling up, and the thought that out of our fleshly girations . . . should come this ripening fruit, this new life partaking of us both, and breaking out of its cocoon. . . . It gave a point to every touch and caress and heave and groan. . . . How beautiful are the Magnificats, the songs of birth!

Which takes us, naturally, to our next heading.

MEN IN RELATION TO THEIR CHILDREN

To repeat: Our authors tell us that men are, to their children, distant, unloving, non-nurturant. Well—since this author has started to quote, let him quote once more, this time from William Gibson,[19] writing of

> . . . a feverish time, it was the most exhiliarating of my life . . . I scribbled the last pages (of my novel) in the hours after midnight in a rocker with my newborn son on my shoulder, a sleepless brat, and a writing board on my thigh. I had my witness, I wrote now in his service too, and I would never again fail to earn a living . . . I was drunk with fatherhood. . . . as my wife suckled our firstborn, the meeting of blind mouth and great mothering breast was the point it seemed on which the world itself turned . . .

Yes, men need to be fathers, quite as almost all women need to be mothers, though they are aware of this to varying degrees, and their awareness comes to them rather later than to women, not in the third but more commonly in the fourth decade of life. Yes, there are bad fathers quite as there are bad mothers and all parents know how easy it is not to be as good, competent, and effective as one thinks one should or might have been. But the fathers the author sees in his practice (mostly upper middle class, now living in the West, but from all areas) are deeply involved with their children, in every possible way, from their inception. They *want* children to begin with, and these days, often want them more than their wives do. They prepare, with their wives, for the great event of the birth, attend classes in baby care, and practice the Lamaze technique. They wish to be and frequently are present at the delivery. They participate in bottle feeding, cleaning, and diapering. They pace the floor in the small hours of the night with the restless, perhaps colicky, perhaps ill child nestled against their chests, with its feverish cheek resting against their stubbly cheek. There is, in all this, nothing that has ever struck any good man as unmanly, nothing that requires him to become more feminine. The icon that most touchingly conveys the part a man plays with his infant is that of Saint Christophorus, the burly giant gently and securely balancing the tiny toddler on his shoulders: the tiny child, so small and light, that yet burdens him with all the cares of the world, and in imposing himself as a burden also bestows upon him the meaning and mission of his life.

It has been said that we live in an age of existential despair. It should also be said that all the famous existentialist writers were childless. (In his latest novel, *The Scheme of Things,* Allen Wheelis[20] has his existentialist psychoanalyst protagonist give in to despair at the point where an adopted child, having grown, moves out of his life.) A man relating to his child—with the supportive backbone of obligations that cannot be shirked, with all that he owes, and gives, and gets: such a man is too busy, too involved, too stimulated to experience the nothingness of the self, the existential loneliness of the narcissist.

What does he get? For one, a chance to regress in the most joyful way, to become a boy again, to create and vicariously to relive a boyhood perhaps better than his own. It is true that nursery schools and kindergartens are almost entirely run by women; but it is also generally true that at home, fathers play and rough-house and let go with their little children more than do the mothers, who are by and large more involved with the daily duties of child care. Life, which is so often unfair, often unfairly gives fathers a much greater chance to have fun and good times with their children than is given to the mothers. Men as disparate as Hans Christian Andersen[21] and Kierkegaard[22] had their fantasies and imaginations fired up in play with their fathers, and Sherwood Anderson[23] gives a loving account of how his father's story-telling inspired his own eventual story-writing.

What does a father owe? For one, he owes his children such conduct as will permit them to look up to him, to admire him:

> A boy wants something very special from his father. You are always hearing it said that fathers want their sons to be what they feel they cannot themselves be but I tell you it also works the other way. I know that, as a small boy, I wanted my father to be . . . a proud, silent, dignified one. When I was with other small boys and he passed along the street, I wanted to feel in my breast the glow of pride. "There he is. That is my father."[23]

For another, and particularly as the child grows older, fathers become, whether they want to or not, teachers to the child of what the world is like, how one is to act in it, what is good and what is bad. The author has elaborated elsewhere the importance of strong fathers for the genesis of positive superego functions,[24] and the inevitable, necessary, and, on the whole, beneficial stresses and antagonisms between the father as the protagonist (the dragon) of the old order and the son as the champion (the hero) of the new.[9,25] But the old does not only have to be defended, it must in the first place and above all be taught. So fathers have a necessary and legitimate role as authority figures and teachers. (This is so obvious that one feels foolish to have to say it, but luckily the matter has recently been buttressed by a study which, being statistical, should weigh heavily, and which shows that children of divorce who do not maintain close contact with their fathers develop poorly and have more trouble than those who continue a relationship with him.[26])

What may be worth stating, in view of some of the androgynous advocacy of the preceding chapters, is that fathers and teachers need, in that capacity, to be quite strict and demanding, that in this role they need to be hard and tough in a manner traditionally associated with men (though of course good women teachers, without thereby undergoing virilization, may be just as exacting, and just as effective, at least for girls, and for students of either sex at higher levels of learning). Boys have trouble accepting learning if it is presented to them by women teachers or mothers and seems a "woman-thing" to be avoided by a "real man" (which explains why in this country, but not in countries where men teach grade school, girls are at first the better students). But above all, boys and girls, men and women students, need a teacher so tough that meeting his standards really means something and gives cause for pride and self-respect. A few years ago, a highly popular movie about law school, "The Paper Chase," presented such a "bastard of a teacher," a meticulous, biting, sarcastic law professor who would tolerate nothing but the best from each student, who is feared at first and ends up not only being respected, but loved. The same actor played a similar role, with similar results, in a sure-to-become-a-classic TV play by John Korty, "Christmas Without Snow," in which, as a choir director, he bullies, intimidates, and inspires an amateur church group into giving a first-rate rendition of Handel's "Messiah." Unconditional, all-accepting, all-forgiving, undemanding love is, typically and in its essence, maternal. Fathers, as Erikson[27] has pointed out, love "more dangerously": they set standards, demand performance, and condition respect (not love) on achievement; and it is necessary for the good of the next generation that they should do so. The indiscriminate "love" of the "flower children" of the 1960s demonstrated disastrously to what extent lack of standards leads to nonperformance and abdication.

WHO WANTS WHAT?

The issue of "changing male roles" seems to involve three parties, each with their own needs, wishes, and methods: the men, the women, and the therapists. A fourth party, the children, is very much involved, but has no voice of its own.

WHAT DO THE MEN WANT?

To believe our authors, they want to be "liberated from male role restrictions" (Bernardez), relieved of their guilt concerning dominance over women (Bernardez), to be less like men and more like women; in short, they want to be androgynous. One must believe our authors when they say that there are men who make such demands. But drawing on the author's own experience of over 25 years of full-time psychotherapy, he does not recall a single man who ever set for himself the goals just described. Oh yes, many of them felt the burdens of work and responsibility to be heavy, many of the young ones were hesitating to assume them, many of the fully grown had daydreams of chucking it all. But far from wishing to become less manly, they by and large were anxious to become better men. As to their supposed inexpressiveness, it was totally absent in the therapeutic setting. Once they had acquired and tested a measure of trust in the therapist, they quite freely and skillfully expressed, in words and gesture, their intimate anxieties and yearnings, their weaknesses, their fatigue. But it is true that many of them did not feel they could show themselves as openly to their wives or girl friends and their reluctance was often based on experience; for while many a good woman can and does support her man in times of danger, distress, and discouragement, many others are rendered acutely anxious by any sign of weakness in their men and likely to respond either with additional despair of their own, or with resentment, hostility, and contempt. So it was, in the author's experience (admittedly with a narrow social stratum), never a question of a man's ability to show feelings, but often a matter of difficult judgment as to whether a given man could reveal specific worries or weaknesses to a given woman without burdening her excessively or provoking her into doubts and hostile reactions damaging to the relationship.

As to the burdens of manliness and the wish to "chuck it all," the author has indeed heard many a professional, businessman, or academic proclaim that this job was "a killer" and that he would never wish his sons or daughters to follow so onerous a path. But these same men, given a chance, would not dream of changing their occupations and most of them would not retire or do so only reluctantly. The griping that men do about their work is generally nothing but a rather transparent appeal for recognition, admiration, and praise, quite compatible with pride in the job and with complete acceptance of work as a man's proper lot. Men want to be able to choose whom and what they serve, but they want to serve. Some labor in the service of an idea, ideal, or ideology, but most of them find their greatest satisfaction in the service of their families. The domineering, tyrannical role which the authors ascribe to men in the family context is in fact rare indeed. Some men are tyrants and so are some women. Few and far between are the men who can simply order their wives what to do, and with rare exceptions it is only in a state of extreme provocation, frustration, and overall impotence that a man will become physically assaultive. Much more commonly there is a tug of strength, fully justified by debatable issues, between personalities with idiosyncratic strengths and weaknesses that are more determined by character than by sex. In summary: what do men want? They want to be good men: good workers, good husbands, good fathers.

WHAT DO WOMEN WANT OF MEN?

Essentially the same. To listen to the radical feminists, they would as lief get rid of men altogether, or at the very least they would wish to topple them from their position of "dominance." But that is not at all what the author hears from his women patients. What he hears is this: They want men, or better, a man. They want a man who knows what he wants and who knows that he wants to choose this one of them as his woman and wants to devote and commit himself to her, predictably, conscientiously, faithfully, loyally, and for life. And some of the professionally most accomplished women add that they would like the man to be at least as bright and successful, if not a little more so, than themselves. In other words, despite the sexual acrimony dispensed in today's bestsellers and the dubious opportunities and freedoms of "sexual liberation," what women want of men is today what it has always been: that they be strong: strong in character, strong in occupational competence, strong in gentleness and love, steadfast, solid, and reliable.

WHAT DO OUR AUTHORS WANT?

They are quite clear about it: they want to help men and women by helping men become more androgynous (Solomon).

The author must admit that he does not understand their term as they use it. That we are all androgynous, that each and every human being has elements of the characteristics of both sexes, has always been known, and has been stated by Plato, Freud, and Jung, by all mythologies, and by good writers and poets of all times. To sort things out and to define what a proper man is, "primitive" people had to institute, "rites of passage"; Brahmin need to be "twice-born"[28] and Jews undergo the Bar Mitzvah ceremony, all to make sure that a boy has moved out of the realm of the mother and into that of the men. All this is well established and well known.

Presumably, our authors mean that this process has gone too far, that men should regain some of their original androgyny by acquiring or by reacquiring those qualities they label as "feminine," such as gentleness, affection, openness of emotion, the ability to communicate, sensitivity, and closeness to children. But with this suggestion they are slandering masculinity in the most outrageous manner, for men have always possessed these qualities though, like women, to a varying degree.

If on the other hand, what they really mean by androgyny is something like unisex, that men and women should be as much alike as possible, presumably in order to understand each other better, then they are caught in a sorry misunderstanding of what makes for solid bonding and are willing to surrender the infinite richness and strength of complementarity in favor of the dreary indifference of sameness.

May,[8] in the introduction to his stimulating book and research report, *Sex and Fantasy*, puts the matter very well indeed:

> . . . there is a tendency, at least in America these days, that anyone who raises the question of sex differences is at best mean-spirited and at worst a reactionary bigot.

It is his (and this author's) point of view that "each of us comes to a level of humanness *through* our maleness and femaleness." Far from considering sex differences "a *problem*, an affront to human dignity and social progress," we should strive for ". . . a language . . . in which to talk about the distinguishing characteristics of men and women without its being demeaning to either."

Pertinently, in a recent article, Barbara Tuchman[29] discusses the nature and current decline of *quality*. The word, she points out, has two meanings: the nature and essential characteristic of something, as in "His voice has the quality of command," or, a condition of excellence implying fine quality as contrasted to poor quality, and resulting from investment of the best skill and effort possible to produce the finest and most admirable result possible. In this perspective, the essential characteristic of a man is surely that which makes him more manly, not more feminine, that which essentially characterizes his sex, not that which he shares with the other; his efforts at excellence must involve an effort to be the best *man* he can be. In other words, is it best for the individual and for society if the differences between men and women are as much as possible effaced, or on the contrary, should they be encouraged to become the sources of special achievement and pride, of gender-linked accomplishments the sexes may offer each other to their mutual admiration and satisfaction? "The new egalitarians," writes Tuchman, "would like to make the whole question of quality vanish by adopting a flat philosophy of the equality of everything." It would be the death of quality, hence of excellence, if they ever had their way. Let therefore a man excel at what is manly, and let him differ from women for the salvation and the glory of men *and* of women.

But the author has been totally carried away. He is not to give his own opinion at this point, nor that of men and women of renown who seem to support his position; he is to address the goals of his fellow authors in this book. And so, to restate, their object is androgyny, and they are to achieve it—how? Why, by "consciousness-raising" (Stein).

Now there is a fancy term for you! As unassailable as motherhood! Surely, raising anything is a noble deed, and consciousness far to be preferred to being unconscious. And in the present context, as far as the author can gather, it suggests that men, dolts that they are, have been unconscious of their cruel oppression of women and must be "raised" out of their ignorance to a more enlightened understanding of such matters. Their only salvation lies in admitting their guilt, in confessing their chauvinist piggishness with a repentant heart, and in joining the formerly oppressed by means of cultivating their own femininity.

Many of us are burdened by enough amorphous guilt to welcome any kind of confessional, a fact to which the popularity of certain preachers amply testifies. And so it is to be expected that a number of men will gladly admit the misdeeds the androgynists accuse them of, even though those who thus confess themselves are, as the penitents in a church, the least likely to have committed real crimes. What is deplorable about this procedure is not that they confess, but that they are permitted and encouraged to confess the wrong guilt. The true crime, in our day, is not likely male oppression, but male delinquency, an excessive preoccupation with the self, a reluctance to assume responsibility toward others and for one's own actions. And it is the crime and guilt of the androgynists that they tend to aid and abet this preoccupation with moods and feelings and with the self, rather than turning the mind of the man toward his actions and responsibilities.

Attitudes and therapies have their fashions. Self-absorption and existential doubt flourish during the aimlessness of defeat (as in World War II France) or the confusion of opulence (as in the United States following World War II). The whole pitiful concern for the expression of "feelings" springs out of the contemporary, relative absence of urgent challenges and purposes. In fact, it is already obsolete, for the problems of ecology, the energy shortage, overpopulation, famine, and the threat of atomic war are increasingly demanding and getting the attentions of youth. It is quite likely that the sentimental journey of the 1970s will be totally irrelevant to the men and women of the 1980s.

The pendulum, the author believes, has swung its farthest, our opulence is fading, and new struggles are upon us. And if men are going to change it is most likely that they will move, not towards androgyny, but back, back to the way they were over and over again in history during the worst of times which, in terms of the manly virtues they elicited, were over and over again, for men, the best of times.

REFERENCES

1. Korner A: Sex differences in newborns with special reference to differences in the organization of oral behavior. J Child Psychol Psychiatry 14:27, 1973
2. Bardwick J, Douvan E: Ambivalence: The socialization of women, in Readings on the Psychology of Women. Edited by Bardwick J. New York, Harper and Row, 1972
3. Burton RF: Personal Narrative of Pilgrimage to Al-Madinah and Meccah (1893), Vol I. New York, Dover, 1964, p 149
4. Matthiessen P: The Snow Leopard. New York, Viking, 1978
5. Johnson RA: HE; Understanding Masculine Psychology, New York, Harper and Row, 1977
6. Shaw GB: Man and Superman (1903), Baltimore, Penguin Books, 1952, p 61
7. Lederer W: Man's dream: Myth and reality, in Women and Men: Roles, Attitudes and Power Relationships, Edited by Zuckerman EL New York, Radcliffe Club of New York, 1975, pp 70–80
8. May R: Sex and Fantasy, Patterns of Male and Female Development. New York, Norton, 1980
9. Lederer W: Oedipus and the serpent. Psychoanal Rev 51:619–644, 1965
10. Heidel A: The Gilgamesh Epic and Old Testament Parallels. Chicago, University of Chicago Press, 1946
11. Lederer W: The Fear of Women. New York, Grune and Stratton, 1968, Harcourt, Brace & Jovanovitch, 1970
12. Johnson RA: SHE, Understanding Feminine Psychology. New York, Harper and Row, 1977
13. Anderson S: in A Book of Men. Edited by Firestone R. New York, Stonehill, 1975, p 128
14. Anderson S: in A Book of Men. Edited by Firestone R. New York, Stonehill, 1975, p 184
15. de Montherlant H: in A Book of Men. Edited by Firestone R. New York, Stonehill, 1975, p 139
16. Williams WC: in A Book of Men. Edited by Firestone R. New York, Stonehill, 1975, p 202
17. Chandler R: in A Book of Men. Edited by Firestone R. New York, Stonehill, 1975, p 246
18. Muggeridge M: in A Book of Men. Edited by Firestone R. New York, Stonehill, 1975, p 256
19. Gibson W: in A Book of Men. Edited by Firestone R. New York, Stonehill, 1975, p 268
20. Wheelis A: The Scheme of Things. New York, Harcourt, Brace and Jovanovitch, 1980
21. Andersen HC: The True Story of My Life. Trans by Howitt M. New York, American–Scandinavian Foundation, 1926
22. Kierkegaard S: in A Book of Men. Edited by Firestone R. New York, Stonehill, 1975, p 21
23. Anderson S: in A Book of Men. Edited by Firestone R. New York, Stonehill, 1975, p 30–39
24. Lederer W: Dragons, Delinquents and Destiny, Psychological Issues No 15. New York, International Universities Press, 1965
25. Lederer W: Historical consequences of father–son hostility. Psychoanal Rev 54:248–276, 1967
26. Wallerstein JS, Kelly JB: Effects of divorce on the visiting father–child relationship. Am J Psychiatry 137:1534–1539, 1980
27. Erikson EH: Young Man Luther. New York, Norton, 1958
28. Carstairs GM: The Twice Born. Bloomington, Indiana University Press, 1961
29. Tuchman B: Quality and non-quality. San Francisco Chronicle, This World Section, November 16, 1980

Author Index

Subject Index